John Brick, PhD
Editor

Handbook of the Medical Consequences of Alcohol and Drug Abuse
Second Edition

Pre-publication
REVIEWS,
COMMENTARIES,
EVALUATIONS . . .

"**A** comprehensive and detailed analysis and reference textbook for the physician, clinician, or expert interested in the use and consequences of use for the most commonly abused drugs today. Drug abuse is a challenging and continuously evolving field, but this book has consolidated decades of the best information into an easily accessible source. . . . One-stop shopping for information related to drugs of abuse. . . . Invaluable because of its ability to quickly identify the medical consequences and effects of drug abuse. An asset for health care professionals and the general public because of its easy-to-follow structure, index, and extensively researched comprehensive sections. . . . A very useful guide for medical and other health professions students who need to have this type of information at their fingertips as they try to evaluate and intervene or just give advice and counseling. Anyone who purchases this book will gain a much deeper appreciation of the range of consequences that accompany use of these drugs."

Mark S. Gold, MD
Distinguished Professor,
University of Florida College of Medicine
Departments of Psychiatry, Neuroscience,
Anesthesiology and Community
Health & Family Medicine

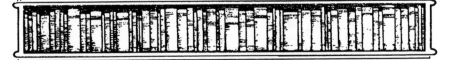

More pre-publication
REVIEWS, COMMENTARIES, EVALUATIONS . . .

"This is an excellent reference source; a must for practitioners. Dr. Brick covers issues relevant to one's everyday clinical practice. It is a necessity for anyone involved in patient care. I feel this book is a progressive, up-to-date addition to my medical library."

William P. Stanell, MD, FACOG
Lawrence OB/GYN Associates, PC,
Lawrenceville, New Jersey

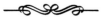

"This handbook presents a thorough and sequential review of the consequences of alcohol, tobacco, and drug abuse. It is a time-saving resource that I will keep on my bookshelf for quick reference. The text provides scientific data as well as layperson terminology and street lingo, and it is full of current and pertinent information organized for fast and easy access. This handy reference book is a must-have for the health care provider."

Elaine Torres-Melendez, DMD
Prosthodontist

"This book presents a vast compendium of data about alcohol and drug addiction. Substance abuse is covered from a global through gross anatomical to a cellular and enzymatic point of view. This book is truly a job well done and worthy of all students of substance abuse."

Gerald Ente, MD, FAAP, FICP, FRSH
Assoc. Clin. Prof. Peds. Emeritus,
SUNY Stonybrook Medical School;
Chief Surgeon, New York State Fraternal
Order of Police

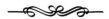

"Remains an indispensable reference tool for medical practitioners and other professionals who may encounter addiction problems in their clients."

Penny Booth Page, MLS
Director of Information Services,
Rutgers University Center of Alcohol Studies

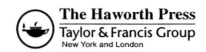

The Haworth Press
Taylor & Francis Group
New York and London

Handbook of the Medical Consequences of Alcohol and Drug Abuse

Second Edition

THE HAWORTH PRESS Series
in Neuropharmacology
John Brick, PhD, MA, FAPA
Senior Editor

Handbook of the Medical Consequences of Alcohol and Drug Abuse, Second Edition edited by John Brick

Titles of Related Interest

Drug Abuse and Social Policy in America: The War That Must Be Won by Barry Stimmel

Pain and Its Relief Without Addiction: Clinical Issues in the Use of Opioids and Other Analgesics by Barry Stimmel

Drugs, the Brain, and Behavior by John Brick and Carlton K. Erickson

Living on the Edge: Understanding and Coping with Alcoholism and Other Addictions by Barry Stimmel

Handbook of the Medical Consequences of Alcohol and Drug Abuse

Second Edition

John Brick, PhD
Editor

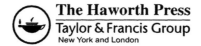

The Haworth Press
Taylor & Francis Group
New York and London

For more information on this book or to order, visit
http://www.haworthpress.com/store/product.asp?sku=6039

or call 1-800-HAWORTH (800-429-6784) in the United States and Canada
or (607) 722-5857 outside the United States and Canada

or contact orders@HaworthPress.com

Published by

The Haworth Press, Taylor & Francis Group, 270 Madison Avenue, New York, NY 10016.

PUBLISHER'S NOTE
The development, preparation, and publication of this work has been undertaken with great care.
However, the Publisher, employees, editors, and agents of The Haworth Press are not responsible
for any errors contained herein or for consequences that may ensue from use of materials or information contained in this work. The Haworth Press is committed to the dissemination of ideas and
information according to the highest standards of intellectual freedom and the free exchange of
ideas. Statements made and opinions expressed in this publication do not necessarily reflect the
views of the Publisher, Directors, management, or staff of The Haworth Press, or an endorsement
by them.

Cover design by Jennifer Gaska.

Library of Congress Cataloging-in-Publication Data

Handbook of the medical consequences of alcohol and drug abuse / John Brick, editor.—2nd ed.
    p. cm.
  Includes bibliographical references and index.
  ISBN 978-0-7890-3573-8 (hard : alk. paper)
  ISBN 978-0-7890-3574-5 (soft : alk. paper)
  1. Substance abuse—Pathophysiology—Handbooks, manuals, etc. I. Brick, John, 1950-
  [DNLM: 1. Substance-Related Disorders—physiopathology. WM 270 H2365 2007]

  RC564.H3585 2007
  616.86—dc22

                                                                        2007026488

CONTENTS

ABOUT THE EDITOR

John Brick, PhD, MA, FAPA, a scientist and educator specializing in alcohol and drug studies for more than twenty-five years, is Executive Director of Intoxikon International, a company that provides multidisciplinary education, training and consulting in alcohol and drug studies to governmental and other agencies. As a member of the research faculty of the Rutgers University Center of Alcohol studies for fourteen years, he held positions as Chief of Research at the Rutgers Center of Alcohol Studies, Education and Training Division, Chairman of the Graduate Curriculum on the Biology of Alcohol, Lab Director of the Alcohol Behavior Research Laboratory, and Associate Director of both the Rutgers Summer School of Alcohol Studies and the Advanced School of Alcohol and Drug Studies. He taught courses in neuropharmacology and related courses at Rutgers and elsewhere for twenty years.

Dr. Brick is the author of over 100 scientific treatises, including the *President's Commission of Model State Drug Laws–Socioeconomic Evaluation of Addictions Treatment; Drugs and the Brain; Drugs, the Brain and Behavior: The Pharmacology of Alcohol and Drug Abuse* (Haworth) and is co-editor of *Stress and Alcohol Use and Alcohol and Aggression* and has authored numerous book chapters and original research on the biobehavioral effects of alcohol and other drugs.

In 1990, Dr. Brick was one of six Americans invited to address the Soviet National Academy of Medicine on their centenary anniversary and the only American alcohol research scientist to receive this distinct honor. In 1992, he co-organized and chaired the International Conference of Alcohol and Aggression and was promoted to Fellow of the American Psychological Association for his outstanding contributions to the science of psychology. In 2002, Dr. Brick was a visiting faculty member at Peking University Institute of Mental Health/International Center of Health Concerns in Beijing, China. Dr. Brick taught Medical Consequences of Alcohol Abuse and addiction-related topics to physicians as part of the first WHO medical educa-

Handbook of the Medical Consequences of Alcohol and Drug Abuse
© 2008 by The Haworth Press, Taylor & Francis Group. All rights reserved.
doi:10.1300/6039_a

tion initiative in China. He is currently Senior Editor for the Haworth Medical Press Neuropharmacology Book Program and has an appointment as a consultant in Biological Psychology and Psychopharmacology for the Rockland County Medical Examiner's Office in New York. Dr. Brick has been in private practice in Yardley, Pennsylvania, since 1985.

CONTRIBUTORS

Neal Benowitz, MD, Clinical Psychiatry and Biopharmaceutical Sciences, University of California, San Francisco, California.

Alan J. Budney, PhD, Center for Addiction Research, Department of Psychiatry, University of Arkansas for Medical Sciences, Little Rock, Arkansas.

Sasha J. Carr, Postdoctoral Resident, Ciminero and Associates, Miami, Florida.

Claire D. Coles, PhD, Emory University School of Medicine, Department of Psychiatry—Genetics, Georgia Mental Health Institute, Atlanta, Georgia.

Fulton T. Crews, PhD, Director, the Bowles Center for Alcohol Studies, University of North Carolina at Chapel Hill, Chapel Hill, North Carolina.

Cristine Delnevo, PhD, MPH, University of Medicine and Dentistry of New Jersey—School of Public Health, Tobacco Surveillance, Evaluation and Research Program, New Brunswick, New Jersey.

Carlton K. Erickson, PhD, Director, Addiction Science Research and Education Center, and Pfizer Centennial Professor of Pharmacology, University of Texas at Austin, College of Pharmacy, Austin, Texas.

Jonathan Foulds, PhD, Professor and Director, Tobacco Dependence Program, University of Medicine and Dentistry of New Jersey—School of Public Health, New Brunswick, New Jersey.

Corinne E. Frantz, PhD, Clinical Neuropsychologist, Private Practice, Ithaca, New York.

Thomas Hildebrandt, Center of Alcohol Studies, Rutgers University, Piscataway, New Jersey.

Karen K. Howell, PhD, Maternal Substance Abuse and Child Development Project, Emory University School of Medicine, Department of Psychiatry—Genetics, Georgia Mental Health Institute, Atlanta, Georgia.

Julie A. Kable, PhD, Emory University School of Medicine, Department of Psychiatry—Genetics, Georgia Mental Health Institute, Atlanta, Georgia.

Paul Kolecki, MD, Assistant Professor Department of Surgery, Division of Emergency Medicine, Thomas Jefferson University, Philadelphia, Pennsylvania.

Mary Jeanne Kreek, MD, Professor and Head, The Rockefeller University, The Laboratory of the Biology of Addictive Diseases, New York, New York.

James Langenbucher, PhD, Center of Alcohol Studies, Rutgers University, Piscataway, New Jersey.

Robert A. Levine, DDS, Diplomate of the American Board of Periodontology, Private Practice, Philadelphia, Pennsylvania.

William J. Lorman, PhD, MSN, PsyNP, Clinical Director, Livengrin Foundation, Bensalem, Pennsylvania.

Pauline F. McHugh, MD, Assistant Research Professor, Department of Psychiatry, New York University School of Medicine, Center for Brain Health, New York, New York.

Brent A. Moore, PhD, University of Vermont, Treatment Research Center, South Burlington, Vermont.

Rosemarie Scolaro Moser, PhD, ABPN, Director, RSM Psychology Center LLC, Lawrenceville, New Jersey.

Adolf Pfefferbaum, MD, Department of Psychiatry and Behavioral Sciences, Stanford University School of Medicine, Stanford, Connecticut.

Terry D. Rees, DDS, Private Practice, Dallas, Texas.

Margaret J. Rosenbloom, Neuroscience Program, SRI International, Menlo Park, California.

Aaron B. Schneir, MD, Medical Toxicology Fellow/Assistant Professor of Emergency Medicine, San Diego Division, California Poison Control System and Division of Medical Toxicology, Department of Emergency Medicine, University of California San Diego Medical Center, San Diego, California.

Richard Shih, MD, Emergency Medicine, Residency Director, Morristown Memorial Hospital, Morristown, New Jersey, and Medical Toxicologist, New Jersey Poison Information and Education Systems, Newark Beth Israel Medical Center, Newark, New Jersey.

Karen E. Simone, PharmD, ABAT, Northern New England Poison Center, Portland, Maine.

Michael B. Steinberg, MD, MPH, University of Medicine and Dentistry of New Jersey—School of Public Health, New Brunswick, New Jersey, Robert Wood Johnson Medical School, Department of Medicine, New Brunswick, New Jersey.

Edith V. Sullivan, PhD, Department of Psychiatry and Behavioral Sciences, Stanford University School of Medicine, Stanford, Connecticut.

Dung Thai, MD, PhD, Clinical Psychiatry and Biopharmaceutical Sciences, University of California, San Francisco, California.

Ryan Vandrey, Behavioral Pharmacology Research Unit, Johns Hopkins University, Baltimore, Maryland.

Mark C. Wallen, PhD, Medical Director, Livengrin Foundation, Inc., Bensalem, Pennsylvania.

Tara S. Wass, PhD, Alcohol Research Center, The Scripps Research Center, La Jolla, California.

Timothy Wiegand, MD, Fellow, Medical Toxicology and Clinical Pharmacology, UCSF, and California Poison Control Center, San Francisco, California.

Douglas M. Ziedonis, MD, MPH, Professor, University of Center for Mental Health Services Research, Massachusetts Medical School, Worcester, Massachusetts.

Foreword

When I wrote the foreword to the first edition of the *Medical Consequences of Alcohol and Drug Abuse,* I stated that the information in the book would remain current "for many years to come." Not satisfied with such currency, Dr. John Brick, editor, has chosen to update and expand upon the topics presented earlier, plus add a number of new and unique chapters. Thus, this edition has almost twice as many chapters as the first edition, with eight new ones and updated versions of the previous topics. To the editor's credit, most of the original authors agreed to update and expand their chapters and he has recruited a number of additional expert scientists to write on specific critical issues of the day regarding medical issues associated with drug use and overuse.

In addition to the original chapters on alcohol pharmacology and toxicology, neuropsychological consequences of alcohol and drug abuse, and alcohol effects on the brain neurochemistry, a new chapter on the consequences of chronic alcohol consumption on brain structure and function has been added. This chapter, written by experienced researchers in the field, provides the latest information on the microstructure and macrostructure of the brain after chronic alcohol use, magnetic resonance imaging (MRI) studies, how brain function changes are related to what is seen in MRIs, and longitudinal studies relating to recovery of function with abstinence.

Updated chapters from the first edition include important topics such as consequences of prenatal alcohol and other drug exposure (two chapters), health consequences of marijuana use, medical consequences of acute and chronic alcohol use, medical consequences of cocaine and other stimulant use and abuse, and consequences of inhalant abuse. These chapters have all been updated and remain significant sources of established and new information on topics mentioned previously. Of special importance, of course, is the information on stimulants, including cocaine, methamphetamine, and other stimulants that always seem to be in the news and are of interest because of their great dependence potential. I still find the chapter on mari-

Handbook of the Medical Consequences of Alcohol and Drug Abuse
doi:10.1300/6039_c

juana to be very important because of its fair and balanced discussions on current topics and the medical aspects of marijuana use.

The remaining seven chapters of the *Handbook of the Medical Consequences of Alcohol and Drug Abuse* are perhaps even more unique and exciting, mainly because they are brand new. It is difficult to find synthesized easy-to-read reviews of contemporary drug problems involving steroids, over-the-counter (OTC) medications, and street drugs such as Ecstasy, LSD, PCP, and mescaline. However, this book has them. Although steroids are not generally considered to be "addicting," medical consequences associated with their use are significant. Furthermore, steroids are always in the news, yet few athletes or others on steroid-enhancing drugs realize or they apparently ignore the enormous risks associated with the use of these chemicals: effects on the endocrine system, the gastrointestinal system, the liver, the circulatory and musculoskeletal systems, and of course the central nervous system. The chapter on steroids clearly lays out all these medical risks and concludes with a discussion of problems associated with routes of supply and methods of administration.

The chapter on problems with the use of OTC medications is unexpectedly comprehensive, given the wide array of OTC medications that can be abused. Medications covered include antihistamines, "cold remedies," caffeine, cough medicines, decongestants, and nicotine replacement products. In this chapter, one can find answers to questions such as "What are the side effects of dextromethorphan on the liver, heart, and skin?" and "What are the medical consequences of caffeine?" This is a unique chapter on an important topic that readers will find fascinating.

Ecstasy and other "hallucinogens" are dealt with in another comprehensive chapter, and of course include "street" and "club" drugs that are so dangerous to adolescents and others who do not recognize their medical dangers. The psychological and physiological effects of these drugs are significant and are outlined with great clarity in this chapter. The coverage includes a history of the use of these drugs, drug interactions and pharmacokinetics of some of the drugs, and complete listings of the effects of these drugs on the major organ systems of the body.

Always contemporary and significant are the health effects of tobacco, nicotine, and exposure to tobacco smoke pollution, dealt with in another of the new chapters. I think this must have been a difficult chapter to write, since there is so much scientific literature on nicotine and smoking. However, the authors have done a fine job sorting out contemporary articles and mixing them with classic information. For example, the nature and history of tobacco use leads to a discussion of diseases caused by tobacco. The health effects of "light" (quotation marks intended) versus regular cigarettes and noncigarette tobacco products (cigars, pipe smoking, and smokeless tobacco) are all included. Where else would you find a scientific discussion of beedis and kreteks, two other forms of noncigarette tobacco products? I was especially impressed with the topics having to do with the benefits of smoking cessation, the effects of smoking on the fetus and early child development, and exposure to tobacco smoke pollution, including second-hand smoke.

Nearing the end of Dr. Brick's book, one finds a highly significant chapter on the interaction of alcohol with medications and other drugs. Does alcohol interact with anticonvulsant medications? With antibiotics? With antidepressants? Of course, and the reasons are spelled out in this chapter. Two general types of interactions, pharmacodynamic and pharmacokinetic, are explained, along with the classical descriptions of additive, synergistic, potentiation, and antagonism types of interactions that are so common with many drugs, but especially with alcohol. As my favorite pharmacist would say, "Where was this information when I was going to school?" This is a wonderful listing of drugs that interact with alcohol that every medical professional should be aware of, along with explanations of the pharmacological mechanisms of those interactions.

The chapter on the little-considered adverse effects of alcohol and drug abuse in the oral cavity is very interesting. Many of us have heard of "meth mouth," but how many of us think about the oral effects of cannabis, Ecstasy, or even alcohol? What is the dental management of the patient who abuses alcohol or other drugs? This chapter, written by dental specialists, is an unusual and welcome addition to this second edition.

The final chapter concerns a very difficult topic, special issues in patients with comorbid psychiatric and chemical dependency disorders. Most clinicians knowingly or unknowingly deal with such patients every day, yet know very little about how to help them. It takes special skills, not only to diagnose individuals with comorbid (co-occurring) disorders, but also to find ways to reduce their suffering. Complex issues such as whether chemical dependency leads to psychiatric illness or whether psychiatric symptoms lead to drug abuse or dependency are considered in some detail. Other questions about which symptoms relate to "true" comorbid disorders and which symptoms are less serious and temporary are dealt with head-on in this chapter. Included are assessment tools, treatment models of comorbid disorder, post–acute withdrawal syndrome, comorbid disorders and suicide, and alcoholism treatment medications and comorbid disorders. Clinicians who read this chapter will not only begin to understand the enormity of the problem but also will find some answers to the difficult question "How do I deal with such patients?" There is hope!

One person could never have written such a comprehensive book. The editor and the authors have done an outstanding job of updating previous chapters and covering some topics that are hard to find anywhere else. I still believe, as I said in my previous foreword, that this book is worth taking the time to read in its entirety. On the other hand, with today's busy professionals, cherry-picking the chapters of greatest importance to the reader is also very easy in such a well-organized book. Either way, John Brick's *Handbook of the Medical Consequences of Alcohol and Drug Abuse* is an excellent addition to anyone's resource library.

Carlton K. Erickson, PhD
Pfizer Centennial Professor of Pharmacology
The University of Texas, Austin

Preface

In formulating the second edition of this book, I was again reminded of the magnitude of alcohol and drug abuse in everyday lives. The addition of many new chapters will hopefully expand the appreciation of this problem. As previously noted, the philosopher Thomas Hobbes (1588-1679) described the condition of humanity as "nasty, brutish and short." Interestingly, he was among the first proponents to write about the biological basis of behavior. In the ensuing 250 years or so, the great human condition and the quality of life have improved in most societies. Life is less nasty, less brutish, and far longer than it has ever been. With few exceptions, life as Hobbes knew it has changed dramatically, although then, as now, alcohol and other drugs were available and abused. Today, highly sophisticated neuroscientific research techniques enable scientists to study the neurophysiological and molecular changes that produce acute intoxication, and the increased longevity provided by advances in medical science allows the long-term consequences of alcohol and drug abuse to be more fully appreciated. Centuries ago, one was more likely to die from infectious diseases, other ailments, or occupational injuries before the pernicious medical consequences of alcohol or drug abuse presented themselves. This assumption is no longer true.

Handbook of the Medical Consequences of Alcohol and Drug Abuse is part of The Haworth Medical Press series in neuropharmacology and is written with the goal of bringing the most recent findings to scientists, physicians, other clinicians, and advanced students of this fascinating and important topic. Alcohol scientists know more about the long-term consequences of alcohol and other drugs than at any other time in our history. Basic and clinical research in this area must continue, as must the efforts to educate physicians and other health care professionals, and increase public education and awareness of this problem. Included in this book are those drugs that generate the most interest and greatest consequences. In the second edition of this book, I am pleased to include eight new and important additional chapters that offer cutting-edge insights into the medical consequences of alcohol and other drugs, as well as updates in a field that is constantly evolving. No special significance should be given to the use of the phrase "alcohol and other drugs," which appears throughout this book. Alcohol is a drug and the use of the phrase is for heuristic convenience only.

Acknowledgments

The contributors have made this a pleasant and worthwhile endeavor and I thank them for taking time from their busy schedules to share their perspectives on this complicated problem. Several others, whose names do not appear in the list of contributors, have nonetheless been influential in this endeavor. Thanks to my first mentor, Dr. Mary E. Reuder, who instilled in me the value of academic excellence and encouraged my pursuit of knowledge; to colleagues Drs. Zelig Dolinsky and Carlton Erickson for their thoughtful comments throughout various stages of this book; and to Drs. Larissa Pohorecky and David Lester for stimulating my interest in alcohol studies. Special appreciation and thanks go to my secretary, Jacquelyn Kaizar. Her steadfast navigation through the seas of revisions made for clear sailing through both editions and was invaluable.

I have been extremely fortunate to have always the encouragement, understanding, and fresh perspective of my wife, Laurie Stockton, and my daughters, Stephanie and Kyla, who remind me every day what life is all about. Thank you. And last but not least, my thanks to Violet Holmes, without whom none of this would be possible. Thank you for providing a lifetime of optimism and hard work and for encouraging me to think with my head, not with my feet.

Handbook of the Medical Consequences of Alcohol and Drug Abuse
© 2008 by The Haworth Press, Taylor & Francis Group. All rights reserved.
doi:10.1300/6039_e

Chapter 1

Characteristics of Alcohol:
Definitions, Chemistry, Measurement,
Use, and Abuse

John Brick

We begin this textbook with an overview of alcohol, one of the oldest and most widely used psychoactive drugs on earth. In an effort to provide a foundation for the interpretation of terms related to alcohol and its use throughout this text and elsewhere, this introductory chapter will define alcohol both as a chemical and as a drug, explain the scientific notation for reporting alcohol in blood or serum, and present an overview of the use of alcohol: how we currently define alcohol use, abuse, and dependence in American society.

WHAT IS ALCOHOL?

The term "alcohol" is used to define several types of alcohol, including the three most common: ethyl alcohol (ethanol), methyl alcohol (methanol), and isopropyl alcohol (isopropanol). All alcohols have a similar chemical structure and contain a hydroxyl group, OH, attached to a saturated carbon molecule. Methyl alcohol, also known as methanol or wood alcohol, is so highly toxic that even small amounts (less than an ounce) may cause retinal damage. Methanol's toxicity is the result of its metabolism to formaldehyde and then to formic acid, a cellular toxin that is about six times more poisonous than methanol. The accumulation of formic acid produces severe metabolic acidosis and more than 6 to 7 ounces of methanol are lethal for most adults.

Handbook of the Medical Consequences of Alcohol and Drug Abuse
© 2008 by The Haworth Press, Taylor & Francis Group. All rights reserved.
doi:10.1300/6039_01

Isopropyl alcohol, also known as isopropanol or common rubbing alcohol, is also highly toxic. Small amounts, as little as a few ounces, can cause permanent damage to the visual system, and 8 ounces is considered a lethal dose. Some alcoholics may consume methanol or isopropanol, intentionally or unknowingly, and of the three alcohols with potentially lethal consequences discussed here, methanol and isopropanol are the most dangerous.

The alcohol that is the subject of this review and the alcohol consumed as a beverage by most people, is ethanol, a clear, relatively odorless chemical. The lethal dose (LD:50) of acute ethanol is estimated to be a blood alcohol concentration of about 0.40 percent, although death may occur at higher or lower concentrations depending upon factors such as tolerance or the presence of other drugs. Given reasonable alcohol pharmacokinetics, a 150-pound male would reach LD:50 after consuming about four to five drinks per hour over a four-hour period. Sublethal doses are more insidious and are the primary focus of this review. Throughout this chapter and throughout this book, the term alcohol will be synonymous with ethanol.

Whether we are discussing alcohol as a chemical or psychoactive drug, alcohol is a relatively simple molecule, $CH_3–CH_2–OH$, formed during a process of fermentation that occurs when yeast combines with water and sugar. The yeast recombines carbon, hydrogen, oxygen, and water to form alcohol and carbon dioxide. Different types of alcoholic beverages are derived from the use of different fermenting ingredients. Wine manufacturing, for example, may utilize grapes, apricots, berries, and other fruits that are rich in sugars and provide the necessary oxygen for fermentation. Fermentation continues until a maximum alcohol concentration of about 15 percent is reached, at which point, the concentration of alcohol is so high the yeast dies. Beers are manufactured with a *different* source of sugar, namely, the starch found in cereal grains, which is enzymatically converted to sugar through a malting process. This process involves sprouting cereal, such as barley, in water. The dried sprouts are then mixed with water. The enzymes formed during sprouting convert starch to sugar, which allows fermentation to proceed. For beers, the process of fermentation is stopped when the alcohol concentration reaches about 3 to 6 percent by volume, although some specialty beers may contain significantly more alcohol. For wines, the process is stopped, or found to be self-limiting, at higher concentrations (typically 11-13 percent by volume). Distillation of fermented beverages allows exceptionally high alcohol concentrations (typically 50-60 percent by volume in some beverages and up to nearly 100 percent in other products) to be obtained.

The range of alcohol concentration in alcoholic beverages is determined by biological processes, manufacturing design, or some combination of the two. Alcoholic beverage contents are usually expressed as a percentage of alcohol by volume, as in the case of beers and wines, or as "proof," an archaic term that is twice the alcohol concentration by volume. From a scientific perspective, the total amount of alcohol in a measured drink should be standardized so that for all practical purposes it is the same from drink to drink. However, the differences in alcohol concentrations among beverages may have medical consequences because of the direct action of alcohol on the tissues with which it comes in contact. The concentration of alcohol in beverages varies widely from about 3 percent in the case of light beers to about 50 percent or more in some liquors. Outside the laboratory, the amount of alcohol in a serving varies due to many factors (e.g., container or serving size, drink formulation, etc.). As alcohol absorption to maximum concentration in blood takes from about 30 to 90 minutes in most social-drinking cases, and total absorption takes even longer; beverage type and beverage concentration may be a factor in determining some of the medical consequences of alcohol use (Brick, 2006). Therefore, studies regarding the acute effects of alcohol should be conducted, and the results interpreted with this fact in mind.

SCIENTIFIC NOTATION
FOR ALCOHOL CONCENTRATIONS

Throughout this book, alcohol concentrations are expressed using various scientific notations. When comparing the results within these chapters with other references, it may be necessary to convert from one scientific notation to another. The concentration of alcohol in blood, serum, water, or any other liquid is the quantity of absolute alcohol by weight in a fixed volume of fluid. When alcohol is measured in breath, most breath-testing instruments are calibrated to take a fixed breath sample size. Instruments are designed on the basis of certain physiological assumptions and calibrated so that the results are reported as whole blood equivalents (e.g., 0.10 percent). In some literature, alcohol concentrations are reported as grams/2,100 cc air, and in blood or other tissues or fluids, they are more commonly reported in milligrams per deciliter (mg/dl). In molecular biological studies of how alcohol affects tissues, alcohol is sometimes reported in millimolar concentrations (mM). In those studies, mg/dl alcohol = mM alcohol $\times$ 4.6 provides a good conversion to a more identifiable concentration. This will be helpful for interpreting some of the data presented in Chapter 5, for example, ethanol concentrations of more than 50 mM (about 230 mg/dl) affect certain brain receptors but in some neurons, concentrations of more than

100 mM (about 460 mg/dl) were necessary to inhibit certain neuronal actions. These are relatively high doses.

When alcohol is measured in blood, the reported blood alcohol concentration (BAC) is the amount of alcohol by weight in a fixed volume of blood, which is usually 100 ml in the United States. BAC is usually expressed in g/100 ml or mg/100 ml of whole blood or serum. The following BAC notations are identical with regard to the amount of alcohol expressed: 0.10 percent, 0.10 g percent, 0.10 g/100 ml, 0.10 g/dl, 100 mg/dl, 100 mg percent, 100 mg/100 cc or ml.

Clinical Measurement of Alcohol

Most hospital clinical laboratories measure alcohol in serum, rather than in whole blood. As alcohol is distributed throughout the water-containing compartments of the body including the blood, serum alcohol is not the equivalent of a blood alcohol concentration because serum contains more water than the whole blood from which it is derived. Therefore, the concentration of alcohol in whole blood is less than that of the serum in proportion to their respective water contents. This may have important implications for scientists comparing test results. Early studies reported that the plasma: whole blood ethanol ratio ranged from 1.10 to 1.35 with an average of 1.18 (Payne, Hill, and Wood, 1968). Payne's average value of 1.18 has found acceptance in the literature (Baselt, 2000) and corresponds as well as our observations comparing serum alcohol measured by the alcohol dehydrogenase (ADH) method with gas chromatography analyses of the same sample (unpublished observations). Other studies suggest the ratio of serum: whole blood alcohol ranges from about 1.1 to 1.18 (Winek and Carfagna, 1987) to 1.25 (Hodgson and Shajani, 1985). Individual differences between subjects or within the same subject after some medical interventions, for example, may alter the water content of blood. Various mathematical models have been proposed when interpreting BACs particularly in patients with hemodilution or hemoconcentration (Brick, 2006; Brick and Erickson, 1999).

DEFINING ALCOHOL USE

Alcohol has been consumed for thousands of years, but the medical consequences of alcohol abuse have come to the attention of the medical/scientific community only in the last 150 years or so. Alcohol consumption and related problems have been well documented (Dufour, 1999). In the United States, for example, nearly half the adult population consumes alcohol, and alcohol-related medical problems account for a disproportionate number of hospital admissions. Data from the National Longitudinal Epidemiologic Survey indicate that nearly 9 percent of adults in the United States consume, on average, more than two drinks per day (Dawson et al., 1995), and the results of an ongoing national survey of high school students recently reported that among twelfth graders, about 3 percent consume alcohol daily and about half of them had consumed alcohol within the last month of the survey (Johnston, O'Malley, and Bachman, 1999). The use of alcohol and other drugs also has a profound economic impact. Estimates place the cost of addiction at more than $200 billion per year from the effect of alcohol on families and society through lost wages, absent or ineffectual parental models, and shared exposure to high risks and resulting injuries associated with intoxication.

Alcohol use is not always associated with deleterious medical consequences. In fact, some research suggests that alcohol use under some conditions is beneficial to health. How alcohol exerts such biphasic effects has been the subject of considerable research and debate. However, we can define alcohol use in two ways: first, through current definitions of use, abuse, and dependence and, second, by defining what constitutes "a drink." The social use of alcohol is now generally described as a cold beer after a ball game, a glass of wine with meals, or a glass of champagne at festive occasions. Alcohol consumption is often defined as drug abuse (or misuse) whenever it places the drinker or others affected by the drinker's behavior at increased risk for injury. The term "moderate" drinking is sometimes used by clinicians, and often used by laypersons, to describe consumption that is neither abusive nor very infrequent, or that describes a constellation of behavioral or other factors that *differentiate* it from "light" or "heavy." However, these terms are relative. For example, a "moderate" drinker may drink heavily (e.g., more than six drinks a day on some days) but not be classified as a "heavy" drinker. On the other hand, the U.S. Department of Agriculture (USDA) and the U.S. Department of Health and Human Services in the *Dietary Guidelines for Americans* defines moderate drinking as one drink per day or less for women and two or fewer drinks per day for men (USDA, 1995). In addition, the National Institute on Alcohol Abuse and Alcoholism (NIAAA, 2000) further recommends that people aged 65 and older limit their consumption of alcohol to one drink per day. The terms light, moderate, and heavy should be interpreted carefully based on the operational definition of the study as the definitions of these terms vary. Similarly, there is considerable variation in terms of defining "a drink" (Case, Destefano, and Logan, 2000; Kerr et al., 2005).

The *Diagnostic and Statistical Manual of Mental Disorders* (DSM-IV) (American Psychiatric Association, 1994) defines two types of problem drinkers: (1) abusers, who intentionally drink too much, too often, and make wrong choices about their use of alcohol, and (2) dependent users (i.e., alcoholics), who lack control over their use of alcohol in lifestyle situations in which abusers would generally stop drinking. Voluntary alcohol abuse is a significant problem that contributes to accidents, medical expenses, lost productivity, family problems, and, of course, a host of direct and indirect medical consequences. Drug dependence, whether the drug is alcohol or some other psychoactive substance, is a brain disease caused by a neurochemical imbalance. The addict has no control of his or her alcohol or other drug use (see Erickson and Wilcox, 2001, for a review). Both types of drinkers are overly represented as inpatients and as patients in hospital emergency rooms.

What Constitutes a Drink?

We can also define what is meant by a drink by standardizing this definition across beverage types so that the interpretation is meaningful and useful. Many epidemiological and empirical research studies define alcohol consumption in terms of the number of drinks consumed or the number of grams of absolute alcohol. Often the precise definition of what constitutes a drink is not included in studies or the range of definitions makes it difficult to compare results across studies. Equating commonly consumed beverages, a drink can be defined as 1.5 ounces of 80-proof alcohol, 5 ounces of 12 percent wine, or a 12-ounce standard beer (~4.8 percent v/v) (Brick, 2006). Each of these contains approximately 14 grams of alcohol, 0.6 ounces of absolute alcohol, and about 100 kilocalories. Outside of the laboratory, a mixed drink may contain more or less than 1.5 ounces of 80-proof alcohol (or the equivalent) and wine may be served in volumes larger or smaller than 5 ounces. Similarly, the concentration of alcohol in beers varies from an average of about 3.8 percent (v/v) for "light" beers to about 5 percent (v/v) for most beers. Imported or specialty beers may contain significantly more alcohol by volume (Case et al., 2000).

Regardless of the type of alcoholic beverage consumed, it is the psychoactive drug ethanol that produces the effects on the brain, virtually all cells within the body, and behavior. The degree of those effects is determined by the concentration, amount, and time of consumption, bioavailability due to factors such as absorption and biotransformation of alcohol, and drinking experience. All of these factors ultimately result in the exposure and response of various cells to concentrations of alcohol.

REFERENCES

American Psychiatric Association (1994). *Diagnostic and Statistical Manual of Mental Disorders,* Fourth Edition. Washington, DC: American Psychiatric Association.

Baselt, R.C., ed. (2000). *Disposition of Toxic Drugs and Chemicals in Man.* Foster City, CA: Chemical Toxicology Institute.

Brick, J. (2006). Standardization of alcohol calculations in research. *Alcoholism Clinical and Experimental Research* 30(8).

Brick, J. and Erickson, C. (1999). *Drugs, the Brain, and Behavior: The Pharmacology of Abuse and Dependence.* Binghamton, NY: The Haworth Medical Press, p. 67.

Case, G.A., Destefano, S., and Logan, B.K. (2000). Tabulation of alcohol content of beer and malt beverages. *Journal of Analytical Toxicology* 24:202-210.

Dawson, D.A., Grant, B.F., Chou, S.P., and Pickering, R.P. (1995). Subgroup variation in U.S. drinking patterns: Results of the 1992 national longitudinal alcohol epidemiologic study. *Journal of Substance Abuse* 7(3):331-344.

Dufour, M.C. (1999). What is moderate drinking? *Alcohol Research & Health*: Winter 1999. Available at: http://www.findarticles.com/p/articles/mim()CXH/is123/ai57050104. Accessed January 18, 2006.

Erickson, C. and Wilcox, R. (2001). Neurobiological causes of addiction. *Journal of Social Work Practice in the Addictions* 1(3):7-22.

Hodgson, B.T. and Shajani, N.K., (1985). Distribution of ethanol: Plasma to the whole blood rations. *Canadian Society of Forensic Science Journal* 18:73

Johnston, L.D., O'Malley, P.M., and Bachman, J.G. (1999). Drug trends in 1999 are mixed. Retrieved from the University of Michigan Web site: http://www.monitoringthefuture.org.

Kerr, W.C., Greenfield, T.K., Tujague, J., and Brown, S.E. (2005). A drink is a drink? Variation in the amount of alcohol contained in beer, wine and spirits drinks in the US methodological sample. *Alcoholism Clinical and Experimental Research* 29(1):2015-2021.

National Institute on Alcohol Abuse and Alcoholism (2000). *Tenth Special Report to the U.S. Congress on Alcohol and Health.* Washington, DC: U.S. Department of Health and Human Services.

Payne, J.P., Hill, D.W., and Wood, D.G.L. (1968). Distribution of ethanol between plasma and erythrocytes in whole blood. *Nature* 217:963-964.

Pieters, J., Wedel, M., and Schaafsma, G. (1990). Parameter estimation in a three-compartment model for blood alcohol curves. *Alcohol and Alcoholism* 25:17-24.

U.S. Department of Agriculture and U.S. Department of Health and Human Services (1995). *Home and Garden Bulletin* No. 232, Fourth Edition. Washington, DC: U.S. Department of Agriculture.

Winek, C.L. and Carfagna, M. (1987). Comparison of plasma, serum and whole blood ethanol concentrations. *Journal of Analytical Toxicology* 11:267-278.

Chapter 2

Medical Consequences of Acute and Chronic Alcohol Abuse

John Brick

INTRODUCTION AND OVERVIEW

More has been written about alcohol and its diverse effects than any other drug. Alcohol is one of the oldest drugs known and it affects virtually every organ system in the body. The number of physiological systems affected by alcohol is staggering both in the scope of medical consequences and in terms of the economics of medical treatment of alcohol-related disorders. Alcohol damages the heart and can elevate blood pressure, increasing the risk of heart failure and stroke. Excessive alcohol consumption can injure various tissues, produce diverse physiological changes, and impair and interfere with the hormonal and biochemical regulation of a variety of cellular and metabolic functions. Chronic alcohol exposure increases the risk for certain forms of cancer, and both acute and chronic alcohol use significantly increase the risk for accidental injuries and impairs the recovery from those injuries. However, not all of the medical consequences of alcohol use are deleterious. Substantial research indicates the beneficial effects of this drug. Nonetheless, the economic and psychosocial costs of alcohol use in American society alone are estimated at more than $200 billion per year. This chapter will review the most significant and well-known medical consequences of alcohol use and abuse in four basic areas: accidental injuries, the skeletal system, the gastrointestinal system, the hepatic system, and the cardiovascular system.

Handbook of the Medical Consequences of Alcohol and Drug Abuse
© 2008 by The Haworth Press, Taylor & Francis Group. All rights reserved.
doi:10.1300/6039_02

ALCOHOL AND ACCIDENTAL INJURIES

Accidental injuries are a direct medical consequence of alcohol intoxication and it is well known that alcohol increases the risk of injuries through impairment of cognitive and psychomotor functioning while performing or engaging in a variety of behavioral activities. Among these, the effects of alcohol on automobile, bicycle, motorcycle, boating, aquatic, and pedestrian injuries, as well as homicide, suicide, and death from fire have been examined.

Impaired Driving

Driving while intoxicated is probably the most well-studied injurious consequence of drinking. Whereas the older scientific literature on drinking and driving focused on the effects of high blood alcohol levels on simple reaction time, on the visual system, and on gross impairment, it is now known that the effects of alcohol are much broader and occur at relatively low blood alcohol levels. For example, alcohol use is coupled with increased risk taking and impulsivity, at least among young males (Cherpitel, 1993), and decreased seat belt use (Centers for Disease Control [CDC], 1991), which invariably places drinkers at increased risk of injury. It is now known that very low levels of alcohol (0.02-0.03 percent) impair the performance of complex divided attention tasks, at least in laboratory studies. Divided attention is believed to be a critical factor in a variety of tasks outside the laboratory, and divided attention failure is the most likely cause of motor vehicle collisions at blood alcohol levels above 0.05 percent, for it is at this level that impairment translates into actual highway statistics (in which the intoxicated driver is the cause of the accident). At higher blood alcohol levels (e.g., 0.15 percent or more), impairment in proprioception, visual perception, and lengthened simple reaction time are additional significant contributing factors to motor vehicle accidents. Most people who present obvious symptoms of intoxication are driving impaired and at increased risk for a fatal crash. Unfortunately, the lack of obvious intoxication does not mean lack of impairment. Most subjects do not appear visibly intoxicated, even though they are intoxicated according to law in regard to motor vehicle operation (Brick and Carpenter, 2001; Brick et al., 1992; Wells et al., 1997; Langenbucher and Nathan, 1983). When most people appear obviously intoxicated, their blood alcohol concentration (BAC) is probably well in excess of any legal definition of intoxication (Hobbs, Rall, and Verdoorn, 1996).

Regardless of which functions are affected by alcohol, impaired drivers clearly present a public health risk because of the increased number of accidental injuries due to intoxication. About 16,000 people are killed each year as a result of drunken driving (National Institute on Alcohol Abuse and Alcoholism [NIAAA], 2000), and about 10 percent of all personal injury accidents and at least 180,000 to 200,000 property and personal injury crashes, respectively, are caused by alcohol intoxication per year (Wieczorek, 1995). The risk of injury as well as the responsibility for causing a collision when driving while intoxicated is proportional to the blood alcohol level. With the current legal definition of driving while intoxicated (0.08 percent), the relative risk for a crash is conservatively estimated to be about six to seven times greater than driving while sober (see Table 2.1). When the interaction between blood alcohol level, gender, and single versus multiple vehicle collisions is considered, the relative risk is many times greater than previously believed. For example, one recent study suggests that the relative risk of a single car collision for a 16- to 20-year-old male with a blood alcohol level of about 0.10 to 0.15 percent is about 82 to 735 times greater when compared with controls. Older subjects (21- to 34-year-olds) have less risk than younger less experienced drinkers, but it is still significantly high—about 18 to 58 times greater compared with controls (Zador, Krawchuk, and Voas, 2000).

Pedestrian and Fall-Down Injuries

The relationship between alcohol intoxication and automobile accidents is by far the most well-studied of alcohol-caused injuries, the investigation of the role of alcohol intoxication in other types of injuries is growing. Earlier studies estimated that about one-third of all fatally injured pedestrians had a BAC of 0.10 percent or more at the time of their death. As driving and pedestrian activity rely on divided attention and visual motor processes, it is reasonable to infer that they share similar alcohol-induced changes in relative risk, although, driving is obviously a more challenging task than walking. Blomberg et al. (1979) reported that the relative risk of involvement in a fatal pedestrian injury did not begin to rise significantly until the pedestrians reached a BAC of 0.15 percent or higher. More research is needed, particularly on the relative risk of nonfatal injuries in intoxicated pedestrians. Driving is a more complex task than pedestrian activity but both behaviors require divided attention, vigilance, and other cognitive skills that are sensitive to the impairment produced by alcohol, often at very low BACs (*Alcohol World,* 1990; NIAAA, 1988; Surgeon General's Workshop on Drunk Driving, 1988).

TABLE 2.1 Alcohol Intoxication, Behavior, and Relative Risk for a Single Vehicle Fatal Crash

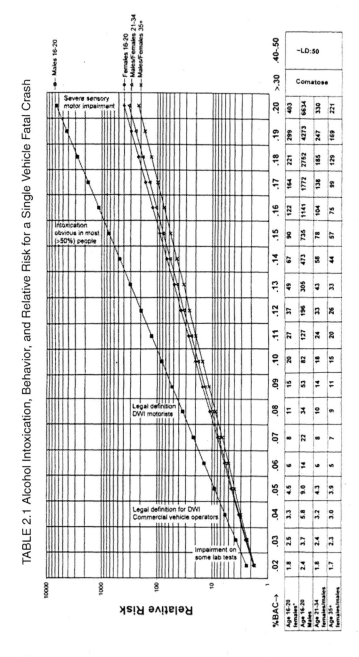

Note: Line graph shows relative risk (log) as a function of BAC, age, and gender. Data derived from stepwise logistic regression coefficients for relative risk is presented in tabularized form below graph. Coefficients are rounded to nearest tenth or whole number. These coefficients apply to single vehicle fatalities. Note that for women age 16-20, a coefficient of 0.03 (range 0.044-0.014) was used. *Source:* Based on Zador et al., 2000, *J Stud Alc* 61(3): 387-395, Zador et al., 2000, USDOT. NHTSA DOT HW 809 051. Also included are biobehavioral descriptors from Brick and Erickson, 1999.

With regard to pedestrian activity, the person must divide their attention between many different tasks. When sober, many of these tasks are performed without difficulty or conscious effort. However, alcohol intoxication may interfere with the ability to walk, in which it is necessary to lift the leg, flex the foot, step forward, rotate the hip, redistribute the weight to the load bearing leg, and repeat this sequence while also allowing for changes in the road surface, and so on. When an intoxicated individual must attend to the many components involved in walking and attend simultaneously to highway, roadway, or structural challenges, that person is at increased risk for an accident, much like the motor vehicle operator.

Injuries related to falls are the second leading cause of accidents in the United States, and account for about 13,000 deaths per year. Most studies suggest that alcohol increases the risk for injuries due to falls, but one study in particular included a control group that allowed researchers to analyze increases in relative risk for a fall due to alcohol intoxication. Honkanen et al. evaluated 313 emergency room patients, more than half of whom had blood alcohol levels greater than 0.20 percent, and compared them with pedestrians who were at the same location of the accident one week later at the same time of day (Honkanen et al., 1983). The comparison revealed the relative risk for a fall was three times greater for patients with blood alcohol levels between 0.05 and 0.10 percent, ten times greater for patients with blood alcohol levels between 0.10 and 0.15 percent, and 60 times greater for patients with BACs 0.16 percent or higher (Honkanen et al., 1983). More than two-thirds of drivers, pedestrians, and bicyclists (see the following) who are killed each year are intoxicated (National Highway Traffic Safety Administration [NHTSA], 1994).

Bicycling

Intoxication is believed to be a factor in nonmotorized vehicle injuries as well. According to NHTSA, there are about 200 fatalities and 7,000 injuries from alcohol-related bicycle crashes each year, and that bicyclists who died at the scene were four times as likely as those who died at hospitals to be legally intoxicated which may be due to the effects of alcohol on injury outcome (discussed later in this chapter). Olkkonen and Honkanen (1994) used a case-control study method, to estimate the relative risk of an alcohol-related bicycle crash. The study involved 200 bicycle victims who were injured fatally in road traffic accidents during the years 1982-1988, and 700 cyclists who were used as unmatched controls for these cases. The study found that alcohol was involved in 25 percent of the collision accidents and in 63 percent of the single accidents involving cyclists aged 15 to 64 years and whose blood alcohol was measured. Only 4 percent of the controls were under the influence of alcohol. A relative risk was of the order of 3 overall, and 58 for the collisions related to alcohol use. Li et al. reported that fatally injured bicyclists were about twice as likely to be intoxicated as cyclists treated for nonfatal injuries (Li et al., 1996).

Fires and Burns

Alcohol intoxication is a contributing factor in injuries from fires and burns, which account for an estimated 5,000 fatalities and about 1.4 million injuries a year, and is a leading cause of accidents and deaths in the United States (Baker, O'Neill, and Karpf, 1992). Howland and Hingson (1987) reviewed studies on alcohol and burn injuries published between 1947 and 1986 and reported on the percentage of the victims who were intoxicated from alcohol. In the overwhelming majority of studies, it was concluded that alcohol exposure was more likely among those who died in fires ignited by cigarettes than from other causes. Although the evidence is not definitive, it strongly suggests that alcohol plays a role in the cause of fires and of subsequent burn injuries and is overly represented in burn victims. It is noteworthy that in a study of deaths due to fire, Hingson and Howland found that one-third to two-thirds of these victims had blood alcohol levels greater than 0.10 percent, which at the time of the study, represented the blood alcohol level that defined intoxicated driving in most states. The authors concluded from these data that alcohol intoxication is a risk factor for fire deaths (Hingson and Howland, 1993). Later studies further revealed that alcohol was a factor in about 22 percent (Cherpitel, 1989) to 26 percent (Jones et al., 1991) of burn injuries. Overall, intoxicated patients have a significantly higher fatality rate in severe burn cases. These data are more thoroughly reviewed in the Ninth Special Report to the U.S. Congress on Alcohol and Health (NIAAA, 1997).

Impairment from alcohol is one of several risk factors found in a substantial percentage of burn victims. For example, Brezel and Kassenbrock (1988) examined drug and alcohol abusers, psychiatric patients, and those with neurological dysfunction to determine whether this group had more complications, more surgical procedures, and longer hospital stays than burn patients without these disorders. However, alcohol abuse (defined as six or more cans of beer or the equivalent, per day) was the most common form of impairment. Although impaired patients had more complications and required a longer period of hospitalization, alcohol intoxication was only one of several contributory factors.

In a study of 1,074 patients admitted to a medical center burn unit, McGill et al. (1995) found that the 40 percent who were positive for alcohol were more likely to have a greater proportion of bodily burns and greater incidence of smoke inhalation than controls. Chronic alcoholics also seem to have a higher fatality rate than do patients without a history of chronic alcohol abuse (Haum et al., 1995). Interestingly, the authors found no significant differences between sober and acutely intoxicated alcoholics suggesting that neurological or other long-lasting consequences of alcohol abuse and acute intoxication produce risk. The authors conclude that alcohol intake prior to burn injury is an independent risk factor in this population.

In a review on the epidemiology and toxicological complications of burn cases involving alcohol and other drugs, Brick (2006a) concluded that there is a clear relationship between alcohol or drug intoxication and the risk for thermal injury. For example, alcohol-intoxicated persons may be at increased risk for accidental injury because of impaired judgment or psychomotor coordination while engaging in normal fire-starting activities (e.g., cooking), but psychomotor impairment is one part of the problem. Neuropsychological status while intoxicated may impair various domains of cognitive functioning decreasing the ability to anticipate problems, lower inhibitions, and increase risky behaviors. Once a fire has started, mental confusion and failure to recognize risk or danger may lead to an inability to anticipate or respond to danger, particularly at high levels of intoxication. This evolving literature shows that the interaction between burn injuries and intoxication is often complex and includes many variables in addition to intoxication.

Water Sports

The relationship between alcohol intoxication and leisure activities, such as swimming and boating, has been a subject of scientific interest for some time. For example, it can be reasonably predicted that because alcohol impairment causes errors in judgment, disorientation, hypothermia, impaired psychomotor skills, and a decrease in the ability to hold one's breath, it would increase drowning accidents. However, studies published prior to 1985 did not establish a causal relationship between these effects of alcohol intoxication and drowning. Hoxie et al. reported that 45 percent of drowning victims had some alcohol in their system and 22 percent were intoxicated with blood alcohol levels of 0.10 percent or more at the time of death (Hoxie et al., 1988). More recent studies suggest that alcohol consumption significantly increases risk for boating fatalities. In a review of the Boating Accident Report Files in Ohio from 1983 to 1986, Molberg et al. found that alcohol consumption was a factor in up to 21 percent of reported boating accidents (Molberg et al., 1993). As alcohol deleteriously impairs balance, motor function, and judgment, intoxicated passengers, as well as vessel operators, are probably at risk for injury (Hingson and Howland, 1993).

In another water sport activity, diving, alcohol intoxication contributes to and aggravates spinal cord injuries that frequently follow diving accidents. In this context, Perrine et al. examined the effects of alcohol on the ability to perform shallow-water entry dives under experimental conditions (Perrine, Mundt, and Winer, 1994). The data revealed a progressive and significant impairment of specific aspects of diving performance at blood alcohol levels of 0.04 percent and higher. Interestingly, this study also correlated diving performance with psychomotor performance using the same standardized field sobriety tests used by many police to detect drunk drivers. Impaired diving correlated well with subjects who failed the validated scoring criteria for the detection of drivers with a blood alcohol level of more than 0.10 percent (Perrine, Mundt, and Winer, 1994).

Aircraft Operation

One of the more complex divided attention tasks to challenge persons outside of the laboratory is flying an aircraft. Pilots must attend to an array of instrumentation and make perceptual and cognitive decisions based on a large amount of information in an environment that changes in more than one plane. Although there have been few cases of fatal airline crashes due to pilot intoxication, sufficient data is available to raise concern about this issue of airline safety. For example, it is known from research in other fields that alcohol impairs skills such as divided attention that are believed necessary for safe motor vehicle operation. It is also known that alcohol deleteriously influences the ability of pilots to evaluate their performance (Morrow et al., 1991) and that low levels of alcohol (0.025-0.04 percent) impair performance of trained pilots in flight simulators (Billings et al., 1991; Ross, Yeazel, and Chau, 1992).

The effects of alcohol on piloting skills may exceed the direct pharmacological action of alcohol. It has also been suggested that alcohol can impair performance on flight simulators many hours after blood alcohol levels have returned to zero (Yesavage, Dolhert, and Taylor, 1994). Although these studies are based on known biobehavioral effects or on flight simulator results, rather than epidemiological data, it is clear more research is needed to understand this important relationship.

Suicide

Suicide or attempted suicide is an often undiagnosed medical consequence of alcohol use. Yet suicide is the eleventh leading cause of death, and for those aged 15-34, the third leading cause of death in the United States (National Center for Health Statistics, 2003).

In a recent review of 16 studies of acute intoxication and suicide attempts, Cherpitel et al. (2004) found that that the mean percentage of alcohol use was 40 percent but the range varied from 10 to 73 percent for attempted suicide and 10 to 69 percent for completed suicides. Although it is generally accepted that there is a relationship between alcohol use and suicide, existing data are often incomplete. For example, Cherpitel et al., in their excellent review, point out that definitions of intoxication in suicide reports included both subjective or objective alcohol data. Nevertheless, the relationship between intoxication and suicide is not difficult to understand. Acute intoxication reduces inhibitions, narrows attention, impairs the ability to appreciate the consequences of behavior, and may promote depressive thoughts and hopelessness, whereas chronic alcohol abuse is often complicated by mental illness, including depression (Cheng, 1995; Conner, Beautrais, and Conwell, 2003; see Waller and Lomer, this volume). In both acute and chronic intoxication, impaired psychomotor and cognitive skill, enhanced aggression including self-aggression, or the use of alcohol in combination with medications may be other biopsychological pathways mediating this behavior (Cherpital, Borges, and Wilcox, 2004). Although, it is unlikely that normally adjusted people commit or attempt to commit suicide simply because they are intoxicated, premorbid suicidal ideology is more likely to be acted upon while under the influence of alcohol. However, there is some evidence that acute intoxication is a greater risk factor for suicide than the previous drinking history (Borges and Rosovsky, 1996) but the causal mechanism for the relationship between alcohol and suicide is simply not known (Hufford, 2001). For more information, see Chiapella and Conner (2004).

Miscellaneous Injuries

In a recent case-control study, Dawson examined the relationship between intoxication and the risk of death from external causes (e.g., suicide, homicide, and accidental injuries) and found that relative to lifetime abstainers and infrequent drinkers, the risk of death from external causes increased logarithmically among infrequent binge drinkers (Dawson, 2001). There was no evidence of reduced risk of death among light or moderate drinkers. The group at highest risk of death from external causes were drinkers who drank less than once a month, but when they did drink, consumed five or more drinks. Within this group, older subjects (defined as 65-plus years) were at the highest risk, but younger drinkers (defined as 18 to 24 years of age) were also at high risk of death. Middle-aged drinkers (25 to 64 years of age) did not show the same increased mortality risk, which the author suggested was related to tolerance and experience. Although these data suggest that infrequent binge drinking, as defined, increases risk as a function of age, possible tolerance, and age-related experience, the blood alcohol level that would result from five drinks would be relatively low, allowing the other variables to have a measurable impact.

Intoxication and Injury Outcome

Not only does alcohol intoxication produce direct medical consequences as a result of injuries (e.g., fractures, traumatic amputations, etc.) sustained in a motor vehicle crash, for example, it may also affect injury outcome, particularly head injuries. This is highly significant as up to half of traumatic brain-injured patients have BACs of 0.10 percent or more at the time of injury (Zink et al., 2001). For example, motorcycle riders with head injuries are about twice as likely to have fatal head injuries if they are intoxicated than similarly injured riders who are sober (Luna et al., 1984), and contrary to popular misconception, drunk drivers are more likely to be seriously or fatally injured than sober drivers (Waller et al., 1986). Alcohol-intoxicated accident victims with central nervous system injuries were more than twice as likely to die sooner than anatomically matched controls (Zink, Maoi, and Chen, 1996).

The mechanisms of the exacerbating effects of alcohol on central nervous system injuries are intriguing, but not well understood. Animal studies suggest that the mechanism may be due to the inhibition of free radical scavengers such as dimethyl sulfoxide (Albin and Bunegin, 1986), alcohol-induced cerebral edema as a result of lipid peroxidation (DeCrescito et al., 1974), or increases in plasma osmolality (Elmer, Goransson, and Zoucas, 1984; Steinbok and Thompson, 1978). However, Ward, Flynn, and Miller (1982) found that hospitalized major trauma victims with average blood alcohol levels of about 0.15 percent were significantly less likely to die from injuries than victims in the sober control group. Similarly, Kraus et al. (1989) found that contrary to expectations, injury severity and mortality were inversely related to blood alcohol levels. This may imply that the mechanisms through which alcohol exacerbates some injuries may be related to metabolic by-products as well as the direct pharmacological actions of alcohol itself. In any case, these older study results support the commonly held belief that being intoxicated somehow protects against injuries. However, such a belief is not supported by the majority of more current research on this topic (e.g., Fell and Hertz, 1993). Recent studies suggest that the severity of hemorrhagic shock is greater when intoxicated and results in a higher mortality rate compared with sober controls (Molina et al., 2002). Hemorrhagic shock also induces acidosis with marked hypercarbia. In such cases, alcohol-induced acidosis would likely increase morbidity and mortality (Chen et al., 2000; Kinkaid et al., 1998; Molina et al., 2002) possibly because of the effects of acidosis on ventilatory responses. Although the literature is complex, some evidence suggests that the effects of alcohol on respiration are mediated through an opioid system. Zink et al. (and others) found that the opiate antagonist naloxone can improve hemodynamics and cerebral infusion following traumatic brain injury and hemorrhagic shock but not in alcohol-treated animals. However, alcohol-induced depression of hypercapnic (carbon monoxide) ventilatory drive was reversed by naltrexone (Zink et al., 2001). As previously discussed, alcohol abuse also increases risk for death in burn patients (Brick, 2006a).

ALCOHOL AND THE SKELETAL SYSTEM

Although it is not difficult to appreciate the positive and causal relationship between alcohol intoxication and skeletal fractures—one need only look at the large number of motor vehicle and slip-and-fall injuries involving alcohol intoxication—this relationship is more complex and certainly did not start with current epidemiological studies. In fact, the relationship between alcohol abuse and increased risks for skeletal fractures was observed by the ancient Egyptians (Conn, 1985; Mathew, 1992; Seller, 1985). This relationship has since been confirmed by research that suggests alcoholics suffer from a generalized skeletal fragility and are prone to fracture.

Alcohol-Induced Fractures

Much of the current scientific research on the prevalence of fractures in alcoholic subjects is based on epidemiological studies. Those results are complex and are often generally inconsistent. Even so, there is some evidence of a positive association between alcohol intake and fracture occurrence. For example, men hospitalized for alcohol-related problems are four times more likely to have rib fractures than nondrinking patients (Lindsell, Wilson, and Maxwell, 1982) and up to 14 times more likely to have spinal-crush fractures (Crilly et al., 1988; Israel et al., 1980).

Women

In a prospective study, Tuppurainen et al. (1995) found alcohol intake higher among 3,140 perimenopausal women who experienced fractures than among those without fractures. Women who drank alcohol had a risk of a fracture that was about 50 percent higher than among women who did not drink. In another study, increased weekly alcohol intake was associated with greater risks for osteoporotic fractures in postmenopausal women (Paganini-Hill, Ross, and Gerkins, 1981). In the Paganini-Hill study, osteoporotic fractures in women who consumed more than eight drinks per week were almost twice as likely as in nondrinkers. Similarly, a survey of 84,500 U.S. women (ages 34 to 59) who consumed 25 grams of alcohol per day was associated with a 133 percent increase in risk for hip fractures and a 38 percent increase in risk for wrist fractures (Hernandez-Avila et al., 1991). This effect is less common in other populations where the consumption of seven or more standard drinks per week was associated with a twofold increased risk of hip fractures in Japanese women (Fujiwara et al., 1997) and a 4.6-fold increased risk of fractures in a study of black women (Grisso et al., 1994).

In the studies described previously, investigators often compare the relationship between drinking quantity and frequency (e.g., drinks per day) with some medical outcome. The definition of what constitutes "a drink" varies between studies, or in some cases, is not well defined. Therefore, the results from such studies should be viewed in relative rather than absolute terms (Brick, 2006b; Miller, Heather, and Hall, 1991).

Men

Alcohol also increases the risk for fractures in men. In men under the age of 65, two to six drinks per week significantly increased the risk of fractures compared with the same injuries in subjects who consumed less than two drinks per week. For male heavy drinkers younger than age 65, there was almost ten times the risk of hip fractures as men in the same age group who drank lightly (Felson et al., 1988). As sobering as the results for men may be, other investigators have not identified any significant association between alcohol intake and risks for various fractures in women (Cumming and Klineberg, 1994; Diaz, O'Neill, and Silman, 1997; Huang et al., 1996; Johnell et al., 1995; O'Neill et al., 1996). Thus, evidence suggests that excessive alcohol intake increases the risk of fracture but the results are not unanimous. Further, the consequences of low levels of alcohol consumption on skeletal integrity are not well understood.

Age

Studies involving older or intoxicated patients, two groups at high risk for fractures, have methodological limitations including but not limited to defining and quantifying alcohol use due to memory impairment. Despite these problems, including a host of confounding environmental factors such as diet, exercise, and general health, a thorough scientific investigation of the relationship between (moderate) alcohol intake and fracture risks would still have enormous public health implications.

Alcohol-Induced Osteoporosis

In addition to the risk of falls and related injuries previously reviewed, some evidence suggests that alcoholics may also suffer from a generalized skeletal fragility. Bone density is a predictor of fractures and the term "osteoporosis" is synonymous with low bone density or osteopenia (NIAAA, 2000). Saville was the first to demonstrate the association of osteopenia with alcohol abuse (Saville, 1965). Studying the bone mass of cadavers, Saville found marked reductions in the bone mass of persons with a history of alcoholism and further noted that the bone mass of young alcoholic males were comparable to elderly, postmenopausal females. Since those initial observations, numerous studies have confirmed this effect (Peris et al., 1995; Spencer et al., 1986). In a prospective case-control analysis of risk factors for the development of osteoporosis, Blaauw et al. found that average alcohol consumption was two to three times higher in both osteoporotic men and women than in age-matched controls (Blaauw et al., 1994). A similar finding was made in an earlier study in which premenopausal women who consumed more than two standard drinks per day exhibited 13 percent lower bone density of the hip, compared with women who consumed less than one standard drink per week (Gonzalez-Calvin et al., 1993).

Alcohol-reduced bone density is not universally reported within or between studies. Some studies have suggested that increasing alcohol consumption was positively, but anatomically and selectively correlated with bone density (Holbrook and Barrett-Connor, 1993; Lairinen, Valimaki, and Keto, 1991; Lairinen et al., 1993). The Study of Osteoporotic Fractures (7,963 ambulatory, nonblack women ages 65 and older) revealed that modest alcohol intake, less than one drink per day in about 85 percent of the subjects, was associated with higher bone density (Orwoll et al., 1996).

Alcohol's contribution to osteopenia in the overall population is not known, although it is tempting to speculate that lower levels of consumption are less likely to be associated with low bone density and may even be associated with higher bone density. However, the evidence for a protective effect of moderate alcohol consumption is not entirely compelling and should be interpreted with caution as many confounding factors exist in and between studies.

Microscopic Changes in Bone

Microscopic examination of bone (bone histomorphometry) from alcoholics has been helpful in understanding the etiology of skeletal disorders induced by alcohol. Bone mass is controlled by a remodeling cycle that begins with bone breakdown by cells called osteoclasts. This initial period of resorption is coupled with an equal amount of new bone formation by cells called osteoblasts. Bone mass remodeling is an ongoing process throughout most of the life cycle, but one that can be disrupted by alcohol. Alcoholics generally show a reduction in new bone formation with varying reports of increases (Schnitzler and Soloman, 1984) or no changes in bone resorption (Diamond et al., 1989). Overall, these studies suggest that alcoholic bone disease is characterized by considerable suppression of bone formation.

Although alcohol can disrupt the modeling cycle, these changes are reversible. Rapid recovery of osteoblast function occurs within two weeks of abstinence (Diamond et al., 1989; Feitelberg et al., 1987; Lairinen et al., 1992). Evidence also suggests that lost bone tissue is recovered following abstinence (Peris et al., 1994).

Potential Mechanisms of Alcohol-Induced Bone Disease

The normal growth of bone cells depends upon a variety of orchestrated factors, including adequate nutrition and the function and interaction of various hormones and intercellular regulating factors. Research in this area suggests that, although the exact mechanism through which alcohol affects the integrity of the skeleton is not known, much has been learned. Even so, likely candidates have not been clearly identified.

Chronic consumption of relatively low amounts of alcohol (one to two drinks per day for women; three to four drinks per day for men) can interfere with the normal metabolism of nutrients. As a result of poor diets, impaired nutrient absorption, or increased renal excretion, alcoholics often have deficiencies in minerals such as calcium, phosphate, and magnesium (Bikle et al., 1985; Kalbfleisch et al., 1963; Lairinen et al., 1992; Tetrito and Tanaka, 1974), as well as low levels of vitamin D, which is necessary for the absorption of calcium from the intestinal system (Lalor et al., 1986; Mobarhan et al., 1984). However, there is little histomorphometric evidence that nutritional deficiencies related to alcohol use are a major cause of alcohol-induced bone disease.

Another agent that may contribute to alcohol-induced bone disease is calcitonin, a peptide produced by the thyroid gland. Calcitonin inhibits bone resorption, in effect protecting bone. Some evidence suggests that the acute administration of alcohol (equal to about four drinks in a 150-pound male) increases calcitonin levels by about 38 percent three hours after consumption by nonalcoholic males (Williams et al., 1978). Such hypercalcitoninemia might explain why moderate intake of alcohol is associated with higher bone density. However, little is known about repeated alcohol use or how chronic alcohol affects calcitonin.

Blood calcium levels are regulated primarily through parathyroid hormone (PTH). When blood calcium levels drop, PTH induces the release of calcium from bone and reduces renal excretion of calcium. In nonalcoholic subjects, acute alcohol consumption decreased PTH levels three hours after drinking, but prolonged drinking for three weeks increased PTH levels as well as serum calcium (Lairinen, Valimaki, and Keto, 1991). It is still unclear how alcohol might affect PTH and calcium in a clinical population where decreases in bone density are typically observed.

Gonadal hormones may also play a role in alcohol-induced bone disease since impaired gonadal function is a well-known risk factor for osteoporosis. Moreover, alcohol abuse has long been associated with impotence, sterility, testicular atrophy (Valimaki, Salaspuro, and Ylikahri, 1982), and low testosterone (Van Thiel, Lester, and Sherins, 1974) in men, and menstrual disturbances, spontaneous abortions and miscarriages, impaired fertility, sexual function, and premature menopause in women (Gavaler, 1991; Hugues et al., 1980; Mello, Mendelson, and Teoh, 1993; Valimaki et al., 1984). Studies in women have yielded inconsistent results. Alcohol increases estradiol, a potent form of estrogen, but this effect has only been reported in postmenopausal women who are undergoing hormone replacement therapy. Nonetheless, if moderate alcohol consumption increases estrogen, it could explain the positive relationship between alcohol use and increased bone density in women (Holbrook and Barrett-Connor, 1993; Orwoll et al., 1996).

Chronic heavy drinking alters the growth and proliferation of many different cell types. In alcoholics, biochemical and histomorphometric studies reveal a significant impairment in osteoblastic, but not osteoclastic activity, suggesting that alcohol's primary adverse effects on bones is through osteoblasts. Since bone remodeling and mineralization both are dependent on osteoblasts, chronic heavy alcohol consumption will ultimately reduce bone mass and consequently lead to fractures.

Alcohol may decrease osteoblast proliferation through a direct toxic mechanism or by the inhibition of intracellular signaling processes that regulate cell replication. Preprogrammed cell death (apoptosis) of some cells is enhanced by alcohol (De et al., 1994; Ewald and Shao, 1993).

Alcohol reduces cell protein and deoxyribonucleic acid (DNA) synthesis in normal osteoblasts (Chavassieux et al., 1993; Friday and Howard, 1991) and impairs the induction of compounds called polyamines (Klein and Carlos, 1995), which regulate the synthesis of DNA. By disrupting the intracellular process that normally stimulates polyamine biosynthesis vital to osteoblast proliferation, alcohol even at low blood alcohol levels (0.04 percent range) may inhibit cell division. Exogenous polyamines antagonize the inhibitory effect of alcohol on cell proliferation (NIAAA, 2000). Osteocalcin is a small peptide synthesized by osteoblasts. When released into the circulation, osteocalcin levels are positively correlated with histomorphometric parameters of bone formation in healthy individuals (Garcia-Carrasco, Gruson, and De Vernejoul, 1988) and patients with metabolic bone disease (Delmas et al., 1985). Alcohol produces a dose-dependent decrease in osteocalcin levels and chronic alcoholic patients have significantly lower osteocalcin levels than controls (Labib et al., 1989).

CANCERS

Gastrointestinal Diseases

Not all of the effects of alcohol occur rapidly, as in the cases of motor vehicle crashes, pedestrian falls, subsequent skeletal injuries, or suicide. Some medical consequences of alcohol are more insidious, taking years to unfold before any significant medical consequence is detected. Among these are cell damage caused by the direct or indirect toxic effects of alcohol. The first tissue that alcohol comes into contact with is, in most instances, the upper gastrointestinal system.* With the exception of minute quantities of alcohol that are directly absorbed through membranes in the buccal cavity and esophagus, when swallowed, alcohol goes directly to the stomach in high concentrations. As the toxic effects of alcohol are directly related to dose and concentrations, one might reasonably predict that high concentrations of

---

* The author has received anecdotal reports from clinicians and recovering alcoholics about intravenous and rectal administration of alcohol, but it is believed that such experimental drug use is rare.

alcohol have potentially deleterious effects throughout the cells of the gastro-intestinal system.

Alcohol inhibits smooth muscle contractions in the lower esophagus (Keshavarzian et al., 1994), which may cause chronic esophageal inflamma-tion. Impaired contraction of the smooth muscles in the esophagus and in the stomach can also precipitate gastric acid reflux, resulting in a range of symptoms from the relatively benign but very uncomfortable heartburn, to severe esophagitis (inflammation of the esophagus). Prolonged gastric reflux may lead to permanent tissue alteration, or metaplasia, of the esophageal lining that may progress to esophageal adenocarcinoma (Gray, Donnelly, and Kingsnorth, 1993).

The relationship between alcohol consumption and various cancers of the gastrointestinal and other systems has been the subject of considerable research. For example several studies have demonstrated a positive rela-tionship between alcohol and esophageal cancer. People who consume more than three drinks per day (21 drinks per week) have almost a tenfold higher risk of esophageal cancer than those who drink less than one drink per day (Vaughan et al., 1995). Esophageal cancers include adenocarcinomas as well as cancers that are derived from normal esophageal cells (i.e., squamous cell carcinomas). Both types of carcinomas are related by the local effects of alcohol metabolites or alcohol-metabolizing enzymes such as alcohol dehydrogenase (ADH) on esophageal cells (Yin et al., 1993). For example, acetaldehyde may alter normal DNA repair mecha-nisms in esophageal cells and lead to gene alterations and tumor formation (Wilson et al., 1994). Alcohol also increases levels of the CYP2E 1 isozyme in the esophageal mucosa, which can activate dietary carcinogens such as nitrosamines (Shimizu et al., 1990).

Even though high concentrations of alcohol reach the stomach from the esophagus, and in spite of the effects of alcohol consumption or alcohol me-tabolites on DNA, alcohol use is not clearly associated with a risk of stom-ach cancer (Franceschi and La Vecchia, 1994). Alcohol can cause gastritis, but other factors, such as bacterium, may be responsible for inflammation of the stomach. For example, gastritis and ulcer disease in nonalcoholics is often caused by *Helicobacter pylori*. Heavy drinkers have a higher inci-dence of *H. pylori* and gastritis, than do light drinkers (Paunio et al., 1994). As alcoholic gastritis is not readily cured by abstinence but is improved by treatment with antibiotics, it has been quite reasonably suggested that gas-tritis is caused by bacterium (Uppal et al., 1991).

The nexus between gastritis and increased risk for stomach cancer is not well established, and the mechanism that leads the progression from chronic gastritis to neoplasia probably involves many factors besides alcohol. For example, nutritional factors, and in particular the deleterious effects of alcohol on the bioavailability of nutrients, probably play a role in alcohol-related colon cancer in humans. Alcohol in combination with diets low in essential nutrients such as methionine and folate, measurably increases the risk for colon cancer (Giovannucci and Willett, 1994; Giovannucci et al., 1995). Alcohol also induces the formation of benign hyperplastic polyps in the colon and rectum in humans (Kearney et al., 1995).

The association between alcohol and cancers of the colon and rectum is positive, but weak (Doll et al., 1993; Longnecker, 1992; Longnecker et al., 1990; Seitz and Pöschl, 1997). Again, although alcohol probably plays some role, other mechanisms are probably involved. Recent studies indicate that smoking tobacco coupled with drinking alcohol may serve as a triggering mechanism for colon cancer (Yamada et al., 1997). Acetaldehyde may also have a role as a cocarcinogen in cases of rectal cancer (Seitz and Pöschl, 1997). See NIAAA (2000) for further discussion on this topic.

Does Alcohol Increase the Risk for Breast Cancer?

Despite decades of research suggesting that alcohol increases the risk for breast cancer, reviews of this relationship suggest that the evidence for this relationship is not compelling (English et al., 1995; International Agency for Research on Cancer, 1988; Longnecker, 1992, 1994, 1995; McPherson, Engelsman, and Conning, 1993; Smith-Warner et al., 1998). For example, in a meta-analysis of epidemiological studies, alcohol sometimes showed a one- to twofold fold increase in risk for breast cancer (Longnecker, 1994). One factor may be that a complex alcohol-endocrine interaction exists that may be related to postmenopause hormone replacement therapy (Colditz, 1990; Gapstur et al., 1992; Schatzkin and Longnecker, 1994; Zumoff, 1997). As breast cancers are estrogen dependent and androgen and estrogen levels are both increased by alcohol, and in women with breast cancer, the weak relationship between alcohol and this form of cancer may be obscured by other risk factors (Beard, 1996).

ALCOHOL-INDUCED PANCREATIC INJURY

It is well known that alcohol abuse can lead to chronic pancreatic inflammation, atrophy, and fibrosis, although only a small proportion of alcoholics develop pancreatic injury. Specific risk and mechanisms that lead to alcoholic pancreatitis have been difficult to identify (Doll et al., 1993; Haber et al., 1995), but research from animal models suggests that acetaldehyde may play some role in the development of alcoholic pancreatitis, as may diets high in polyunsaturated fat. Although alcohol is believed to be a cause of pancreatitis, a link between alcohol and pancreatic cancer has not been made (NIAAA, 2000).

ALCOHOL-INDUCED LIVER INJURY

As a major portion of the alcohol consumed leaves the gastrointestinal tract, it travels via the hepatic portal vein from the small intestines to the liver, the largest organ in the body and the primary site of alcohol metabolism. As some alcohol metabolites are toxic, and because the concentration of alcohol reaching the liver is so high, and the liver is the primary site of alcohol metabolism, liver damage may be among the most likely and most serious physiological consequences of alcohol abuse. This is particularly significant because of the central role the liver plays in so many physiological activities. Epidemiological data clearly reveals that alcohol abuse is by far the leading cause of liver-related mortality in the United States. Excessive alcohol consumption leads to three serious types of liver injuries: fatty liver, hepatic inflammation (alcoholic hepatitis), and progressive liver scarring (fibrosis or cirrhosis). Chronic heavy drinking can alter normal metabolism and lead to an accumulation of fat in the liver. As a result, the liver cells become infiltrated and the liver itself becomes enlarged. The bad news is that extensive lipid infiltration may damage cells. The good news is that fatty liver condition is reversible with abstinence.

Hepatitis is a more serious medical condition, characterized by prolific inflammation and tissue damage. Hepatitis is life threatening but there can be significant recovery following abstinence. The most serious form of liver damage is cirrhosis. This irreversible liver disease is characterized by scarring and cell death. Impaired liver functioning can cause primary hepatic encephalopathy, a brain disorder characterized by altered psychomotor, intellectual, and behavioral functioning.

Although chronic, heavy drinking may produce metabolic tolerance and unusually high rates of alcohol elimination, hepatitis and fibrosis will ultimately impair liver function and produce a reverse metabolic tolerance and impaired oxidation of alcohol. Underreporting of alcohol consumption makes the exact prevalence of alcoholic liver disease in the United States difficult to measure, but health statistics suggest that some form of alcoholic liver disease affects more than 2 million drinkers (Dufour, Stinson, and Caces, 1993). It is estimated that 900,000 Americans have cirrhosis, and of the 26,000 who die each year, 40 to 90 percent have a history of alcohol abuse (Dufour, Stinson, and Caces, 1993).

It is clear that the development of alcoholic liver disease is due to a combination of factors, most notably, prolonged alcohol consumption. One commonly asked question by both scientists and concerned drinkers is "How much alcohol does one need to drink before liver damage occurs?" Epidemiological studies suggest that reliable signs of injury begin after a "threshold" dose of alcohol is reached. Although there are always individual exceptions, the evidence suggests that the threshold is equal to a cumulative dose of about 600 kilograms for men, and between 150 and 300 kilograms for women. To place this in perspective, at the high end (for men), this is roughly equivalent to the average consumption of 10 to 12 drinks a day for ten years, and at the low end (for women), about three drinks per day (see Chapter 1). Below these doses, it is difficult (but certainly not impossible) to reliably detect liver injury (Lelbach, 1975; Marbet et al., 1987; Mezey et al., 1988; Tuyns and Pequignot, 1984), or the damage is not significant enough to warrant medical attention. The differences in threshold doses between men and women cannot be accounted for by anthropometrics or pharmacokinetics. In addition, many individuals who consume these amounts of alcohol never develop liver disease and less than one-half of heavy drinkers develop alcoholic hepatitis or liver fibrosis (Lelbach, 1975). This suggests that alcohol does not produce its effects independently and that hereditary and/or environmental factors interact with alcohol to affect the natural history of liver injury (Marbet et al., 1987). Marbet et al. suggested that other factors contribute to the pathogenesis of liver disease in alcoholics because even though a substantial amount of alcohol is required to induce liver injury, alcohol dose alone is not a good predictor of the severity of liver injury (Marbet et al., 1987).

Numerous possible mechanisms may affect the susceptibility of certain people to alcohol-induced liver damage, but the exact mechanisms by which chronic alcohol abuse leads to liver disease are unknown. A number of mechanisms have been suggested which will be briefly reviewed in following text.

Mechanisms of Liver Injury

The metabolism of alcohol by hepatocytes requires oxygen, a process that produces free radicals, such as hydroxyl and 1-hydroxyethyl radicals and superoxide anions (Kukielka, Dicker, and Cederbaum, 1994; Rashba-Step, Turro, and Cederbaum, 1993; Reinke et al., 1994). These highly reactive compounds can interact with proteins, lipids, and DNA to cause damage or death to liver cells (Fromenty et al., 1995; Nordmann, Rjbiere, and Rouach,

1992). Chronic alcohol consumption also causes white blood cells (neutro-phils) to migrate to the liver where they are activated by an inflammatory sub-stance to release large amounts of superoxides, which may contribute to liver pathology (Bautista et al., 1992).

Normal liver cells contain antioxidants that can neutralize free radicals. Chronic alcohol consumption decreases antioxidant levels in the liver re-sulting in a state of oxidative stress that makes liver cells more susceptible to free-radical-induced injury. One such antioxidant is glutathione, which is present at high concentrations in liver cytosol and mitochondria. Alcohol inhibits glutathione transport from the cytosol to the mitochondria of the cell, causing impaired mitochondrial functioning, which is believed to cause necrosis (Fernandez-Checa et al., 1991; Garcia-Ruiz et al., 1994).

Acetaldehyde is another highly reactive compound that may promote he-patic injury as high concentrations of this metabolite can become a substrate for aldehyde oxidase and other enzymes which produce free radicals as by-products of this reaction (Kato et al., 1990; Shaw and Jayatilleke, 1990; Tsukamoto et al., 1995). Since earlier studies have demonstrated that alco-holics accumulate high levels of acetaldehyde (Baraona et al., 1987), acetaldehyde may be part of the process by which the production of free radicals increase and injure liver cells. Acetaldehyde also can react with specific amino acid residues on cellular proteins to form acetaldehyde-pro-tein adducts (Holstege et al., 1994; Niemela, Juvonen, and Parkkila, 1991), which tend to be localized in sites of greatest liver injury. Acetaldehyde-protein adducts may also stimulate liver cells to produce collagen, which may result in fibrosis and, ultimately, cirrhosis (Bedossa et al., 1994; Casini et al., 1993). Eriksson (2001) recently pointed out that the most compelling evidence that acetaldehyde plays a role in alcoholic liver disease comes from a study of alcoholics who carry the ALDH2*2 and ADH2*2 alleles. In Asian, but not Caucasian alcoholics, there is an association between ADH2*2 alleles and cirrhosis. Interestingly, people with this allele drink less than those without it but are not protected from alcoholic liver disease. In fact, they may develop liver disease (i.e., cirrhosis) at lower levels of alcohol consumption (Eriksson, 2001).

Chronic alcohol use also depletes hepatic levels of vitamin A and E antioxidants (Hagen et al., 1989; Leo, Rosman, and Lieber, 1993), which enhance alcohol-induced lipid peroxidation and exacerbates liver injury in animals (Kawase, Kato, and Lieber, 1989; Sadrzadeh and Nanji, 1994). However, health-supplement drinkers should note that neither vitamin A nor E has been shown to have any significant preventative effects against alcoholic liver injury (Ahmed, Leo, and Lieber, 1994; Leo et al., 1992; Sadrzadeh et al., 1995).

Cytokines are a diverse group of substances with inflammatory, fibrogenic, and growth-promoting properties. Many cytokines associated with alcohol-related liver disease are also believed to be mediators of liver injury because patients with alcohol-related hepatitis frequently have high circulating levels of cytokines such as interleukin-1 (IL-1), interleukin-6 (IL-6), interleukin-8 (IL-8), and tumor necrosis factor–alpha (TNF-alpha) (Bird et al., 1990; Hill et al., 1992, 1993; Khoruts et al., 1991; Ohlinger et al., 1993; Sheron et al., 1993; Tilg et al., 1992). Cytokines IL-8 and TNF-alpha, in particular, correlate negatively with prognosis of liver disease (Felver et al., 1990; Hill et al., 1992, 1993; Sheron et al., 1993). Another cytokine transforming growth factor-beta (TGF-beta), which is found in the livers of alcoholics, is believed to be critical in the development of hepatic fibrosis.

Cirrhosis

Chronic alcohol consumption induces liver fibrosis (scarring) by stimulating the fat-storing cells of the liver to differentiate into collagen-producing stellate cells. It is believed this leads to irreversible cirrhosis. Alcoholic liver fibrosis may occur indirectly through acetaldehyde-protein adducts that can enhance collagen synthesis by stellate cells in vitro (Bedossa et al., 1994; Casini et al., 1993; Moshage, Casini, and Lieber, 1990). Products of lipid peroxidation also increase collagen synthesis which may lead to fibrosis (Maher, Tzagarakis, and Gimenez, 1994; Parola et al., 1993; Tsukamoto, 1993).

Though there are a variety of biomechanical mechanisms through which alcohol or alcohol metabolites may cause liver damage, the problem is more complex. Hereditary variations in enzymes may explain why only a small proportion of alcoholics develop serious liver disease. Although generic variants, polymorphisms in ADH, CYP2E1 isozyme, and aldehyde dehydrogenase (ALDH) result in various rates of alcohol metabolism among different ethnic groups, no single ADH allele has been causally linked to alcoholic liver injury (Chao et al., 1994; Day et al., 1991; Poupon et al., 1992).

ALDH polymorphisms may also play a role in the development of alcoholic liver injury. ALDHY, an allele which is present in about half of all Chinese and Japanese, encodes an enzyme that is completely nonreactive toward acetaldehyde. ALDHY homozygotic individuals (those who have two copies of this allele) generally have an aversion to alcohol because of the accumulation of acetaldehyde. However, chronic drinkers who are ALDHY heterozygotes (those who have one copy of the ALDHY allele) do not have an alcohol aversion and develop liver injury more frequently and at lower cumulative doses than people with normal ALDH (Enomoto et al., 1991; see Eriksson, 2001).

Finally, gender may also play a role in the development of alcohol-induced liver damage. Some evidence indicates that women are more susceptible than men to the cumulative effects of alcohol on the liver, even though women drink less than men (Becker et al., 1996; Gavaler and Arria, 1995; Hisatomi et al., 1997; Naveau et al., 1997; NIAAA, 1997). Compared with men, women who have alcoholic liver injuries remain at higher risk of disease progression even with abstinence (Galambos, 1972; Pares et al., 1986). This curious gender difference suggests that gastric ADH may be a causative factor. ADH is present at high levels in the liver in both men and women, but differences in gastrointestinal ADH between men and women may affect its bioavailability. Women have lower levels of gastric ADH activity than men (Frezia et al., 1990; Seitz et al., 1992) so their livers receive more concentrated levels of alcohol from the gut, thereby placing women a greater risk for liver damage. Although this is an interesting concept, other investigators have found no such gender differences in gastric ADH activity (Thuluvath et al., 1994), and some researchers question the significance of the stomach in the first-pass metabolism of alcohol (Levitt and Levitt, 1994).

Gender differences in alcohol-induced liver injury may be related to gender differences in the metabolism of fatty acids rather than alcohol itself. The accumulation of nonmetabolized fatty acids in the liver through alcohol inhibition of the oxidation of fatty acids by hepatic mitochondria has long been known to be part of the alcoholic disease process (Lieber and DeCarli, 1970; Lieber, Jones, and DeCarli, 1965). It is believed the infiltration of fat impairs intracellular functioning and causes cell injury (NIAAA, 1997).

CARDIOVASCULAR DISEASES

Cardiovascular disease is the leading cause of death among Americans, followed by cancer and stroke (U.S. Department of Health and Human Services [USDHHS], 1995). The role of alcohol as both a risk factor and a potential protective factor for cardiovascular disease has been the focus of intense investigation for many years (see NIAAA, 1997; Zakhari and Wassef, 1996). The results are clear: alcohol has both deleterious and beneficial effects, but the conditions under which alcohol exerts these unusual behavior effects and the mechanisms involved are complex at best.

Alcohol and Heart Disease

It has been known for nearly 80 years that heavy drinking decreases longevity. Pearl noted that moderate drinkers lived longer than either abstainers or heavy drinkers (Pearl, 1926). Over the life span, total alcohol consumption is inversely associated with heart damage. The deterioration of heart muscle, a condition known as alcoholic cardiomyopathy, is one of the most serious consequences of chronic heavy drinking. As cardiac cells deteriorate, the unique ability of these cells to contract is impaired. This is particularly significant in the heart's left ventricle, which pumps freshly oxygenated blood throughout the body. Compensatory mechanisms result in an enlarged heart, but any benefit from such cardiac hypertrophy is temporary. Eventually the heart is unable to meet the body's demand for oxygen. Alcoholic cardiomyopathy is the most common cause of nonischemic cardiomyopathy in Western societies and is a major source of heart failure and death (NIAAA, 1997, 2000).

As with other diseases, women may also be more sensitive to the toxic effects of alcohol on the heart, even though women drink less, or report drinking less, than men (Fernandez-Sola et al., 1997; Urbano-Marquez et al., 1995).

Possible Beneficial Effects of Alcohol on Coronary Heart Disease (CHD)

Several prospective studies have reported a reduced risk of death from CHD across a wide range of alcohol consumption. These include studies among men in the United Kingdom (Doll et al., 1994), Germany (Keil et al., 1997), Japan (Kitamura et al., 1998), and the United States (Fuchs et al., 1995). The definitions of moderate drinking vary among studies; however, most, if not all, of the apparent protective effect against CHD was realized at low to moderate levels of alcohol consumption. For example, in the Fuchs study of more than 85,000 U.S. women, "light to moderate" drinking ranging from one to three drinks per week to one to two drinks per day was associated with a reduced risk of death from cardiovascular diseases.

A meta-analysis of data from 19 cohort studies and six case-control studies found that the risk of death from CHD was reduced at all levels of alcohol consumption, but the maximum reduction in risk occurred when alcohol consumption was low (English et al., 1995). Other studies have suggested that the protective effects of alcohol are greatest in people already at risk for cardiovascular diseases. For example, an analysis of data from a nine-year follow-up of 490,000 Americans in the Cancer Prevention Study II (Thun et al.,

1997) found that both men and women who consumed alcohol had a 30 to 40 percent lower risk of death from all cardiovascular diseases compared with those who abstained from drinking. This effect was greatest among people diagnosed as at risk and was not related to the amount of alcohol consumed.

Similarly, another large U.S. survey, the National Health and Nutrition Examination Survey I, found that the incidence of CHD in men who drank was lower across all levels of consumption than in nondrinkers (Rehm et al., 1997). CHD was also reduced among women, but only in those who consumed low to moderate levels of alcohol. In fact, an increased risk was observed in subjects who consumed more than 28 drinks per week, a finding that is not unique (see Hanna, Chou, and Grant, 1997).

An association between moderate drinking and lower risk for CHD does not necessarily mean that alcohol itself is the protective agent. For example, a review of population studies indicates that the higher mortality risk among abstainers may be attributable to shared traits—socioeconomic and employment status, mental health, overall health, and health habits such as smoking—rather than participants' nonuse of alcohol (Fillmore et al., 1998).

It is also important to note that the apparent benefits of moderate drinking on CHD mortality are offset at higher drinking levels by increased risk of death from other types of heart disease, cancer, liver cirrhosis, and trauma (USDHHS, 1999). For these and other reasons, the U.S. Department of Agriculture (USDA) and the USDHHS have defined moderate drinking as one drink per day or less for women and two or fewer drinks per day for men (USDA, 1995). In addition, the NIAAA further recommends that people aged 65 and older limit their consumption of alcohol to one drink per day (NIAAA, 2000). Definitions of what constitutes a standard drink vary considerably and should be taken into consideration in interpreting such data (Brick, 2006b).

Beverage Type and Medical Risks/Benefits

The National Longitudinal Alcohol Epidemiological Survey (NLAES) is a measure of the prevalence of alcohol use disorders and associated physical and psychological disorders. Chou, Grant, and Dawson (1998) reasoned that nonalcoholic components of beer, wine, or liquor might produce different effects on health and may explain the "French Paradox" (relatively low mortality despite high saturated fat diets among the French) and examined NLAES data to determine the relationship, if any, between a broad range of diseases associated with alcohol abuse and beverage preference. Compared with abstainers, beer and wine drinkers had reduced morbidity rates from cardiovascular disease and hypertension. However, liquor drinkers were at increased risk for multiple disorders including diseases of the digestive track, coronary diseases, and arthritis (Chou, Grant, and Dawson, 1998). The authors note that since the nature of the observed effects are unclear and as there are many other factors including amount of alcohol consumed, and interactions with other medications and breast cancer, all of which are associated with moderate drinking, the results should be interpreted with extreme caution. Nevertheless, this study adds to the interesting but complex interrelationship between the protective effects of alcohol use in some people, under some conditions.

How Does Alcohol Protect Against Heart Disease?

The mechanisms through which alcohol may protect against CHD are diverse. Animal studies suggest that alcohol may impede uptake of fatty acids into the heart (Brick, Pohorecky, and DeTurck, 1987), the accumulation of fatty deposits, or atherosclerotic plaques in coronary arteries (Dai, Miller, and Lin, 1997). Furthermore, alcohol consumption may increase links of high-density lipoproteins (HDL), or "good cholesterol," that is clinically associated with lower risk of CHD (Fumeron et al., 1995).

Other studies have indicated that alcohol consumption increases HDL cholesterol levels by decreasing the activity of cholesteryl ester transfer protein (CETP), which transfers cholesterol molecules from HDL particles to low density lipoproteins (LDL) or very low density lipoproteins (VLDL) density lipoprotein particles. High levels of LDL and VLDL are associated with increased risk of CHD (Fumeron et al., 1995). Drinking alcohol seems to alter the gene functioning to increase HDL cholesterol. Researchers have confirmed the association between alcohol consumption and increased HDL cholesterol in people through several large epidemiological studies (e.g., Huijbregts, Freskens, and Kromhout, 1995; Marques-Vidal et al., 1995; Sonnenberg et al., 1996). However, these changes in HDL cholesterol and LDL-cholesterol levels contribute only about half of the observed protection against CHD with alcohol consumption. This suggests that other mechanisms may be contributory to the protective effects of alcohol. For example, alcohol may have antithrombotic effects, and may reduce platelet activation and clotting factor activity (Rubin and Rand, 1994). Indeed, evidence suggests that drinking 30 grams of alcohol (just over two drinks) per day for four weeks causes a reduction of platelet aggregation and a decrease in blood levels of fibrinogen, which stimulates clot formation (Pellegrini et al., 1996). Moderate alcohol consumption may have other antithrombic effects by increasing blood levels of tissue plasminogen activator, an enzyme that breaks down blood clots (Ridker et al., 1994), or it may suppress the production of substances that promote clotting (Booyse, Aiken, and Grenett, 1999).

Beverage Type and Pattern of Consumption

Wine may confer special protection against CHD (Goldberg, Hahn, and Parkes, 1995) or this protective effect may be due to the alcohol itself (Doll, 1997; Rimm et al., 1996). Reviews of lipid-reducing effects of wines are available (see Chadwick and Goode, 1998; Goldberg, Hahn, and Parkes, 1995) and at least one recent study of Chinese men revealed no additional reduction in overall mortality associated with drinking rice-fermented wine (Yuan et al., 1997). However, other factors besides wine may contribute to this effect. The pattern of drinking, rather than the type of alcohol consumed, may help explain how drinking wine might protect against CHD (Doll, 1997; Grønboek et al., 1995; Klatsky and Armstrong, 1993). For example, wine drinkers tend to consume small amounts of alcohol daily rather than consume larger amounts of alcohol on weekends. It has been suggested that the pattern of frequent drinking may confer some protection against CHD and that large amounts are not needed to achieve a beneficial effect (Bondy, 1996). Similarly, alcohol consumed with meals was found to reduce the postprandial elevations of blood lipids (Beenstra et al., 1990; Rubin and Rand, 1994). Other studies have reported a reduced risk of coronary death or acute myocardial infarction with moderate, regular drinking and an increased risk associated with binge drinking (Kauhanen et al., 1991, 1997; McElduff and Dobson, 1997).

Finally, because many of the epidemiological studies from which much of the evidence is derived have involved middle-aged or older persons in stable social situations, the findings may not necessarily apply to younger drinkers, whose risk of CHD is low to begin with, or to other social groups.

In summary, lowered CHD risk is most closely associated with a consistent pattern of drinking small amounts of alcohol. The apparent CHD benefit is largely, if not wholly, attributable to alcohol itself and not to specific beverages or to other constituents of particular beverages such as red wine. Future research should help bring clarity to this body of literature (Klatsky, Armstrong, and Friedman, 1997; Rimm et al., 1996).

Alcohol and Blood Pressure

There is a well-documented association between heavy alcohol consumption and hypertension (Ascherio et al., 1996; Campbell et al., 1999; Seppa, Laippala, and Sillanaukee, 1996; York and Hirsch, 1997). Heavy alcohol consumption elevates blood pressure and causes or exacerbates hypertension (Puddey et al., 1995; Ueshima et al., 1993). It is estimated that one drink per day can chronically increase blood pressure by one millimeter of mercury in aged individuals, and even more in the elderly and people with preexisting hypertension (Beilin, Puddey, and Burke, 1996). Controversy remains as to whether moderate alcohol consumption has any beneficial effects on blood pressure, but reducing alcohol intake may be one means of reducing blood pressure in people with hypertension (Lang et al., 1995; World Health Organization, 1996).

Despite the well-recognized association between alcohol and hypertension, the cellular mechanisms of alcohol's effect on blood pressure are not well understood and are made confusing by the fact that, initially, drinking alcohol dilates blood vessels, which lowers blood pressure. Studies looking to explain how long-term, heavy alcohol consumption reverses this effect and leads to elevated blood pressure have generally concluded that this effect is due to the action of alcohol on the autonomic nervous system. For example, heavy alcohol consumption has been associated with increased release of the stress hormones adrenaline and norepinephrine, which constrict the blood vessels, increase blood pressure, and decrease the sensitivity of baroreceptors. This may be one mechanism through which alcohol leads to hypertension.

Moderate alcohol consumption (about one to three drinks per day) is associated with a slight reduction in blood pressure and may protect against age-related development of hypertension (Gillman et al., 1995; Palmer et al., 1995). The significance of these findings may be offset by an increased risk of death from causes unrelated to cardiovascular disease (e.g., accidental injuries, liver disease, etc.). Heavy alcohol consumption also may alter peripheral regulation of blood pressure by affecting smooth muscle cells in the walls of blood vessels (see Altura and Altura, 1996).

Evidence indicates that the increased blood pressure associated with alcohol use is related to alcohol withdrawal rather than a direct effect of alcohol. Kawano et al. found that a single drink of alcohol depresses the blood pressure of patients with hypertension for several hours (Kawano et al., 1996). However, patients who consume one drink each evening for seven days have blood pressure that seesaws; it is low in the evening and increases in the morning, suggesting that regular consumption of alcohol can raise blood pressure during the hours that alcohol is not consumed (Abe et al., 1994). These findings are consistent with observations that sympathetic-nervous-system-induced increases in blood pressure occur during alcohol withdrawal (Denison et al., 1997).

Stroke Risk

There are two relevant forms of stroke: ischemic and hemorrhagic. Ischemic stroke occurs when a blood vessel in the brain is blocked. Hemorrhagic stroke occurs when a blood vessel in the brain ruptures. Alcohol-related hypertension, or high blood pressure, may increase the risk of both forms of stroke. Yet in people with normal blood pressure, the risk of ischemic stroke may be decreased due to the apparent ability of alcohol to lessen damage to blood vessels due to lipid deposits and to reduce blood clotting. However, whereas alcohol's anticlotting effects may decrease the risk of ischemic stroke, alcohol-induced hypertension may increase the risk of hemorrhagic stroke (Hillbom and Juvela, 1996).

Two relatively recent reviews of the relationship between alcohol consumption and stroke risk revealed no differences in the risk patterns for ischemic or hemorrhagic stroke. One study found clear evidence that heavy drinking was associated with increased stroke risk, particularly in women. This evidence was inconsistent regarding a protective effect of low doses of alcohol against stroke (English et al., 1995). In the second review, the author concluded that although moderate drinking (defined in this review as usual consumption of fewer than two drinks daily for men and less than one drink daily for women) does not appear to increase the risk of ischemic stroke, it is not clear whether moderate drinking protects against this type of stroke (Camargo, 1996). Other studies also fail to offer clear evidence that moderate drinking protects against stroke (Knuiman and Vu, 1996; Yuan et al., 1997) and there is evidence, albeit inconsistent, that moderate drinking may actually increase the risk of hemorrhagic stroke (Camargo, 1996).

In contrast, the Cancer Prevention Study II found that all levels of drinking were associated with a significant decrease in the risk of stroke death in men, but in women, the decreased risk was significant only among those who consumed one drink or less per day (Thun et al., 1997). The Physicians' Health Study reported that male physicians who consumed more than one drink per week had a reduced overall risk of stroke compared with participants who had less than one drink per week (Berger et al., 1999). The authors concluded that the benefit was apparent with as little as one drink per week.

Among young people, long-term heavy alcohol consumption has been identified as an important risk factor for stroke (You et al., 1997). Very recent alcohol intoxication has also been found to be associated with a significant increase in the risk of ischemic stroke, especially in both men and women aged 16 through 40 (Hillbom et al., 1995). For example, researchers in another study reported that recent consumption of alcohol was associated with the onset of stroke in young people during weekends and holidays, possibly reflecting an association with heavy drinking (Haapaniemi, Hillbom, and Juvela, 1996).

In summary, heavy drinking appears to increase the risk of hypertension and, although the evidence is not entirely consistent, may also increase the risk of stroke. It remains uncertain whether lower levels of alcohol can help prevent ischemic stroke. In addition to examining how much alcohol is consumed, it may be important to consider drinking patterns in determining stroke risk.

Peripheral Vascular Disease

The possibility that alcohol may protect against CHD has led researchers to hypothesize that alcohol may also protect against peripheral vascular disease. In a 1985 analysis of data from the Framingham Heart Study, alcohol was not found to have a significant relationship, either harmful or protective, with regard to peripheral vascular disease (Kannel and McGee, 1985). Other studies have failed to find a significant relationship between alcohol consumption and the narrowing of blood vessels that define peripheral vascular disease as well. However, a recent study produced much more encouraging results. In an analysis of the 11-year follow-up data from more than 22,000 men enrolled in the Physicians' Health Study, researchers found that daily drinkers who consumed seven or more drinks per week had a 26 percent reduction in risk of peripheral vascular disease (Camargo et al., 1997). This study took into account the effects of smoking, exercise, diabetes, and parental history of myocardial infarction.

Two other studies found inconsistent results with regard to gender. One study of middle-aged and older men and women in Scotland showed that as alcohol consumption increased, the prevalence of peripheral vascular disease declined in men, but not in women (Jepson et al., 1995). In contrast, among people with non-insulin-dependent diabetes, alcohol was associated with a lower prevalence of peripheral vascular disease in women but not in men (Mingardi et al., 1997). Clearly, the relationship of alcohol consumption to peripheral vascular disease requires further study.

SUMMARY AND CONCLUSIONS

As a pharmacological agent, alcohol is a relatively simple compound. The ubiquitous nature of this drug on most, if not all major organ systems is consistent with its simple molecular structure and its widespread use. Alcohol affects the gastrointestinal, hepatic, cardiovascular, and skeletal systems included in this chapter, but these effects extend to the organism as a whole when accidental injuries due to intoxication are considered.

From the available alcohol research, several conclusions may be drawn regarding the medical consequences of alcohol use. Most notably and across physiological systems, alcohol's effects are multiphasic. Although the nature of the deleterious and possible protective effects of alcohol continue to emerge, the conditions under which these medical consequences present themselves is complex and will, in all probability, remain elusive for several years. Variables such as gender, diet, environment, lifestyle, genetics, dose and frequency of alcohol use, other drugs, and age interact in complex but sometimes visible ways. The majority of studies suggest that, overall, higher doses of alcohol are deleterious to many physiological systems and precipitate a range of psychosocial and biobehavioral problems. In some individuals and under some conditions, alcohol use seems to have a beneficial effect on health. Both experimental and clinical studies suggest that the protective effects of alcohol, when they do occur, are most often associated with low doses (the equivalent of about one to two drinks per day).

There are many other medical consequences beyond those selected for this chapter, some of which are presented elsewhere in this book. The exclusion of that body of literature was a function of the enormity of the topic and not the significance of that research. Also, while the research relied upon in this chapter focused on clinical studies, preclinical research has been helpful in testing and identifying many of the underlying mechanisms through which alcohol use and abuse causes pernicious as well as beneficial medical consequences. Finally, the importance of continued multidisciplinary research to identify the conditions under which, and the subjects in whom, alcohol produces medical consequences cannot be overstated.

REFERENCES

Abe, H.; Kawano, Y.; Kojima, S.; Ashida, T.; Kuramochi, M.; Matsuoka, H.; Omae, T. (1994). Biphasic effects of repeated alcohol intake on 24-hour blood pressure in hypertensive patients. *Circulation* 89(6):2626-2633.

Ahmed, S.; Leo, M.A.; Lieber, C.S. (1994). Interactions between alcohol and betacarotene in patients with alcoholic liver disease. *Am Clin Nutr* 60(3):430-436.

Albin, M.; Bunegin, L. (1986). An experimental study of craniocerebral trauma during ethanol intoxication. *Crit Care Med* 14(10):841-846.

Alcohol World (1990). Vol. 14(1).

Altura, B.M.; Altura, B.T. (1996). Mechanisms of alcohol-induced hypertension: Importance of intracellular cations and magnesium. In: Zakhari, S. and Wassef, M. (eds.), *Alcohol and the Cardiovascular System* (pp. 591-614). National Institute on

Alcohol Abuse and Alcoholism Research Monograph No. 31, Pub. No. 96-4133. Bethesda, MD: NIAAA.

Ascherio, A.; Hennekens, C.; Willett, W.C.; Sacks, F.; Rosner, B.; Manson, J.; Witteman, J.; Stampfer, M.J. (1996). Prospective study of nutritional factors, blood pressure, and hypertension among U.S. women. *Hypertension* 27(5): 1065-1072.

Baker, S.P.; O'Neill, B.; Karpf, R. (1992). *The Injury Fact Book*, Second Edition. New York: Oxford University Press.

Baraona, E.; DiPadova, C.; Tabasco, I.; Lieber, C.S. (1987). Transport of acetaldehyde in red blood cells. *Alcohol Alcohol Suppl* 1:203-206.

Bautista, A.P.; D'souza, N.B.; Lang, C.H.; Spitzer, I.I. (1992). Modulation of Fmetleu-phe induced chemotactic activity and superoxide production by neutrophils during chronic ethanol intoxication. *Alcohol Clin Exp Res* 16(4):788-794.

Beard, J. (1996). Reports of the Joint Scientific Meeting of the Research Society in Alcoholism and the International Society for Biomedical Research on Alcoholism. In: Singletary, K.W. (ed.), Alcohol and breast cancer: Interactions between alcohol and other risk factors. *Alcohol Clin Exp Res* 20(8 Suppl):57A-61A.

Becker, U.; Deis, A.; Sorensen, T.I.; Grønbaek, M.; Borch-Johnsen, K.; Muller, C.F.; Schnohr, P.; Jensen, G. (1996). Prediction of risk of liver disease by alcohol intake, sex, and age: A prospective population study. *Hepatology* 23(5):1025-1029.

Bedossa, P.; Houglum, K.; TrautWein, C.; Holstege, A.; Chojkier, M. (1994). Stimulation of collagen alpha 1 (I) gene expression is associated with lipid perioxidation in hepatocellular injury: A link to tissue fibrosis? *Hepatology* 19(5):1262-1271.

Beenstra, J.; Ockhuizen, T.; Van de Pol, H.; Wedel, M.; Schaafsma, G. (1990). Effects of a moderate dose of alcohol on blood lipids and lipoproteins postprandially and in the fasting state. *Alcohol Alcohol* 25(4):371-377.

Beilin, L.J.; Puddey, I.B.; Burke, V. (1996). Alcohol and hypertension—Kill or cure? [Review]. *J Hum Hypertens* 10 (Suppl 2):S1-S5.

Berger, K.; Ajani, U.A.; Kase, C.S.; Gaziano, M.; Buring, J.E.; Glynn, R.J.; Hennekens, C.H. (1999). Light-to-moderate alcohol consumption and the risk of stroke among U.S. male physicians. *N Engl J Med* 341(21):1557-1564.

Bikle, D.D.; Genant, H.K.; Cann, C.E.; Recker, R.R.; Halloran, B.P.; Strewler, G.J. (1985). Bone disease in alcohol abuse. *Ann Intern Med* 103:42-48.

Billings, C.; Demosthesen, T.; White, T.; O'Hara, D. (1991). Effects of alcohol on pilot performance in simulated flight. *Aviat Space Environ Med* 62(3):2323-2335.

Bird, G.L.A.; Sheron, N.; Goka, A.K.; Alexander, G.J.; Williams, R.S. (1990). Increased plasma tumor necrosis factor in severe alcoholic hepatitis. *Ann Intern Med* 112(12):917-920.

Blaauw, R.; Albertse, E.C.; Beneke, T.; Lombard, C.J.; Laubscher, R.; Hough, F.S. (1994). Risk factors for the development of osteoporosis in a South African population: A prospective analysis. *S Afr Med J* 84:328-332.

Blomberg, R.D.; Preusser, D.F.; Hale, A.; Ulmer, R.G. (1979). A comparison of alcohol involvement in pedestrians and pedestrian casualties. DOT HS 805 249. Washington, DC: National Highway Traffic Safety Administration.

Bondy, S. (1996). Overview of studies on drinking patterns and consequences. *Addiction* 91(11):1663-1674.

Booyse, F.M.; Aikens, M.L.; Grenett, H.E. (1999). Endothelial cell fibrinolysis: Transcriptional regulation of fibrinolytic protein gene expression (t-PA, u-PA, and PAI-1) by low alcohol. *Alcohol Clin Exp Res* 23(6):1119-1124.

Borges, G.; Rosovsky, H. (1996). Suicide attempts and alcohol consumption in an emergency room sample. *J Stud Alcohol* 57:543-548.

Brezel, B.S.; Kassenbrock, M. (1988). Burns in substance abusers and in neurologically and mentally impaired patients. *J Burn Care Rehabil,* Mar-Apr; 9(2): 169-191.

Brick, J. (2006a) Interaction between toxicology and burn victim physiology. In: Alan Clark (ed.), *Burns: The Medical and Forensic Model* (pp. 221-256). Lawyers & Judges Publishing Company.

Brick, J. (2006b). Standardization of alcohol calculations in research. *Alcohol Clin Exp Res* 30(8):1276-1287.

Brick, J.; Adler, J.; Cocco, K.; Wesrick, E. (1992). Alcohol intoxication: Pharmacokinetic prediction and behavior in humans. Current topics. *Pharmacol* 1:57-67.

Brick, J.; Carpenter, J.A. (2001). The identification of alcohol intoxication by police. *Alcohol Clin Exp Res* 25(6):850-855.

Brick, J.; Erickson, C. (1999). *Drugs, the Brain, and Behavior: The Pharmacology of Abuse and Dependence.* Binghamton, NY: The Haworth Medical Press, p. 72.

Brick, J.; Pohorecky, L.; DeTurck, K. (1987). Effect of ethanol and stress on cardiac lipase activity. *Life Sciences* 40:1897-1901.

Camargo, C.A., Jr. (1996). Case-control and cohort studies of moderate alcohol consumption and stroke. *Clin Chim Acta* 246(1-2):107-119.

Camargo, C.A., Jr.; Stampfer, M.J.; Glynn, R.J.; Gaziano, J.M.; Manson, J.E.; Goldhaber, S.Z.; Hennekens, C.H. (1997). Prospective study of moderate alcohol consumption and risk of peripheral arterial disease in U.S. male physicians. *Circulation* 95(3):577-580.

Campbell, N.R.; Ashley, M.J.; Carruthers, S.G.; Lacourciere, Y.; McKay, D.W. (1999). Lifestyle modifications to prevent and control hypertension. 3. Recommendations on alcohol consumption. Canadian Hypertension Society, Canadian Coalition for High Blood Pressure Prevention and Control, Laboratory Centre for Disease Control at Health Canada, Heart and Stroke Foundation of Canada. *Can Med Assoc J* 160 (Suppl 9):S13-S20.

Casini, A.; Galli, G.; Salzano, R.; Rotella, C.M.; Surrenti, C. (1993). Acetaldehydeprotein adducts, but not lactate and pyruvate, stimulate gene transcription of collagen and fibronectin in hepatic fat-storing cells. *Hepatology* 19(3):385-392.

Centers for Disease Control (1991). *Morbidity and Mortality Weekly Report,* June 21.

Chadwick, D.J.; Goode, J.A. (eds.) (1998). *Alcohol and Cardiovascular Diseases. Novartis Foundation Symposium 216.* New York: John Wiley & Sons.

Chao, Y.C.; Liou, S.R.; Chung, Y.Y.; Tang, H.S.; Hsu, C.T.; Li, T.K.; Yin, S.J. (1994). Polymorphism of alcohol and aldehyde dehydrogenase genes and alcoholic cirrhosis in Chinese patients. *Hepatology* 19(2):360-366.

Chavassieux, P.; Serre, C.M.; Vernaud, P.; Delmas, P.D.; Meunier, P.J. (1993). In vitro evaluation of dose-effects of ethanol on human osteoblastic cells. *Bone Miner* 22:95-103.

Chen, R.J.; Fang, J.F.; Lin, B.C.; Hsu, Y.P.; Kao, J.L.; Chen, M.F. (2000). Factors determining operative mortality of grade V blunt hepatic trauma. *J Trauma* 49: 886-891.

Cherpitel, C.J. (1989). Breath analysis and self reports as measures of alcohol-related emergency room admissions. *J Stud Alcohol* 50(2):155-161.

Cherpitel, C.J. (1993). Alcohol, injury, and risk-taking behavior: Data from a national sample. *Alcohol Clin Exp Res* 17(4):762-766.

Cherpital, C.J.; Borges, G.L.G.; Wilcox, H.C. (2004). Acute alcohol use and suicidal behavior: A review of the literature. *Alcohol Clin Exp Res* 28(s1):18S-28S.

Cheng, A.T.A. (1995). Mental illness and suicide. *Br J Psychiatry* 170:441-446.

Chou, S.P.; Grant, B.F.; Dawson, D.A. (1998). Alcoholic beverage preference and risks of alcohol-related medical consequence: A preliminary report from the National Longitudinal Alcohol Epidemiologic Survey. *Alcohol Clin Exp Res* 22(7): 1450-1455.

Colditz, G.A. (1990). A prospective assessment of moderate alcohol intake and major chronic diseases. *Ann Epidemiol* 1(2):167-177.

Conn, H.O. (1985). Natural history of complications of alcoholic liver disease. *Acta Med Scand* 703(Suppl):127-134.

Conner, K.R.; Beautrais, A.L.; Conwell, Y. (2003). Risk factors for suicide and medically serious suicide attempts among alcoholics: Analyses of Canterbury Suicide Project Data. *J Stud Alcohol* 64:551-554.

Crilly, R.G.; Anderson, C.; Hogan, D.; Delaquerriére-Richardson, L. (1988). Bone histomorphometry, bone mass, and related parameters in alcoholic males. *Calcif Tissue Int* 43:269-276.

Cumming, R.G.; Klineberg, R.J. (1994). Case-control study of risk factors for hip fractures in the elderly. *Am J Epidemiol* 139:493-503.

Dai, J.; Miller, B.A.; Lin, R.C. (1997). Alcohol feeding impedes early atherosclerosis in low-density lipoprotein receptor knockout mice: Factors in addition to high-density lipoprotein-apolipoprotein A1 are involved. *Alcohol Clin Exp Res* 21(1): 11-18.

Dawson, D. (2001). Alcohol and mortality from external cues. *J Stud Alcohol* 62:790-797.

Day, C.P.; Bashir, R.; James, O.F.; Bassendine, M.F.; Crabb, D.W.; Thomasson, H.R.; Li, T.K.; Edenberg, H.J. (1991). Investigation of the role of polymorphisms at the alcohol and aldehyde dehydrogenase loci in genetic predisposition to alcohol-related end-organ damage. *Hepatology* 14(5):798-801.

De, A.; Boyadjieva, N.I.; Pastorcic, M.; Reddy, B.V.; Sarkar, D.K. (1994). Cyclic AMP and ethanol interact to control apoptosis and differentiation in hypothalamic-endorphin neurons. *J Biol Chem* 269:26697-26705.

DeCrescito, V.; Demopoulos, H.; Flamm, E.; Ransohoff, J. (1974). Ethanol potentiation of traumatic cerebral edema. *Surgical Forum* 25:438-440.

Delmas, P.D.; Malaval, L.; Arlot, M.E.; Meunier, P.J. (1985). Serum bone Glaprotein compared to bone histomorphometry in endocrine diseases. *Bone* 6:339-341.

Denison, J.; Jern, S.; Jagenburg, R.; Wandestam, C.; Wallerstedt, S. (1997). STsegment changes and catecholamine-related myocardial enzyme release during alcohol withdrawal. *Alcohol and Alcoholism* 32(2):185-194.

Diamond, T.; Stiel, D.; Lunzer, M.; Wilkinson, M.; Posen, S. (1989). Ethanol reduces bone formation and may cause osteoporosis. *Am J Med* 86:282-288.

Diaz, M.N.; O'Neill, T.W.; Silman, A.J. (1997). The influence of alcohol consumption on the risk of vertebral deformity. *Osteoporos Int* 7:65-71.

Doll, R. (1997). Cochrane and the benefits of wine. In: Maynard, A.C. (ed.), *Nonrandom Reflections on Health Services Research on the 15th Anniversary of Archie Cochrane's Effectiveness and Efficiency.* London, UK: BMJ Publishing Group.

Doll, R.; Foreman, D.; La Vecchia, D.; Woutersen, R. (1993). Alcoholic beverages and cancers of the digestive tract and larynx. In: Verschuren, P.M. (ed.), *Health Issues Related to Alcohol Consumption* (pp. 125-166). Washington, DC: International Life Sciences Institute Press.

Doll, R.; Peto, R.; Hall, E.; Wheatley, K.; Gray, R. (1994). Mortality in relation to consumption of alcohol: 13 years' observations on male British doctors. *BMJ* 309(6959):911-918.

Dufour, M.C.; Stinson, F.S.; Caces, M.F. (1993). Trends in cirrhosis morbidity and mortality: United States, 1979-1988. *Semin Liver Dis* 13(2):109-125.

Elmer, O.; Goransson, G.; Zoucas, E. (1984). Impairment of primary hemostasis and platelet function after alcohol ingestion in man. *Haemostasis* 14:223-228.

English, D.R.; Holman, C.D.J.; Milne, E.; Winter, M.J.; Hulse, G.K.; Codde, G.; Bower, C.I.; et al. (1995). *The Quantification of Drug-Caused Morbidity and Mortality in Australia, 1992.* Canberra, Australia: Canberra Commonwealth Department of Human Services and Health.

Enomoto, N.; Takase, S.; Takada, N.; Takada, A. (1991). Alcoholic liver disease in heterozygotes of mutant and normal aldehyde dehydrogenase-2 genes. *Hepatology* 13(6):1071-1075.

Eriksson, C.J. (2001). The role of acetaldehyde in the actions of alcohol (update 2000). *Alcohol Clin Exp Res* 25(5):15S-33S.

Ewald, S.J.; Shao, H. (1993). Ethanol increases apoptotic cell death of thymocytes in vitro. *Alcohol Clin Exp Res* 17(2):359-365.

Feitelberg, S.; Epstein, S.; Ismail, F.; D'Amanda, C. (1987). Deranged bone mineral metabolism in chronic alcoholism. *Metabolism* 36:322-326.

Fell, J.; Hertz, E. (1993). The effects of blood alcohol concentration on time of death for fatal crash victims. *Alcohol Drugs and Driving* 9(2):97-106.

Felson, D.T.; Kiel, D.P.; Anderson, J.J.; Kannel, W.B. (1988). Alcohol consumption and hip fractures: The Framingham Study. *Am J Epidemiol* 128:1102-1110.

Felver, M.E.; Mezey, I.; McGuire, M.; Mitchell, M.C.; Herlong, H.F.; Veech, G.A.; Veech, R.L. (1990). Plasma tumor necrosis factor alpha predicts decreased long-term survival in severe alcoholic hepatitis. *Alcohol Clin Exp Res* 14(2):255-259.

Fernandez-Checa, I.C.; Garcia-Ruiz, C.; Ookhtens, M.; Kaplowitz, N. (1991). Impaired uptake of glutathione by hepatic mitochondria from chronic ethanol-fed rats: Tracer kinetic studies in vitro and in vivo and susceptibility to oxidant stress. *J Clin Invest* 87(2):397-405.

Fernandez-Sola, J.; Estruch, R.; Nicholas, J.M.; Pare, JC; Sacanella, E.; Antunex, E.; Urbano-Marquez, A. (1997). A comparison of alcohol cardiomyopathy in women versus men. *Am J Cardiol* 80(4):481-485.

Fillmore, K.M.; Golding, J.M.; Graves, K.L.; Kniep, S.; Leino, E.V.; Romelsjo, A.; Shoemaker, C.; Ager, C.R.; Allebeck, P.; Ferrer, H.P. (1998). Alcohol consumption and mortality. I. Characteristics of drinking groups. *Addiction* 93(2):183-203.

Franceschi, S.; La Vecchia, C. (1994). Alcohol and the risk of cancers of the stomach and colon-rectum. *Dig Dis* 12(5):276-289.

Frezia, M.; di Padova, C.; Pozzato, G.; Terpin, M.; Baraona, E.; Lieber, C.S. (1990). High blood alcohol levels in women: The role of decreased gastric alcohol dehydrogenase activity and first-pass metabolism. *N Engl J Med* 322(2):95-99.

Friday, K.; Howard, G.A. (1991). Ethanol inhibits human bone cell proliferation and function in vitro. *Metabolism* 40:562-565.

Fromenty, B.; Grimbert, S.; Mansouri, A.; Beaugrand, M.; Erlinger, S.; Rotig, A.; Pessayre, D. (1995). Hepatic mitochondrial DNA deletion in alcoholics: Association with microvesicular steatosis. *Gastroenterology* 108(1):193-200.

Fuchs, C.S.; Stampfer, M.J.; Colditz, G.A.; Giovannucci, E.L.; Manson, J.E.; Kawachi, I.; Hunter, D.J.; Hankinson, S.E.; Hennekens, C.H.; Rosner, B. (1995). Alcohol consumption and mortality among women. *N Engl J Med* 332(19): 1245-1250.

Fujiwara, S.; Kasagi, F.; Yamada, M.; Kodama, K. (1997). Risk factors for hip fracture in a Japanese cohort. *J Bone Miner Res* 12:998-1004.

Fumeron, F.; Betoulle, D.; Luc, G.; Behague, I.; Ricard, S.; Poirier, O.; Jemaa, R.; et al. (1995). Alcohol intake modulates the effect of a polymorphism of the cholesteryl ester transfer protein gene on plasma high density lipoprotein and the risk of myocardial infarction. *J Clin Invest* 96(3):1664-1671.

Galambos, I.T. (1972). Natural history of alcoholic hepatitis. 3: Histological changes. *Gastroenterology* 63(6):1026-1035.

Gapstur, S.M.; Potter, J.D.; Sellers, T.A.; Folsom, A.R. (1992). Increased risk of breast cancer with alcohol consumption in postmenopausal women. *Am J Epidemiol* 136(10):1221-1231.

Garcia-Carrasco, M.; Gruson, M.; De Vernejoul, C. (1988). Osteocalcin and bone histomorphometric parameters in adults without bone disease. *Calcif Tissue Int* 42:13-17.

Garcia-Ruiz, C.; Morales, A.; Ballesta, A.; Rodes, I.; Kaplowitz, N.; Fernandez-Checa, I.C. (1994). Effect of chronic ethanol feeding on glutathione and functional integrity of mitochondria in periportal and perivenous rat hepatocytes. *J Clin Invest* 94(1):193-201.

Gavaler, J.S. (1991). Effects of alcohol on female endocrine function. *Alcohol Health Res World* 15:104-109.

Gavaler, J.S.; Arria, A.M. (1995). Increased susceptibility of women to alcoholic liver disease: Artifactual or real? In: Hall, P.M. (ed.), *Alcoholic Liver Disease*:

Pathology and Pathogenesis, Second Edition (pp. 123-133). London, UK: Edward Arnold.

Gillman, M.W.; Cook, N.R.; Evans, D.A.; Rosner, B.; Hennekens, C.H. (1995). Relationship of alcohol intake with blood pressure in young adults. *Hypertension* 25(5):1106-1110.

Giovannucci, E.; Rimm, E.B.; Ascherio, A.; Stampfer, M.J.; Colditz, G.A.; Willett, W.C. (1995). Alcohol, low-methionine, low-folate diets, and risk of colon cancer in men. *J Natl Cancer Inst* 87(4):265-273.

Giovannucci, E.; Willett, W.C. (1994). Dietary factors and risk of colon cancer. *Ann Med* 26(6):443-452.

Goldberg, D.M.; Hahn, S.E.; Parkes, J.G. (1995). Beyond alcohol beverage consumption and cardiovascular mortality. *Clin Chim Acta* 237(1-2):155-187.

Gonzalez-Calvin, J.L.; Garcia-Sanchez, A.; Bellot, V.; Munoz-Torres, M.; Raya-Alvarez, E.; Salvatierra-Rios, D. (1993). Mineral metabolism, osteoblastic function, and bone mass in chronic alcoholism. *Alcohol and Alcoholism* 28:571-579.

Gray, M.R.; Donnelly, R.I.; Kingsnorth, A.N. (1993). The role of smoking and alcohol in metaplasia and cancer risk in Barrett's columnar lined oesophagus. *Gut* 34(6):727-731.

Grisso, J.A.; Kelsey, J.L.; Strom, B.L.; O'Brien, L.A.; Maislin, G.; LaPann, K.; Samelson, L.; Hoffman, S. (1994). Risk factors for hip fracture in black women. The Northeast Hip Fracture Study Group. *N Engl J Med* 330:1555-1559.

Grønboek, D.A.; Deis, A.; Sørensen, T.I.; Becker, U.; Schnohr, P.; Jensen, G. (1995). Mortality associated with moderate intake of wine, beer, or spirits. *BMJ* 310(6988):1165-1169.

Haapaniemi, H.; Hillbom, M.; Juvela, S. (1996). Weekend and holiday increase in the onset of ischemic stroke in young women. *Stroke* 27(6):1023-1027.

Haber, P.; Wilson, I.; Apte, M.; Korsten, M.; Pirola, R. (1995). Individual susceptibility to alcoholic pancreatitis: Still an enigma. *J Lab Clin Med* 125(3):305-312.

Hagen, B.F.; Bjorneboe, A.; Bjorneboe, G.E.; Drevon, C.A. (1989). Effect of chronic ethanol consumption on the content of alpha-tocopherol in subcellular fractions of rat liver. *Alcohol Clin Exp Res* 13(2):246-251.

Hanna, F.Z.; Chou, S.P.; Grant, B.F. (1997). The relationship between drinking and heart disease morbidity in the United States: Results from the National Health Interview Survey. *Alcohol Clin Exp Res* 21(1):111-118.

Haum, A.; Perbix, W.; Hack, H.J.; Stark, G.B.; Spilker, G.; Doehn, M. (1995). Alcohol and drug abuse in burn injuries. *Burns* May 21(3):194-199.

Hernandez-Avila, M.; Colditz, G.A.; Stampfer, M.J.; Rosner, B.; Speizer, F.E.; Willett, W.C. (1991). Caffeine, moderate alcohol intake, and risk of fractures of the hip and forearm in middle-aged women. *Am J Clin Nutr* 54:157-163.

Hill, D.B.; Marsano, L.; Cohen, D.; Allen, I.; Shedlofsky, S.; McClain, C.I. (1992). Increased plasma interleukin-6 concentrations in alcoholic hepatitis. *J Lab Clin Med* 119(5):547-552.

Hill, D.B.; Marsano, L.S.; McClain, C.I. (1993). Increased plasma interleukin-8 concentrations in alcoholic hepatitis. *Hepatology* 18(3):576-580.

Hillbom, M.; Haapaniemi, H.; Juvela, S.; Palomaki, H.; Numminen, H.; Kaste, M. (1995). Recent alcohol consumption, cigarette smoking, and cerebral infarction in young adults. *Stroke* 26(1):40-45.

Hillbom, M.; Juvela, S. (1996). Alcohol and risk for stroke. In: Zakhari, S. and Wassef, M. (eds.), *Alcohol and the Cardiovascular System* (pp. 63-83). NIAAA Research Monograph No. 31. Bethesda, MD: NIAAA.

Hingson, R.; Howland, J. (1993). Alcohol and non-traffic unintended injuries. *Addiction* 88(7):877-883.

Hisatomi, S.; Kumashiro, R.; Sata, M.; Ishii, K.; Tanikawa, K. (1997). Gender difference in alcoholic and liver disease in Japan: An analysis based on histological findings. *Hepatol Res* 8(2):113-120.

Hobbs, W.R., Rall, T.W., and Verdoorn, T.A. (1996). Hypnotics and sedatives; Ethanol. In: J.G. Hardman, J.G. and Limbird, L.E. (eds.), *Goodman and Gilman's The Pharmacological Basis of Therapeutics* (pp. 361-396). New York: McGraw-Hill.

Holbrook, T.L.; Barrett-Connor, E. (1993). A prospective study of alcohol consumption and bone mineral density. *BMJ* 306:1506-1509.

Holstege, A.; Bedossa, P.; Poynard, T.; Kollinger, M.; Chaput, J.C.; Houglum, K.; Chojkier, M. (1994). Acetaldehyde-modified epitopes in liver biopsy specimens of alcoholic and nonalcoholic patients: Localization and association with progression of liver fibrosis. *Hepatology* 19(2):367-374.

Honkanen, R.; Ertoma, L.; Kuosmanen, P.; Linnoina, M.; Alah, A.; Visori, T. (1983). The role of alcohol in accident falls. *J Stud Alcohol* 44:231-245.

Howland, J.; Hingson, R. (1987). Alcohol as a risk factor for injuries or death due to fires and burns: Review of the literature. *Public Health Rep* 102:475-483.

Hoxie, P.; Cardosi, K.; Stearns, M.; Mengert, P. (1988). *Alcohol in Fatal Recreational Boating Accidents.* Pub. No. DOT CGD 0488. Washington, DC: U.S. Department of Transportation, U.S. Coast Guard.

Huang, Y.S.; Chan, C.Y.; Wu, J.C.; Pai, C.H.; Chao, Y.; Lee, S.D. (1996). Serum levels of interleukin-8 in alcoholic liver disease: Relationship with disease stage, biochemical parameters, and survival. *J Hepatol* 24(4):377-384.

Hufford, M.R. (2001). Alcohol and suicidal behavior. *Clin Psychol Rev* 21:797-811.

Hugues, J.N.; Coste, T.; Perret, G.; Jayle, M.F.; Sebaoun, J.; Modigliani, E. (1980). Hypothalamopituitary ovarian function in thirty-one women with chronic alcoholism. *Clin Endocrinol* 12:543-551.

Huijbregts, P.P.; Freskens, E.J.; Kromhout, D. (1995). Dietary patterns and cardiovascular risk factors in elderly men: The Zutphen Elderly Study. *Int J Epidemiol* 24(2):313-320.

International Agency for Research on Cancer (1988). *Alcohol Drinking.* Lyon, France: IARC.

Israel, Y.; Orrego, H.; Holt, S.; Macdonald, D.W.; Meema, H.E. (1980). Identification of alcohol abuse: Thoracic fractures on routine chest x-rays as indicators of alcoholism. *Alcoholism* 4:420-422.

Jepson, R.G.; Fowkes, F.G.; Donnan, P.T.; Housley, E. (1995). Alcohol intake as a risk factor for peripheral arterial disease in the general population in the Edinburgh Artery Study. *Eur J Epidemiol* 11(1):9-14.

Johnell, O.; Gullberg, B.; Kanis, J.A.; Allander, E.; Elffors, L.; Dequeker, J.; Dilsen, G.; et al. (1995). Risk factors for hip fracture in European women: The MEDOS study. *J Bone Miner Res* 10:1802-1815.

Jones, J.D.; Barber, B.; Engrav, L.; Heimbach, D. (1991). Alcohol use and burn injury. *J Burn Care Rehabil* 12(2):148-152.

Kalbfleisch, J.M.; Lindeman, R.D.; Ginn, H.E.; Smith, W.O. (1963). Effects of ethanol administration on urinary excretion of magnesium and other electrolytes in alcoholic and normal subjects. *J Clin Invest* 42:1471-1475.

Kannel, W.B.; McGee, D.L. (1985). Update on some epidemiologic features of intermittent claudication: The Framingham study. *J Am Geriatr Soc* 33(1):13-18.

Kato, S.; Kawase, T.; Alderman, J.; Inatomi, N.; Lieber, C.S. (1990). Role of xanthine oxidase in ethanol-induced lipid peroxidation in rats. *Gastroenterology* 98(1):203-210.

Kauhanen, J.; Kaplan, G.A.; Goldberg, D.D.; Cohen, R.D.; Lakka, T.A.; Salonen, J.T. (1991). Frequent hangovers and cardiovascular mortality in middle-aged men. *Epidemiology* 8(3):310-314.

Kauhanen, J.; Kaplan, G.A.; Goldberg, D.E.; Salonen, J.T. (1997). Beer binging and mortality: Results from the Kuopio ischaemic heart disease risk factor study, a prospective population based study. *BMJ* 315(7112):846-851.

Kawano, Y.; Abe, H.; Imanishi, M.; Kojima, S.; Yoshimi, H.; Takishita, S.; Omae, T. (1996). Pressor and depressor hormones during alcohol-induced blood pressure reduction in hypertensive patients. *J Hum Hypertens* 10(9):595-599.

Kawase, T.; Kato, S.; Lieber, C.S. (1989). Lipid peroxidation and antioxidant defense systems in rat liver after chronic ethanol feeding. *Hepatology* 10(5):815-821.

Kearney, J.; Giovannucci, E.; Rimm, E.B.; Stampfer, M.J.; Colditz, G.A.; Ascherio, A.; Bleday, R.; Willett, W.C. (1995). Diet, alcohol, and smoking and the occurrence of hyperplastic polyps of the colon and rectum (United States). *Cancer Causes Control* 6(1):45-56.

Keil, U.; Chambless, L.E.; Doring, A.; Filipiak, B.; Stieber, J. (1997). The relation of alcohol intake to coronary heart disease and all-cause mortality in a beer drinking population. *Epidemiology* 8(2):150-156.

Keshavarzian, A.; Zorub, O.; Sayeed, M.; Urban, G.; Sweeney, C.; Winship, D.; Fields, J. (1994). Acute ethanol inhibits calcium influxes into esophageal smooth but not striated muscle: A possible mechanism for ethanol-induced inhibition of esophageal contractility. *J Pharmacol Exp Ther* 270(3):1057-1062.

Khoruts, A.; Stahnke, L.; McClain, C.J.; Logan, G.; Allen, J.I. (1991). Circulating tumor necrosis factor, interleukin-1, and interleukin-6 concentrations in chronic alcoholic patients. *Hepatology* 13(2):267-276.

Kinkaid, E.H.; Miller, P.R.; Meredith, J.W.; Rahman, N.; Change, M.C. (1998). Elevated arterial base deficit in trauma patients: A marker of impaired oxygen utilization. *J Am Coll Surg* 187:384-392.

Kitamura, A.; Iso, H.; Sankai, T.; Naito, Y.; Sato, S.; Kiyama, M.; Okamura, T.; Nakagawa, Y.; Iida, M.; Shimamoro, T.; Komachi, Y. (1998). Alcohol intake and premature coronary heart disease in urban Japanese men. *Am J Epidemiol* 147(1):59-65.

Klatsky, A.L.; Armstrong, M.A. (1993). Alcoholic beverage choice and risk of coronary artery disease mortality: Do red wine drinkers fare best? *Am J Cardiol* 71(5):467-469.

Klatsky, A.L.; Armstrong, M.A.; Friedman, G.D. (1997). Red wine, white wine, liquor, beer, and risk for coronary artery disease hospitalization. *Am J Cardiol* 80(4):416-420.

Klein, R.F.; Carlos, A.S. (1995). Inhibition of osteoblastic cell proliferation and ornithine decarboxylase activity by ethanol. *Endocrinology* 136:3406-3411.

Knuiman, M.W.; Vu, H.T. (1996). Risk factors for stroke mortality in men and women: The Busselton Study. *J Cardiovasc Risk* 3(5):447-452.

Kraus, J.; Morgenstern, H.; Fife, D.; Conroy, C.; Nourjah, P. (1989). Blood alcohol tests, prevalence of involvement and outcomes following brain injury. *Am J Pub Health* 79(3):294-299.

Kukielka, E.; Dicker, E.; Cederbaum, A.I. (1994). Increased production of reactive oxygen species by rat liver mitochondria after chronic ethanol treatment. *Arch Biochem Biophys* 309(2):377-386.

Labib, M.; Abdel-Kader, M.; Ranganath, L.; Teale, D.; Marks, V. (1989). Bone disease in chronic alcoholism: The value of plasma osteocalcin measurement. *Alcohol and Alcoholism* 24:141-144.

Lairinen, K.; Karkkainen, M.; Lalla, M.; Lambergallardt, C.; Tunninen, R.; Tahtela, R.; Valimaki, M. (1993). Is alcohol an osteoporosis-inducing agent for young and middle-aged women? *Metabolism* 42(7):875-881.

Lairinen, K.; Lamberg-Allardt, C.; Tunninen, R.; Harkonen, M.; Valimaki, M. (1992). Bone mineral density and abstention-induced changes in bone and mineral metabolism in noncirrhotic male alcoholics. *Am J Med* 93:642-650.

Lairinen, K.; Valimaki, M.; Keto, P. (1991). Bone mineral density measured by dual-energy X-ray absorptiometry in healthy Finnish women. *Calcif Tissue Int* 48:224-231.

Lalor, B.C.; France, M.W.; Powell, D.; Adams, P.H.; Counihan, T.B. (1986). Bone and mineral metabolism and chronic alcohol abuse. *Q J Med* 59:497-511.

Lang, T.; Nicaud, V.; Darne, B.; Rueff, B. (1995). Improving hypertension control among excessive alcohol drinkers: A randomised controlled trial in France. The WALPA Group. *J Epidemiol Comm Health* 49(6):610-616.

Langenbucher, J.; Nathan, P. (1983). Psychology, public policy and the evidence for intoxication. *American Psychologist* 38:1070-1077

Lelbach, W.K. (1975). Cirrhosis in the alcoholic and its relation to the volume of alcohol abuse. *Ann NY Acad Sci* 252:85-105.

Leo, M.A.; Kim, C.; Lowe, N.; Lieber, C.S. (1992). Interaction of ethanol with betacarotene: Delayed blood clearance and enhanced hepatotoxicity. *Hepatology* 15(5):883-891.

Leo, M.A.; Rosman, A.S.; Lieber, C.S. (1993). Differential depletion of carotenoids and tocopherol in liver disease. *Hepatology* 17(6):977-986.

Levitt, M.D.; Levitt, D.G. (1994). The critical role of the rate of ethanol absorption in the interpretation of studies purporting to demonstrate gastric metabolism of ethanol. *Pharmacol Exp Ther* 269(1):297-304.

Li., G.; Baker, S.P.; Sterling, S.; Smialek, J.E.; Dischinger, P.C.; Soderstron, C. (1996). A comparative analysis of alcohol in fatal and non-fatal bicycling injuries. *Alcohol Clin Exp Res* 20:1553-1559.

Lieber, C.S.; DeCarli, L.M. (1970). Quantitative relationship between amount of dietary fat and severity of alcoholic fatty liver. *Am Clin Nutr* 23(4):474-478.

Lieber, C.S.; Jones, D.P.; DeCarli, L.M. (1965). Effects of prolonged ethanol intake: Production of fatty liver despite adequate diets. *Clin Invest* 44(6):1009-1021.

Lindsell, D.R.; Wilson, A.G.; Maxwell, J.D. (1982). Fractures on the chest radiograph in detection of alcoholic liver disease. *BMJ* 285:597-599.

Longnecker, M.P. (1992). Alcohol consumption in relation to risk of cancers of the breast and large bowel. *Alcohol Health Res World* 16:223-229.

Longnecker, M.P. (1994). Alcoholic beverage consumption in relation to risk of breast cancer: Meta-analysis and review. *Cancer Causes Control* 5(1):73-82.

Longnecker, M.P. (1995). Alcohol consumption and risk of cancer in humans: An overview. *Alcohol* 12(2):87-96.

Longnecker, M.P.; Orza, M.J.; Adams, M.E.; Vioque, J.; Chalmers, T.C. (1990). A meta-analysis of alcoholic beverage consumption in relation to risk of colorectal cancer. *Cancer Causes Control* 1(1):59-68.

Luna, G.K.; Maier, R.V.; Sowder, L.; Copass, M.K.; Oreskovich, M.R. (1984). The influence of ethanol intoxication on outcome of injured motorcyclists. *J Trauma* 24(8):695-700.

Maher, J.J.; Tzagarakis, C.; Gimenez, A. (1994). Malondialdehyde stimulates collagen production by hepatic lipocytes only upon activation in primary culture. *Alcohol and Alcoholism* 29(5):605-610.

Marbet, U.A.; Bianchi, L.; Meury, U.; Stalder, G.A. (1987). Long-term histological evaluation of the natural history and prognostic factors of alcoholic liver disease. *J Hepatol* 4(3):364-372.

Marques-Vidal, P.; Cambou, J.P.; Nicaud, V.; Luc, G.; Evans, A.; Arveiler, D.; Bingham, A.; Cambien, F. (1995). Cardiovascular risk factors and alcohol consumption in France and Northern Ireland. *Atherosclerosis* 115(2):225-232.

Mathew, V.M. (1992). Alcoholism in biblical prophecy. *Alcohol and Alcoholism* 27:89-90.

McElduff, P.; Dobson, A.J. (1997). How much alcohol and how often? Population based case-control study of alcohol consumption and risk of a major coronary event. *BMJ* 314(7088):1159-1164.

McGill, V.; Kowal-Vern, A.; Kahn, S.; Gamelli, R.L. (1995). The impact of substance use on mortality and morbidity from thermal injury. *J. Trauma* Jun 38(6):931-934.

McPherson, K.; Engelsman, E.; Conning, D. (1993). Breast cancer. In: Verschuren, P. (ed.), *Alcoholic Beverages and European Society: Annex 3. Health Issues Related to Alcohol Consumption* (pp. 221-244). Brussels, Belgium: International Life Sciences Institute.

Mello, N.K.; Mendelson, I.H.; Teoh, S.K. (1993). An overview of the effects of alcohol on neuroendocrine function in women. In: Zakhari, S. (ed.), *Alcohol and the Endocrine System* (pp. 139-169). NIAAA Research Monograph No.23, National Institutes of Health Pub. No.93-3533. Bethesda, MD: NIH, NIAAA.

Mezey, E.; Kolman, C.I.; Diehl, A.M.; Mitchell, M.C.; Herlong, H.F. (1988). Alcohol and dietary intake in the development of chronic pancreatitis and liver disease in alcoholism. *Am Clin Nutr* 48(1):148-151.

Miller, W.R.; Heather, N.; Hall, W. (1991). Calculating standard drink units: International comparisons. *Br J Addict* 86:43-47.

Mingardi, R.; Avogaro, A.; Noventa, F.; Strazzabosco, M.; Stocchiero, C.; Tiengo, A.; Erie, G. (1997). Alcohol intake is associated with a lower prevalence of peripheral vascular disease in non-insulin-dependent diabetic women. *Nutr Metab Cardiovasc Dis* 7(4):301-308.

Mobarhan, S.A.; Russell, R.M.; Recker, R.R.; Posner, D.B.; Iber, F.L.; Miller, P. (1984). Metabolic bone disease in alcoholic cirrhosis: A comparison of the effect of Vitamin D2, 25-hydroxy vitamin D, or supportive treatment. *Hepatology* 4:266-273.

Molberg, P.; Hopkins, R.; Paulson, J.; Gunn, R. (1993). Fatal incident risk factors in recreational boating in Ohio. *Pub Health Rep* 108(3):340-346.

Molina, P.E.; McClain, C.; Valla, D.; Guidot, D.; Diehl, A.M.; Lang, C.H.; Neuman, M. (2002). Molecular pathology and clinical aspects of alcohol-induced tissue injury. *Alcohol Clin Exp Res* 26(1):120-128.

Morrow, D.; Leirer, V.; Yesavage, J.; Tinklenberg, J. (1991). Alcohol, age, and piloting: Judgment, mood, and actual performance. *Int J Addict* 26(6):669-683.

Moshage, H.; Casini, A.; Lieber, C.S. (1990). Acetaldehyde selectively stimulates collagen production in cultured rat liver fat-storing cells but not in hepatocytes. *Hepatology* 12(3):511-518.

National Center for Health Statistics (2003). National Vital Statistics Records, Vol. 52, No. 3, U.S. Department of Health and Human Services, Washington, DC. Available at http://www.cdc.gov/nchs/data/nvsr/nvsr54_03.pdf.

National Highway Traffic Safety Administration (1994). *Traffic Safety Facts 1993: Alcohol*. Washington, DC: U.S. Department of Transportation, National Center for Statistics and Analysis.

National Institute on Alcohol Abuse and Alcoholism (1988). U.S. Department of Health and Human Services. *Effects of Alcohol on Driving Performance, Effects of Low Doses of Alcohol on Driving-related Skills: A Review of the Evidence.* U.S. Department of Transportation/National Highway Traffic Safety Administration DOT HS 807 280.

National Institute on Alcohol Abuse and Alcoholism (1997). *Ninth Special Report to the U.S. Congress on Alcohol and Health.* NIH Publication No. 97-4017. Bethesda, MD: NIAAA.

National Institute on Alcohol Abuse and Alcoholism (2000). *Tenth Special Report to the U.S. Congress on Alcohol and Health.* Washington, DC: U.S. Department of Health and Human Services.

Naveau, S.; Giraud, V.; Borocto, E.; Aubert, A.; Capron, F.; Chaput, J.C. (1997). Excess weight risk factor for alcoholic liver disease. *Hepatology* 25(1):108-111.

Niemela, O.; Juvonen, T.; Parkkila, S. (1991). Immunohistochemical demonstration of acetaldehyde-modified epitopes in human liver after alcohol consumption. *J Clin Invest* 87(4):1367-1374.

Nordmann, R.; Rjbiere, C.; Rouach, H. (1992). Implication of free radical mechanisms in ethanol-induced cellular injury. *Free Radical Biol Med* 12(3):219-240.

Ohlinger, W.; Dinges, H.P.; Zatloukal, K.; Mair, S.; Gollowitsch, F.; Denk, H. (1993). Immunohistochemical detection of tumor necrosis factor-alpha, other cytokines, and adhesion molecules in human livers with alcoholic hepatitis. *Virchows Arch A Pathol Anat Histopathol* 423(3):169-176.

Olkkonen, S.; Honkanen, R. (1994) The role of alcohol in non-fatal bicycle injuries. *Accid Anal Prev* 22:89-96.

O'Neill, T.W.; Marsden, D.; Adams, J.E.; Silman, A.J. (1996). Risk factors, falls, and fracture of the distal forearm in Manchester, UK. *J Epidemiol Comm Health* 50:288-292.

Orwoll, E.S.; Bauer, D.C.; Vogt, T.M.; Fox, K.M. (1996). Axial bone mass in older women: Study of osteoporotic fracture research group. *Ann Intern Med* 124:187-196.

Paganini-Hill, A.; Ross, R.K.; Gerkins, V.R. (1981). Menopausal estrogen therapy and hip fractures. *Ann Intern Med* 95:28-31.

Palmer, A.J.; Fletcher, A.E.; Bulpitt, C.J.; Beevers, D.G.; Coles, E.C.; Ledingham, J.G.; Petrie, J.C.; Webster, J.; Dollery, C.T. (1995). Alcohol intake and cardiovascular mortality in hypertensive patients: Report from the Department of Health Hypertension Care Computing Project. *J Hypertens* 13(9):957-964.

Pares, A.; Caballeria, J.; Bruguera, M.; Torres, M.; Rodes, J. (1986). Histological course of alcoholic hepatitis: Influence of abstinence, sex and extent of hepatic damage. *J Hepatol* 2(1):33-42.

Parola, M.; Pinzani, M.; Casini, A.; Albano, E.; Poli, G.; Gentilini, A.; Gentilini, P.; Dianzani, M.U. (1993). Stimulation of lipid peroxidation or 4-hydroxynonenal treatment increases procollagen alpha 1 (I) gene expression in human liver fat-storing cells. *Biochem Biophys Res Commun* 194(3):1044-1050.

Paunio, M.; Hook-Nikanne, J.; Kosunen, T.U.; Vainio, U.; Salaspuro, M.; Makinen, J.; Heinonen, O.P. (1994). Association of alcohol consumption and *Helicobacter pylori* infection in young adulthood and early middle age among patients with gastric complaints: A case-control study on Finnish conscripts officers and other military personnel. *Eur J Epidemiol* 10(2):205-209.

Pearl, R. (1926). *Alcohol and Longevity.* New York: Alfred Knopf.

Pellegrini, M.; Pareti, F.I.; Stabile, F.; Brusamolino, A.; Simonetti, P. (1996). Effects of moderate consumption of red wine on platelet aggregation and haemostatic variables in healthy volunteers. *Eur J Clin Nutr* 50(4):209-213.

Peris, P.; Guanabens, N.; Parés, A.; Pons, F.; Del Rio, L.; Monegal, A.; Suris, X.; Caballeria, J.; Rodes, J.; Munoz-Gómez, J. (1995). Vertebral fractures and osteopenia in chronic alcoholic patients. *Calcif Tissue Int* 57:111-114.

Peris, P.; Pares, A.; Guanabens, N.; Del Rio, L.; Pons, F.; Deosaba, M.J.M.; Monegal, A.; Caballeria, J.; Rodes, J.; Munoz-Gómez, J. (1994). Bone mass improves in alcoholics after 2 years of abstinence. *J Bone Miner Res* 9(10):1607-1612.

Perrine, M.W.; Mundt, J.C.; Winer, R.I. (1994). When alcohol and water don't mix: Diving under the influence. *J Stud Alcohol* 55:517-524.

Poupon, R.E.; Nalpas, B.; Coutelle, C.; Fleury, B.; Couzigou, P.; Higueret, D. (1992). Polymorphism of alcohol dehydrogenase, alcohol and aldehyde dehydrogenase activities: Implication in alcoholic cirrhosis in white patients. The French Group for Research on Alcohol and Liver. *Hepatology* 15(6):1017-1022.

Puddey, I.B.; Beilin, L.J.; Vandongen, R.; Rouse, I.L.; Rogers, P. (1995). Evidence for a direct effect of alcohol consumption on blood pressure in normotensive men: A randomized controlled trial. *Hypertension* 7(5):707-713.

Rashba-Step, J.; Turro, N.J.; Cederbaum, A.I. (1993). Increased NADPH- and NADH-dependent production of superoxide and hydroxyl radical by microsomes after chronic ethanol treatment. *Arch Biochem Biophys* 300(1):401-408.

Rehm, J.T.; Bondy, S.J.; Sempos, C.T.; Vuong, C.V. (1997). Alcohol consumption and coronary heart disease morbidity and mortality. *Am J Epidemiol* 146(6): 495-501.

Reinke, L.A.; Moore, D.R.; Hague, C.M.; McCay, P.B. (1994). Metabolism of ethanol to I-hydroxyethyl radicals in rat liver microsomes: Comparative studies with three spin trapping agents. *Free Radic Res Commun* 21(4):213-222.

Ridker, P.M.; Vaughan, D.E.; Stampfer, M.J.; Glynn, R.J.; Hennekens, C.H. (1994). Association of moderate alcohol consumption and plasma concentration of endogenous tissue-type plasminogen activator. *JAMA* 272(12):929-933.

Rimm, E.B.; Klatsky, A.; Grobbee, D.; Stampfer, M.J. (1996). Review of moderate alcohol consumption and reduced risk of coronary heart disease: Is the effect due to beer, wine, or spirits? *BMJ* 312(7033):731-736.

Ross, L.; Yeazel, L.; Chau, A. (1992). Pilot performance with blood alcohol concentrations below 0.04 percent. *Aviat Space Environ Med* 63(11):951-956.

Rubin, R.; Rand, M.L. (1994). Alcohol and platelet function. *Alcohol Clin Exp Res* 18(1):105-110.

Sadrzadeh, S.M.; Meydani, M.; Khettry, U.; Nanji, A.A. (1995). High-dose vitamin E supplementation has no effect on ethanol-induced pathological liver injury. *J Pharmacol Exp Ther* 273(1):455-460.

Sadrzadeh, S.M.; Nanji, A.A. (1994). Detection of lipid peroxidation after acute alcohol administration is dependent on time of sampling. *Int J Vitam Nutr Res* 64(2):157-158.

Saville, P.D. (1965). Changes in bone mass with age and alcoholism. *J Bone Joint Surg* 47A:492-499.

Schatzkin, A.; Longnecker, M.P. (1994). Alcohol and breast cancer: Where are we now and where do we go from here? *Cancer* 74(Suppl 3):1101-1110.

Schnitzler, C.M.; Solomon, L. (1984). Bone changes after alcohol abuse. *S Afr Med J* 66:730-734.

Seitz, H.; Pöschl, G. (1997). Alcohol and gastrointestinal cancer: Pathogenic mechanisms. *Addict Biol* 2(1):19-33.

Seitz, H.K.; Simanowski, U.A.; Egerer, G.; Waldherr, R.; Oertl, U. (1992). Human gastric alcohol dehydrogenase: In vitro characteristics and effect of cimetidine. *Digestion* 51(2):80-85.

Seller, S.C. (1985). Alcohol abuse in the Old Testament. *Alcohol* 20:69-76.

Seppa, K.; Laippala, P.; Sillanaukee, P. (1996). High diastolic blood pressure: Common among women who are heavy drinkers. *Alcohol Clin Exp Res* 20(1):47-51.

Shaw, S.; Jayatilleke, E. (1990). The role of aldehyde oxidase in ethanol-induced hepatic lipid peroxidation in the rat. *Biochem* 268(3):579-583.

Sheron, N.; Bird, G.; Koskinas, I.; Portmann, B.; Ceska, M.; Lindley, I.; Williams, R. (1993). Circulating and tissue levels of the neutrophil chemotaxin interleukin8 are elevated in severe acute alcoholic hepatitis, and tissue levels correlate with neutrophil infiltration. *Hepatology* 18(1):41-46.

Shimizu, M.; Lasker, I.M.; Tsutsumi, M.; Lieber, C.S. (1990). Immunohistochemical localization of ethanol-inducible P450IIE1 in the rat alimentary tract. *Gastroenterology* 99(4):1044-1053.

Smith-Warner, S.A.; Spiegelman, D.; Yaun, S.-S.; van den Brandt, P.A.; Folsom, A.R.; Goldbohm, R.A.; Graham, S.; et al. (1998). Alcohol and breast cancer in women: A pooled analysis of cohort studies. *JAMA* 279(7):535-540.

Sonnenberg, L.M.; Quatromoni, P.A.; Gagnon, D.R.; Cupples, L.A.; Franz, M.M.; Ordovas, J.M.; Wilson, P.W.; Schaefer, E.J.; Millen, B.E. (1996). Diet and plasma lipids in women. II. Macronutrients and plasma triglycerides, highdensity lipoprotein, and the ratio of total to high-density lipoprotein cholesterol in women: The Framingham Nutrition Studies. *J Clin Epidemiol* 49(6):665-672.

Spencer, H.; Rubio, N.; Rubio, E.; Indreika, M.; Seitam, A. (1986). Chronic alcoholism: Frequently overlooked cause of osteoporosis in men. *Am J Med* 80:393-397.

Steinbok, P.; Thompson, G.B. (1978). Metabolic disturbances after head injury: Abnormalities of sodium and water intoxication. *Neurosurgery* 3:9-15.

Surgeon General's Workshop on Drunk Driving (1988). U.S. Department of Health and Human Services, Office of the Surgeon General, Washington.

Tetrito, M.C.; Tanaka, K.R. (1974). Hypophosphatemia in chronic alcoholism. *Arch Intern Med* 134:445-447.

Thuluvath, P.; Wojno, K.; Yardley, J.H.; Mezey, E. (1994). Effects of *Helicobacter pylori* infection and gastritis on gastric alcohol dehydrogenase activity. *Alcohol Clin Exp Res* 18(4):795-798.

Thun, M.J.; Peto, R.; Lopez, A.D.; Monaco, J.H.; Henley, S.J.; Heath, C.W.; Doll, R. (1997). Alcohol consumption and mortality among middle-aged and elderly U.S. adults. *N Engl J Med* 337(24):1705-1714.

Tilg, H.; Wilmer, A.; Vogel, W.; Herold, M.; Nolchen, B.; Judmaier, G.; Huber, C. (1992). Serum levels of cytokines in chronic liver diseases. *Gastroenterology* 103(1):264-274.

Tsukamoto, H. (1993). Oxidative stress, antioxidants, and alcoholic liver fibrogenesis. *Alcohol* 10(6):465-467.

Tsukamoto, H.; Horne, W.; Kamimura, S.; Niemela, O.; Parkkila, S.; Yla-Herttuala, S.; Brittenham, G.M. (1995). Experimental liver cirrhosis induced by alcohol and iron. *J Clin Invest* 96(1):620-630.

Tuppurainen, M.; Kroger, H.; Honkanen, R.; Puntial, E.; Huopia, J.; Saarikoski, S.; Alhave, E. (1995). Risks of perimenopausal fractures: A prospective population-based study. *Acta Obstet Gynecol Scand* 74:624-628.

Tuyns, A.; Pequignot, G. (1984). Greater risk of ascitic cirrhosis in females in relation to alcohol consumption. *Int J Epidemiol* 13(1):53-57.

Ueshima, H.; Mikawa, K.; Baba, S.; Sasaki, S.; Ozawa, H.; Tsushima, M.; Kawaguchi, A.; Omae, T.; Katayama, Y.; Kayemori, Y. (1993). Effect of reduced alcohol consumption on blood pressure in untreated hypertensive men. *Hypertension* 21(2):248-252.

Uppal, R.; Lateef, S.K.; Korsten, M.A.; Paronetto, F.; Lieber, C.S. (1991). Chronic alcoholic gastritis: Roles of alcohol and *Helicobacter pylori*. *Arch Intern Med* 151(4):760-764.

Urbano-Marquez, A.; Estruch, R.; Ferandez-Sola, J.; Nicolas, J.M.; Pare, J.C.; Rubin, E. (1995). The greater risk of alcoholic cardiomyopathy and myopathy in women compared with men. *JAMA* 274(2):149-154.

U.S. Department of Agriculture; U.S. Department of Health and Human Services (1995). *Home and Garden Bulletin* No. 232, Fourth Edition. Washington, DC: U.S. Department of Agriculture.

U.S. Department of Health and Human Services (1995). *Healthy People 2000. Midcourse Review and 1995 Revisions.* Washington, DC: U.S. Department of Health and Human Services, U.S. Public Health Service.

U.S. Department of Health and Human Services (1999). *Alcohol and Coronary Heart Disease.* Alcohol Alert No. 45. Washington, DC: U.S. Department of Health and Human Services.

Valimaki, M.; Salaspuro, M.; Ylikahri, R. (1982). Liver damage and sex hormones in chronic male alcoholics. *Clin Endocrinol* 17:469-477.

Valimaki, M.; Pelkonen, R.; Salaspuro, M.; Harkonen, J.; Hirvonen, E.; Ylikahri, R. (1984). Sex hormones in amenorrheic women with alcoholic liver disease. *J Clin Endocrinol Metab* 59:133-138.

Van Thiel, D.H.; Lester, R.; Sherins, R.J. (1974). Hypogonadism in alcoholic liver disease: Evidence for a double defect. *Gastroenterology* 67:1188-1199.

Vaughan, T.I.; Davis, S.; Kristal, A.; Thomas, D.B. (1995). Obesity, alcohol, and tobacco as risk factors for cancers of the esophagus and gastric cardia: Adenocarcinoma versus squamous cell carcinoma. *Cancer Epidemiol Biomarkers Prev* 4(2):85-92.

Waller, P.; Steward, J.; Hansen, A.; Stutts, J.; Popkin, C.; Rodgman, E. (1986). The potentiating effects of alcohol on driver injury. *JAMA* 256(11):1461-1466.

Ward, R.; Flynn, T.; Miller, P. (1982). Effects of ethanol ingestion on the severity and outcome of trauma. *Am J Surg* 144:153-157.

Wells, J.; Greene, M.; Foss, R.; Ferguson, S.; Williams, A. (1997). Drinking drivers missed at sobriety checkpoints. *J Studies Alcohol* 58:513-517.

Wieczorek, W.F. (1995). The role of treatment in reducing alcohol-related accidents involving DWI offenders. In Watson, R.R. (ed.), *Alcohol, Cocaine and Accidents. Drug Alcohol Abuse Rev* 7:105-129.

Williams, G.A.; Bowser, E.N.; Hargis, G.K.; Kukreja, S.C.; Shah, J.H.; Vora, N.M.; Henderson, W.J. (1978). Effect of ethanol on parathyroid hormone and calcitonin secretion in man. *Proc Soc Exp Biol Med* 159:187-191.

Wilson, D.M. III; Tenrler, J.J.; Carney, J.P.; Wilson, T.M.; Kelley, M.R. (1994). Acute ethanol exposure suppresses the repair of O6-methylguanine DNA lesions in castrated adult male rats. *Alcohol Clin Exp Res* 18(5):1267-1271.

World Health Organization (1996). Report of the Ad Hoc Committee on Health Research Relating to Future Intervention Options. *Investing in Health Research and Development.* Geneva, Switzerland: WHO.

Yamada, K.; Araki, S.; Tamura, M.; Sakai, I.; Takahashi, Y.; Kashihara, H.; Kono, S. (1997). Case-control study of colorectal carcinoma in situ and cancer in relation to cigarette smoking and alcohol use. *Cancer Causes Control* 8(5):780-785.

Yesavage, J.; Dolhert, N.; Taylor, J. (1994). Flight simulator performance of younger and older aircraft pilots. Effects of age and alcohol. *J Am Geriat Soc* 42(6): 577-582.

Yin, S.J.; Chou, F.J.; Chao, S.F.; Tsai, S.F.; Liao, C.S.; Wang, S.L.; Wu, C.W.; Lee, S.C. (1993). Alcohol and aldehyde dehydrogenases in human esophagus: Comparison with the stomach enzyme activities. *Alcohol Clin Exp Res* 17(2): 376-381.

York, J.L.; Hirsch, J.A. (1997). Association between blood pressure and lifetime drinking patterns in moderate drinkers. *J Stud Alcohol* 58(5):480-485.

You, R.X.; McNeil, J.J.; O'Malley, H.M.; Davis, S.M.; Thrift, A.G.; Donnan, G.A. (1997). Risk factors for stroke due to cerebral infarction in young adults. *Stroke* 28(10):1913-1918.

Yuan, J.-M.; Ross, R.K.; Gao, Y.-T.; Henderson, B.E.; Yu, M.C. (1997). Follow up study of moderate alcohol intake and mortality among middle-aged men in Shanghai, China. *BMJ* 314(7073):18-23.

Zador, P.L.; Krawchuk, S.A.; Voas, R.B. (2000). Alcohol-related risk of driver fatalities and driver involvement in fatal crashes in relation to driver age and gender: An update using 1996 data. *J Stud Alcohol* 61:387-395.

Zador, P.L; Krawchuk, S.A.; Voas, R.B. (2000) Relative risk of fatal crash involvement by BAC, age and gender. U.S. Department of Transportation, National Highway Traffic Safety Administration DOT HS 809 050

Zakhari, S.; Wassef, M. (eds.) (1996). Alcohol and the Cardiovascular System. NIAAA Research Monograph No. 31, Pub. No. 96-4133. Bethesda, MD: NIAAA.

Zink, B.; Maoi, R.; Chen, B. (1996). Alcohol, central nervous system injury, and time to death in fatal motor vehicle crashes. *Alcohol Clin Exp Res* 20(9):1518-1522.

Zink, B.J.; Schultz, C.H.; Stern, S.A.; Mertz, M.; Wang, X.; Johnston, P.; Keep, R.F. (2001). Effects of ethanol and naltrexone in a model of traumatic brain injury with hemorrhagic shock. *J Clin Exp Res* 25(6):916-923.

Zumoff, B. (1997). The critical role of alcohol consumption in determining the risk of breast cancer with postmenopausal estrogen administration. *J Clin Endocrinol Metab* 82(6):1656-1658.

Chapter 3

The Neuropsychological Consequences of Alcohol and Drug Abuse

Rosemarie Scolaro Moser
Corinne E. Frantz
John Brick

INTRODUCTION AND OVERVIEW

Scientific and public interest in the nature of alcohol and drug action and addiction on the human body, and the psychosocial impact of substance abuse continues to evolve. Insight into the process of addiction and how the rewarding effects of certain substances are a result of dysregulation of the brain reward circuit (Leshner and Koob, 1999), and research linking the physical effects of substances of abuse to cognitive or neuropsychological functioning continues to expand, leading to a better understanding of how physical changes in the brain due to substance abuse may lead to acute, transient, and permanent alterations in the way one thinks and processes information.

In this chapter, we survey the research identifying the documented relationships between alcohol and drug abuse and neuropsychological functioning. Clearly, a significant portion of the research in this area has focused on alcohol abuse and this chapter will begin with an understanding of that body of research. This is followed by a review of the research on polydrug abuse in which population samples are not distinguished by a particular drug, as is often the case. It is for this group of drug abusers that neurotoxicity has been most frequently observed (Hartman, 1995).

Few abusers commit to one substance alone, so it is difficult to find formidable research that represents each substance of abuse (Miller, 1985).

Handbook of the Medical Consequences of Alcohol and Drug Abuse
© 2008 by The Haworth Press, Taylor & Francis Group. All rights reserved.
doi:10.1300/6039_03

Nonetheless, some specific research is available for a few drugs. The illegal drugs that have been more typically represented in neuropsychological research, including cannabinoids (e.g., marijuana), cocaine, lysergic acid diethylamide (LSD), and phencyclidine (PCP), are reviewed here. Opiates, solvents, and new designer drugs are also mentioned despite the dearth of neuropsychological research pertaining to them.

Neuropsychology is the scientific study of brain-behavior relationships and more specifically how physiological brain function impacts neuropsychological processes such as "memory, language skills, sensory/perceptual/motor skills, visual/spatial skills, mental speed/efficiency/flexibility, physical and mental coordination, listening skills, attention and concentration, problem solving, and reasoning" (Moser, 1999, p. 2). Neuropsychologists, or cognitive scientists, utilize a variety of assessment tools to measure neuropsychological processes, a number of which will be referred to in this chapter.

When alcohol and other drugs have an effect on the brain, the effect tends not to be clear, lateralized, and focal in nature as seen in strokes, tumors, or other localized brain disorders. Rather, a more generalized, pervasive effect on the brain, with perhaps particular areas of concentration of dysfunction, may be observed. Thus, some drugs may specifically affect certain neuropsychological functions, although these functions may not be specific to a certain area of the brain. Effects may be immediate and acute, or long lasting and chronic.

Much controversy exists regarding the effects of repeated use of nonprescription drugs because of problems in the experimental design of the existing studies. With this in mind, the reader is cautioned to consider the limitations of current research in the area of the neuropsychology of alcohol and drug abuse. Nonetheless, the promise of future research may lie in the complementary use of neuroimaging and neuropsychological assessments that will offer greater insight into brain-behavior relationships. For example, Chapter 6 discusses neuroanatomical changes associated with alcohol exposure and the resultant behavioral correlates.

BRAIN IMPAIRMENT AND ALCOHOL ABUSE

Alcohol ranks as one of the most serious substances of abuse due to the prevalence of alcohol abuse in the general population and the severity of its toxic effects. It has been estimated that between 5 and 12 million individuals abuse alcohol, with a significantly greater proportion being male (Hartman, 1995; Thompson, 2000). The acute effects of alcohol intoxication are well known and include changes in psychomotor and cognitive functioning, as well as changes in affect. Some of the effects of chronic alcohol abuse are also well known and have been extensively reviewed, particularly the dramatic effect of alcohol on memory in the case of Korsakoff's syndrome (Butters, 1984; Butters and Miliotis, 1985). Less clear and still somewhat controversial are answers to the following questions:

1. What are the cognitive effects of chronic alcohol abuse in the absence of Korsakoff's syndrome?
2. What, if any, are the direct toxic effects of alcohol on brain tissue?
3. Are there cognitive predictive factors for individuals at high risk for alcohol abuse?
4. What is known about the recovery of cognitive functions after abstinence from chronic alcohol abuse?

As with all drugs of abuse, alcohol is initially sought out for its pleasurable effects which are mediated in the brain by its impact on the mesolimbic reward system (Leshner, 1997).

Recent evidence, however, points to alcohol's impact on the gamma-aminobutyric acid (GABA) receptor complex embedded in the membrane of neurons; in particular, the barbiturate site on the $GABA_A$ receptors (Thompson, 2000). Converging evidence from a variety of sources indicates that much like other anxiolytics such as benzodiazepines, alcohol significantly alters GABA neurotransmission; GABA may mediate many of the acute behavioral effects, such as alcohol-induced motor incoordination, anxiolysis, and sedation; and GABA plays an important role in the development of alcohol tolerance and susceptibility to alcohol dependence (Grobin et al., 1998; Mihic and Harris, 1997). Thus, in addition to its common effects on the brain's reward system, which are shared by all substances of abuse, alcohol also affects those brain regions outside of the pleasure system that utilize GABA (Leshner, 1997; Thompson, 2000; see Chapter 4 for additional information).

Acute Effects of Alcohol Intoxication

Alcohol is rapidly absorbed from the gastrointestinal tract into the circulation and easily crosses the blood-brain barrier to produce various effects of acute intoxication. The effects of alcohol are generally believed to be dose-dependent across many variables (Brick and Erickson, 1999; Hartman, 1995). General diagnostic criteria for acute intoxication include, but are not limited to, slurred speech, incoordination, unsteady gait, nystagmus, impairment in attention or memory, stupor or coma (American Psychiatric

Association [APA], 1994). Studies of neuropsychological performance associated with acute alcohol intake have found impairments on a variety of cognitive tasks. Alcohol is known to impair judgment, increase risk taking, decrease perceived negative consequences of risk-taking behavior, and alter perception (Burian, Liguori, and Robinson, 2002). Minocha et al. (1985), for example, found impairments in fine motor coordination, attention, concentration, auditory-verbal skills, and visuospatial skills. In a study comparing the acute effects of alcohol and temazepam ingestion on the formation of new semantic and episodic memories, Tiplady et al. (1999) found that the acquisition of new semantic and episodic memories, assessed with a test of learning-invented facts and by a measure of long-term learning of words on the Buschke test, were impaired by ingestion of both drugs. The effects of ethanol were more marked than the effects of temazapam on new learning. Psychomotor speed, assessed with the digit symbol subtest of the Wechsler Adult Intelligence Scale, was equally impaired by both drugs. Semantic memory refers to recall of general knowledge that is not tagged to specific life experiences (e.g., knowledge of vocabulary and overlearned facts). Episodic memory, in contrast, refers to recall of events or facts that are related to an individual's specific life experiences. Both types of memory are considered to be declarative in nature, which will be defined later.

GABA exerts a prominent inhibitory effect on brain systems which it subserves. As already noted, this may account for the anxiolytic effect of alcohol intake. Similarly, the agitation and convulsions observed during alcohol withdrawal may be due to neuronal hypersensitivity. This is the hypersensitivity theory of withdrawal and addiction (Thompson, 2000).

Not all effects of alcohol are due to acute intoxication. Some research suggests a dose-response relationship between alcohol consumption and neuropsychological test performance in social drinkers (Parker et al., 1983). Although such performance may not rise to the level of clinical impairment, neuropsychological performance deficits are measurable. Parsons (1986) concluded that in sober social drinkers, cognitive impairment from alcohol use was inconclusive. However, alcoholics present a significant, albeit complicated range of neuropsychological deficits.

The negative effect of chronic heavy drinking is well documented in the alcohol literature and as indicated in this and other chapters (e.g., Chapters 2 and 5), neuropsychological and anatomical consequences are of particular interest in understanding recovery of function. Recovery of function is variable for many reasons, not the least of which is that many factors such as age, medical status, or lack of baseline can affect the interpretation of the results.

Neuropsychological Findings in Chronic Alcoholism with Korsakoff's Amnesia

Considerable neuropsychological attention has been focused on the cognitive features of Korsakoff's syndrome, a somewhat rare but profound consequence of chronic heavy drinking. Afflicted individuals first undergo an acute encephalopathic crisis called Wernicke's encephalopathy that resolves into a persistent and severe amnesia referred to as Korsakoff's amnesia. The characteristics of this amnesia include a severe anterograde loss of memory during which the afflicted individual is unable to learn new verbal or nonverbal information that is declarative and episodic in nature. Declarative memory refers to knowledge of facts or events that can be consciously stated or declared by the individual. Episodic memory, as noted earlier, refers to recall of facts or events that occurred at a specific time in a person's life, such as recalling what one ate for breakfast in the morning. The anterograde amnesia in Korsakoff's syndrome is often accompanied by normal or near normal intellectual functions and a milder retrograde amnesia. Retrograde amnesia refers to difficulty in retrieving facts or events from long-term memory that occurred before the onset of the illness. It is usually more pronounced for events that occurred just prior to the onset of the illness, while remote events, such as childhood memories, are relatively well preserved (Albert, Butters, and Brandt, 1981; Butters and Miliotis, 1985).

It has been known for some time that the damaging effects to the central nervous system, or brain, which give rise to Korsakoff's syndrome occur as an indirect effect of alcohol on the brain, namely, a severe nutritional deficiency that accompanies increasingly severe and protracted alcohol intake and results in a complete absence of thiamine in the diet. The immediate treatment for an individual suffering from Wernicke's encephalopathy is administration of large doses of thiamine. Although considered to be rare, there is evidence that Wernicke's encephalopathy is significantly underdiagnosed among chronic alcoholics (Hartman, 1995). Autopsy studies of individuals who have been afflicted with Wernicke-Korsakoff syndrome revealed pronounced damage to several limbic system structures, including the mammillary bodies of the hypothalamus and the medialis dorsalis nucleus of the thalamus. In addition, damage has been reported to the vermis of the cerebellum, the oculomotor nucleus which controls eye movements, and association areas in the cerebral cortex. Damage to the hippocampus has not been consistently reported (Butters and Miliotis, 1985). However, the mammillary bodies and the medialis dorsalis nucleus of the thalamus are known to have strong anatomical connections with the hippocampus, which is involved with memory functions.

Early investigations found that individuals with Korsakoff's syndrome were impaired in their retention of new information after delays of only a few seconds (Butters and Cermak, 1975; Kinsbourne and Wood, 1975; Piercy, 1978). Analysis of the nature of errors made in recall by Korsakoff patients revealed a high incidence of intrusions rather than errors of omission, suggesting that Korsakoff patients were highly vulnerable to distraction; in particular, they were vulnerable to the effects of proactive interference on recall (Butters, 1979; Butters and Miliotis, 1985). Proactive interference refers to the inability to acquire new information because of interference from previously learned material. As distributed practice of new information has been known to be effective in reducing the effects of interference on recall, Butters et al. (1976) trained Korsakoff patients on new learning with distributed practice and found that patients' recall of new information was similar to that of control subjects who learned new information under conditions of mass practice.

Other studies have pointed to the possibility that the severe retention difficulties of Korsakoff patients reflect a failure to encode a sufficient number of attributes of the new information at the time of storage in order to facilitate adequate retrieval, thus making the new information more vulnerable to the effects of interference (Butters, 1979; Butters and Miliotis, 1985). In an early study, for example, Butters and Cermak (1974) found that semantic cues did not help Korsakoff patients retrieve new verbal information, even though phonemic cues did. They suggested that Korsakoff patients might be deficient in their ability to semantically analyze the material, which would limit the stored attributes of the material for later recall. This is consistent with studies in which patients were found to respond to irrelevant paraphernalia such as hats, and so, in attempting to recall faces in a facial matching task (Diamond and Carey, 1977; Dricker et al., 1978). These studies suggested that difficulty with retention and recall may be related to limited perceptual analysis. Additional work led to the formulation of the contextual encoding theory that posits that Korsakoff patients exhibit a specific failure to encode the contextual attributes of new information which gives rise to retrieval impairments (Butters, 1979; Butters and Miliotis, 1985).

Studies of the role of hippocampal neurons in memory and learning conducted with patients suffering from Korsakoff's amnesia and with animals have interesting points of convergence.

The mammillary bodies, an important site of damage in Korsakoff's syndrome, have strong anatomical connections to the hippocampus within the limbic system, a site known to be important in memory functions. For example, studies have found that rats with damaged hippocampi can learn which of two arms in a maze to run down for water in a conditioned brightness discrimination task, but have great difficulty unlearning it if the stimulus conditions change (Kimble, 1968). The animals appear to show behavioral perseveration which is similar to the phenomenon of proactive interference in the memory performance of Korsakoff patients. Other rat studies involving single cell recordings from the hippocampus have led to the discovery of "place cells" which appear to respond to particular locations in space (Thompson, 2000). This is consistent with decades of research indicating that the hippocampus plays a role in various learning paradigms (Graham, 1990). These findings suggest that the hippocampus may play an important role in laying down contextual cues for the facilitation of recall of new information, and lend support to the clinical findings of vulnerability to distraction and interference due to a failure of the contextual encoding of new information in Korsakoff patients.

It has been noted that Korsakoff patients demonstrate relative preservation of intellectual functions in the presence of their specific memory disturbance. Through extensive reviews of clinical research literature, Butters et al. (Butters, 1979; Butters and Miliotis, 1985) have noted that although overall IQ scores are indistinguishable from matched controls, Korsakoff patients manifest a number of specific cognitive deficits during formal neuropsychological testing. These deficits include (1) a low symbol subtest score on the Wechsler Adult Intelligence Scale–Revised (WAIS-R), and (2) severely depressed Wechsler Memory Scale scores on logical memory (verbal passage recall), figural memory, and paired associate learning subtests. Hartman (1995) notes that Korsakoff patients also have difficulty in cognitive tasks such as the Halstead-Reitan Tactual Performance Test, which involves the ability to create and utilize a visuospatial internal representation of the location of target stimuli through tactile-kinesthetic sensory input. Additional deficits are reported to be found in tests involving visuospatial and constructional abilities, and tests involving categorization, rule learning, and set shifting or mental flexibility (e.g., Wisconsin Card Sorting Test and Halstead-Reitan Category Test) (Hartman, 1995).

Despite the severity of impairment for new declarative memory in Korsakoff patients, these individuals are able to learn new motor tasks involving implicit, procedural memory (Butters and Miliotis, 1985). Support for this finding comes from a study by Beaunieux et al. (1998) who discovered a Korsakoff patient who was able to learn to solve the Tower of Hanoi puzzle, a test that involves cognitive procedural memory. Procedural memory is also known as nondeclarative or implicit memory and refers to the memory of how a task is accomplished.

Neuropsychological Findings in Nonamnesic Chronic Alcoholics

Neuropsychological interest has focused on documenting the chronic effects of alcoholism in the absence of Wernicke-Korsakoff syndrome. Ryback (1971) proposed the continuity hypothesis, which posits that Korsakoff's syndrome is the end product of a gradual decline associated with chronic alcoholism (Hartman, 1995). In addition, chronic alcoholics without Korsakoff's syndrome have often been used as control subjects in studies on Korsakoff patients without a full understanding of the nature of their specific cognitive deficits.

About 45 to 70 percent of alcoholics have deficits in problem solving, abstract thinking, psychomotor performance, and memory tasks during treatment (Eckardt and Martin, 1986). By some estimates, about 25 percent of alcoholics do not exhibit neuropsychological deficits (Tarter and Edwards, 1986) suggesting that despite a myriad of neurological and neuropathological deficits produced by excessive alcohol abuse, not all alcoholics develop these pathologies (Tarter and Edwards, 1986).

Studies that have looked directly at the question of similarities or differences in cognitive functioning between Korsakoff amnesics and nonamnesic chronic alcoholics do not, in general, support the continuity hypothesis. In one study, Wilkinson and Carlen (1980) compared Korsakoff patients with non-Korsakoff alcoholics and found significant differences between the two groups on most subtests of the Wechsler Memory Scale, the digit symbol subtest of the Wechsler Adult Intelligence Scale (WAIS), and the memory score of the Halstead-Reitan Tactual Performance Test. Krabbendam et al. (2000) looked at neuropsychological data and magnetic resonance imaging (MRI) brain structure volumes in a group of Korsakoff patients and compared their findings with a group of chronic alcoholics and a normal control group. Significant differences in performance were found between the Korsakoff patients and the other two groups on tests of memory, visuoperceptual and executive functions, as well as in brain structure volumes, leading the investigators to conclude that the cognitive deficits seen in Korsakoff patients were unlikely to be accounted for by the mere chronic consumption of alcohol. In keeping with these findings, Hartman (1995) points out that cognitive deficits in Korsakoff patients favor an additive model of acute traumatic effects arising out of avitaminosis superimposed on more chronic traumatic effects associated with long-term alcoholism. In a recent review of studies that have found positive neuropsychological test results associated with chronic alcoholism, Hartman (1995) identified a number of important areas of demonstrable cognitive impairment. These areas include abstract thinking or flexible problem solving, visuospatial processing, and memory. A number of studies have found deficits on tests that assess conceptual problem solving and mental flexibility (e.g., Halstead-Reitan Category Test, Raven's Progressive Matrices Test, and Wisconsin Card Sorting Test) (Hartman, 1995). Impairments in visuospatial abilities have been repeatedly found throughout the literature. In addition, memory deficits in chronic alcoholics without Korsakoff's syndrome have been demonstrated through neuropsychological testing (Hartman, 1995).

Factors that appear to influence neuropsychological test performance include age at onset of drinking, pattern of drinking (i.e., frequency and amount consumed), handedness, predisposing risk factors such as family history, genetic vulnerability, and history of head injury (Hartman, 1995). In one study, DeBellis et al. (2000) used MRI to ascertain hippocampal volume in a group of 12 adolescents with adolescent-onset alcohol abuse. A matched control group was also studied. DeBellis et al. found that both left-hemispheric and right-hemispheric hippocampal volumes were significantly smaller in adolescents who abused alcohol than in the control group. Other volume indices measured by MRI in this study, including intracranial, cerebral, cortical gray and white matter, as well as measures of the midsagittal area of the corpus callosum, were *not* significantly different between the two groups. Total hippocampal volume correlated positively with age at onset (i.e., younger age of onset of drinking was associated with smaller total hippocampal volumes), and correlated negatively with the duration of the alcohol-use disorder (i.e., shorter duration of alcohol-use disorder was associated with larger total hippocampal volumes). These results suggest that during adolescence, the hippocampus, an important site for memory functions, may be particularly vulnerable to the adverse effects of alcohol. Other studies suggest that older alcoholics may be more vulnerable to the negative impact of alcohol on brain-behavior functions than younger adult alcoholics. Pfefferbaum et al. (1997), for example, found that a younger group of alcoholic men (ages 26 to 44) had significant cortical gray matter volume deficits and sulcal and ventricular enlargement on MRI when compared with a group of age-matched controls. However, a group of older alcoholic men (ages 45 to 63) showed volume deficits in both cortical gray and white matter in addition to sulcal and ventricular enlargement. When Pfefferbaum et al. looked closer at six cortical areas for MRI volume deficits, they found that the older alcoholic group had selectively more severe deficits in prefrontal gray matter compared with the younger alcoholic group. The two groups *differed* in age, but not in disease duration or estimated lifetime alcohol consumption.

Ambrose, Bowden, and Whelan (2001) examined working memory (temporary storage where information can be accessed and manipulated or processed) using a delayed reaction task in alcoholics. The delayed alternation tasks in this study required subjects to figure out the correct alternating sequence of targets on a computer monitor, one of which would lead to a reward. More complicated alternations increased the working memory demand. Alcohol dependent subjects required more trials to learn the delayed alternation sequences. Performance declined in all subjects as task complexity increased but the deficits in alcohol dependent subjects were greater with moderate as compared with extremely complex memory demands. These investigators noted that they tested subjects after a relatively brief period of abstinence. Previous reviews of cognitive impairment in detoxified alcoholics suggest that many of the impairments noted in the present study and by others (e.g., Parsons, 1994) are relatively stable during the first few weeks of abstinence and that recovery of cognitive deficits may take months or years. However, other investigators have reported significant cognitive improvement shortly after acute withdrawal with improved neuropsychological functioning within weeks of entry into treatment (Goldman, 1995; Goldman et al., 1983).

Regarding pattern of drinking, at least one study found that a pattern of daily drinking, compared with "bout" drinking, was associated with lower scores on age-corrected Wechsler Adult Intelligence Scale Performance IQ measures, as well as on the Mental Control and Digit Span subtests of the Wechsler Memory Scale. "Bout" drinking refers to a pattern of periods of abstinence in between episodes of drinking for days, weeks, or months, compared with a pattern of drinking five or more days a week (Tarbox, Connors, and McLauglin, 1986).

Some studies have suggested that left-handedness may be more highly represented among alcohol abusers than is seen in the general population. The exact significance of this finding, however, is uncertain in the absence of more carefully controlled, replicative studies (Hartman, 1995). Handedness has important implications for the interpretation of certain neuropsychological test findings and may represent a sign, in some cases, of coexisting vulnerability to other disorders that may contribute to or may be part of a predisposing risk factor.

Given the high correlation between alcohol abuse and a family history of alcoholism, a number of studies have looked at children in an effort to identify possible patterns of preexisting neuropsychological vulnerabilities in family members of alcoholics (Hartman, 1995). These studies have been able to *differentiate* the sons of alcoholics from control subjects on the basis of poorer performance on selected neuropsychological tests such as the Rey-

Osterreith Complex Figure Test, the hard (unfamiliar) paired associates from the Wechsler Memory Scale, and the information subtest of the WAIS-R (Peterson, Finn, and Pihl, 1992), as well as on tasks of verbal and nonverbal abstraction and perceptual-motor skill (Schaeffer, Parsons, and Yohman, 1984). Insufficient research exists to form a clear consensus about the interpretation or significance of these findings; however, the strong possibility of preexisting cognitive vulnerabilities in certain individuals who may be at risk for developing an alcohol-use disorder represents an important direction for future research.

Demographic data point to a high association between alcohol abuse and head injury (see Chapter 2 for a review). Dikmen et al. (1993) note:

> Alcohol use shortly before injury is the most commonly cited and best established predisposing factor in head trauma, having a high level of direct and indirect involvement in motor vehicle accidents, falls, and assaults, which represent the most common causes of such injuries. (p. 296)

According to a variety of sources cited by Dikmen et al. (1993), "Up to two thirds of head trauma victims have a detectable alcohol level . . . and from a third to a half are intoxicated when they arrive at the emergency room; . . . a third of head trauma victims [are] diagnosed as alcohol dependent" (p. 296). (For more information on alcohol-related head injuries, see Chapter 2.) The latter data indicate a much higher percentage of chronic alcohol abuse in the premorbid history of head trauma victims than in the general population. Thus, chronic alcohol abuse represents a serious complicating factor in the neuropsychological profile of head trauma patients, and vice versa. Dikmen et al. (1993) studied the question of whether a premorbid history of alcohol abuse leads to an increase in neuropsychological deficits associated with head injuries in a group of diverse head-injured patients compared with a group of demographically matched and preexisting-condition-matched body trauma controls. They found that severity of head injury and degree of alcohol problems were both related to neuropsychological test performance; however, an interaction between head injury and alcohol problems was could not be demonstrated. In other words, a head injury sustained by an individual who had a history of heavy drinking was not more detrimental on neuropsychological test performance than a head injury sustained in the absence of a history of heavy drinking (Dikmen et al., 1993). A subgroup of head-injured patients seen in this study was characterized by lower levels of education, poor neuropsychological test performance (including lower verbal/intellectual skills), and a lifestyle pattern of heavy drinking. Dikmen et al. raised the possibility that this subgroup may be similar to another subgroup that has been identified in the literature as meeting diagnostic criteria for antisocial personality disorder with a high incidence of alcohol abuse, a history of poorer verbal cognitive abilities possibly associated with premorbid attention deficit disorder or minimal brain dysfunction, and an increased risk for head injuries (Malloy et al., 1990; Tarter, 1988; Tarter and Edwards, 1988).

According to Hartman (1995), three neuropathological possibilities have been proposed in the literature to account for neurological and cognitive findings associated with nonamnesic chronic alcoholism. The first neuropathological explanation is that chronic alcoholism gives rise to *diffuse* brain injury. Neuroradiological studies, for example, have found bilateral enlargement of the lateral ventricles, the third ventricle, and cerebral sulci (Hartman, 1995), suggesting the presence of widespread cerebral atrophy. The second neuropathological explanation is that chronic alcoholism gives rise to lateralized damage involving the right hemisphere. This is based on observations of visuospatial and constructional deficits in the test performances of chronic alcoholics. However, the localizing value of these findings and the lack of consistent clinical research support for this neuropathological conclusion have called this explanation into question (Hartman, 1995). The third neuropathological explanation is that chronic alcoholism gives rise to brain damage or neural compromise in frontal-limbic-diencephalic brain regions. In a recent study, Dao-Castellana et al. (1998) used MRI and positron emission tomography (PET) scans to examine a group of chronic alcoholics with no known neurological or psychiatric complications. They found metabolic abnormalities in the mediofrontal and left dorsolateral prefrontal cortex, which correlated with impairment on neuropsychological tests assessing verbal fluency and mental flexibility (Stroop test: Interference condition). In another study, Ratti et al. (1999) looked at standard computerized axial tomography (CAT) scan data in a group of male alcoholic inpatients and a matched control group. Atrophy of the frontal region was found significantly more frequently among the alcoholic inpatient group than among the controls. Davila et al. (1994) looked at MRI images of the mammillary bodies, cerebellar hemispheres, and cerebellar vermis in a group of middle-aged and older chronic alcoholics (ages 40 to 65 years), who had no history of Korsakoff's amnesia, alcoholic dementia, or diagnosed cerebellar degeneration. Tissue volume ratings were evaluated along with performance on neuropsychological tests of long-term declarative memory and measures of balance. They found that the alcoholics were more impaired on measures of balance than they were on measures of declarative memory, and that the difficulty with balance (in particular, ataxia while eyes are closed) showed a modest relationship with volume reduction in cerebellar vermis tissue. A high percentage of the alcoholic group also showed clinically abnormal mammillary body tissue ratings despite a relative absence of significant deficits on measures of declarative memory, consistent with expectations for nonamnesic chronic alcoholics. Evidence of compromise to the mammillary bodies is in keeping with the hypothesis of frontal-limbic-diencephalic brain involvement in chronic alcohol abuse. Davila et al. noted that brain tissue volume reductions might not represent atrophy (i.e., cell loss), but rather tissue shrinkage due to possible intracellular fluid shifts or other factors that may be partly or totally reversible (Davila et al., 1994).

In summary, individuals who present with nonamnesic chronic alcohol abuse have been found to exhibit a significant picture of neuropsychological deficit affecting abstract thinking, perceptual processing, memory and learning, attention and concentration, and psychomotor skills. Neuropsychological deficits are well documented but the relationship between these deficits with the amount of alcohol consumed over time is complex.

Bates et al. observed a variety of risk factors which correlated with neuropsychological impairment in executive function, memory, verbal ability, and verbal processing (Bates, Labouvie, and Voelbel, 2002) in subjects with alcohol or drug use disorders. Bates points out that variability in the relationship between abstinence and cognitive recovery is complicated when testing occurs, by definitions of abstinence, family history, and the wide range of neuropsychological tests as well as the statistical analysis used. In a recent study, Bates et al., administered neuropsychological tests to subjects six weeks after they entered treatment and found that cognitive recovery of memory improved. However, while executive function, verbal ability, and information processing speed improved, the change was of limited clinical significance. Cognitive recovery of memory deficits does occur in the first six weeks of treatment but other changes are relatively minor (Bates et al., 2005).

Di Sclafani et al. (1995) examined brain atrophy and cognitive function in older abstinent alcoholic men and found that in comparison to controls, abstinent alcoholics exhibited cognitive impairments in memory and visual-spatial-motor skills. However, global cerebral atrophy was not significant between groups, even though recovering alcoholics were significantly more impaired in delayed memory tests and visual-spatial-motor skills tests.

Mechanisms of Indirect and Direct Toxic Effects from Alcohol Abuse

Several studies have noted the indirect toxic effects of alcohol on brain memory systems due to severe nutritional depletion. Marchiafava-Bignami syndrome, a rare condition associated with severe malnourishment in chronic alcoholism involves demyelination or necrosis of the corpus callosum with accompanying damage to pericallosal white matter. Symptoms include dementia, dysarthria, spasticity, and inability to ambulate (Hartman, 1995). One of the many consequences of chronic alcohol abuse is cirrhosis (see Chapter 2). Liver disease represents an additional indirect toxic effect of alcohol that can give rise to hepatic encephalopathy and can account for a significant portion of neuropsychological performance deficits (Hartman, 1995). Hepatic encephalopathy is associated with brain damage in widespread areas including the basal ganglia, thalamus, red nucleus, pons, and cerebellum (Charness, 1994; cited in Hartman, 1995; also see Chapter 4 for additional review). Hepatic encephalopathy can produce impairment in multiple domains of behavior. Symptoms of hepatic encephalopathy include but are not limited to: forgetfulness, confusion, disorientation, delirium, loss of memory, intellectual changes, reasoning changes, and mood changes.

Since neuropsychological impairment is relatively common among some alcoholics and some percentage of alcoholics have liver damage, interest in the role of hepatic encephalopathy in alcoholics as a cause of neuropsychological impairment has been a logical extension. To examine this relationship further, Tarter et al. (1988) compared alcoholics and nonalcoholics in whom cirrhosis was confirmed by biopsy to determine the extent to which alcoholism with liver disease impacts on neuropsychological test performance. The results were quite interesting. Advanced liver disease is a more significant factor than alcoholism as a determinant of neuropsychological deficits. Nonalcoholics with cirrhosis and alcoholics with cirrhosis performed similarly, in comparison with normal controls on trail-making, symbol digit, digit span forward, visual retention, memory, Stroop test, and a grooved pegboard test. This finding led to the conclusion that neuropsychological performance of alcoholics with cirrhosis is no different from nonalcoholics with cirrhosis. In other words, medically healthy alcoholics (no liver disease) were not impaired on neuropsychological tests suggesting that impaired neuropsychological performance strongly correlated with liver disease, not alcoholism, per se. Tarter et al. (Tarter et al., 1990) have found that alcoholics who also suffer liver damage are more compromised than alcoholics without demonstrated liver damage on tasks involving short-term memory, visual tracking, and eye-finger coordination (cited in Hartman, 1995). Clearly, although, it is likely that other factors contribute to neuropsychological impairment, such results have important implications in treatment and in understanding treatment outcome. It is interesting to note that although hepatic encephalopathy is a well known and recognized phenomena, it has received relatively little attention in the more recent studies within alcohol literature.

In addition to indirect toxic effects, growing evidence suggests that alcohol is also a direct neurotoxin in the central nervous system. Various studies have documented important neurochemical changes affecting the functioning of cell membranes, neurotransmission, and the availability of certain neurotransmitter substances necessary for the integrity of important brain circuits (Hartman, 1995). Numerous studies have documented cerebral atrophy, including loss of both cortical gray matter and subcortical white matter (Jernigan et al., 1991; Pfefferbaum et al., 1992). Korbo (1999) studied the total number of neuron and glial cells in the hippocampus in a small group of severely affected alcoholics and a group of controls. A statistically significant loss of glial cells, but not neurons, *differentiated* the severe alcoholics from the controls. Glial cells provide important support functions to help maintain the health of neurons. These functions include taking up excess chemical transmitters, cleaning away cellular debris after neuronal damage or death, myelinating axons for effective neurotransmission along the axon, and establishing the blood-brain barrier. In addition, recent discoveries indicate that some glial cells can transmit information between themselves within the immediate environment and may play a role in certain memory processes (Thompson, 2000). Thus, the finding that hippocampal glial cell loss is associated with severe alcoholism may have important implications for the cognitive finding of memory loss in afflicted individuals.

Risk Factors for Alcohol Abuse and Neuropsychological Dysfunction

The issue of predicting risk among adolescent boys for future drug involvement was raised by Aytaclar et al. (1999) who looked at the predictive value of executive cognitive functioning deficiency, measured by neuropsychological tests, and high levels of behavioral activity in a group of high risk preadolescent boys whose fathers had a history of lifetime psychoactive substance-abuse disorder. The boys were compared with a low-to-average risk control group of boys whose fathers had neither psychoactive substance-abuse disorder nor a history of any other psychiatric diagnosis. Total number of drugs ever tried, severity of drug involvement, and presence of tobacco and cannabis use two years later were predicted by the presence of measurable executive cognitive dysfunction but not by behavioral activity levels. Another study, conducted by Hammoumi et al. (1999), looked at the relationship of alcohol dependence and dysfunction of the serotonin 5-hydroxytryptamine (5-HT) system based on recent research that suggests that the serotonin system's transporter chemical and receptor may be important in the etiology of alcohol dependence (Lovinger, 1997). Hammoumi et al.

(1999) found a significant difference between alcohol-dependent patients and control subjects in the frequency of a genetic variant of serotonin transmission that might be predictive of a genetic vulnerability for alcohol dependence.

Recovery of Function After Chronic Alcohol Abuse

The importance of abstinence for the recovery of functions in chronic alcohol abusers cannot be more strongly emphasized, given the severity of the risk for permanent brain damage associated with long-term, protracted abuse and given recent studies that show some recovery of neuropsychological functioning is possible in abstinent chronic alcohol abusers who have not suffered Korsakoff's syndrome, cerebellar degeneration, or irreversibly damaging encephalopathic conditions. Rourke and Grant (1999) found that chronic male alcoholics who maintained interim abstinence for a period of two years following initial detoxification showed improvement on neuropsychological tests of abstracting ability compared with a group of chronic male alcoholics who resumed drinking during the two-year postdetoxification period, and compared with a control group of long-term abstinent alcoholics and a control group of nonalcoholics. The latter two groups were comparable in their neuropsychological performances on measures of abstracting ability, complex perceptual-motor integration, and simple motor skills. The group of relapsed chronic male alcoholics showed deterioration in their performance on the motor tests.

In another study that looked at perfusion images in frontal brain systems of abstinent long-term alcoholics using single photon emission computerized tomography (SPECT), Gansler et al. (2000) found an increased level of perfusion in the left inferior frontal brain region associated with greater years of sobriety in recovering alcoholics. Alcoholics with less than four years of sobriety showed a significantly reduced left inferior-frontal perfusion when compared with a group of nonalcoholic controls and a group of recovering alcoholics who had been abstinent for a longer period of time. These findings not only support the hypothesis of the negative impact of chronic alcohol intake on frontal-limbic-diencephalic brain systems, but also the possibility for some recovery of function in these brain systems with prolonged abstinence. More recent neuropsychological studies have noted improvement in memory, visual, spatial, and motor functioning during abstinence, although there is variability in the speed of recovery in different domains of functioning (Rosenbloom, Pfefferbaum, and Sullivan, 2004; Sullivan et al., 2000).

Studies which have looked at the recovery of cognitive functions have found that maintaining prolonged abstinence is a crucial requirement for any recovery of cognitive functions. However, even with abstinence, not all cognitive functions show recovery or recover to levels equal to those of the control subjects. Age at onset of drinking, premorbid intellectual status, history of head injury, and age at which abstinence begins appear to be important modifying factors in determining cognitive function recovery (Hartman, 1995).

Despite evidence that chronic alcohol abuse, even in the absence of an amnesic syndrome, is associated with neuropsychological deficits that are indicative of moderate to severe cerebral dysfunction (Morris and Lawson, 1998), few treatment programs for recovering alcoholics routinely include neuropsychological evaluation and consultation as a standard treatment modality or offer rehabilitation for cognitive deficits as an integral part of their treatment program. Such deficits can present a significant obstacle to an individual's ability to fully participate and benefit from various aspects of the prescribed treatment program. The need for further research into the efficacy of such an integrated treatment program for recovering alcoholics has been recently called for (Allen, Goldstein, and Seaton, 1997).

BRAIN IMPAIRMENT AND ILLICIT DRUG ABUSE

Studies of General and Polydrug Abuse

Our more recent understanding of how drug addiction occurs involves the interference of brain reward circuits, resulting in an increase in the desire to use. In particular, it is posited that the amygdala and subregions of the basal forebrain are involved in a mesolimbic dopamine system that activates mesolimbic dopamine function. Repeated use alters dopamine production, resulting in a dysregulation of the brain reward circuitry. The result is a biological addiction to the drug (Leshner and Koob, 1999).

With such brain involvement and alteration of the brain circuitry, alterations in neuropsychological functioning are likely. A preliminary report of neuropsychological functioning in polydrug abusers by Grant et al. (1977) noted a study in which 15 polydrug users were administered a comprehensive neuropsychological battery including neuropsychological tests from the Halstead-Reitan Neuropsychological Test Battery, as well as the Wechsler Adult Intelligence Scale, and the Minnesota Multiphasic Personality Inventory (MMPI). The 15 polydrug users were compared with a group of 66 psychiatric inpatients. Although both groups demonstrated severe psychopathology, as measured by the MMPI, the patterns of neuropsychological impairment that were observed in both groups were diverse. The pattern of impairment suggested *differences* between the two groups in terms of sensory, motor, perceptual, and verbal abilities. Although no significant difference occurred in the *level* of neuropsychological functioning, there were significant *differences* in the *pattern* of functioning in those ability areas. The polydrug group appeared to rely upon spatial/perceptual/motor abilities in problem solving and exhibited weakness in verbal abilities. The converse was true for the psychiatric patients whose *pattern* of neuropsychological functioning, although impaired, resembled that of normal adults. Further results from this research suggested that greater neuropsychological impairment was related to the use of opiates and depressants rather than to alcohol, stimulants, or marijuana.

In a later study of polydrug users, Carlin et al. (1980) sought to discern whether any differences occurred in neuropsychological functioning between two groups of polydrug users: "streetwise" users "whose lifestyle and value orientation reflect the drug culture underworld" (p. 229) and "straight" users whose lifestyle was more associated with traditional values. Seventy-nine polydrug users were studied and grouped into one of the two categories. The Halstead-Reitan Neuropsychological Test Battery was administered and neuropsychological impairment was statistically related to heavy alcohol and opiate abuse in the streetwise abusers. In contrast, straight abusers who were identified with neuropsychological dysfunction tended to use fewer drugs in general with the exception of depressants. These straight abusers were also found to have more medical problems that were associated with greater events of drug toxicity. It was suggested that neuropsychological impairment in the straight abusers could be associated with medical risk that is secondary to developmental history or greater vulnerability to drug toxicity, and that for the streetwise users, impairment could be associated with heavy drug intake resulting in toxicity. The meaning of these results is not very clear although the authors also posited that alcohol, opiates, and "perhaps the depressants" were most related to brain impairment.

Cognitive or neuropsychological impairment clearly affects behavioral functioning in polysubstance abusers. Schafer, Birchler, and Fals-Stewart (1994) observed that the emotional and marital functioning of male polysubstance abusers was directly related to their level of neuropsychological impairment. In a study of 31 married couples, the cognitive functioning of the husband was related to a pattern of negative communication behaviors, fewer positive behaviors, and increased events of violence.

Traditional testing of neuropsychological or cognitive performance has been called into question in a recent study by Beatty and Borrell (2000). It was suggested that some of the deficits identified by testing drug abusers could be accounted for by the knowledge these abusers acquire due to their lifestyle, and that this knowledge may be *different* from the knowledge acquired by nondrug abusers. Beatty and Borrell compared the test results of 63 methadone clinic clients with 24 nonabusing participants. They devised a task that included identifying the title, artist, year, and meaning of a song. There were no significant differences in task performance between the abusers and nonabusers except that the abusers tended to relate the song to drug addiction. Beatty and Borrell (2000) offered an interesting hypothesis, although the extent of cognitive assessment in their study was both narrow and limited.

Not surprisingly, drug abusers have been shown to demonstrate impaired decision-making skills. An interesting study employed a gambling task to assess decision-making skills, choice, and planning (Grant, Contoreggi, and London, 2000). Thirty polysubstance abusers and 24 nonabusers were compared using the Wisconsin Card Sorting Task, a measure of executive functioning and planning, as well as on the gambling task, which assesses judgment regarding short-term and long-term losses. There was no significant difference between the two groups on the Wisconsin Card Sorting Test. However, the groups demonstrated *differences* on the gambling task, suggesting that the drug abusers were more likely to use poor decision-making skills.

The questions of whether drug abuse results in deficits in executive functioning and whether individuals with such deficits are predisposed to substance abuse was investigated by Giancola and Tarter (1999). Giancola and Tarter (1999) identified children who were at high risk for drug abuse by selecting those children whose parents exhibited a substance-use disorder. High-risk children tended to exhibit greater dysfunction of the prefrontal cortex as identified through electrophysiological studies that documented attenuated amplitudes of the P300 event-related potential. Since the attenuated amplitude measure has been associated with the prefrontal cortex, which is believed to be involved in executive cognitive functioning, the authors hypothesized that individuals with dysfunction in the prefrontal cortex tend to experience deficits in executive cognitive functioning that would then leave them more vulnerable to substance-use disorders. This finding is important to consider when attempting to infer causality from correlational data regarding drug abusers' cognitive functioning.

The comorbidity of substance abuse, neuropsychological dysfunction, and violent behavior have been identified as mediated by executive functioning and the prefrontal cortex (Fishbein, 2000). Bauer and Hesselbrock (1999) related the decrease in P300 amplitude in teenagers to a coincidence of family alcohol/drug dependence and the prevalence of conduct disorder problems. In this study, 57 participants (15 to 20 years old) were evaluated.

Smaller P300 amplitudes in the posterior region were associated with increased conduct problems in the teenagers who were younger than 16.5 years. For older teenagers, the effect was seen in the frontal region.

The more recent use of imaging of the brain has been helpful in relating neuropsychological findings to structural and anatomic functioning in the substance-abuse population. Gatley and Volkow (1998) noted the value of PET and SPECT in research designs that employ neuropsychological measures. Indeed, functional-imaging and brain-imaging studies have contributed to the understanding of maladaptive behavior as it is associated with orbitofrontal cortex connections (London et al., 2000). Studies such as Liu et al.'s (1998) have documented the reduced volume of prefrontal lobe area in polysubstance abusers through the use of magnetic resonance imaging.

Cognitive functioning is especially important in the patient's ability to benefit from rehabilitation. In a study by Blume, Davis, and Schmaling (1999), 22 dually diagnosed inpatients were administered intellectual-executive, and memory-functioning tests, as well as an assessment of their readiness to change. The authors reported that, especially for those who are dually diagnosed with both a substance-abuse and psychiatric disorder, cognitive impairment was related to a lowered likelihood of motivation to change their substance abuse behaviors.

Drug abuse may leave its mark on brain functioning. However, the synergistic effect of drug abuse on an individual who already suffers from a history of traumatic brain injury can be devastating. The interaction of traumatic brain injury and substance abuse has been documented. In a study of 119 participants with severe closed-head traumatic brain injuries (Kelly et al., 1997), those who tested positively for drug use at the time of head injury performed significantly lower on testing than those patients with a normal drug screening at the time of trauma. It is suggested that there is an additive effect of substance abuse on the neuropsychological outcome of those with traumatic brain injuries (Kelly et al., 1997).

Cocaine

Cocaine, a derivative of the coca plant, was first noted for its use among South American Indians sometime between 3000 and 1500 BC. (Bolla, Cadet, and London, 1998; Hartman, 1995). Cocaine became popular for pharmacological use in medicine in the late 1800s as it offered both anesthetic and mood-altering properties. In the 1980s, the estimated use of cocaine on at least one occasion affected more than 22 million Americans (Washton and Gold, 1984). With the introduction of "crack" in 1985, a resurgence of cocaine use was observed. By the mid-1990s, it was estimated that 1.5 million Americans used cocaine (Bolla, Cadet, and London, 1998).

The effects of chronic cocaine use include irritability, fatigue, depression, impotence, and loss of libido. Neurotoxic reactions resulting in cardiac arrhythmia, convulsions, and respiratory failure have also been noted. Cocaine has been documented for its powerful psychologically addictive qualities with a question as to the extent to which there is an actual physical addiction or associated withdrawal syndrome (Brick and Erickson, 1999; Washton and Gold, 1984). The neuropsychological studies that have focused on cocaine use have not been as forthcoming as the studies that have focused on neuroimaging (Hartman, 1995). Although neuropsychological impairment has been documented in cocaine abusers, studies have not been able to support differential diagnoses of specific structural abnormalities (Hartman, 1995). Thus, the mechanism for the impairment, whether vascular, metabolic, and so on, is not clear. In adults under the age of 45, cocaine abuse has been reported as a significant risk factor for stroke (Lacayo, 1995). Many of these medical consequences of cocaine are reviewed in Chapter 10, so we will focus on more specific neuropsycholgical consequences of cocaine abuse. Particular subgroups of cocaine abusers may reveal abnormalities in brain perfusion that are related to cognitive deficits (Strickland and Stein, 1995).

In a review by Strickland et al. (1998), the authors noted how cerebral metabolic and hypoperfusion irregularities are seen in the neuroimaging of the cocaine abuser. In particular, techniques such as CAT and MRI may show significant cerebral events, although newer techniques such as PET, SPECT, and quantitative electroencephalography (QEEG) are able to reveal a greater frequency of changes in brain functioning that may have initially gone unnoticed.

Findings of these neuroimaging studies have been validated by neuropsychological evaluations. For example, in a study of eight long-term cocaine abusers who were abstinent for six months, the use of SPECT revealed significant differences between abusers and normal subjects. Neuropsychological impairment was documented in users, particularly in the areas of learning, memory, and executive functioning. Interestingly, the use of MRI was unremarkable for seven out of the eight patients. The pattern of multifocal hypoperfusion seen on SPECT exam was associated with deficits in neuropsychological test performance (Strickland et al., 1993).

In another study pairing diagnostic imaging with neuropsychological testing, Bolla, Cadet, and London (1998) revealed that use of PET and MRI with neuropsychological evaluation revealed that those who abuse cocaine, experience specific difficulties in executive functioning, judgment, and decision making. It is suggested that structures of the prefrontal, orbitofrontal, and anterior cingulate gyrus are affected in cocaine abusers (Bolla, Cadet, and London, 1998).

The use of MRI to determine premorbid brain size or intracranial volume in abstinent crack/cocaine and crack/cocaine and alcohol-dependent individuals has been studied (Di Sclafani et al., 1998). Findings concluded that crack- and crack-and-alcohol-dependent individuals appeared similar both in neuropsychological performance and in brain size. However, intracranial volume appeared to account for the variability in neuropsychological test performance. It was suggested that individuals with larger brains are better able to maintain cognitive functioning in spite of substance abuse or other cerebral insult. Thus, it appears that the more brain reserves one has, the more one can afford to lose.

Although cocaine use has been related to numerous structural brain complications including seizure, stroke, hemorrhage, transient ischemic attacks, and cerebral vasculitis/spasms, as well as changes in cerebral blood flow and metabolism, we are still beginning to explore the specific ways in which cocaine abuse affects neuropsychological or cognitive functioning (Horner, 1999). In a study of 37 crack abusers, Ardila, Rosselli, and Strumwasser (1991) observed overall lower neuropsychological test performance in abusers with regard to short-term verbal memory and attention abilities. In particular, the "lifetime amount" of cocaine use was related to neuropsychological test performance, implicating a direct relationship between cognitive impairment and long-term use of cocaine.

A subsequent study by Mittenberg and Motta (1993) also examined attention and learning. Sixteen chronic abstinent cocaine abusers were tested on tasks of verbal learning, word knowledge, and nonverbal visual-motor perceptual reasoning. When compared with controls, the cocaine abusers demonstrated significantly greater problems with learning and recall of words. However, there was no significant difference regarding intellectual ability. The authors concluded from their findings that cognitive impairment related to chronic cocaine use may be associated more with memory storage difficulties than with problems of attention or general intellectual functioning.

A study by Horner (1997) further explored memory abilities. An examination of the neuropsychological functioning of 32 cocaine-dependent alcoholic patients versus 52 alcoholic patients who did not engage in cocaine abuse supported poor performance on tests of immediate and delayed verbal memory for the cocaine-dependent individuals. Although all the patients in the study abused alcohol, those who also abused cocaine demonstrated specific deficits in the area of verbal memory. An assessment of attention, visual-spatial abilities, and reasoning and judgment skills revealed no significant differences between the groups. This study supports the review by Horner

(1999) in which he reported that in seventeen research studies examining attention skills in cocaine abusers, he observed inconsistent findings and insufficient evidence regarding the implication of impaired attention in cocaine abusers. This study also appears to support the previously discussed findings of Mittenberg and Motta (1993) with regard to inconsiderable impairment of attention.

Instead of examining alcohol abusers with and without cocaine abuse, Robinson, Heaton, and O'Malley (1999) studied cocaine abusers with and without alcohol dependence. Overall, subjects who abused both cocaine and alcohol demonstrated few differences on neuropsychological testing measures when compared with nonabusers. However, mild cognitive dysfunction was noted in those individuals who abused cocaine. Importantly, those young abusers of both alcohol and cocaine appeared to be less neuropsychologically impaired than those who abused cocaine only. These findings may well be a function of the mediating factor of age.

Few studies have been able to follow substance abusers on a long-term basis. However, the chronicity of abnormal QEEG profiles in crack cocaine users has been noted even after six months of abstinence (Alper et al., 1998). Five to ten days, one month, and six months after last cocaine use, QEEG measures of seventeen subjects revealed no significant changes over time. The implications of these findings are not clear. Relating such electrophysiological studies to neuropsychological test data may provide greater insight into the functional long-term effects of cocaine abuse.

Marijuana

Although the use of marijuana became especially popular during the 1960s, its use since then has appeared to decline significantly (Hartman, 1995). Tetrahydrocannabinol (THC) is the psychoactive ingredient in marijuana that is now used for experimental medical use and for its antiemetic and appetite-enhancing effects in cancer patients. As with cocaine, neuropsychological research has been mixed regarding the effects of marijuana use on long-term cognitive functioning. An early study of long-term effects (Carlin and Tupin, 1977) examined a group of ten individuals who smoked marijuana daily for an average of five years. The authors concluded that when compared with nonusers, minimal differences in cognitive functioning were observed with no support for any differences between groups on complex cognitive tasks.

As with most substance-abuse research, the short-term effects of marijuana have received greater attention in the research literature. The allegation that marijuana in some way enhances creative or associational thinking was tested by Tinklenberg et al. (1978). In this study, 16 male subjects were tested while under the influence of marijuana. Contrary to myth and popular belief, the authors concluded that marijuana did not increase fluency, flexibility, elaboration, or uniqueness in responses to a creative thinking task.

Other popular beliefs of enhanced attention and greater access to long-term memory have also been explored and challenged. Some studies support that speed in visual scanning is negatively affected in those who begin use of cannabis at an early age (Ehrenreich et al., 1999). Casswell and Marks (1973) documented problems with attention on a visual task testing both experienced and nonexperienced users who were under the influence of cannabis. The authors reported that the results of this study were similar to those that would be found in one of alcohol intoxication, and that there was no evidence to support the idea that experienced cannabis users are better able to negotiate visual stimuli (such as during driving) than nonusers.

Similarly, the idea that marijuana may enhance access to information in long-term memory has not received much scientific support. To the contrary, impairment of memory has been noted as the "single most consistently reported psychological deficit produced by cannabinoids" (Miller and Branconnier, 1983, p. 453).

The phenomenon of thought disorder and memory intrusions during marijuana intoxication was tested during a word list learning task (Pfefferbaum et al., 1997). Sixteen males were each evaluated under intoxicated and nonintoxicated conditions. Results suggested that while under the influence of marijuana, one may be subjected to memory intrusions. Marijuana use was associated with poor correctly called list items and increased intrusions, or incorrect word recall. These findings suggested the possibility that marijuana results in disinhibition or intrusive thoughts.

Melges et al. (1970) discussed a similar phenomenon called "temporal incoordination," suggesting that marijuana use disorganizes sequential thought and cognitive processes. Eight male graduate students were tested on four different days while under the influence of marijuana extract or a placebo. Performance on serial subtraction of sevens did not appear to be impaired by THC consumption. However, performance on forward and backward digit span revealed *differences* in short-term memory related to THC. A more complicated goal-directed serial alternation task, which required more complex serial addition and subtraction, was administered to assess for temporal disintegration. Significant *differences* in performance, with greater disorganization and disintegration while under the influence of THC, were observed. This increased disorganization is reminiscent of the problems with complex attention and concentration described earlier.

Indeed, discontinuity of thought and disorganization were related to marijuana in a study where the thought processes of 72 male volunteers were analyzed based on their responses to the Thematic Apperception Test (TAT) (Roth et al., 1975). The TAT is a projective test in which pictures of scenes are presented to the subject and the subject provides a response in the form of a story. Subjects' written stories were evaluated with regard to three components: (1) events preceding the scene in the picture, (2) a description of what was happening in the picture, and what each of the characters was thinking and feeling, and (3) the resolution or outcome of the story. The researchers concluded that while subjects were under the influence of marijuana, greater discontinuity of thought and contradictory ideas were observed, as well as a tendency toward unusual ideas.

Neuroimaging has also begun to help researchers understand the effects of marijuana use. In a recent study, 18 young adult (mean age of 22 years) frequent marijuana users were compared with nonusers with regard to evidence of tissue volume on MRI (Block et al., 2000). No significant differences or abnormalities in MRIs were noted between the two groups. Interestingly, ventricular cerebrospinal fluid volumes were lower in marijuana users despite there being no differences in tissue volume and composition.

The neuroimaging procedure, SPECT, has also been used to study marijuana users with attention-deficit/hyperactivity disorder (ADHD) (Amen and Waugh, 1998). Thirty heavy marijuana users with ADHD were compared with ten nonusers with ADHD who served as the control group. The authors concluded that chronic marijuana use results in decreased cerebral perfusion particularly in the temporal lobe areas of the brain. The temporal lobe has been commonly associated with memory abilities.

LSD

Lysergic acid diethylamide (LSD-25) is a natural substance and hallucinogen that made its appearance in modern times during the mid-1900s. Its use peaked in the American culture in the 1950s and 1960s. LSD became most popular for its mind altering effects, which include visual distortion and hallucinations, a distorted sense of time, feelings of detachment, alterations in sensory perception, emotional liability, and mystical experiences (Strassman, 1984). There has been a question as to whether LSD use results in organic brain damage. An early study by McGlothlin et al. (1969) examined sixteen subjects who had received LSD in either an experimental or psychotherapeutic setting. These subjects and controls, who were matched for sex, age, and education, were administered a number of spatial and visual tests including the Trail Making Test, which assesses the speed and accuracy of visual scanning and cognitive flexibility. Also, a measure of general intelligence, a verbal fluency test, and tests from the Halstead-Reitan Neuropsychological Test Battery were administered. Results revealed that only the category test, which assesses nonverbal reasoning and abstract problem solving, demonstrated a significant difference in performance between the two groups. Otherwise, there was no support for generalized brain damage related to the amount of LSD ingestion. Although mean performances for the LSD group on a number of visual perception tests was lower, none of the differences reached statistical significance. The authors noted limitations to their research with concern that premorbid factors might have accounted for the *difference* in category test scores between the two groups.

A later study by Wright and Hogan (1972) concluded that there was no significant difference between a group of 20 LSD users and a control group matched for age, sex, education, and intelligence when compared on the Halstead-Reitan Neuropsychological Test Battery. A more comprehensive evaluation of LSD users was conducted by Culver and King (1974) who studied undergraduate seniors over a period of two years, comparing a control group with a marijuana-using group and an LSD-using group. Subjects were matched on intellectual and personality dimensions, as well as comparative drug use. Although LSD users performed within normal limits on the Trail Making Test, their performances were statistically significantly lower than either the marijuana users or normal controls. The authors concluded that although such differences were observed, a clear argument for organic dysfunction could not be made.

PCP

Phencyclidine was originally synthesized for use as an anesthetic agent in the late 1950s (Burns et al., 1975). However, it was taken off the market due to its side effects that include disorientation, hallucinations, and excitatory activity. Insufflation or "snorting" low doses of PCP (also called angel dust or crystal) can produce mild agitation, catatonic rigidity, and possible lack of verbal communication. Higher doses can result in coma, apnea, hypertension, and fatality.

The possibility that PCP produces organic mental impairment was studied by Carlin et al. (1979). PCP abusers who had been abstinent for an average length of 27 months were compared on a number of neuropsychological measures with polydrug users who had never used PCP and to controls who were neither alcohol nor substance abusers. Neuropsychological impairment was demonstrated for 6 of the 12 PCP users, 5 of the 12 polydrug users, and none of the controls. Neuropsychological test protocols of the Halstead-

Reitan Neuropsychological Test Battery and MMPI were rated on overall level of performance on a scale of 1 to 6. Subjects were matched for age, education, sex, and ethnicity. The authors found that 50 percent of the PCP users demonstrated neuropsychological deficits in the range of mild organic mental impairment.

A comprehensive review by Ellison (1995) documented animal studies that revealed the neurotoxic effects in, and neuronal degeneration of, limbic structures. Increased glucose metabolism in the areas of degeneration was noted. These changes in the limbic circuit with degeneration and alteration in glucose metabolism appeared to be similar to that seen in "some schizophrenics and most Alzheimer's patients" (Ellison, 1995, p. 250). Thus, increased glucose utilization and neuronal degeneration from neurotoxicity in the limbic structures is seen as the reason for memory disturbances in schizophrenics, Alzheimer's patients, and chronic PCP users. Animal studies have also suggested that PCP is involved in a number of different brain neurotransmitter systems (Sircar and Li, 1994). Compared with the illegal drug studies already discussed, the PCP research seems to demonstrate most clearly its deleterious effects.

Amphetamines and MDMA (Ecstasy)

Although amphetamine use can result in neurological findings such as hypertension, stroke, brain hemorrhage, or other neuropathy, neuropsychological findings in human subjects have not been well documented, except in the cases of infant and developmental exposure (Hartman, 1995). With the increase of methamphetamine use in the United States, patients are presenting with chronic psychotic illnesses likely to be related to vasoconstriction and neurotoxicity resulting in brain damage (Buffenstein, Heaster, and Ko, 1999).

The decision-making abilities of chronic amphetamine abusers were studied by Rogers et al. (1999). In a computerized decision-making task, chronic amphetamine abusers tended to exhibit longer response times before making their decisions when compared with opiate abusers. In general, the research data suggested that decision-making performances of chronic amphetamine abusers was similar to the performances of patients with focal damage of the prefrontal cortex. In addition, it was found that the chronic amphetamine abusers' performances were also similar to that of the performances of normal volunteers with induced decreases in plasma tryptophan. This finding suggests amphetamine abusers may experience reduced levels of serotonin (5-hydroxytryptamine, 5-HT) in the orbital regions of the brain. The authors suggested that the results supported the likelihood that amphetamines affect the orbitofrontal/prefrontal cortex.

Recently, Volkow, Chang, Wang, Fowler, Leonido-Yee, et al. (2001) and Volkow, Chang, Wang, Fowler, Franceschi, et al. (2001) examined the effects of methamphetamine on motor skills and memory in former methamphetamine abusers who were abstinent for at least two months, using PET. The PET was used to detect chemical markers that bind to dopamine transporters in the brain to measure transporter levels. Compared with subjects who never used methamphetamine, the abstinent abuser subjects had a 24 percent reduction in dopamine transporters in the striatum, a dopamine rich brain area that is responsible, in part, for the control of movement, attention, motivation, and reward. Fine (timed peg insertion task) and gross (walking a straight line) motor skills, and memory (work recall) were also different between subjects. Abstinent methamphetamine abusers had impaired memory and motor skills proportional to levels of dopamine transporters. In other words, lower dopamine transporters were associated with poor neuropsychological performance on the various tests (Volkow, Chang, Wang, Fowler, Leonido-Yee, et al., 2001; Volkow, Chang, Wang, Fowler, Franceschi, et al., 2001).

With the introduction of "designer drugs," there seems to have been a shift in the research focus with fewer investigations into the effects of classic amphetamines per se. One of these new designer drugs is Ecstasy (3,4-methylenedioxymethamphetamine or MDMA). MDMA is considered a psychedelic compound that is chemically related to methamphetamine and results in problems similar to those found in amphetamine and cocaine usage (Campagna, 1986). This synthetic amphetamine derivative has been shown to produce effects such as cerebral venous sinus thrombosis (Rothwell and Grant, 1993) and Parkinsonism (Mintzer, Hickenbottom, and Gilman, 1999). The neurotoxicity of MDMA has been well documented (McCann and Ricuarte, 1995). Despite the frightening popularity of MDMA in the U.S. college student population, insidious effects of serotonin toxicity are likely to go unnoticed until significant brain damage has occurred.

With the benefit of neuroimaging, the effects of MDMA can be more critically documented. In a study of 21 abstinent MDMA users and 21 age- and gender-matched nonusers, both SPECT and MRI studies were reviewed to detect any changes in cerebral blood flow (Chang et al., 2000). Abstinent MDMA users initially demonstrated no significant differences in cerebral blood flow when compared with nonusers. Overall results indicated that persistent changes in cerebral blood flow were not observed in low-dose users. However, higher dosages of MDMA resulted in decreased regional cerebral blood flow within three weeks post-MDMA administration, in the visual cortex, the caudate, and the superior parietal and dorsolateral frontal regions of the brain. In a study of long-term effects on the brain, PET was employed for seven Ecstasy users and seven controls (Obrocki et al., 1999). The authors concluded that users' glucose metabolic uptake was altered within the areas of the amygdala, hippocampus, and Brodmann's area II (part of the primary somatosensory cortex on the postcentral gyrus) when compared with control subjects. Thus, it is possible that cerebral glucose metabolic rate is altered by MDMA.

A computerized cognitive performance test battery was administered to 22 MDMA users and 23 control subjects to assess differences in cognitive performance (McCann et al., 1999). Although controls and MDMA users performed similarly on some neuropsychological tasks, MDMA users demonstrated weaker sustained attention, short-term memory, and verbal reasoning. Results were thought to support "subtle but significant" neuropsychological deficits.

Memory disturbances are also noted in a study by Reneman et al. (2000). To assess for memory disturbance in five abstinent MDMA users versus nine nonusers, the Rey Auditory Verbal Learning Test was administered. SPECT studies of the subjects were compared revealing preliminary results that suggested altered functioning of the occipital cortex associated with memory impairment. A previous study conducted by Bolla, McCann, and Ricuarte (1998) documented memory impairment associated with greater MDMA use. In particular, immediate verbal memory and delayed visual memory were most affected. The authors concluded that even abstinent users could show these pervasive cognitive effects and that impairment was correlated with serotonin neurotoxicity and degree of exposure to MDMA. Thus, the research confirms the clear toxicity and deleterious effects of MDMA, especially in the area of memory.

Other Illegal Drug Use

Although the research on neuropsychological (neurophysiological) consequences of polysubstance abuse, cocaine, marijuana, LSD, phencyclidine, and amphetamines is, on the whole, quite limited, research on the remaining illicit drugs is even more sparse.

Inhalants

The use of solvent inhalants, such as toluene, has been demonstrated to result in dementia and cerebral white-matter deterioration (Filley, Heaton, and Rosenberg, 1990). Idiopathic Parkinsonism in a case of solvent abuse has also been documented (Uitti et al., 1994).

Solvent abuse is one of the most rapidly rising forms of abuse in the United States, particularly among children and young adults and are associated with a variety of medical consequences (Chapter 11). In addition, solvent abuse has been reported to produce various neurological deficits including impaired cognitive functioning. There is, however, the potential for solvent exposure in industrial settings where workers are exposed to solvents every day and in whom "painter's syndrome" from chronic low-level exposure has been reported. Neurological abnormalities in this population may also include cognitive deficits. However, this is a somewhat controversial area since much of the research is based upon self-reports and is often without controls, and rarely with direct anatomical evidence of brain damage.

Rosenberg et al. (2002) examined toluene abusers with regard to neuropsychological performance and MRI data. Performance was measured through general cognitive ability (IQ test), working memory (word recall and visual nonverbal stimuli recall), short-term memory and visual recall, delayed recall, speed and capacity of information processing (Trail Making Test, Stroop Color Test, alternating alpha-numeric sequence test), speech and language (name common objects), and executive functions (planning, active problem solving, organizing work directing attention and controlling behavior). Compared with subjects with extensive histories of other drug use, solvent abusers were significantly impaired in working memory and executive functions. Overall, about 44 percent of the solvent abusers in this study had MRI abnormalities. In comparison to other drug users (e.g., alcohol, cocaine, marijuana), the most significant findings were abnormalities in the basal ganglia (22 percent of subjects), cerebellum (21 percent), and pons (40 percent). The authors (Rosenberg et al., 2002) note it was difficult to rule out premorbid cognitive deficits even though the MRI findings coupled with the neuropsychological impairment and the known neurotoxic effects of solvents might suggest a causal relationship. Of particular interest was the finding of significant neuropsychological impairment and MRI abnormalities in many of the comparison (non-solvent-abusing) subjects and the lack of dose-response relationship between solvent abuse and neuropsychological testing. The latter observation suggests that extreme caution should be used in relying solely on neuropsychological testing in assessing neurological injury from solvents (Rosenberg et al., 2002).

Amyl nitrite may have an extensive body of literature associated with documentation of physiological changes, however, neuropsychological investigation has not been very forthcoming. Amyl nitrite inhalation has been found to be related to increases in cerebral blood flood (Mathew, Wilson, and Tant, 1989). It also has been employed in medical applications as a coronary vasodilator (Hartman, 1995). Its recreational use has been documented in male homosexuals to facilitate intercourse and heighten sexual experience.

Neuropsychological deficits from chronic use of heroin and other opiates have not been consistently demonstrated (Hartman, 1995). Furthermore, it is not clear whether these substances result in any medical neurotoxicity.

SUMMARY AND CONCLUSIONS

With regard to the neuropsychological consequences of alcohol abuse, the research indicates that chronic alcohol abuse gives rise to not only severe indirect toxic effects on brain and behavior functioning, but it is also a source of direct toxic effects on brain functions. In addition to the well known and extensively studied syndrome of Korsakoff amnesia arising from severe nutritional depletion associated with chronic alcoholism, a history of nonamnesic chronic alcohol abuse is also associated with well documented evidence of neuropsychological deficits which include impairments in abstraction and mental flexibility, perceptual skills, memory and learning functions, attention and concentration, and fine motor skills. Evidence appears to favor the hypothesis of dysfunction in the frontal-limbic-diencephalic brain regions in addition to involvement of the cerebellum, even in the absence of evidence of cerebellar degeneration. With prolonged abstinence, some recovery of cognitive functioning can occur for some individuals. Because of the high prevalence of neuropsychological deficits indicative of moderate to severe cerebral dysfunction in individuals who chronically abuse alcohol and because of the impediment that such cognitive deficits can present in an individual's ability to benefit from certain aspects of an alcohol treatment or rehabilitation program, neuropsychological evaluation, consultation, and rehabilitation of cognitive deficits is strongly recommended to form an integral part of such intervention programs.

Research regarding the neuropsychological consequences of illegal drug use is especially sparse, limited, or in some cases, nonexistent. A review of the literature indicates some type of neuropsychological impairment in polydrug abusers, memory difficulties in cocaine abusers, attention and disorganizational problems in users of marijuana, and more serious brain consequences in those who abuse amphetamines and newer, synthetic drugs. However, available studies tend to be inconclusive, small in size, unable to control for, or take into account, premorbid functioning or other factors, or tend to be focused on immediate rather than long-term effects. It is well known that some neuropsychological effects may be possible with abuse of any type of drug, especially depending on the dosage administration. However, the identification of enduring, long-term effects is complicated by the lack of well-controlled research as well as a myriad of subject and research factors. Much of the research is correlational, and therefore, it is difficult to determine causality and the role of premorbid predisposition to substance abuse.

In the assessment of neuropsychological/cognitive functioning of any individual, it is important to identify and recognize preexisting or constitutional factors that may account, in part or in whole, for the individual's symptoms and test performance. The value of a thorough developmental, intellectual, academic, medical, vocational, social, and psychiatric history cannot be underestimated in the interpretation of current cognitive impairment.

REFERENCES

Albert, M. S.; Butters, N.; and Brandt, J. (1981). Patterns of remote memory in amnesic and demented patients. *Archives of Neurology,* 38, 495-500.

Allen, D. N.; Goldstein, G.; and Seaton, B. E. (1997). Cognitive rehabilitation of chronic alcohol abusers. *Neuropsychology Review,* 7(1), 21-39.

Alper, K. R.; Prichep, L. S.; Kowalik, S.; Rosenthal, M. S.; and John, E. R. (1998). Persistent QEEG abnormality in crack cocaine users at 6 months of drug abstinence. *Neuropsychopharmacology,* 19(1), 1-9.

Ambrose, M. L.; Bowden, S. C.; and Whelan, G. (2001). Working memory impairments in alcohol-dependent participants without clinical amnesia. *Alcoholism: Clinical and Experimental Research,* 25(2), 185-191.

Amen, D. G. and Waugh, M. (1998). High resolution brain SPECT imaging of marijuana smokers with AD/HD. *Journal of Psychoactive Drugs,* 30(2), 209-214.

American Psychiatric Association (1994). *Diagnostic and Statistical Manual of Mental Disorders,* Fourth Edition. Washington, DC: American Psychiatric Association.

Ardila, A.; Rosselli, M.; and Strumwasser, S. (1991). Neuropsychological deficits in chronic cocaine abusers. *International Journal of Neuroscience,* 57, 73-79.

Aytaclar, S.; Tarter, R. E.; Kirisci, L.; and Lu, S. (1999). Association between hyperactivity and executive cognitive functioning in childhood and substance use in early adolescence. *Journal of the American Academy of Child and Adolescent Psychiatry,* 38(2), 172-178.

Bates, M. E.; Labouvie, E. W.; and Voelbel, G. T. (2002). Individual differences in latent neuropsychological abilities in addictions treatment entry. *Psychology of Addictive Behaviors,* 16, 35-46.

Bates, M. E.; Voelbel, G. T.; Buckman, J. F.; Labouvie, E. W.; and Gbarry, D. (2005). Short term neuropsychologial recovery in clients with substance use disorders. *Alcoholism: Clinical and Experimental Research,* 29(3), 367-377.

Bauer, L. O. and Hesselbrock, V. M. (1999). P300 decrements in teenagers with conduct problems: Implications for substance abuse risk and brain development. *Biological Psychiatry,* 46(2), 263-272.

Beatty, W. W. and Borrell, G. K. (2000). Forms of knowledge, cognitive impairment, and drug abuse: A demonstration. *Progress in Neuropsychopharmacology and Biological Psychiatry,* 24(1), 17-22.

Beaunieux, H.; Desgranges, B.; LaLevee, C.; de la Sayette, V.; Lechevalier, B.; and Eustache, F. (1998). Preservation of cognitive procedural memory in a case of Korsakoff's syndrome: Methodological and theoretical insights. *Perceptual and Motor Skills,* 86(3), 1267-1287.

Block, R. I.; O'Leary, D. S.; Ehrhardt, J. C.; Augustinack, J. C.; Ghoneim, M. M.; Arndt, S.; and Hall, J. A. (2000). Effects of frequent marijuana use on brain tissue volume and composition. *Neuroreport: For Rapid Communication of Neuroscience Research,* 11(3), 491-496.

Blume, A. W.; Davis, J. M.; and Schmaling, K. B. (1999). Neurocognitive dysfunction in dually-diagnosed patients: A potential roadblock to motivating behavior change. *Journal of Psychoactive Drugs,* 31(2), 111-115.

Bolla, K. I.; Cadet, J.; and London, E. D. (1998). The neuropsychiatry of chronic cocaine abuse. *Journal of Neuropsychiatry and Clinical Neurosciences,* 10(3), 280-289.

Bolla, K. I.; McCann, U. D.; and Ricuarte, G. A. (1998). Memory impairment in abstinent MDMA (Ecstasy) users. *Neurology,* 51(6), 1532-1537.

Brick, J. and Erickson, C. (1999). *Drugs, the Brain, and Behavior: The Pharmacology of Abuse and Dependence.* Binghamton, NY: The Haworth Medical Press.

Buffenstein, A.; Heaster, J.; and Ko, P. (1999). Chronic psychotic illness methamphetamine. *American Journal of Psychiatry,* 156(4), 662.

Burian, S. E.; Liguori, A.; and Robinson, J. H. (2002). Effects of alcohol on risk-taking during simulated driving. *Human Psychopharmacology—Clinical and Experimental,* 17, 141-150.

Burns, R. S.; Lerner, S. E.; Corrado, R.; James, S.; and Schnoll, S. (1975). Phencyclidine: States of acute intoxications and fatalities. *The Western Journal of Medicine,* 123, 345-349.

Butters, N. (1984). Alcoholic Korsakoff's syndrome: An update. *Seminars in Neurology,* 4(2), 229-247.

Butters, N. and Cermak, L. S. (1974). The role of cognitive factors in the memory disorder of alcoholic patients with the Korsakoff syndrome. *Annals of the New York Academy of Science,* 233, 61-75.

Butters, N. and Cermak, L. S. (1975). Some analyses of amnesic syndromes in brain-damaged patients. In: Pribram, K. and Isaacson, R. (Eds.), *The Hippocampus* (pp. 377-410). New York: Plenum Press.

Butters, N. and Miliotis, P. (1985). Amnestic disorders. In: Heilman, K. and Valenstein, E. (Eds.), *Clinical Neuropsychology,* Second Edition (pp. 403-451). New York: Oxford University Press.

Butters, N.; Tarlow, S.; Cermak, L. S.; and Sax, D. (1976). A comparison of the information processing deficits of patients with Huntington's chorea and Korsakoff's syndrome. *Cortex,* 12, 134-144.

Campagna, K. D. (1986). Drug information forum: What are designer drugs? *U.S. Pharmacist,* 11(5), 16-17.

Carlin, A. S.; Grant, I.; Reed, R.; and Adams, K. (1979). Is phencyclidine (PCP) abuse associated with organic mental impairment? *American Journal of Drug and Alcohol Abuse,* 6, 273-281.

Carlin, A. S.; Stauss, F. F.; Grant, I.; and Adams, K. M. (1980). Drug abuse style, drug use type, and neuropsychological deficit in polydrug users. *Addictive Behaviors,* 5(3), 229-234.

Carlin, A. S. and Tupin, E. W. (1977). The effect of long-term chronic marijuana use on neuropsychological functioning. *International Journal of the Addictions,* 12(5), 617-624.

Casswell, S. and Marks, D. (1973). Cannabis induced impairment of performance of a divided attention task. *Nature,* 241, 60-61.

Chang, L.; Grob, C. S.; Ernst, T.; Itti, L.; Mishkin, F. S.; Jose-Melchor, R.; and Poland, R. (2000). Effect of ecstasy 3,4-methylenedioxymethamphetamin (MDMA) on cerebral blood flow: A co-registered SPECT and MRI study. *Psychiatry Research: Neuroimaging,* 98(1), 15-28.

Charness, M. E. (1994). Brain lesions in alcoholics. *Alcoholism: Clinical and Experimental Research,* 17, 2-11.

Culver, C. M. and King, F. W. (1974). Neuropsychological assessment of undergraduate marihuana and LSD users. *Archives of General Psychiatry,* 31, 707-711.

Dao-Castellana, M. H.; Samson, Y.; Legault, F.; Martinot, J. L.; Aubin, H. J.; Crouzel, C.; Feldman, L. et al. (1998). Frontal dysfunction in neurologically normal chronic alcoholic subjects: Metabolic and neuropsychological findings. *Psychological Medicine,* 28(5), 1039-1048.

Davila, M. D.; Shear, P. K.; Lane, B.; Sullivan, E. V.; and Pfefferbaum, A. (1994). Mammillary body and cerebellar shrinkage in chronic alcoholics: An MRI and neuropsychological study. *Neuropsychology,* 8(3), 433-444.

DeBellis, M. D.; Clark, D. B.; Beers, S. R.; Soloff, P. H.; Boring, A. M.; Hall, J.; Kersh, A.; and Keshavan, M. S. (2000). Hippocampal volume in adolescent-onset alcohol use disorders. *American Journal of Psychiatry,* 157(5), 737-744.

Diamond, R. and Carey, S. (1977). Developmental changes in the representation of faces. *Journal of Experimental Child Psychology,* 23, 1-22.

Dikmen, S. S.; Donovan, D. M.; Loberg, T.; Machamer, J. E.; and Temkin, N. R. (1993). Alcohol use and its effects on neuropsychological outcome in head injury. *Neuropsychology,* 7(3), 296-305.

Di Sclafani, V.; Clark, H. W.; Tolou-Shams, M.; Bloomer, C. W.; Salas, G. A.; Norman, D.; and Fein, G. (1998). Premorbid brain size is a determinant of functional reserve in abstinent crack-cocaine and crack-cocaine-alcohol dependent adults. *Journal of the International Neuropsychological Society,* 4(6), 559-565.

Di Sclafani, V.; Ezekiel, F.; Meyerhoff, D. J.; MacKay, S.; Dillion, W. P.; Weiner, M. W.; and Fein, G. (1995). Brain atrophy and cognitive function in older abstinent alcoholic men. *Alcoholism: Clinical and Experimental Research,* 19(5), 1121-1126.

Dricker, J.; Butters, N.; Berman, G.; Samuels, I.; and Carey, S. (1978). Recognition and encoding of faces by alcoholic Korsakoff and right hemisphere patients. *Neuropsychologia,* 16, 683-695.

Eckardt, M. J. and Martin R. P. (1986). Clinical assessment of cognition in alcoholism. *Alcoholism: Clinical Experimental and Research,* 19(2), 123-127.

Ehrenreich, H.; Rinn, T.; Kunert, H. J.; Moeller, M. R.; Poser, W.; Schilling, L.; Gigerenzer, G.; and Hoehe, M. R. (1999). Specific attentional dysfunction in adults following early start of cannabis use. *Psychopharmacology,* 142(3), 295-301.

Ellison, G. (1995). The *N*-methyl-D-aspartate antagonists phencyclidine, ketamine, and dizocilpine as both behavioral and anatomical models of the dementias. *Brain Research Reviews,* 20(2), 250-267.

Filley, C. M.; Heaton, R. K.; and Rosenberg, N. L. (1990). White matter dementia in chronic toluene abuse. *Neurology,* 40(3), 532-534.

Fishbein, D. (2000). Neuropsychological function, drug abuse, and violence: A conceptual framework. *Criminal Justice and Behavior,* 27(2), 139-159.

Gansler, D. A.; Harris, G. J.; Oscar-Berman, M.; Streeter, C.; Lewis, R. F.; Ahmed, I.; and Achong, D. (2000). Hypoperfusion of the inferior frontal brain regions in abstinent alcoholics: A pilot SPECT study. *Journal of Studies on Alcohol,* 61(1), 32-37.

Gatley, S. J. and Volkow, N. D. (1998). Addiction and imaging of the living human brain. *Drug and Alcohol Dependence,* 51(1-2), 97-108.

Giancola, P. R. and Tarter, R. E. (1999). Executive cognitive functioning and risk for substance abuse. *Psychological Science,* 10(3), 203-205.

Goldman, M. S. (1983). Cognitive impairment in chronic alcoholics: Some cause for optimism. *The American Psychologist,* 38, 1045-1054.

Goldman, M. S. (1995). Recovery of cognitive functioning in alcoholics—the relationship to treatment. *Alcohol Health and Research World,* 19, 148-154.

Graham, R. B. (1990). *Physiological Psychology.* Belmont, CA: Wadsworth Publishing Company.

Grant, I.; Adams, K. M.; Carlin, A. S.; and Rennick, P. M. (1977). Neuropsychological deficit in polydrug users. A preliminary report of the findings of the collaborative neuropsychological study of polydrug users. *Drug and Alcohol Dependence,* 2(2), 91-108.

Grant, S.; Contoreggi, C.; and London, E. D. (2000). Drug abusers show impaired performance in a laboratory test of decision making. *Neuropsychologia,* 38(8), 1180-1187.

Grobin, A. C.; Matthews, D. B.; Devaud, L. L.; and Morrow, A. L. (1998). The role of GABA(A) receptors in the acute and chronic effects of ethanol. *Psychopharmacology,* 139(1-2), 2-19.

Hammoumi, S.; Pyen, A.; Favre, J.-D.; Balmes, J.-L.; Bernard, J.-Y.; Husson, M.; Ferrand, J.-P.; Martin, J.-P.; and Daoust, M. (1999). Does the short variant of the serotonin transporter linked polymorphic region constitute a marker of alcohol dependence? *Alcohol,* 17(2), 107-112.

Hartman, D. E. (1995). *Neuropsychological Toxicology.* New York: Plenum Press.

Horner, M. D. (1997). Cognitive functioning in alcoholic patients with and without cocaine dependence. *Archives of Clinical Neuropsychology,* 12(7), 667-676.

Horner, M. D. (1999). Attentional functioning in abstinent cocaine abusers. *Drug and Alcohol Dependence,* 54(1), 19-33.

Jernigan, T. L.; Butters, N.; DiTraglia, G.; Schafer, K.; Smith, T.; Irwin, M.; Grant, I.; Schuckit, K.; and Cermak, L. (1991). Reduced cerebral gray matter observed in alcoholics using magnetic resonance imaging. *Alcoholism: Clinical and Experimental Research,* 15(3), 418-427.

Kelly, M. P.; Johnson, C. T.; Knoller, N.; and Drubach, D. A. (1997). Substance abuse, traumatic brain injury, and neuropsychological outcome. *Brain Injury,* 11(6), 391-402.

Kimble, D. P. (1968). Hippocampus and internal inhibition. *Psychological Bulletin,* 70, 285-295.

Kinsbourne, M. and Wood, F. (1975). Short-term memory processes and the amnesic syndrome. In: Deutsch, D. and Deutsch, J. A. (Eds.), *Short-Term Memory* (pp. 288-291). New York: Academic Press.

Korbo, L. (1999). Glial cell loss in the hippocampus of alcoholics. *Alcoholism: Clinical and Experimental Research,* 23(1), 164-168.

Krabbendam, L.; Visser, P. J.; Derix, M. M. A.; Verhey, F.; Hofman, P.; Verhoeven, W.; Tuinier, S.; and Jolles, J. (2000). Normal cognitive performance in patients with chronic alcoholism in contrast to patients with Korsakoff's syndrome. *Journal of Neuropsychiatry and Clinical Neurosciences,* 12(1), 44-50.

Lacayo, A. (1995). Neurologic and psychiatric complications of cocaine abuse. *Neuropsychiatry, Neuropsychology, and Behavioral Neurology,* 8(1), 53-60.

Leshner, A. I. (1997). Addiction is a brain disease, and it matters. *Science,* 278 (5335), 45-47.

Leshner, A. I. and Koob, G. F. (1999). Drugs of abuse and the brain. *Proceedings of the Association of American Physicians,* 111(2), 99-108.

Liu, X.; Matochik, J. A.; Cadet, J.; and London, E. D. (1998). Smaller volume of prefrontal lobe in polysubstance abuser: A magnetic resonance imaging study. *Neuropsychopharmacology,* 18(4), 243-252.

London, E. D.; Ernst, M.; Grant, S.; Bonson, K.; and Weinstein, A. (2000). Orbitofrontal cortex and human drug abuse: Functional imaging. *Cerebral Cortex,* 10(3), 334-342.

Lovinger, D. M. (1997). Serotonin's role in alcohol's effects on the brain. *Alcohol Health and Research World,* 21(2), 114-120.

Malloy, P.; Noel, N.; Longabaugh, R.; and Beattie, M. (1990). Determinants of neuropsychological impairment in anti-social substance abusers. *Addictive Behaviors,* 15, 431-438.

Mathew, R. J.; Wilson, W. H.; and Tant, S. R. (1989). Regional cerebral blood flow changes associated with amyl nitrite inhalation. *British Journal of Addiction,* 84(3), 293-299.

McCann, U. D. and Ricuarte, G. A. (1995). On the neurotoxicity of MDMA and related amphetamine derivatives. *Journal of Clinical Psychopharmacology,* 15(4), 295-296.

McCann, U. D.; Mertl, M.; Eligulashvili, V.; and Ricuarte, G. A. (1999). Cognitive performance in 3,4-methylenedioxymenthamphetamine (MDMA, ecstasy) users: A controlled study. *Psychopharmacology,* 143(4), 417-425.

McGlothlin, W. H.; Arnold, D. O.; and Freedman, D. X. (1969). Organicity measures following repeated LSD ingestion. *Archives of General Psychiatry,* 21(6), 704-709.

Melges, F. T.; Tinklenberg, J. R.; Hollister, L. E.; and Gillespie, H. K. (1970). Marihuana and temporal disintegration. *Science,* 168, 1118-1120.

Mihic, S. J. and Harris, R. A. (1997). GABA and the GABA (A) receptor. *Alcohol Health and Research World,* 21(2), 127-131.

Miller, L. (1985). Neuropsychological assessment of substance abusers: Review and recommendations. *Journal of Substance Abuse Treatment,* 2, 5-17.

Miller, L. L. and Branconnier, R. J. (1983). Cannabis: Effects on memory and the cholinergic limbic system. *Psychological Bulletin,* 93, 441-456.

Minocha, A.; Barth, J. T.; Roberson, D. G.; Herold, D. A.; and Spyker, D. A. (1985). Impairment of cognitive and psychomotor function by ethanol in social drinkers. *Veterinary and Human Toxicology,* 27, 533-536.

Mintzer, S.; Hickenbottom, S.; and Gilman, S. (1999). Parkinsonism after taking ecstasy. *New England Journal of Medicine,* 340(18), 1443.

Mittenberg, W. and Motta, S. (1993). Effects of chronic cocaine abuse on memory and learning. *Archives of Clinical Neuropsychology,* 8, 477-483.

Morris, J. A. and Lawson, W. M. (1998). Neuropsychological deficits in patients with alcohol and other psychoactive substance abuse and dependency: A pilot study. *Alcoholism Treatment Quarterly,* 16(4), 101-111.

Moser, R. S. (1999). *Practice Information Clearinghouse of Knowledge (PICK 42): Clinical Neuropsychology.* Washington, DC: American Psychological Association.

Obrocki, J.; Buchert, R.; Vaeterlein, O.; Thomasius, R.; Beyer, W.; and Shiermann, T. (1999). Ecstasy—long-term effects on the human central nervous system revealed by positron emission tomography. *British Journal of Psychiatry,* 175, 186-188.

Parsons, O. A. (1986). Cognitive functioning in sober social drinkers: A review and critique. *Journal of Studies on Alcohol* 47, 387-404.

Parsons, O. A. (1994). Determinants of cognitive deficits in alcoholics: The search continues. *Clinical Neuropsychologist,* 8, 39-589.

Parsons, O. A. (1998). Neurocognitive deficits in alcoholics and social drinkers: A continuum? *Alcoholism: Clinical and Experimental Research* 22(4), 954-961.

Peterson, J. B.; Finn, P. R.; and Pihl, R. O. (1992). Cognitive dysfunction and inherited predisposition to alcoholism. *Journal of Studies on Alcohol,* 53, 154-160.

Pfefferbaum, A.; Lim, K. O.; Zipursky, R. B.; Mathalon, D. H.; Lane, B.; Ha, C. N.; Rosenbloom, M. J.; and Sullivan, E. V. (1992). Brain gray and white matter volume loss accelerates with aging in chronic alcoholics: A quantitative MRI study. *Alcoholism: Clinical and Experimental Research,* 16, 1078-1089.

Pfefferbaum, A.; Sullivan, E. V.; Mathalon, D. H.; and Lim, K. O. (1997). Frontal lobe volume loss observed with magnetic resonance imaging in older chronic alcoholics. *Alcoholism: Clinical and Experimental Research,* 21(3), 521-529.

Piercy, M. F. (1978). Experimental studies of the organic amnesic syndrome. In: Whitty, C. W. M. and Zangwill, O. L. (Eds.), *Amnesia,* Second Edition (pp. 1-51). London: Butterworths.

Ratti, M. T.; Soragna, D.; Sibilla, L.; Giardini, A.; Albergati, A.; Savoldi, F.; and Bo, P. (1999). Cognitive impairment and cerebral atrophy in "heavy drinkers." *Progress in Neuro-Psychopharmacology and Biological Psychiatry,* 23(2), 243-258.

Reneman, L.; Booij, J.; Schmand, B.; van der Brink, W.; and Gunning, B. (2000). Memory disturbances in Ecstasy users are correlated with an altered brain serotonin neurotransmission. *Psychopharmacology,* 148(3), 322-324.

Robinson, J. E.; Heaton, R. K.; and O'Malley, S. S. (1999). Neuropsychological functioning in cocaine abusers with and without alcohol dependence. *Journal of International Neuropsychological Society,* 5(1), 10-19.

Rogers, R. D.; Everitt, B. J.; Baldacchino, A.; Blackshaw, A. J.; Swainson, R.; Wynne, K.; Baker, N. B. et al. (1999). Dissociable deficits in the decision-making cognition of chronic amphetamine abuser, opiate abusers, patients with focal damage to prefrontal cortex, and tryptophan-depleted normal volunteers: Evidence for monoaminergic mechanisms. *Neuropsychopharmacology,* 20(4), 322-339.

Rosenberg, N. L.; Grigsby J.; Dreisbach J.; Busenbark D.; Grigsby P. (2002). Neuropsychologic impairment and MRI abnormalities associated with chronic solvent abuse. *Journal of Toxicology: Clinical Toxicology,* 40, 21-34.

Rosenbloom, M. J.; Pfefferbaum, A.; and Sullivan, E. V. (2004). Recovery of short-term memory and psychomotor speed but not postural stability with long-term sobriety in alcoholic women. *Neuropsychology,* 18(3), 589-597.

Roth, W. T.; Rosenbloom, M. J.; Darley, C. F.; Tinklenberg, J. R.; and Kopell, B. S. (1975). Marihuana effects on TAT form and content. *Psychopharmacologia,* 43(3), 261-266.

Rothwell, P. M. and Grant, R. (1993). Cerebral venus sinus thrombosis induced by "ecstasy." *Journal of Neurology, Neurosurgery, and Psychiatry,* 56(9), 1035.

Rourke, S. B. and Grant, I. (1999). The interactive effects of age and length of abstinence on the recovery of neuropsychological functioning in chronic male alcoholics: A 2-year follow-up study. *Journal of the International Neuropsychological Society,* 5(3), 234-246.

Ryback, R. (1971). The continuum and specificity of the effects of alcohol on memory: A review. *Quarterly Journal of Studies on Alcohol,* 32, 995-1016.

Schaeffer, K. W.; Parsons, O. A.; and Yohman, J. R. (1984). Neuropsychological differences between male familial and nonfamilial alcoholics and nonalcoholics. *Alcoholism: Clinical and Experimental Research,* 8, 347-351.

Schafer, J.; Birchler, G. R.; and Fals-Stewart, W. (1994). Cognitive affective, and marital functioning of recovering male polysubstance abusers. *Neuropsychology,* 8(1), 100-109.

Sircar, R. and Li, C. (1994). PCP/NMDA receptor-channel complex and brain development. *Neurotoxicology and Teratology,* 16(4), 369-375.

Strassman, R. J. (1984). Adverse reactions to psychedelic drugs. *Journal of Nervous and Mental Disease,* 172, 577-595.

Strickland, T. L.; Mena, I.; Villanueva-Meyer, J.; Miller, B.; Cummings, J.; Mehringer, C. M.; Satz, P.; and Myers, H. (1993). Cerebral perfusion and neuropsychological consequences of chronic cocaine use. *Journal of Neuropsychiatry and Clinical Neurosciences,* 5, 419-427.

Strickland, T. L.; Miller, B. L.; Kowell, A.; and Stein, R. (1998). Neurobiology of cocaine-induced organic brain impairment: Contributions from functional neuroimaging. *Neuropsychology Review,* 8(1), 1-9.

Strickland, T. L. and Stein, R. (1995). Cocaine-induced cerebrovascular impairment: Challenges to neuropsychological assessment. *Neuropsychology Review,* 5(1), 69-79.

Sullivan, E. V.; Rosenbloom, N. M.; Lim, K. O.; and Pfefferbaum, A. (2000). Longitudinal changes in cognition, gait, and balance in abstinent and relapsed alcoholic men: Relationships to changes in brain structure. *Neuropsychology,* 14(2) 178-188.

Tarbox, A. R.; Connors, G. J.; and McLauglin, E. J. (1986). Effects of drinking pattern on neuropsychological performance among alcohol misusers. *Journal of Studies on Alcohol,* 47, 176-179.

Tarter, R. E. (1988). Are there inherited behavioral traits that predispose to substance abuse? *Journal of Consulting and Clinical Psychology,* 56, 189-196.

Tarter, R. E. and Edwards, K. L. (1986). Multifactorial etiology of neuropsychological impairment in alcoholics. *Alcoholism: Clinical and Experimental Research,* 10(2), 128-135.

Tarter, R. E. and Edwards, K. (1988). Psychological factors associated with the risk for alcoholism. *Alcoholism: Clinical and Experimental Research,* 12, 471-480.

Tarter, R. E.; Moss, H.; Arria, A.; and Van Thiel, D. (1990). Hepatic, nutritional, and genetic influences on cognitive processes in alcoholics. *National Institute on Drug Abuse Research Monograph Series: 1990 Research Monograph,* 101, 124-135.

Tarter, R. E.; Van Thiel, D. H.; Arria, A. M.; Carra, J.; and Moss, H. (1988). Impact of cirrhosis on the neuropsychological test performance of alcoholics. *Alcoholism: Clinical and Experimental Research,* 12(5), 619-621.

Thompson, R. F. (2000). *The Brain: A Neuroscience Primer,* Third Edition. New York: Worth Publishers.

Tinklenberg, J. R.; Darley, C. F.; Roth, W. T.; Pfefferbaum, A.; and Kopell, B. S. (1978). Marijuana effects on associations to novel stimuli. *Journal of Nervous and Mental Disease,* 166(5), 362-364.

Tiplady, B.; Harding, C.; McLean, D.; Ortner, C.; Porter, K.; and Wright, P. (1999). Effects of ethanol and temazepan on episodic and semantic memory: A dose-response comparison. *Human Psychopharmacology—Clinical and Experimental,* 14(4), 263-269.

Uitti, R. J.; Snow, B. J.; Shinotoh, H.; Vingerhoets, F. J.; Hayward, M.; Hashimoto, S.; Richmond, J.; Markey, S.; Markey, C.; and Calne, D. (1994). Parkinsonism induced by solvent abuse. *Annals of Neurology,* 35, 616-619.

Volkow, N. D.; Chang, L.; Wang, G.-J.; Fowler, J. S.; Franceschi, D.; Sedler, M.; Gatley, S. J. et al. (2001). Loss of dopamine transporters I methamphetamine abusers recovers with protracted abstinence. *Journal of Neuroscience,* 21(23), 9414-9418.

Volkow, N. D.; Chang, L.; Wang, G.-J.; Fowler, J. S.; Leonido-Yee, M.; Franceschi, D.; Sedler, M. J. et al. (2001). Association of dopamine transporter reduction with psychomotor impairment in methamphetamine abusers. *American Journal of Psychiatry,* 158(3), 377-382.

Washton, A. and Gold, M. (1984). Chronic cocaine abuse. *Psychiatric Annals,* 14, 733-743.

Wilkinson, D. A. and Carlen, P. L. (1980). Relationship of neuropsychological test performance to brain morphology in amnesic and non-amnesic chronic alcoholics. *Acta Psychiatrica Scandinavica,* 62 (Suppl. 286), 89-101.

Wright, M. and Hogan, T. (1972). Repeated LSD ingestion and performance on neuropsychological tests. *Journal of Nervous and Mental Disease,* 154(6), 432-438.

Chapter 4

Consequences of Excessive Chronic Alcohol Consumption on Brain Structure and Function

Margaret J. Rosenbloom
Edith V. Sullivan
Adolf Pfefferbaum

INTRODUCTION AND OVERVIEW

People with alcohol use disorders consume alcohol to excess despite being aware of its harmful effects on their behavior, and these harmful behavioral effects are mediated through the brain where changes in structure, function, and basic physiology occur and underlie the development of tolerance and dependence. These changes can persist for years, even after sobriety is maintained, although neuroadaptation with sobriety enables some restoration of function in a damaged brain. Thus, the consequences of chronic excessive alcohol use include not only the structural damage apparent shortly after sobriety is attained, but also persistent functional deficits that reflect diminished functional reserve and plasticity, and contribute to the self-sustaining nature of alcoholism.

In this chapter, we review evidence provided by four magnetic resonance imaging (MRI) modalities on the consequences of excessive chronic alcohol consumption for brain macrostructure, microstructure, chemistry, and function. To assess the immediate effects of chronic excessive drinking on the brain and cognitive and motor performance, investigators most commonly

Authors' note: Support in the preparation of this chapter was provided by the National Institute on Alcohol Abuse and Alcoholism (AA10723, AA05965, AA12388).

compare treatment-seeking alcoholics, tested shortly after entering a treatment program, to low-alcohol-consuming controls, matched to the alcoholics on factors that affect brain and cognition, including age, sex, and education. To determine the persistent consequences of excessive alcohol consumption, cross-sectional studies compare alcoholics with different durations of sobriety while longitudinal studies retest alcoholics after varying periods of sobriety. All studies of the consequences of excessive alcohol consumption on the brain must be interpreted in full recognition of the multifaceted etiology and consequences of this disease (Tarter and Edwards, 1986). Many conditions associated with alcoholism, such as liver disease, malnutrition, and head trauma have their own consequences on the brain (see Chapter 2). Thus, potential participants in brain imaging research studies must be carefully screened and other unavoidable factors that may influence the brain thoroughly described. Socioeconomic status, premorbid mental status, family history of alcoholism, comorbid psychiatric conditions (Grant et al., 2004; Mathalon et al., 2003; Sullivan, Deshmukh, Desmond, Mathalon, et al., 2000; Sullivan, Rosenbloom, et al., 2003), nonalcohol substance abuse (Bjork, Grant, and Hommer 2003; Di Sclafani et al., 1998; Nixon, Paul, and Phillips, 1998), infection from HIV (for review, see Pfefferbaum, Adalsteinsson, and Sullivan, 2005a), and Hepatitis C virus can each exacerbate or mitigate the consequences of alcohol on the brain in ways that are not yet fully understood. Furthermore, total lifetime alcohol consumption, as well as recency and pattern of exposure must be quantified, even though the complex etiology of alcohol-related damage often obscures simple dose-response effects. Despite the challenges of conducting in vivo imaging studies of the consequences of excessive alcohol consumption on the brain, there is a growing consensus regarding the pattern of disruption that builds upon a large literature of postmortem pathological findings.

Brain imaging can detect abnormalities on both macrostructural and microstructural levels, alterations in some of the biochemical elements present in brain tissue, and in the efficiency with which blood flow serves neuronal activation called forth by experimental cognitive tasks. In this chapter, we summarize a number of cross-sectional studies of the consequences of excessive alcohol consumption on the brain, consider the contributions of age, sex, and amount of alcohol consumed to the findings, and conclude that although few regions of the brain appear entirely immune to the untoward consequences of excessive alcohol, the regions most at risk include frontal cortex and subjacent white matter, cerebellar sites, and white matter structures and tracts, including the corpus callosum. These observations provide the basis for an integrative hypothesis for the mechanisms of functional impairment. Then we present available evidence regarding the brain consequences of excessive alcohol consumption that appear to be reversible in the first weeks and months of sobriety and those that persist even with extended sobriety. We provide evidence from four different MRI methods—structural MRI, diffusion tensor imaging (DTI), magnetic resonance spectroscopy (MRS), and functional MRI (fMRI)—and present a brief introduction to each method before presenting findings from that modality. The reader is referred elsewhere for fuller descriptions of the MRI methods, quantification approaches, as well as artifactual considerations that limit the usefulness of brain imaging data (Adalsteinsson, Sullivan, and Pfefferbaum, 2002; Hennig et al., 2003; Pfefferbaum, Adalsteinsson, and Sullivan, 2006; Rosenbloom, Sullivan, and Pfefferbaum, 2003).

CROSS-SECTIONAL STUDIES OF THE CONSEQUENCES OF CHRONIC EXCESSIVE ALCOHOL USE ON THE BRAIN

Macrostructure: Volumes of Cortical Regions, Cerebellum and Subcortical Structures Observed with Structural MRI

Conventional structural MRI takes advantage of the water-based composition of the brain comprising gray matter (about 80 percent water), white matter (about 70 percent water), and cerebrospinal fluid (CSF) (100 percent water) to reveal the size, shape, and tissue composition (gray versus white matter) of the brain and its constituent parts. Gray matter consists of neurons and surrounding glial cells. White matter is made up of long, thin, nerve cell fibers called axons that carry information between neurons. White matter is paler in color than gray matter because the axons are surrounded by myelin, which is a system of cell bodies (oligodendrocytes) that wind around the axon and augment neural transmission. The axons form fiber tracts linking near and distant neurons across different brain regions (i.e., white matter tracts). Structural MRI enables the identification of differences in brain tissue types and structures by manipulating the way in which water protons are excited, yielding intensity differences between tissue types that enable gross brain neuroanatomy (macrostructure) to be mapped. Typically these structural images are segmented to differentiate gray matter, white matter, and CSF the liquid that fills inner spaces and surrounds the brain within the skull. Volumes of gray matter, white matter, and CSF can then be measured in different regions of the brain. In addition, specific neuroanatomic structures such as the corpus callosum, hippocampus, and basal ganglia can be outlined and their volumes measured.

Cross-sectional MRI studies, comparing patients with chronic alcoholism to people without a history of excessive alcohol use, typically reveal smaller volumes of both gray matter (Fein et al., 2002; Jernigan et al., 1991) and white matter (Pfefferbaum et al., 1992) in the cerebral cortex, the folded outer layer of the brain. Older alcoholics show greater volume deficits relative to age-matched controls than younger alcoholics, especially in the frontal lobes (Pfefferbaum et al., 1997) This is evident even in samples where older alcoholics have drunk equivalent amounts over their lifetime as younger alcoholics. This age-alcoholism interaction suggests that as people age, their brains become more vulnerable to the effects of excessive alcohol (Pfefferbaum et al., 1992). MRI of the cerebral cortex also shows that temporal lobe white matter deficits are prevalent in patients with a history of seizure (Sullivan et al., 1996) but the greatest cortical loss in uncomplicated alcoholism occurs in the frontal lobes (Kubota et al., 2001; Pfefferbaum et al., 1997), which subserve reasoning, working memory, and problem solving (Moselhy, Georgiou, and Kahn, 2001; Oscar-Berman and Hutner, 1993) (see Figure 4.1, upper panel).

In addition to affecting the cerebrum, MRI shows that the cerebellum, the "little brain" which lies behind and beneath the cerebral cortex, is also adversely affected, even in patients with uncomplicated alcoholism (Sullivan, Deshmukh, Desmond, Lim, et al., 2000) (see Figure 4.1, middle panel). These findings are consistent with postmortem reports of shrinkage, prominent in large neurons of the anterior superior vermis (Harper, 1998; Phillips, Harper, and Kril, 1987; Torvik and Torp, 1986). Traditionally, the cerebellum was thought to be mainly responsible for controlling balance; alcohol-related damage to this structure is presumed to be responsible for the lower limb motor deficit or ataxia found in patients with the alcohol and nutritionally-based disorder of Wernicke-Korsakoff syndrome (Victor, Adams, and Collins, 1971). More recent studies of the role of the cerebellum and the extensive circuits linking it to subcortical and cortical regions have highlighted its critical role for higher order functions classically associated with the frontal lobes (Schmahmann, 1997). Damage to the vermis (the central portion of the cerebellum) and the cerebellar hemispheres from excessive alcohol consumption thus contributes not only to deficits of balance and gait in chronic alcoholics (Sullivan, Rose, and Pfefferbaum, 2006; Sullivan, Deshmukh, Desmond, Lim et al., 2000), but also to impairment in functions such as problem solving and working memory. We shall elaborate on this at a later point in this chapter.

Structural MRI studies have shown that subcortical and brainstem structures, known to be affected in severe syndromes associated with excessive alcohol consumption or associated nutritional deficiency such as Marchiafava-Bignami disease (a condition involving demyelination of the corpus callosum that leads to a range of neurological problems), central pontine myelinolysis

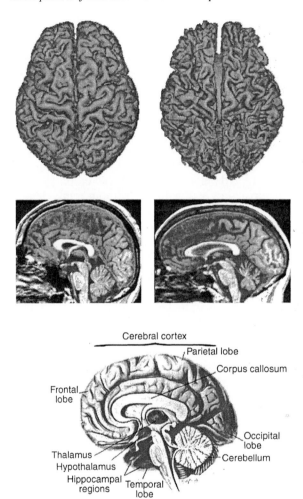

FIGURE 4.1. Upper Panel: Three-dimensional surface of the brain of a healthy (left) and alcoholic (right) man, seen from above. The front of the brain is at the top. Note the shriveled appearance of the alcoholic brain, particularly in the frontal lobes. *Source:* From Sullivan, 2000. Middle Panel: Slice through the middle of the brain and cerebellum of a healthy (left) and alcoholic (right) man viewed from the side. Note severely shrunken folia of the anterior superior vermis in the alcoholic brain. *Source:* From Sullivan, Harding, et al., 2003. Lower Panel: Schematic representation of the brain identifying areas most affected by alcohol. *Source:* From Oscar-Berman and Marinkovic, 2003.

(a condition affecting the pons that can lead to quadriplegia), alcoholic cerebellar degeneration, and Korsakoff's syndrome, are also affected in patients
with uncomplicated alcoholism, albeit to a lesser degree. These structures
include bodies of white matter such as the corpus callosum (Estruch et al.,
1997; Hommer et al., 1996; Pfefferbaum et al., 1996) and pons (Bloomer,
Langleben, and Meyerhoff, 2004; Sullivan and Pfefferbaum, 2001; Sullivan et al., 2005); subcortical basal ganglia structures such as the thalamus
(Sullivan, Rosenbloom et al., 2003), caudate, and putamen (Sullivan et al.,
2005); and memory-related structures such as the mammillary bodies (Davila
et al., 1994; Shear et al., 1996; Sullivan et al., 1999) and right (Laakso et al.,
2000) or anterior (Agartz et al., 1999; Sullivan et al., 1995) hippocampus
that are seen in alcoholics both with and without frank memory disorder.

Microstructure: White Matter Integrity Observed with Diffusion Tensor Imaging

Although neuroanatomically detailed, macrostructual MRI does not
clearly reflect the microstructure of brain tissue and its components, such as
axons, microtubules, and myelin. DTI measures the diffusion of water molecules within brain cells and in extracellular spaces. When unconstrained,
as in the fluid-filled space of the lateral ventricles, molecules move equally
in all directions (isotropic movement). However, in tissue with a regular and
orderly microstructure, such as brain white matter (Hirano and Llena, 1995),
the water molecules are constrained to move mainly in the orientation of
specific fiber tracts (anisotropic movement). Anisotropy is calculated on a
within-voxel basis and is commonly expressed as a percent or fraction, that
is, fractional anisotropy (FA) (Pierpaoli and Basser, 1996), that reflects the
extent to which water molecules are constrained by the microstructure of
white matter tracts. FA can range from 0 for CSF-filled spaces to 1 for highly
organized, parallel bands of white matter such as the corpus callosum,
whereas the amount of diffusion (diffusivity) is high in CSF and much
lower in gray and white matter. With trauma or disease, the axonal cyto-
skeleton, including myelin and the linear orientation of neurofilaments that
lends to high anisotropy in healthy white matter, can be perturbed and result
in diminished anisotropy (Arfanakis et al., 2002). Disease-related accumulation of fluids in the extracellular spaces between fibers provide an avenue
for water movement in white matter, increasing diffusivity. Thus, high FA
and low diffusivity generally reflect healthy white matter. On an FA image,
higher intensity signals denote higher FA and typically highlight the white
matter skeleton (see Figure 4.2). Detailed reviews on DTI methods can be
found elsewhere (Adalsteinsson, Sullivan, and Pfefferbaum, 2002; Hors-

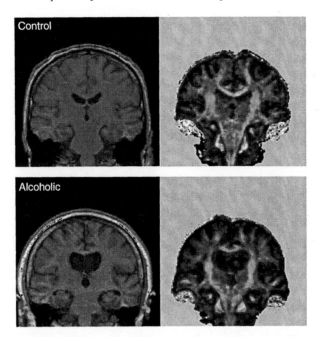

FIGURE 4.2. Slice through the brain of a 61-year-old healthy (upper) and 61-year-old alcoholic (lower) man at the level of the lateral ventricles and hippocampus, viewed from the back. The left column contains structural MR images. The right column contains FA images from a DTI scan, depicting the white matter "skeleton." Higher intensity reflects higher FA. *Source:* From Pfefferbaum and Sullivan, 2005.

field and Jones, 2002; Le Bihan, 2003; Rosenbloom, Sullivan, and Pfefferbaum, 2003).

As with structural MRI, DTI studies must characterize normal aging effects before determining the consequences of alcoholism on the brain, because of the possibility of the interaction of age and alcoholism occurring at the microstructural level. Several DTI studies have demonstrated variability of white matter anisotropy across brain regions in healthy individuals, depending on the linearity and homogeneity of the local fiber structure (Madden et al., 2004; Pfefferbaum, Adalsteinsson, and Sullivan, 2005b; Pierpaoli et al., 2001; Salat et al., 2005; Virta, Barnett, and Pierpaoli, 1999). Normal aging and certain neurological and psychiatric conditions also modulate regional FA and diffusivity (for reviews, see Kubicki et al., 2002; Lim and Helpern, 2002; Moseley, 2003; Pfefferbaum and Sullivan, 2005). A series of neuropathological studies in a monkey model of aging revealed postmortem cross-sectional evidence for fluctuations in the condition of myelin with age including degenerative and regenerative changes (Peters and Sethares, 2002; Peters and Sethares, 2003; Peters, Sethares, and Killiany, 2001). Such evidence from postmortem studies can direct the focus of in vivo DTI to seek sensitive markers of age-related, degenerative and restorative alterations in the structural integrity of axonal constituents.

Age-alcoholism interactions have been observed in the macrostructure of the corpus callosum both postmortem (Wiggins et al., 1988) and in vivo (Pfefferbaum et al., 1996). DTI studies of corpus callosal microstructure confirm these observations. Our first studies reported abnormally low anisotropy in regions of the corpus callosum as well as the supratentorial white matter region termed the centrum semiovale in alcoholic men (Pfefferbaum et al., 2000) and women (Pfefferbaum and Sullivan, 2002). Both men and women show deficits in anisotrophy of the callosal genu and centrum semiovale, and men showed additional deficits in the callosal splenium and pericallosal white matter. These microstructural deficits were seen even though in some cases, structural MRI did not detect size deficits in the corpus callosum.

A more recent study of the corpus callosum in an independent sample found that diffusivity was strikingly higher in alcoholic men and women than controls and showed regionally nonspecific, substantial correlations with macrostructural volume. Furthermore, older alcoholics had greater abnormalities for their age in both diffusivity and FA than younger ones (Pfefferbaum, Adalsteinsson, and Sullivan, 2006). The functional significance of these observations were revealed by selective correlations between regional measures of diffusivity and FA in the corpus callosum and tests of working memory, visuospatial ability, and gait and balance. This is a topic to which we shall return later.

As with MRI studies of the brain's macrostructure, in vivo DTI studies of white matter's microstructure in aging and alcoholism are consistent with postmortem findings (Kemper, 1994). Small connecting fibers of the anterior corpus callosum are especially vulnerable in aging (Aboitiz et al., 1996) and likely contribute to deficits in cognitive processes dependent on prefrontal circuitry (Craik et al., 1990; Gunning-Dixon and Raz, 2003; Raz, 1999).

Proton Metabolites: Biochemical Changes Observed with Magnetic Resonance Spectroscopy

Although DTI provides more detailed information about the microstructural integrity of white matter than can be found from structural MRI, it does not provide information about the chemical composition of brain tissue. For this we turn to proton MRS that can detect the concentration of certain chemical constituents of the brain, especially those with methyl protons that resonate in a certain frequency range, but only when the signal from water, the most prominent constituent, is suppressed. Among the spectroscopically visible metabolites are *N*-acetyl aspartate (NAA), a marker of living, mature neurons and thus a potential indicator of neuronal and axonal integrity; myoinositol (mI) which increases with glial activity or gliosis; choline (Cho) which reflects cell membrane turnover; and creatine + phosphocreatine (Cr), a complex composite that reflects high-energy phosphate metabolism. The concentration of these metabolites is much lower than that of water (neat water is 55 molar while brain metabolite concentrations are 10 millimolar or less—a ratio > 5,000:1). Due to this low signal-to-noise ratio, most clinical MRS studies derive spectra from a few large voxels, or brain samples, located in specific regions of interest such as frontal lobes or cerebellum (see Figure 4.3). Measurement difficulties also motivate the convention of expressing metabolites as a ratio of Cr, for example, NAA/Cr, rather than as an absolute value—a procedure that assumes a stable value for Cr. Despite the technical challenges involved, increasing numbers of studies report absolute metabolite concentrations and image their distribution over broad regions of the brain in chronic alcohol users (e.g., Ende et al., 2005; Meyerhoff et al., 2004). Gray and white matter each have characteristic concentrations of these metabolites, for example, most studies find higher concentrations of NAA in gray matter than in white matter (e.g., Pfefferbaum et al., 1999; Wang and Li, 1998). MRS thus provides another technique with which to assess the integrity and metabolic status of gray and white matter in the brain.

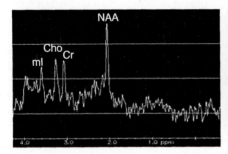
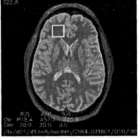

FIGURE 4.3. An axial slice through the brain as viewed from above illustrating a region of interest in the frontal lobe from which metabolites are measured. The box to the left illustrates the proton spectrum with peaks for *N*-acetyl aspartate (NAA), creatine (Cr), choline (Cho), and myoinositol (mI) identified.

Cross-sectional MRS studies generally report abnormally low NAA in frontal (Bendszus et al., 2001; Fein et al., 1994; Jagannathan, Desai, and Raghunathan, 1996) and cerebellar (Bendszus et al., 2001; Jagannathan, Desai, and Raghunathan, 1996; Seitz et al., 1999) regions in alcoholics compared with controls. Studies testing patients soon after abstinence (four weeks) (Schweinsburg et al., 2001), or comparing current heavy drinkers with light drinkers (Meyerhoff et al., 2004), also find lower NAA in frontal white matter as well as higher mI in parietal regions. In one study (Meyerhoff et al., 2004), the NAA white matter effect was more marked when subjects younger than age 38 were excluded, suggesting an interaction between age and the effects of alcohol. A recent MRS study, using stringent statistical criteria, found a trend for reduced NAA in frontal white matter, and strong effects for reduced Ch in frontal white matter and cerebellum (Ende et al., 2005). Abnormally low NAA and high Cr have also been observed in a midbrain region of interest encompassing the pons in high-drinking compared with low-drinking men (Bloomer, Langleben, and Meyerhoff, 2004).

Sex Differences and Dose-Response Effects

An early computerized tomography (CT) study found comparable enlargement of the lateral ventricles (the large fluid-filled spaces in the middle of the brain that increase in size as adjacent brain tissue shrinks) in men and women, even though the women had drunk much less alcohol than the men over their lifetime (Jacobson, 1986). This lead to the proposal that the brains of women were more vulnerable to the consequences of excessive alcohol use than those of men. Several studies have since reported comparable deficits, relative to same sex controls, in alcoholic men and women despite lower alcohol consumption in women. These include MRI studies of cortical white and gray matter and CSF (Hommer et al., 2001), the corpus callosum (Hommer et al., 1996), and hippocampal volumes (Agartz et al., 1999), as well as DTI studies of FA and diffusivity (Pfefferbaum, Adalsteinsson, and Sullivan, 2006) and MRS studies of NAA (Meyerhoff et al., 2004; Schweinsburg et al., 2003). By contrast, some MRI studies found that men had greater abnormalities than women in the size of the lateral ventricles, cortical gray matter (Pfefferbaum et al., 2001) and white matter, corpus callosum, and pons (Pfefferbaum et al., 2002), once differences in head size and amount of alcohol drunk were taken into account. These discrepancies could have been due to methodological differences in technique used to account for the normal sex differences in head size as well as authentic differences in sample characteristics, especially with regard to age, length of illness, and lifetime alcohol consumption relative to body weight. Indeed, in a new samples our group has found comparable thinning of the corpus callosum in men and women (Pfefferbaum, Adalsteinsson, and Sullivan, 2006).

A CT study (Mann et al., 2005) found equivalent brain deficits in a relatively large sample of alcoholic men and women, who were matched in age, scanned after comparable periods of sobriety, and had drunk equivalent amounts of alcohol over their lifetime after accounting for weight differences. However, the women had a significantly shorter mean duration of alcohol dependence (five and a half years) compared to the men (10.4 years). These results were taken to denote a telescoping of the harmful consequences of alcohol on the brain for women. Such telescoping is consistent with studies showing a more rapid emergence of medical and social alcohol-related problems in women than men (Schuckit et al., 1995).

A direct dose-response characterization of the consequences of alcohol consumption on the brain has been elusive. Premorbid factors such as sex, family history of alcoholism, and age combine with postmorbid factors such as nutrition and concurrent illness to establish vulnerability or confer a measure of protection for the individual concerned. Although group differences in brain measures between alcoholics and controls—whose lifetime histories of alcohol use can differ typically by a factor of 10 or more—are regularly observed, dose-response effects linking severity of brain abnormality to lifetime or even recent quantities of drinking among alcoholics are not consistently reported. This failure to detect consistent dose response relationships reflects the complex etiology of the disorder as well as difficulties in accurately assessing histories of alcohol exposure.

COGNITIVE AND MOTOR FUNCTION: THE LINK TO NEUROIMAGING OBSERVATIONS

Neuroimaging studies have documented a range of consequences of chronic excessive alcohol use, including volume deficits in frontal lobes and cerebellum, compromised integrity of white matter, and abnormally low levels of NAA (an index of neuronal viability), principally located in the frontal lobes and cerebellum. What are the practical consequences of these changes in terms of deficits in cognitive and motor function? A significant percentage of recovering chronic alcoholics exhibit mild to moderate deficits in complex cognitive processes. It is worth noting that functions tend to be impaired but not completely lost. Typically, the processes affected are visuospatial abilities, executive functions, and gait and balance (for reviews, see Fein et al., 1990; Moselhy, Georgiou, and Kahn, 2001; Oscar-Berman, 2000; Sullivan, 2000), evidenced in both alcoholic men (Sullivan, Rosenbloom, and Pfefferbaum, 2000) and women (Sullivan, Fama, et al., 2002). The executive functions affected include working memory, problem solving, temporal ordering, response inhibition, and psychomotor speed (Moselhy, Georgiou, and Kahn, 2001; Nixon et al., 2002; Oscar-Berman and Hutner, 1993; Sullivan, 2000).

Despite the multiplicity of behavioral deficits associated with chronic alcohol dependence, only a few studies have been able to demonstrate links between relatively specific component processes and measures of localized deficit in specific brain regions (e.g., Meyerhoff et al., 2004). In contrast, sensory or motor functions that draw on focal rather than multiple brain regions for successful performance have been more readily associated statistically with the relevant brain region. For example, olfactory discrimination ability was correlated with thalamic volumes in one study (Shear et al., 1992), and two other studies showed that postural stability correlated selectively with anterior superior cerebellar vermian volumes (Sullivan, Rose, and Pfefferbaum, 2004; Sullivan, Deshmukh, Desmond, Lim et al., 2000).

The difficulty in finding simple associations between alcohol-related deficits in specific brain structures and specific cognitive functions has lead to the hypothesis that the mechanism underlying alcohol-related cognitive compromise may arise from degradation of selective neural circuitry connecting cortical sites rather than either specific damage at the site or complete disconnection of white matter tracts providing connectivity between the cortical sites (Sullivan, 2003). In this context, DTI evidence of reduced integrity of white matter structures is particularly relevant. In two separate samples of alcoholic men and a sample of alcoholic women (Pfefferbaum and Sullivan, 2002; Pfefferbaum, Adalsteinsson, and Sullivan, 2006; Pfefferbaum et al., 2000), we observed that the level of performance on tests of attention, working memory, and visuospatial ability was related selectively to the regional microstructural integrity of the corpus callosum in alcoholics. The associations observed are consistent with the topographically compartmentalized tracts of the corpus callosum in which the genu connects lateralized frontal sites and the splenium connects lateralized parietal and occipital sites (de Lacoste, Kirkpatrick, and Ross, 1985; Pandya and Seltzer, 1986). In one study (Pfefferbaum, Adalsteinsson, and Sullivan, 2006), we calculated a composite score for working memory, classically considered a "frontal lobe" function, based on Backward Digit Span and Block Spans from the Wechsler Memory Scale–Revised (Wechsler, 1987) and Trail Making Part B (Lezak, 1995), and also assessed visuospatial ability with the Matrix Reasoning subtest of the Wechsler Abbreviated Scale of Intelligence (Wechsler, 1999), performance on which is selectively impaired by lesions of the parietal cortex (Villa et al., 1990). A series of multiple regression analyses identified a double dissociation in alcoholics: low scores on the working memory composite correlated with high diffusivity (an index of white matter tissue compromise) in the genu, whereas low scores on matrix reasoning correlated with high diffusivity in the splenium.

Another source of evidence for the importance of circuitry to performance by alcoholics derives from tasks requiring callosal transfer (Schulte et al., 2005). These tasks are of two types: those naturally requiring processing contributions from both hemispheres and those demanding bihemispheric, distributed processing because of neurological compromise. Regarding the first instance, cognitive and motor tasks typically invoke multiple functions of both hemispheres and require callosal integrity for interhemispheric information exchange (Ellis and Oscar-Berman, 1989; Schulte, Pfefferbaum, and Sullivan, 2003). In groups of controls and alcoholics, we tested whether DTI indices of callosal integrity would predict reaction time measures of interhemispheric processing. The paradigms used were the crossed-uncrossed difference (CUD), testing visuomotor information transfer between the cerebral hemispheres, and the redundant targets effect (RTE), testing parallel, simultaneous processing of visual information by each cerebral hemisphere; a large CUD and a small RTE each indicative of slower interhemispheric transfer. We found that in controls a large CUD correlated with low FA and high diffusivity in the genu and splenium, and that in alcoholics, a small RTE correlated with low FA in genu and splenium and high diffusivity in the callosal body. These results suggest that even subtle degradation of callosal fiber coherence can result in "mild yet detectable disturbance in interhemispheric processing" (Schulte et al., 2005, p. 1390). Regarding the second instance, even when only one cerebral hemisphere is needed for task execution, elderly and compromised individuals (Cabeza et al., 2002), including alcoholics (Pfefferbaum, Desmond, et al., 2001), commonly draw on both hemispheres.

Hemodynamic Activation: Compensatory Shifts in Process Demands Observed with Functional MRI

The techniques described previously—MRI, DTI, and MRS—all provide static representations of the brain. In contrast, fMRI describes the brain at work by measuring brain blood oxygen level as a proxy for the neural activity demanded by specific motor, sensory, or cognitive processes (Logothetis and Pfeuffer, 2004). fMRI locates changes in levels of oxygen in blood vessels, the hemodynamic response, occurring in response to experimental manipulations by measuring the difference between oxygenation time-locked to a specific cognitive or motor operation and oxygenation occurring during a rest period or neutral activity. The regions of the brain showing greatest difference between active and neutral conditions are believed to be those most involved in performing the operation under investigation (Hennig et al., 2003; Toma and Nakai, 2002).

fMRI studies in alcoholics have tested brain activity associated with working memory (Desmond et al., 2003; Pfefferbaum, Desmond et al., 2001) and motor (Parks et al., 2003) tasks. A common finding is that for a given task alcoholics activated different brain regions from controls, suggesting compensatory reorganization. Alcoholics performed more slowly than controls on an index finger tapping task, activated a greater extent of the brain regions examined than controls for dominant hand tapping, and failed to show normal differences in patterns of lateralized cerebellar activation for dominant and nondominant hand tapping (Parks et al., 2003). These results were interpreted as evidence of motor inefficiency and compensatory alterations of cortical-cerebellar circuits. In another study, alcoholics performed a spatial working memory task at an equivalent level to controls but manifest less activation in prefrontal regions than controls and more activation of posterior and inferior regions, suggesting a functional reorganization of the brain (Pfefferbaum, Desmond, et al., 2001). Similarly, alcoholics performing a verbal working memory task performed as fast and as accurately as controls but manifested greater activations in the left prefrontal cortex and the right superior cerebellum (Desmond et al., 2003). These data were interpreted as evidence for the role of the cerebellum in augmenting or compensating for functional impairment of the prefrontal cortex in alcoholics, consistent with well-documented, frontocerebellar circuits (Schmahmann, 1996; Schmahmann and Pandya, 1997).

Findings based on fMRI suggest the importance in alcoholics of cerebellar activation in otherwise frontal lobe functions. This additional activation enabled alcoholics to achieve normal levels of coordinated motor performance despite evidence for cerebellar dysmorphology but at a cost to processing capacity. This functional style observed in alcoholics, although perhaps compensatory, has been characterized as inefficient (Nixon and Parsons, 1991). As noted by Nixon (1993), traditional concepts of processing inefficiency derive from conditions engendering altered speed/accuracy trade-offs. Alcoholics are slower to attain normal accuracy, as we observed in a quantified version of the finger-to-nose test, in which alcoholics achieved equivalent or even smaller trajectory deviations than controls (Sullivan, Desmond, et al., 2002). This performance is symptomatic of cerebellar hemisphere dysfunction, characterized by deliberation of otherwise automatic movements. When automatic processing becomes effortful, it calls on limited processing capacity, which is then unavailable for other tasks. Taken together, these phenomena suggest a common neuropsychological mechanism—processing inefficiency—and perhaps a neural mechanism—degraded white matter microstructure—as underlying these possible instances of impaired neural transmission.

LONGITUDINAL STUDIES:
PROSPECTS FOR RECOVERY WITH ABSTINENCE

The negative consequences of chronic excessive alcohol use on the brain are mitigated to some extent by maintaining sobriety, as was first demonstrated with CT (Carlen et al., 1986). Measuring the extent and time-course of such recovery in humans is a challenging task that typically first takes place while patients are in an alcohol treatment program, tracking effects of withdrawal and short-term sobriety, but then moves out into the community to follow patients after discharge and track effects of longer term sobriety or relapse. Studies of the long-term prospects for recovery take the form of naturalistic rather than controlled experiments because the investigator has no control over which patients will maintain sobriety, who will return to drinking, and what drinking level will be embraced. Furthermore, attrition will take its toll on follow-up sample size. Ideally, a follow-up study must also retest a control sample of low drinkers at the same intervals as the alcoholics in order to measure the changes associated with sobriety or relapse relative to those changes associated with normal aging and other uncontrolled experimental conditions. Another approach for studying long-term prospects for recovery is to compare alcoholics with different lengths of sobriety, cross-sectionally, although that also has its drawbacks.

Longitudinal MRI studies of alcoholics during short-term treatment-related abstinence, followed by continued abstinence or relapse after discharge have found that with short-term (about one month) abstinence from alcohol, cortical gray matter (Pfefferbaum et al., 1995) or overall brain tissue volume (Gazdzinski, Durazzo, and Meyerhoff, 2005) increase in volume. After discharge, those who maintained sobriety (on average 6-12 months) showed reduced volume of the third ventricle (Pfefferbaum et al., 1995), or overall brain tissue increase (Gazdzinski, Durazzo, and Meyerhoff, 2005), but those who relapsed showed expansion of the third ventricle and shrinkage of white matter (Pfefferbaum et al., 1995), or loss of the overall brain tissue gains made during abstinence (Gazdzinski, Durazzo, and Meyerhoff, 2005). Additional studies have highlighted that cortical white matter volume may be particularly amenable to recovery with abstinence (Agartz et al., 2003; Meyerhoff, 2005; O'Neill, Cardenas and Meyerhoff, 2001; Shear, Jernigan, and Butters, 1994) or vulnerable to further decline with continued drinking (Pfefferbaum et al., 1995).

The few studies that have been made of extended sobriety (five years) have differentiated between those who maintained virtual sobriety and those who resumed drinking (Muuronen et al., 1989; Pfefferbaum et al., 1998). Alcoholics who maintained prolonged sobriety showed improvement or stabilization of measures of brain tissue volume, while those who returned to drinking showed increased ventricular volume. Furthermore, the amount of cortical gray matter loss especially in the frontal lobes over the follow-up period was associated with the degree of excessive drinking in retested alcoholics (Pfefferbaum et al., 1998).

Investigators do not yet know the mechanism for either loss of brain tissue volume with drinking or its restoration with abstinence. Changes in both myelination and axonal integrity in white matter and glial and dendritic changes in cortical neuropil are probably involved. Animal studies have revealed neurogenesis in the hippocampus in long abstinent animals (Nixon and Crews, 2004), although no equivalent evidence is currently available in humans. Some longitudinal studies using MRS have revealed significant increases in NAA in frontal lobes over short-term supervised abstinence (Bendszus et al., 2001) and in cerebellum over long-term abstinence (Parks et al., 2002). Both studies also documented associated improvement on cognitive tests. Similar results are suggested by a preliminary report (Meyerhoff, 2005) of an ongoing study that found greatest increase in NAA during the initial month of sobriety. Although NAA concentrations in frontal white and gray matter regions increased further with seven months of abstinence, they did not normalize. Evidence of NAA increases with sobriety is not a universal finding, and the verdict is still out on exactly what spectroscopically visible changes can be expected over the course of withdrawal and sobriety in chronic alcoholics, and in which brain structures and tissue types they may occur. For example, a longitudinal study of recently sober alcoholics tested first on an average of two weeks after withdrawal, and again after three and six months of abstinence (Ende et al., 2005) did not find significant increase in NAA, at either cerebellar or frontal regions. However Cho, which had been significantly reduced in alcoholics at withdrawal, increased significantly between time 1 and time 2. By six months, Cho values in the reduced set of alcoholics who had maintained sobriety were comparable to Cho values seen in controls at time 1. Likewise, a cross-sectional study inferring change by comparing alcoholics with different lengths of sobriety did not find group differences in NAA measures (O'Neill, Cardenas, and Meyerhoff, 2001; Schweinsburg et al., 2000), although one did provide evidence of increased mI (Schweinsburg et al., 2000).

A growing number of longitudinal neuropsychological studies report significantly better scores on tests of working memory, visuospatial abilities, and gait and balance with abstinence from alcohol. Some components of these functional domains recover faster (Rosenbloom, Pfefferbaum, and Sullivan, 2004) or more fully than others (e.g., Becker et al., 1983; Brandt et al., 1983; Mann et al., 1999; Nixon and Glenn, 1995; Parsons, Butters, and Nathan, 1987; Sullivan, Rosenbloom, et al., 2000), but at least a measurable degree of recovery typically accompanies prolonged sobriety, suggesting that the changes observed with neuroimaging have functional consequences.

SUMMARY AND CONCLUSIONS

The chronic, excessive consumption of alcohol has significant consequences for brain structure, physiology, and function. MRI techniques have delineated reduced volume of macrostructure, impaired microstructural integrity of white matter tracts that link functional circuits, alterations in biochemical properties of brain tissue, and alterations in functional response to cognitive challenge in chronic alcoholics.

The brain consequences of alcoholism predominantly affect the frontal lobes and cerebellum. It is now recognized that the cerebellum and its extensive circuitry support functions classically associated with the frontal lobes, including verbal associate learning, word production, problem solving, cognitive planning, attentional set shifting, and working memory (e.g., Courchesne et al., 1994; Schmahmann, 2000). Owing to their far-reaching circuitry, disruption of selective cerebellar loci can have significant effects on remote brain regions, including the prefrontal cortex. To date, our guiding hypothesis that disruption of frontocerebellar circuitry is a principal neural mechanism underlying alcoholism's salient, enduring, and debilitating deficits—ataxia, executive dysfunction, and visuospatial impairment—has been consistently supported by our MRI structural-neuropsychological studies and fMRI experiments. Given the possibility of structural and functional repair and recovery in sober alcoholics, at least a portion of the neuropathology must be transient and the lesions incomplete (Filley, 2001; Sullivan, 2000). This transience of certain aspects of brain pathology may underlie the problem of finding specific brain structural volume-functional relationships in alcoholics. Indeed, the dynamic course of alcoholism presents an important and challenging neuroscience model for understanding mechanisms of functional recovery, compensation, and processing limitations that should be applicable to any neurological condition characterized by a fluctuating course.

REFERENCES

Aboitiz, F.; Rodriguez, E.; Olivares, R.; Zaidel, E. (1996). Age-related changes in fibre composition of the human corpus callosum: Sex differences. *Neuroreport* 7(11):1761-1764.

Adalsteinsson, E.; Sullivan, E.V.; Pfefferbaum, A. (2002). Biochemical, functional and microstructural magnetic resonance imaging (MRI). In: Y. Liu and D.M. Lovinger (Eds.), *Methods in Alcohol-Related Neuroscience Research* (pp. 345-372), Boca Raton, FL, CRC Press.

Agartz, I.; Brag, S.; Franck, J.; Hammarberg, A.; Okugawa, G.; Svinhufvud, K.; Bergman, H. (2003). MR volumetry during acute alcohol withdrawal and abstinence: A descriptive study. *Alcohol and Alcoholism* 38(1):71-78.

Agartz, I.; Momenan, R.; Rawlings, R.R.; Kerich, M.J.; Hommer, D.W. (1999). Hippocampal volume in patients with alcohol dependence. *Arch Gen Psychiatry* 56(4):356-363.

Arfanakis, K.; Haughton, V.M.; Carew, J.D.; Rogers, B.P.; Dempsey, R.J.; Meyerand, M.E. (2002). Diffusion tensor MR imaging in diffuse axonal injury. *Am J Neuroradiol* 23(5):794-802.

Becker, J.T.; Butters, N.; Hermann, A.; D'Angelo, N. (1983). A comparison of the effects of long-term alcohol abuse and aging on the performance of verbal and nonverbal divided attention tasks. *Alcohol Clin Exp Res* 7:213-219.

Bendszus, M.; Weijers, H.G.; Wiesbeck, G.; Warmuth-Metz, M.; Bartsch, A.J.; Engels, S.; Boning, J.; Solymosi, L. (2001). Sequential MR imaging and proton MR spectroscopy in patients who underwent recent detoxification for chronic alcoholism: Correlation with clinical and neuropsychological data. *Am J Neuroradiol* 22(10):1926-1932.

Bjork, J.M.; Grant, S.J.; Hommer, D.W. (2003). Cross-sectional volumetric analysis of brain atrophy in alcohol dependence: Effects of drinking history and comorbid substance use disorder. *Am J Psychiatry* 160(11):2038-2045.

Bloomer, C.W.; Langleben, D.D.; Meyerhoff, D.J. (2004). Magnetic resonance detects brainstem changes in chronic, active heavy drinkers. *Psychiatry Res* 132(3): 209-218.

Brandt, J.; Butters, N.; Ryan, C.; Bayog, R. (1983). Cognitive loss and recovery in long-term alcohol abusers. *Arch Gen Psychiatry* 40(4):435-442.

Cabeza, R.; Anderson, N.D.; Locantore, J.K.; McIntosh, A.R. (2002). Aging gracefully: Compensatory brain activity in high-performing older adults. *Neuroimage* 17(3):1394-1402.

Carlen, P.L.; Penn, R.D.; Fornazzari, L.; Bennett, J.; Wilkinson, D.A.; Wortzman, G. (1986). Computerized tomographic scan assessment of alcoholic brain damage and its potential reversibility. *Alcohol Clin Exp Res* 10:226-232.

Courchesne, E.; Townsend, J.; Akshoomoff, N.A.; Saitoh, O.; Yeung-Courchesne, R.; Lincoln, A.J.; James, H.E.; Haas, R.H.; Schreibman, L.; Lau, L. (1994). Impairment in shifting attention in autistic and cerebellar patients. *Behav Neurosci* 108(5):848-865.

Craik, F.I.M.; Morris, L.W.; Morris, R.G.; Loewen, E.R. (1990). Relations between source amnesia and frontal lobe functioning in older adults. *Psychol Aging* 5(1):148-151.

Davila, M.D.; Shear, P.K.; Lane, B.; Sullivan, E.V.; Pfefferbaum, A. (1994). Mammillary body and cerebellar shrinkage in chronic alcoholics: An MRI and neuropsychological study. *Neuropsychology* 8:433-444.

de Lacoste, M.; Kirkpatrick, J.; Ross, E. (1985). Topography of the human corpus callosum. *J Neuropathol Exp Neurol* 44:578-591.

Desmond, J.E.; Chen, S.H.A.; De Rosa, E.; Pryor, M.R.; Pfefferbaum, A.; Sullivan, E.V. (2003). Increased fronto-cerebellar activation in alcoholics during verbal working memory: An fMRI study. *Neuroimage* 19:1510-1520.

Di Sclafani, V.; Clark, H.W.; Tolou-Shams, M.; Bloomer, C.W.; Salas, G.A.; Norman, D.; Fein, G. (1998). Premorbid brain size is a determinant of functional reserve in abstinent crack-cocaine and crack-cocaine-alcohol-dependent adults. *J Int Neuropsychol Soc* 4(6):559-565.

Ellis, R.J.; Oscar-Berman, M. (1989). Alcoholism, aging, and functional cerebral asymmetries. *Psychol Bull* 106:128-147.

Ende, G.; Welzel, H.; Walter, S.; Weber-Fahr, W.; Diehl, A.; Hermann, D.; Heinz, A.; Mann, K. (2005). Monitoring the effects of chronic alcohol consumption and abstinence on brain metabolism: A longitudinal proton magnetic resonance spectroscopy study. *Biol Psychiatry* 58(12):974-980.

Estruch, R.; Nicolas, J.M.; Salamero, M.; Aragon, C.; Sacanella, E.; Fernandez-Sola, J.; Urbano-Marquez, A. (1997). Atrophy of the corpus callosum in chronic alcoholism. *J Neurol Sci* 146(2):145-151.

Fein, G.; Bachman, L.; Fisher, S.; Davenport, L. (1990). Cognitive impairments in abstinent alcoholics. *West J Med* 152:531-537.

Fein, G.; Di Sclafani, V.; Cardenas, V.A.; Goldmann, H.; Tolou-Shams, M.; Meyerhoff, D.J. (2002). Cortical gray matter loss in treatment-naive alcohol dependent individuals. *Alc Clin Exp Research* 26(4):558-564.

Fein, G.; Meyerhoff, D.; Di Sclafani, V.; Ezekiel, F.; Poole, N.; MacKay, S.; Dillon, W.P.; Constans, J.-M.; Weiner, M.W. (1994). 1H magnetic resonance spectroscopic imaging separates neuronal from glial changes in alcohol-related brain atrophy. In: F. Lancaster (Ed.), *Alcohol and Glial Cells,* NIAAA Research Monograph No. 27 (pp. 227-241), Bethesda, MD, U.S. Government Printing Office.

Filley, C.M. (2001). *The Behavioral Neurology of White Matter* (pp. 247-267), Oxford, Oxford University Press.

Gazdzinski, S.; Durazzo, T.C.; Meyerhoff, D.J. (2005). Temporal dynamics and determinants of whole brain tissue volume changes during recovery from alcohol dependence. *Drug Alcohol Depend* 78(3):263-273.

Grant, B.F.; Stinson, F.S.; Dawson, D.A.; Chou, S.P.; Ruan, W.J.; Pickering, R.P. (2004). Co-occurrence of 12-month alcohol and drug use disorders and personality disorders in the United States: Results from the National Epidemiologic Survey on alcohol and related conditions. *Arch Gen Psychiatry* 61(4):361-368.

Gunning-Dixon, F.M.; Raz, N. (2003). Neuroanatomical correlates of selected executive functions in middle-aged and older adults: A prospective MRI study. *Neuropsychologia* 41(14):1929-1941.

Harper, C. (1998). The neuropathology of alcohol-specific brain damage, or does alcohol damage the brain? *J Neuropathol Exp Neurol* 57(2):101-110.

Hennig, J.; Speck, O.; Koch, M.A.; Weiller, C. (2003). Functional magnetic resonance imaging: A review of methodological aspects and clinical applications. *J Magn Reson Imaging* 18(1):1-15.

Hirano, A. and Llena, J.F. (1995). Morphology of central nervous system axons. In: S.G. Waxman, J.D. Kocsis, and P.K. Stys (Eds.), *The Axon: Structure, Function and Pathophysiology* (p. 67), New York, Oxford University Press.

Hommer, D.W.; Momenan, R.; Kaiser, E.; Rawlings, R.R. (2001). Evidence for a gender-related effect of alcoholism on brain volumes. *Am J Psychiatry* 158(2): 198-204.

Hommer, D.; Momenan, R.; Rawlings, R.; Ragan, P.; Williams, W.; Rio, D.; Eckardt, M. (1996). Decreased corpus callosum size among alcoholic women. *Arch Neurol* 53(4):359-363.

Horsfield, M.A.; Jones, D.K. (2002). Applications of diffusion-weighted and diffusion tensor MRI to white matter diseases—A review. *NMR Biomed* 15(7-8): 570-577.

Jacobson, R. (1986). The contributions of sex and drinking history to the CT brain scan changes in alcoholics. *Psychol Med* 16:547-549.

Jagannathan, N.R.; Desai, N.G.; Raghunathan, P. (1996). Brain metabolite changes in alcoholism: An in vivo proton magnetic resonance spectroscopy (MRS) study. *J Magn Reson Imaging* 14:553-557.

Jernigan, T.L.; Butters, N.; DiTraglia, G.; Schafer, K.; Smith, T.; Irwin, M.; Grant, I.; Schuckit, M.; Cermak, L. (1991). Reduced cerebral grey matter observed in alcoholics using magnetic resonance imaging. *Alcohol Clin Exp Res* 15(3):418-427.

Kemper, T.L. (1994). Neuroanatomical and neuropathological changes during aging and dementia. In: M.L. Albert and J.E. Knoefel (Eds.), *Clinical Neurology of Aging* (pp. 3-67), New York, Oxford University Press.

Kubicki, M.; Westin, C.-F.; Maier, S.E.; Mamata, H.; Frumin, M.; Ersner-Hershfield, H.; Kikinis, R.; Jolesz, F.A.; McCarley, R.; Shenton, M.E. (2002). Diffusion tensor imaging and its application to neuropsychiatric disorders. *Harv Rev Psychiatry* 10:324-336.

Kubota, M.; Nakazaki, S.; Hirai, S.; Saeki, N.; Yamaura, A.; Kusaka, T. (2001). Alcohol consumption and frontal lobe shrinkage: Study of 1432 non-alcoholic subjects. *J Neurol Neurosurg Psychiatry* 71(1):104-106.

Laakso, M.P.; Vaurio, O.; Savolainen, L.; Repo, E.; Soininen, H.; Aronen, H.J.; Tiihonen, J. (2000). A volumetric MRI study of the hippocampus in type 1 and 2 alcoholism. *Behav Brain Res* 109(2):177-186.

Le Bihan, D. (2003). Looking into the functional architecture of the brain with diffusion MRI. *Nat Rev Neurosci* 4(6):469-480.

Lezak, M.D. (1995). *Neuropsychological Assessment* (Third Edition) (pp. 381-384), New York, Oxford University Press.

Lim, K.O.; Helpern, J.A. (2002). Neuropsychiatric applications of DTI—A review. *NMR Biomed* 15(7-8):587-593.

Logothetis, N.K.; Pfeuffer, J. (2004). On the nature of the BOLD fMRI contrast mechanism. *J Magn Reson Imaging* 22(10):1517-1531.

Madden, D.J.; Whiting, W.L.; Huettel, S.A.; White, L.E.; MacFall, J.R.; Provenzale, J.M. (2004). Diffusion tensor imaging of adult age differences in cerebral white matter: Relation to response time. *Neuroimage* 21(3):1174-1181.

Mann, K.; Gunther, A.; Stetter, F.; Ackermann, K. (1999). Rapid recovery from cognitive deficits in abstinent alcoholics: A controlled test-retest study. *Alcohol and Alcoholism* 34(4):567-574.

Mann, K.F.; Ackermann, K.; Croissan, B.; Mundle, G.; Diehl, A. (2005). Neuroimaging of gender differences in alcoholism: Are women more vulnerable? *Alcohol Clin Exp Res* 29:896-901.

Mathalon, D.H.; Pfefferbaum, A.; Lim, K.O.; Rosenbloom, M.J.; Sullivan, E.V. (2003). Compounded brain volume deficits in schizophrenia-alcoholism comorbidity. *Arch Gen Psychiatry* 60(3):245-252.

Meyerhoff, D.J. (2005). Brain spectroscopic imaging, morphometry, and cognition in social drinkers and recovering alcoholics. *Alcohol Clin Exp Res* 29:153-154.

Meyerhoff, D.J.; Blumenfeld, R.; Truran, D.; Lindgren, J.; Flenniken, D.; Cardenas, V.; Chao, L.L.; Rothlind, J.; Studholme, C.; Weiner, M.W. (2004). Effects of heavy drinking, binge drinking, and family history of alcoholism on regional brain metabolites. *Alcohol Clin Exp Res* 28(4):650-661.

Moseley, M. (2003). Diffusion tensor imaging and aging—A review. *NMR Biomed* 15:553-560.

Moselhy, H.F.; Georgiou, G.; Kahn, A. (2001). Frontal lobe changes in alcoholism: A review of the literature. *Alcohol and Alcoholism* 36(5):357-368.

Muuronen, A.; Bergman, H.; Hindmarsh, T.; Telakivi, T. (1989). Influence of improved drinking habits on brain atrophy and cognitive performance in alcoholic patients: A 5-year follow-up study. *Alcohol Clin Exp Res* 13(1):137-141.

Nixon, K.; Crews, F.T. (2004). Temporally specific burst in cell proliferation increases hippocampal neurogenesis in protracted abstinence from alcohol. *J Neurosci* 24(43):9714-9722.

Nixon, S.J. (1993). Application of theoretical models to the study of alcohol-induced brain damage. In: W. Hunt and S.J. Nixon (Eds.), *Alcohol Induced Brain Damage*, NIAAA monograph (pp. 213-228), Rockville, MD, National Institutes of Health.

Nixon, S.J.; Glenn, S.W. (1995). Cognitive, psychosocial performance and recovery in female alcoholics. In: M. Galanter (Ed.), *Recent Developments in Alcoholism, Vol 12. Alcoholism and Women* (pp. 287-308), New York, Plenum Press.

Nixon, S.J.; Parsons, O.A. (1991). Alcohol-related efficiency deficits using an ecologically valid test. *Alcohol Clin Exp Res* 15(4):601-606.

Nixon, S.J.; Paul, R.; Phillips, M. (1998). Cognitive efficiency in alcoholics and polysubstance abusers. *Alcohol Clin Exp Res* 22(7):1414-1420.

Nixon, S.J.; Tivis, R.; Ceballos, N.; Varner, J.L.; Rohrbaugh, J. (2002). Neurophysiological efficiency in male and female alcoholics. *Prog Neuropsychopharmacol Biol Psychiatry* 26(5):919-927.

O'Neill, J.; Cardenas, V.A.; Meyerhoff, D.J. (2001). Effects of abstinence on the brain: Quantitative magnetic resonance imaging and magnetic resonance spectroscopic imaging in chronic alcohol abuse. *Alcohol Clin Exp Res* 25(11): 1673-1682.

Oscar-Berman, M. (2000). Neuropsychological vulnerabilities in chronic alcoholism. In: A. Noronha, M. Eckardt, and K. Warren (Eds.), *Review of NIAAA's Neuroscience and Behavioral Research Portfolio,* NIAAA Research Monograph No. 34 (pp. 437-472), Bethesda, MD, National Institutes of Health.

Oscar-Berman, M.; Hutner, N. (1993). Frontal lobe changes after chronic alcohol ingestion. In: W.A. Hunt and S.J. Nixon (Eds.), *Alcohol-Induced Brain Damage,* NIAAA Research Monographs No. 22 (pp. 121-156), Rockville, MD, National Institutes of Health.

Oscar-Berman, M.; Marinkovic, K. (2003). Alcoholism and the brain: An overview. *Alcohol Res Health* 27(2):125-133.

Pandya, D.N.; Seltzer, B. (1986). The topography of commissural fibers. In: F. Lepore, M. Ptito, and H.H. Jasper (Eds.), *Two Hemispheres—One Brain: Functions of the Corpus Callosum* (pp. 47-74), New York, Alan R. Liss, Inc.

Parks, M.H.; Dawant, B.M.; Riddle, W.R.; Hartmann, S.L.; Dietrich, M.S.; Nickel, M.K.; Price, R.R.; Martin, P.R. (2002). Longitudinal brain metabolic characterization of chronic alcoholics with proton magnetic resonance spectroscopy. *Alcohol Clin Exp Res* 26(9):1368-1380.

Parks, M.H.; Morgan, V.L.; Pickens, D.R.; Price, R.R.; Dietrich, M.S.; Nickel, M.K.; Martin, P.R. (2003). Brain MRI activation associated with self-paced finger-tapping in chronic alcohol dependent patients. *Alcohol Clin Exp Res* 27:704-711.

Parsons, O.A.; Butters, N.; Nathan, P.E. Eds. (1987). *Neuropsychology of Alcoholism: Implications for Diagnosis and Treatment,* New York, Guilford Press.

Peters, A.; Sethares, C. (2002). Aging and the myelinated fibers in prefrontal cortex and corpus callosum of the monkey. *J Comp Neurol* 442(3):277-291.

Peters, A.; Sethares, C. (2003). Is there remyelination during aging of the primate central nervous system? *J Comp Neurol* 460(2):238-254.

Peters, A.; Sethares, C.; Killiany, R.J. (2001). Effects of age on the thickness of myelin sheaths in monkey primary visual cortex. *J Comp Neurol* 435(2):241-248.

Pfefferbaum, A.; Adalsteinsson, E.; Spielman, D.; Sullivan, E.V.; Lim, K.O. (1999). In vivo spectroscopic quantification of the N-acetyl moiety, creatine and choline from large volumes of gray and white matter: Effects of normal aging. *Magn Reson Med* 41(2):276-284.

Pfefferbaum, A.; Adalsteinsson, E.; Sullivan, E.V. (2005a). Cortical NAA deficits in HIV infection without dementia: Influence of alcoholism comorbidity. *Neuropsychopharmacology* 30(7):1392-1399.

Pfefferbaum, A.; Adalsteinsson, E.; Sullivan, E.V. (2005b). Frontal circuitry degradation marks healthy adult aging: Evidence from diffusion tensor imaging. *Neuroimage* 26(3):891-899.

Pfefferbaum, A.; Adalsteinsson, E.; Sullivan, E.V. (2006). Dysmorphology and microstructural degradation of the corpus callosum: Interaction of age and alcoholism. *Neurobiol Aging* 27(7):994-1009.

Pfefferbaum, A.; Desmond, J.E.; Galloway, C.; Menon, V.; Glover, G.H.; Sullivan, E.V. (2001). Reorganization of frontal systems used by alcoholics for spatial working memory: An fMRI study. *Neuroimage* 14:7-20.

Pfefferbaum, A.; Lim, K.O.; Desmond, J.; Sullivan, E.V. (1996). Thinning of the corpus callosum in older alcoholic men: A magnetic resonance imaging study. *Alcohol Clin Exp Res* 20(4):752-757.

Pfefferbaum, A.; Lim, K.O.; Zipursky, R.B.; Mathalon, D.H.; Lane, B.; Ha, C.N.; Rosenbloom, M.J.; Sullivan, E.V. (1992). Brain gray and white matter volume loss accelerates with aging in chronic alcoholics: A quantitative MRI study. *Alcohol Clin Exp Res* 16(6):1078-1089.

Pfefferbaum, A.; Rosenbloom, M.J.; Deshmukh, A.; Sullivan, E.V. (2001). Sex differences in the effects of alcohol on brain structure. *Am J Psychiatry* 158(2): 188-197.

Pfefferbaum, A.; Rosenbloom, M.J.; Serventi, K.; Sullivan, E.V. (2002). Corpus callosum, pons and cortical white matter in alcoholic women. *Alcohol Clin Exp Res* 26:400-405.

Pfefferbaum, A.; Sullivan, E.V. (2002). Microstructural but not macrostructural disruption of white matter in women with chronic alcoholism. *Neuroimage* 15:708-718.

Pfefferbaum, A.; Sullivan, E.V. (2005). Diffusion MR imaging in neuropsychiatry and aging. In: J. Gillard, A. Waldman, and P. Barker (Eds.), *Clinical MR Neuroimaging: Diffusion, Perfusion and Spectroscopy* (pp. 558-578), Cambridge, Cambridge University Press.

Pfefferbaum, A.; Sullivan, E.V.; Hedehus, M.; Adalsteinsson, E.; Lim, K.O.; Moseley, M. (2000). In vivo detection and functional correlates of white matter microstructural disruption in chronic alcoholism. *Alcohol Clin Exp Res* 24(8):1214-1221.

Pfefferbaum, A.; Sullivan, E.V.; Mathalon, D.H.; Lim, K.O. (1997). Frontal lobe volume loss observed with magnetic resonance imaging in older chronic alcoholics. *Alcohol Clin Exp Res* 21(3):521-529.

Pfefferbaum, A.; Sullivan, E.V.; Mathalon, D.H.; Shear, P.K.; Rosenbloom, M.J.; Lim, K.O. (1995). Longitudinal changes in magnetic resonance imaging brain volumes in abstinent and relapsed alcoholics. *Alcohol Clin Exp Res* 19(5):1177-1191.

Pfefferbaum, A.; Sullivan, E.V.; Rosenbloom, M.J.; Mathalon, D.H.; Lim, K.O. (1998). A controlled study of cortical gray matter and ventricular changes in alcoholic men over a five year interval. *Arch Gen Psychiatry* 55(10):905-912.

Phillips, S.C.; Harper, C.G.; Kril, J. (1987). A quantitative histological study of the cerebellar vermis in alcoholic patients. *Brain* 110:301-314.

Pierpaoli, C.; Barnett, A.; Pajevic, S.; Chen, R.; Penix, L.; Virta, A.; Basser, P.J. (2001). Water diffusion changes in Wallerian degeneration and their dependence on white matter architecture. *Neuroimage* 13:1174-1185.

Pierpaoli, C.; Basser, P.J. (1996). Towards a quantitative assessment of diffusion anisotropy. *Magn Reson Med* 36:893-906.

Raz, N. (1999). Aging of the brain and its impact on cognitive performance: Integration of structural and functional findings. In: F.I.M. Craik and T.A. Salthouse (Eds.), *Handbook of Aging and Cognition II* (pp. 1-90), Mahwah, NJ, Erlbaum.

Rosenbloom, M.J.; Pfefferbaum, A.; Sullivan, E.V. (2004). Recovery of short-term memory and psychomotor speed but not postural stability with long-term sobriety in alcoholic women. *Neuropsychology* 18(3):589-597.

Rosenbloom, M.J.; Sullivan, E.V.; Pfefferbaum, A. (2003). Using magnetic resonance imaging and diffusion tensor imaging to assess brain damage in alcoholics. *Alcohol Res Health* 27:146-152.

Salat, D.H.; Tuch, D.S.; Greve, D.N.; van der Kouwe, A.J.W.; Hevelone, N.D.; Zaleta, A.K.; Rosen, B.R. et al. (2005). Age-related alterations in white matter microstructure measured by diffusion tensor imaging. *Neurobiol Aging* 26: 1215-1227.

Schmahmann, J.D. (1996). From movement to thought: Anatomic substrates of the cerebellar contribution to cognitive processing. *Hum Brain Mapp* 4(3):174-198.

Schmahmann, J.D. (1997). *The Cerebellum and Cognition*, San Diego, Academic Press.

Schmahmann, J.D. (2000). The role of the cerebellum in affect and psychosis. *J Neurolinguist* 13:189-214.

Schmahmann, J.D.; Pandya, D.N. (1997). Anatomic organization of the basilar pontine projections from prefrontal cortices in rhesus monkey. *J Neurosci* 17(1):438-458.

Schuckit, M.A.; Anthenelli, R.M.; Bucholz, K.K.; Hesselbrock, V.M.; Tipp, J. (1995). The time course of development of alcohol-related problems in men and women. *J Stud Alcohol* 56(2):218-225.

Schulte, T.; Pfefferbaum, A.; Sullivan, E.V. (2003). Parallel interhemispheric processing in aging and alcoholism: Relation to corpus callosum size. *Neuropsychologia* 42(2):257-271.

Schulte, T.; Sullivan, E.V.; Müller-Oehring, E.M.; Adalsteinsson, E.; Pfefferbaum, A. (2005). Corpus callosal microstructural integrity influences interhemispheric processing: A diffusion tensor imaging study. *Cereb Cortex* 15:1384-1392.

Schweinsburg, B.; Taylor, M.; Videen, J.; Alhassoon, O.; Patterson, T.; Grant, I. (2000). Elevated myo-Inositol in gray matter of recently detoxified but not long-term abstinent alcoholics: A preliminary MR spectroscopy study. *Alcohol Clin Exp Res* 24:699-705.

Schweinsburg, B.C.; Alhassoon, O.M.; Taylor, M.J.; Gonzalez, R.; Videen, J.S.; Brown, G.G.; Patterson, T.L.; Grant, I. (2003). Effects of alcoholism and gender on brain metabolism. *Am J Psychiatry* 160(6):1180-1183.

Schweinsburg, B.C.; Taylor, M.J.; Alhassoon, O.M.; Videen, J.S.; Brown, G.G.; Patterson, T.L.; Berger, F.; Grant, I. (2001). Chemical pathology in brain white matter of recently detoxified alcoholics: A 1H magnetic resonance spectroscopy investigation of alcohol-associated frontal lobe injury. *Alcohol Clin Exp Res* 25(6):924-934.

Seitz, D.; Widmann, U.; Seeger, U.; Nagele, T.; Klose, U.; Mann, K.; Grodd, W. (1999). Localized proton magnetic resonance spectroscopy of the cerebellum in detoxifying alcoholics. *Alcohol Clin Exp Res* 23(1):158-163.

Shear, P.K.; Butters, N.; Jernigan, T.L.; DiTraglia, G.M.; Irwin, M.; Schuckit, M.A.; Cermak, L.S. (1992). Olfactory loss in alcoholics: Correlations with cortical and subcortical MRI indices. *Alcohol* 9(3):247-255.

Shear, P.K.; Jernigan, T.L.; Butters, N. (1994). Volumetric magnetic resonance imaging quantification of longitudinal brain changes in abstinent alcoholics. *Alcohol Clin Exp Res* 18(1):172-176.

Shear, P.K.; Sullivan, E.V.; Lane, B.; Pfefferbaum, A. (1996). Mammillary body and cerebellar shrinkage in chronic alcoholics with and without amnesia. *Alcohol Clin Exp Res* 20(8):1489-1495.

Sullivan, E.V. (2000). Human brain vulnerability to alcoholism: Evidence from neuroimaging studies. In: A. Noronha, M. Eckardt, and K. Warren (Eds.), *Review of NIAAA's Neuroscience and Behavioral Research Portfolio*, NIAAA Research Monograph No. 34 (pp. 473-508), Bethesda, MD, National Institutes of Health.

Sullivan, E.V. (2003). Compromised pontocerebellar and cerebellothalamocortical systems: Speculations on their contributions to cognitive and motor impairment in nonamnesic alcoholism. *Alcohol Clin Exp Res* 27(9):1409-1419.

Sullivan, E.V.; Deshmukh, A.; De Rosa, E.; Rosenbloom, M.J.; Pfefferbaum, A. (2005). Striatal and forebrain nuclei volumes: Contribution to motor function and working memory deficits in alcoholism. *Biol Psychiatry* 57(7):768-776.

Sullivan, E.V.; Deshmukh, A.; Desmond, J.E.; Lim, K.O.; Pfefferbaum, A. (2000a). Cerebellar volume decline in normal aging, alcoholism, and Korsakoff's syndrome: Relation to ataxia. *Neuropsychology* 14(3):341-352.

Sullivan, E.V.; Deshmukh, A.; Desmond, J.E.; Mathalon, D.H.; Rosenbloom, M.J.; Lim, K.O.; Pfefferbaum, A. (2000b). Contribution of alcohol abuse to cerebellar volume deficits in men with schizophrenia. *Arch Gen Psychiatry* 57(9):894-902.

Sullivan, E.V.; Desmond, J.E.; Lim, K.O.; Pfefferbaum, A. (2002). Speed and efficiency but not accuracy or timing deficits of limb movements in alcoholic men and women. *Alcohol Clin Exp Res* 26:705-713.

Sullivan, E.V.; Fama, R.; Rosenbloom, M.J.; Pfefferbaum, A. (2002). A profile of neuropsychological deficits in alcoholic women. *Neuropsychology* 16(1):74-83.

Sullivan, E.V.; Harding, A.J.; Pentney, R.; Dlugos, C.; Martin, P.R.; Parks, M.H.; Desmond, J.E. et al. (2003). Disruption of frontocerebellar circuitry and function in alcoholism. *Alcohol Clin Exp Res* 27:301-309.

Sullivan, E.V.; Lane, B.; Rosenbloom, M.J.; Deshmukh, A.; Desmond, J.; Lim, K.O.; Pfefferbaum, A. (1999). In vivo mammillary body volume deficits in amnesic and nonamnesic alcoholics. *Alcohol Clin Exp Res* 23(10):1629-1536.

Sullivan, E.V.; Marsh, L.; Mathalon, D.H.; Lim, K.O.; Pfefferbaum, A. (1995). Anterior hippocampal volume deficits in nonamnesic, aging chronic alcoholics. *Alcohol Clin Exp Res* 19:110-122.

Sullivan, E.V.; Marsh, L.; Mathalon, D.H.; Lim, K.O.; Pfefferbaum, A. (1996). Relationship between alcohol withdrawal seizures and temporal lobe white matter volume deficits. *Alcohol Clin Exp Res* 20(2):348-354.

Sullivan, E.V.; Pfefferbaum, A. (2001). Magnetic resonance relaxometry reveals central pontine abnormalities in clinically asymptomatic alcoholic men. *Alcohol Clin Exp Res* 25(6):1206-1212.

Sullivan, E.V.; Rose, J.; Pfefferbaum, A. (2004). Postural sway, sensorimotor integration, and the cerebellum (abs). In: *Annual Meeting of the Society for Neuroscience*, San Diego, CA.

Sullivan, E.V.; Rose, J.; Pfefferbaum, A. (2006). Effect of vision, touch, and stance on cerebellar vermian-related sway and tremor: A quantitative physiological and MRI study. *Cereb Cortex* 16(8):1077-1086.

Sullivan, E.V.; Rosenbloom, M.J.; Lim, K.O.; Pfefferbaum, A. (2000). Longitudinal changes in cognition, gait, and balance in abstinent and relapsed alcoholic men: Relationships to changes in brain structure. *Neuropsychology* 14(2):178-188.

Sullivan, E.V.; Rosenbloom, M.J.; Pfefferbaum, A. (2000). Pattern of motor and cognitive deficits in detoxified alcoholic men. *Alcohol Clin Exp Res* 24(5):611-621.

Sullivan, E.V.; Rosenbloom, M.J.; Serventi, K.L.; Deshmukh, A.; Pfefferbaum, A. (2003). The effects of alcohol dependence comorbidity and anti-psychotic medication on volumes of the thalamus and pons in schizophrenia. *Am J Psychiatry* 160:1110-1116.

Tarter, R.E.; Edwards, K.L. (1986). Multifactorial etiology of neuropsychological impairment in alcoholics. *Alcohol Clin Exp Res* 10(2):128-135.

Toma, K.; Nakai, T. (2002). Functional MRI in human motor control studies and clinical applications. *Magn Reson Med Sci* 1(2):109-120.

Torvik, A.; Torp, S. (1986). The prevalence of alcoholic cerebellar atrophy: A morphometric and histological study of an autopsy material. *J Neurol Sci* 75:43-51.

Victor, M.; Adams, R.D.; Collins, G.H. (1971). *The Wernicke-Korsakoff Syndrome*, Philadelphia, PA, F.A. Davis Co.

Villa, G.; Gainotti, G.; De Bonis, C.; Marra, C. (1990). Double dissociation between temporal and spatial pattern processing in patients with frontal and parietal damage. *Cortex* 26(3):399-407.

Virta, A.; Barnett, A.; Pierpaoli, C. (1999). Visualizing and characterizing white matter fiber structure and architecture in the human pyramidal tract using diffusion tensor MR. *J Magn Reson Imaging* 17(8):1121-1133.

Wang, Y.; Li, S.-J. (1998). Differentiation of metabolic concentrations between gray matter and white matter of human brain by in vivo 1H magnetic resonance spectroscopy. *Magn Reson Med* 39:28-33.

Wechsler, D. (1987). *Wechsler Memory Scale—Revised*, San Antonio, TX, The Psychological Corporation.

Wechsler, D. (1999). *The Wechsler Abbreviated Scale of Intelligence*, New York, The Psychological Corporation.

Wiggins, R.C.; Gorman, A.; Rolsten, C.; Samorajski, T.; Ballinger, W.E.; Freund, G. (1988). Effects of aging and alcohol on the biochemical composition of histologically normal human brain. *Metab Brain Dis* 3(1):67-80.

Chapter 5

Effects of Alcohol Abuse on Brain Neurochemistry

Fulton T. Crews

INTRODUCTION AND OVERVIEW

Alcohol is a major drug of use and abuse by Americans. An estimated 15 million Americans are alcohol abusers or are alcohol dependent (Massey et al., 1989). Lifetime prevalence of alcohol dependence is estimated at 13 percent and 4 percent for American men and women over 18 years of age, respectively (Grant and Dawson, 1997). According to the National Drug and Alcoholism Treatment Unit Survey (Massey et al., 1989), 1.8 million individuals were treated for alcoholism in the United States in 1989. It is well established that chronic excessive ethanol consumption produces deficits in cognitive and motor abilities (Crews, 1999; Sullivan, Rosenbloom, and Pfefferbaum, 2000; also see Chapters 2 and 3 of this book). Alcoholic dementia is a leading cause of adult dementia in the United States, accounting for approximately 10 percent of cases (Alzheimer's disease is the leading cause, accounting for 40 to 60 percent of cases) (Martin et al., 1986). Although evidence suggests reversibility of deficits with sobriety (Sullivan et al., 2000), studies report that 50 to 75 percent of sober, detoxified, long-term alcohol-dependent individuals suffer from some degree of detectable cognitive impairment, with approximately 10 percent being seriously demented (Martin et al., 1986). The effects of alcohol appear as a continuum, with moderate deficits in the majority of long-term alcoholics, progressing to the more severe deficits of Wernicke's disease and Wernicke's encephalopathy with Korsakoff's amnestic syndrome (Butterworth, 1995; Pfefferbaum et al., 1996). A variety of lifestyle factors, including nutrition, are implicated in

Handbook of the Medical Consequences of Alcohol and Drug Abuse
© 2008 by The Haworth Press, Taylor & Francis Group. All rights reserved.
doi:10.1300/6039_05

the more severe cases. However, all alcohol-induced deficits appear to be related to alcohol consumption and to the amount of alcohol consumed; that is, the more severe cases of brain damage are associated with more severe and long-term alcoholism (Butterworth, 1995; Pfefferbaum et al., 1996). Thus, alcohol can be neurotoxic when abused. The acute and chronic effects as well as the neurotoxic actions of alcohol appear to be due to changes in neuronal signaling. Our understanding of the effects of ethanol on the brain has increased tremendously in the past decade and will likely continue to increase as researchers investigate the specific sites of action of ethanol on the brain.

Ethanol Effects on Neuronal Signaling

A review of all of the actions of ethanol on neuronal signaling is not addressed in this chapter due to the extensive number of studies and a poor understanding of how changes in neuronal signaling relate to the effects of ethanol. This chapter will focus on the glutamate and GABA (gamma-aminobutyric acid) neurotransmitter systems because they are the major excitatory and inhibitory neurotransmitters in the brain, respectively, and appear to be the predominant neurotransmitters involved in the actions of ethanol on the brain.

ETHANOL EFFECTS ON GLUTAMATE RECEPTOR ION CHANNELS

Glutamate receptors are altered by ethanol and represent major excitatory receptors in the brain. The three classes of ionotropic glutamate receptors include the *N*-methyl-D-aspartic acid (NMDA), kainate, and L-α-amino-3-hydroxy-5-methyl-4-isoxazole proportionate (AMPA) receptor subtypes (Bettler and Mulle, 1995; Hollmann and Heineman, 1994; Sommer and Seeburg, 1992; Sprengel and Seeburg, 1993). There is also a group of metabotropic receptors that couple to secondary messengers, for example, G-protein coupled receptors. Although there is some evidence that ethanol directly or indirectly affects all types of glutamate receptors, overwhelming evidence and a vast literature document ethanol's direct effects on NMDA receptors and the radical changes in neuronal signaling and cognitive function that result. As such, the focus of this section will be on NMDA receptors with a brief discussion of other glutamate receptors.

NMDA Receptors

Late in 1991, a report appeared in *Nature* that an NMDA-receptor complementary DNA (cDNA) had been cloned from a rat brain (Moriyoshi et al., 1991). The protein described by Moriyoshi et al. was designated as NMDAR-1 and had significant sequence homology with previously identified AMPA/kainate receptors (Hollmann et al., 1989). It is now clear that this cDNA was associated with the classic NMDA receptor previously identified pharmacologically (Davies et al., 1981; Watkins, 1962). NMDAR-1 was immediately recognized to have a ubiquitous distribution in the brain (Monyer et al., 1994; Moriyoshi et al., 1991) and later to have eight splice variants generated from the presence of three cassettes—two on the C-terminal and one on the N-terminal (Durand et al., 1992; Nakanishi, Axel, and Shneider, 1992; Sugihara et al., 1992). The discovery of the splice variants for the NMDAR-1 subunit provided the potential for heterogeneity among NMDA receptors. Partial probes of these NMDAR-1 variants showed by in situ hybridization that these variants were differentially distributed in the brain (Laurie and Seeburg, 1994; Monyer et al., 1994; Standaert et al., 1993). Pharmacologically, the type "A" splice variants (lacking the N-terminal cassette) possess greater agonist potencies, lower antagonist associations, and are potentiated by Zn^{2+} (Hollmann et al., 1993). The converse is true for type "B" variants (with the N-terminal insert).

Other NMDA subunits homologous to the NMDAR-1 subunit were subsequently cloned and are referred to as NMDAR-2A, -2B, -2C, and -2D (Meguro et al., 1992; Monyer et al., 1992; Nakanishi, Axel, and Shneider, 1992; Yamazaki et al., 1992), although another classification system based upon cloning from mouse brains refers to these same subunits as ξ1-4 (Kutsuwada et al., 1992; Meguro et al., 1992; Yamazaki et al., 1992). All NMDAR-2 subunits must be expressed with an NMDAR-1 subunit for maximal sensitivity to NMDA (Monyer et al., 1992; Nakanishi, Axel, and Shneider, 1992). As was found for the variants of the NMDAR-1 subunit, the NMDAR-2 subunits have a discrete neuroanatomical localization in the brain (Ishii et al., 1993; Monyer et al., 1992). Comparisons with other ion channel receptors and a variety of other direct NMDA receptor studies have led to the conclusion that endogenous NMDA receptors are heteromeric multisubunit complexes of NMDAR-1 and NMDAR-2 subunits with a wide variety of combinations in *different* brain regions.

NMDA receptor heterogeneity has also been demonstrated with Mg^{2+} (Mayer, Westbrook, and Guthrie, 1984; Nowak et al., 1984), redox manipulations (Sullivan et al., 1994), polyamines (Bowe and Nadler, 1995; Ransom and Stec, 1988; Reynolds, 1990; Reynolds and Miller, 1989; Rock and

Macdonald, 1995), glycine (Igarashi and Williams, 1995; Johnson and Ascher, 1987; Kleckner and Dingledine, 1988; Reynolds, Murphy, and Miller, 1987), Zn^{2+} (Peters, Koh, and Choi, 1987; Westbrook and Mayer, 1987), and noncompetitive NMDA antagonists (Reynolds and Miller, 1989; Williams et al., 1993, 1994). The variants of the NMDAR-1 subunit and the four NMDAR-2 subunits provide the potential for considerable heterogeneity among NMDA receptor isoforms (Buller et al., 1994; Durand et al., 1992; Ishii et al., 1993; Kumar et al., 1991; Meguro et al., 1992; Monaghan, 1991; Monyer et al., 1992, 1994; Moriyoshi et al., 1991; Nakanishi, Axel, and Shneider, 1992; Sugihara et al., 1992). Pharmacological studies of the noncompetitive NMDA antagonist ifenprodil provide evidence that multiple NMDA receptor isoforms exist in the brain (Williams et al., 1993). The action and binding of ifenprodil appear to be selective for the NMDAR-2B subunit (Lovinger, 1995; Nicolas and Carter, 1994; Williams et al., 1993, 1994). Ifenprodil inhibition of NMDA receptors through the NMDAR-2B subunit was hypothesized from research that ifenprodil inhibited NMDA responses from a recombinant receptor formed by the NMDAR-1A and NMDAR-2B subunits, but was found to be relatively inactive against the combination of NMDAR-1A and NMDAR-2A subunits (Lynch et al., 1995; Williams et al., 1993, 1994). When developmental expression of NMDA subunits was evaluated, an association was also found between ifenprodil binding and the presence of the NMDAR-1A and NMDAR-2B subunits, but not the NMDAR-2A subunits (Molinoff et al., 1994; Zhong et al., 1994). As the NMDAR-2B subunit has a variable distribution in the brain (Monyer et al., 1992, 1994), it was presumed that ifenprodil would affect responses to NMDA in vivo in a subset of neurons which expressed the NMDAR-2B subunit, and this was indeed found to be the case (Yang et al., 1996). Although the basic molecular mechanism of ifenprodil antagonism has yet to be determined, evidence is convincing that the NMDAR-2B receptor subunit is important to the action of this drug. The particular importance of ifenprodil to the pharmacological action of ethanol on NMDA responses will become clear later in this chapter.

Ethanol's Physiological Actions Mediated Through Changes in NMDA Receptor Function

Initial evidence that ethanol antagonizes NMDA-induced responses came from electrophysiological studies (Lima-Landman and Albuquerque, 1989; Lovinger, White, and Weight, 1989, 1990; Weight, 1992), as well as in vitro experiments which show that ethanol inhibits NMDA activation of calcium flux and cGMP formation (Dildy and Leslie, 1989; Hoffman, Moses, and

Tabakoff, 1989; Hoffman et al., 1989). Electrophysiological studies performed in vivo (Frohlich, Patzelt, and Illes, 1994) have provided additional evidence that low-to-moderate concentrations of ethanol antagonize NMDA-induced increases in firing rate. Rats trained to discriminate doses of ethanol (1.0, 1.5, and 2.0 g/kg) from water substituted the noncompetitive NMDA antagonists, phencyclidine (PCP) and dizocipline (MK-801) for higher doses of ethanol (Grant and Colombo, 1993). In contrast, the competitive NMDA receptor antagonist, CPPene, did not substitute for ethanol in this paradigm (Grant et al., 1991). It was concluded that antagonism of NMDA receptor function by a channel-blocking NMDA antagonist is perceived by the animal as equivalent to the administration of ethanol (Grant and Colombo, 1993). This latter finding indicates that inhibition of NMDA receptors is an important mechanism by which ethanol affects brain function. Thus, strong evidence supports that moderate concentrations of ethanol antagonize NMDA responses and that this action of ethanol has functional consequences.

Differential Action of Ethanol on NMDA-Stimulated Responses

Following the seminal findings concerning ethanol antagonism of NMDA (Simson, Criswell, and Breese, 1993; Simson et al., 1991), using in vivo recording techniques in anesthetized rats, it was found that systemically administered ethanol antagonized the effect of NMDA on some, but not all, cells in the medial septum. Local application of ethanol onto neurons was later found to reduce NMDA-stimulated responses, eliminating the possibility that systemic administration of ethanol was acting at distant brain sites to inhibit NMDA at the recording site (Criswell et al., 1993; Simson, Criswell, and Breese, 1993). Initial extracellular recordings that found sensitive and insensitive NMDA-stimulated responses in the medial septum and substantia nigra reticulata (SNR) (Breese et al., 1993; Criswell et al., 1993; Simson, Criswell, and Breese, 1993), have been extended to additional sites in the brain including the ventral tegmental area, the deep mesencephalic nucleus, and the red nucleus (Yang et al., 1996). In the hippocampus, ethanol inhibited NMDA responses from all neurons, but did not antagonize NMDA-stimulated responses in the lateral septum, suggesting a degree of brain regional specificity for ethanol's inhibition. Using calcium flux, Wilson, Bosy, and Ruth (1990) also found regional differences in ethanol inhibition of NMDA-stimulated responses that were consistent with earlier findings (Criswell et al., 1993; Simson, Criswell, and Breese, 1993; Simson et al., 1991). Regional differences in NMDA antagonism by ethanol support the hypothesis that these differences were due to regional differences in NMDA receptor isoform expression.

NMDA Receptor Isoforms and Differential Ethanol Sensitivity

The existence of a relationship between the ability of ifenprodil and ethanol to inhibit NMDA-stimulated responses is supported by recent studies. During a four-week period, neocortical neurons in culture showed a decreased sensitivity to both ethanol and ifenprodil inhibition of NMDA-stimulated responses as the neurons matured (Lovinger, 1995). Both ifenprodil and ethanol were found to inhibit recombinant NMDA receptors containing the NMDAR-2B subunit. The ability of ethanol to inhibit NMDA responses was recently compared to ifenprodil (Yang et al., 1996). Whenever ethanol antagonized an NMDA-stimulated response, ifenprodil also inhibited this response. However, neurons were identified to which ifenprodil antagonized NMDA-stimulated responses, but ethanol did not (Yang et al., 1996). Thus, the most likely mechanism of differential ethanol inhibition of NMDA-stimulated responses appears to be related to the expression of different NMDA receptor isoforms; that is, different receptor isoforms are more or less sensitive to ethanol inhibition (Breese et al., 1993; Criswell et al., 1993; Simson, Criswell, and Breese, 1993; Yang et al., 1996).

Several studies support the hypothesis that ethanol has a differential action on NMDA receptor isoforms. As mentioned earlier, ifenprodil most potently inhibits a subset of NMDA receptors that contain the NMDAR-2B subunit (Williams et al., 1993) and inhibits NMDA receptors that are sensitive to ethanol inhibition in cultured neurons (Lovinger, 1995) and in vivo (Yang et al., 1996). Reconstitution studies also suggest that ethanol has selective actions on particular subtypes of NMDA receptors. Several investigators have combined the NMDAR-1A variant with the four NMDAR-2 subunits in *Xenopus* oocytes or HEK-293 cells and examined the action of ethanol on responses to NMDA (Buller et al., 1995; Chu, Anantharam, and Treistman, 1995; Lovinger, 1995; Masood et al., 1994; Mirshahi and Woodward, 1995). Consistent with neuronal studies that suggest NMDAR-2B and ifenprodil predict potent inhibitory actions of ethanol, the ε2 subunit (mouse NMDAR-2B subunit) when expressed with the ζ1 (mouse NMDAR-1A variant) in *Xenopus* oocytes is significantly inhibited by concentrations of ethanol less than 25 mM (Masood et al., 1994). Higher concentrations of ethanol also inhibited ε1 (mouse NMDAR-2A subunit) combined with the ζ1, but concentrations as high as 100 mM had little or no effect on ε3 (mouse NMDAR-2C subunit) and ε4 (mouse NMDAR-2D subunit) combined with ζ1 (mouse NMDAR-1A subunit). Similar studies done by Buller et al. (1995) found both NMDAR-2A and NMDAR-2B in combination with NMDAR-1A to be the NMDA receptor isoforms most sensitive to inhibition by ethanol. All studies agree that the recombinant NMDA receptors containing either the NMDAR-2C or the NMDAR-2D subunits with the NMDAR-1A subunit are not sensitive to ethanol inhibition (Buller et al., 1995; Lovinger, 1995; Masood et al., 1994). Lovinger (1995) found that the NMDA receptor formed from NMDAR-1A and NMDAR-2A was inhibited by ethanol, however, when NMDAR-2B was added, the recombinant NMDA receptor was considerably more sensitive to ethanol inhibition of NMDA than the recombinant receptor containing only the NMDAR-2A subunit. In vivo, NMDA receptors in the cerebral cortex likely contain combinations of NMDAR-1, NMDAR-2A, and NMDAR-2B subunits (Sheng et al., 1994). Taken together, the findings suggest that NMDA receptors containing NMDAR-2B subunits, alone or in combination with NMDAR-2A subunits, are likely to make up the NMDA receptor isoforms most sensitive to ethanol inhibition whereas those containing NMDAR-2C or NMDAR-2D subunits are likely to be relatively insensitive to inhibition by ethanol.

The presence of specific NMDAR-1 subunit variants (Monyer et al., 1992) may also contribute to differential sensitivity of NMDA isoforms to inhibition by ethanol. Koltchine et al. (1993) provided evidence that four of the NMDAR-1 variants had differential sensitivity to ethanol, with the variant containing both the N-terminal and another cassette being the most sensitive to inhibition by ethanol when expressed in oocytes as homomeric assemblies. When the NMDAR-1B subunit, which contains the N-terminal cassette, was combined with the NMDAR-2B or NMDAR-2A subunit, the resulting isoforms were more sensitive to ethanol inhibition of NMDA than isoforms with NMDAR-2C or -2D subunits (Chu, Anantharam, and Treistman, 1995). As NMDAR-1A variants, which lack an N-terminal insert (Durand, Bennett, and Zukin, 1993; Durand et al., 1992), are also sensitive to ethanol when combined with the NMDAR-2B subunit, it is possible that the NMDAR-1 variants in combination with the NMDAR-2 variants indicate that there is a wide spectrum of NMDA receptor isoforms with differential sensitivity to inhibition by ethanol. Thus, for the NMDAR-1 variants investigated, an interaction of both the R-1 splice variant properties combined with the various NMDAR-2 subunits appears to modulate the sensitivity to ethanol, with NMDAR-1 variants containing inserts and NMDAR-2B subunits apparently being the most sensitive to inhibition by ethanol.

NMDA Receptor Modulatory Sites and Differential Sensitivity to Ethanol

Another aspect regarding differential inhibition of NMDA receptors by ethanol could involve an interaction with specific modulatory sites on the NMDA receptor (Johnson and Ascher, 1987; Peters, Koh, and Choi, 1987;

Reynolds and Miller, 1989). Glycine was reported to reverse ethanol inhibition of NMDA-induced calcium flux and cyclic guanosine monophosphate (cGMP) in cerebellar granule cells (Dildy and Leslie, 1989; Hoffman et al., 1989; Rabe and Tabakoff, 1990). However, glycine did not reverse ethanol inhibition of NMDA-stimulated excitotoxicity in cerebral cortical neurons (Chandler et al., 1993) or patch clamp responses in cultured hippocampal neurons (Peoples and Weight, 1992). Studies by Buller et al. (1995) may explain these contradictory results. Buller et al. demonstrated that NMDA-stimulated responses in *Xenopus* oocytes containing the recombinant NMDAR-1A/NMDAR-2B subunits were desensitized by the addition of ethanol when subsaturating concentrations of glycine were present (Buller et al., 1995). Increasing the concentration of glycine reversed this desensitization. However, other aspects of this study clearly demonstrate glycine-independent components. This work suggests that ethanol can have two distinct effects on NMDA-stimulated responses depending on the glycine concentration. Manipulations of various other modulatory sites (e.g., polyamines, Mg^{2+}, Zn^{2+}) or the presence of the drug dithiothreitol (i.e., oxidation and reduction) did not affect ethanol inhibition of NMDA in recombinant systems (Chu, Anantharam, and Treistman, 1995; Matsumoto et al., 1993).

NMDA Receptor Phosphorylation and Differential Sensitivity to Ethanol

Phosphorylation is important in direct and indirect modulation of NMDA receptors and several studies have demonstrated that phosphorylation may contribute to NMDA receptors' *differential* sensitivity to ethanol (Huganir and Greengard, 1990; Wright, Sefland, and Walaas, 1993). The NMDA receptor subunits contain a site that allows for phosphorylation by protein kinase C (PKC) and other kinases (Lieberman and Mody, 1994; Monyer et al., 1992; Nakanishi, Axel, and Shneider, 1992). Snell, Tabakoff, and Hoffman (1994) found that staurosporine or calphostin, PKC inhibitors, reversed the inhibitory effect of ethanol on NMDA-stimulated responses, suggesting that ethanol may facilitate phosphorylation of the NMDA receptor and thereby inhibit NMDA-stimulated responses. Consequently, the proper phosphorylation state of the NMDA receptor may be required for ethanol and ifenprodil inhibition of NMDA. However, Tabakoff (1995) noted that PKC does not appear to have the same role in all cell populations in determining the effect of ethanol on NMDA-stimulated responses, and stated that more investigation is needed to define clearly the role of NMDA receptor phosphorylation in differential sensitivity to ethanol.

Differential Action of Ethanol
on AMPA/Kainate-Stimulated Responses

Initial investigations with low-to-moderate concentrations of ethanol suggested that ethanol did not affect the function of non-NMDA glutamate receptors (Hoffman et al., 1989; Lovinger, White, and Weight, 1989; Simson, Criswell, and Breese, 1993). These reports have given way to data indicating that ethanol can inhibit agonist-stimulated responses, but some controversy and uncertainty still exists about the concentration of ethanol required for this action to occur.

Lovinger, White, and Weight (1989) reported that only high concentrations of ethanol (~100 mM) can antagonize kainate-stimulated responses in cultured neurons from fetal rodent brains. Likewise, ethanol (>100 mM) was shown to inhibit responses from recombinant AMPA-type glutamate receptor subunits expressed in kidney 243 cells (Lovinger, 1993). Based on work with cultured neurons Weight et al. (1993) reported that only ethanol concentrations above 50 mM affected the non-NMDA receptors, suggesting that ethanol's ability to produce general anesthesia could be attributed to inhibition of kainate and AMPA receptor function. High concentrations of ethanol (100 mM) have also been found to inhibit kainate and AMPA responses in vivo in the rat locus coeruleus (Frohlich, Patzelt, and Illes, 1994). Collectively, these data suggested that non-NMDA receptors are considerably less sensitive to ethanol than NMDA receptors, although some regional differences may exist in brain (Gonzales, 1990).

A particularly important observation made by Dildy-Mayfield and Harris (1992a,b) was that ethanol inhibition was potentiated at lower, rather than higher, concentrations of kainate. In fact, the inhibition of a low concentration of AMPA by ethanol was similar to that seen for NMDA. The region of the brain may also be a contributing factor as to whether ethanol affects non-NMDA receptors (Dildy-Mayfield and Harris, 1992a,b). Martin, Tayyeb and Swartzwelder (1995) found that ethanol inhibited agonist responses to the non-NMDA receptors in hippocampal slices, but as noted in earlier studies, this action depended greatly on the concentration of the agonist used. Similarly, Chandler et al. (1994) found that AMPA-stimulated nitrous oxide formation in cerebral cortical cultures was inhibited by ethanol. Thus, there is no question that ethanol can inhibit non-NMDA receptor stimulated responses. However, a complete understanding of the differences observed between the various studies as to the concentration of ethanol required to inhibit kainate- or AMPA-stimulated responses is yet to be resolved. It is possible that the variable effects of ethanol relate to the differing subunit composition of various non-NMDA receptor subtypes. In addition, consensus sites are found on some subunits for protein kinase II and PKC (Keinanen et al., 1990; Wright, Sefland, and Walaas, 1993). Thus, phosphorylation could account for some of the *differences* observed. These potential reasons for the varying observations need to be critically tested.

Until recently there has been much controversy regarding the effect of ethanol on kainate receptors. This was mainly due to the inability of researchers to pharmacologically isolate kainate receptors from other glutamate receptors. The few studies mentioned previously found that ethanol inhibited kainate receptor function in recombinant receptor systems. However, these findings only suggested such an effect was possible, as the characteristics of recombinant kainate receptors *differ* from endogenous receptors.

AMPA receptor antagonists recently became available allowing researchers to characterize endogenous kainate receptors and ethanol's effect upon them. Two groups have since investigated kainate receptors and their sensitivity to ethanol, one in cerebellar granule cells (Valenzuela, Cardoso, et al., 1998) and one in CA3 pyramidal neurons (Weiner, Dunwiddie, and Valenzuela, 1999). Both groups found that intoxicating concentrations of ethanol inhibited kainate currents and Weiner's group also found that ethanol in concentrations as low as 20 mM depressed kainate excitatory postsynaptic currents. Further studies are necessary to more fully characterize ethanol's inhibition of kainate receptors and any behavioral or cognitive consequences that may occur.

ETHANOL EFFECTS
ON GABA$_A$/BENZODIAZEPINE RECEPTORS

Gamma-aminobutyric acid is the most ubiquitous inhibitory neurotransmitter in the brain. GABA interacts with a family of receptors containing recognition sites for the anxiolytic and sedative benzodiazepines, barbiturates, and endogenous neurosteroids. These binding sites are linked allosterically to a GABA recognition site, and each site is involved directly or indirectly in the gating properties of integral chloride channels. GABA receptor-mediated activation of Cl$^-$ conductance results in membrane hyperpolarization and decreased neuronal excitability (Skolnick and Paul, 1982). Ethanol alters the gating properties of this receptor complex; however, ethanol binds with little or no affinity to recognition sites for GABA, benzodiazepines, barbiturates, or cage convulsants (Davis and Ticku, 1981; Greenberg et al., 1984). GABA$_A$ receptor isoforms are heteromeric protein complexes consisting of five distinct, yet homologous, membrane-spanning glycoprotein subunits. These subunits exist in eight major classes: α, β, γ, δ, ϵ, θ, π, and ρ (Levitan et al., 1988; Schofield, 1989; Schofield et al., 1987). Within each class of subunits, there are various isoforms that include α1-6, β1-4, γ1-4, δ, and ρ1-2 (Cutting et al., 1991, 1992). Additional variants are possible due to posttranslational processing (see Macdonald and Olsen, 1994, for review; Seeburg et al., 1990). The structural features of GABA$_A$ receptor channels have been inferred to a large extent by analogy to nicotinic, cholinergic, and glycine receptors, which are members of the superfamily of ligand-gated ion channels (Unwin, 1989). However, the pentameric structure of native GABA$_A$ receptors has been confirmed by electron microscopy and rotational spin analysis of isolated receptors (Nayeem et al., 1994).

The actual subunit composition of GABA$_A$ receptor isoforms in vivo is not yet known. However, it is clear that subunit composition determines the pharmacological and functional properties of GABA$_A$ receptor isoforms.

For example, the coexpression of different β and γ subunits in recombinant expression systems results in GABA$_A$ receptors with *different* pharmacological properties, and may account for the functional heterogeneity of GABA$_A$ receptors (Levitan et al., 1988; Pritchett, Lüddens, and Seeburg, 1989; Pritchett et al., 1989; Puia et al., 1991; Wafford et al., 1990). In transient expression systems, benzodiazepine type I binding characteristics are observed with the expression of α2βxγ2 subunits (where x indicates any β subunit). In contrast, the expression of α2βxγ2, α3βxγ2, or α5βxγ2 subunits results in benzodiazepine type II pharmacology (Pritchett, Lüddens, and Seeburg, 1989). Further diversity of ~2 subunits are created by an 8-aminoacid insertion site of the GABA$_A$ receptor ~2L subunit, which encodes a sequence that can be phosphorylated by PKC (Whiting, McKernan, and Iversen, 1990) and appears to confer ethanol sensitivity to recombinant GABA$_A$ receptors expressed in some circumstances (Wafford and Whiting, 1992; Wafford et al., 1991). There is increasing evidence that all GABA$_A$ receptor subunit combinations contribute to specific functional properties in assembled receptors. The expression of α1, α2, α3, or α5 subunits with β1, β2, or β3 subunits in conjunction with γ2L subunits in frog oocytes results in 12 receptors that exhibit unique pharmacological properties (White and Gurley, 1995). Understanding the heterogeneity of native GABA$_A$ receptors will provide additional insight into heterogeneous signaling in the brain.

The functional properties of GABA$_A$ receptors may also be influenced by posttranslational mechanisms that are presumed to alter receptor conformation. The potential role of phosphorylation in the regulation of GABA responses is controversial. Evidence suggests that GABA receptor phosphorylation is both associated with (Heuschneider and Schwartz, 1989; Leidenheimer et al., 1990; Porter et al., 1990) and prevents (Gyenes, Farrant, and Farb, 1988; Stelzer, Kay, and Wong, 1988) $GABA_A$ receptor desensitization. Artifacts related to the actions of cAMP, which are independent of protein phosphorylation, have been described (Heuschneider and Schwartz, 1989; Leidenheimer et al., 1990) and complicate the interpretation of the results of these studies. In addition, the heterogeneity of $GABA_A$ receptors may explain some of the conflicting results. Another mechanism may involve $GABA_A$ receptor isoforms that are phosphorylated by maximal GABA stimulation, whereas other isoforms are not. $GABA_A$ receptors contain putative phosphorylation sites on $\beta 1$-3 and $\gamma 2L$ subunits (Wang and Burt, 1991; Ymer et al., 1989), but the expression of these subunits varies in different brain regions (Wang and Burt, 1991; Zhang et al., 1995). Thus, the potential role of phosphorylation and other posttranslational processes remains obscure.

Ethanol Interactions with GABA_A Receptors

Ethanol is believed to act at many sites in the brain, but $GABA_A$/benzodiazepine receptors may be the major targets responsible for many of its behavioral effects. GABA-mimetic drugs enhance and prolong the behavioral effects of ethanol, while antagonists shorten ethanol narcosis (Frye and Breese, 1982; Martz, Dietrich, and Harris, 1983). Likewise, benzodiazepines and GABA-mimetics ameliorate the symptoms of ethanol withdrawal (Frye, McCown, and Breese, 1983a; Sellers and Kalant, 1976), while GABA antagonists potentiate these symptoms (Goldstein, 1973). Furthermore, benzodiazepine receptor inverse agonists, such as Ro15-4513 and FG-7142, antagonize many ethanol-induced behaviors in the rat, including intoxication (Koob, Percy, and Britton, 1989; Lister, 1988; Suzdak, Glowa et al., 1986; Suzdak et al., 1988). The behavioral effects of various chain-length alcohols have also been used to establish a link between alcohol interactions with GABA receptors and the production of their behavioral effects. Recent studies have shown that while short-chain alcohols activate $GABA_A$ receptors (Suzdak, Schwartz, and Paul, 1987), long-chain alcohols (greater than ten carbons) no longer activate $GABA_A$ receptors (Dildy-Mayfield et al., 1996). This loss of GABA activation correlates with the effects of various length alcohols on the loss of righting reflex in tadpoles (Dildy-Mayfield et al., 1996). Site-specific effects of ethanol on $GABA_A$ receptors that result in sedation have been demonstrated in the medial septum (Givens and Breese, 1990b).

Direct evidence that ethanol interacts with $GABA_A$ receptors at pharmacologically relevant concentrations has been demonstrated in studies using subcellular brain preparations and cultured embryonic neurons, wherein ethanol and other short-chain alcohols have been shown to stimulate (Suzdak,

Schwartz, and Paul, 1987; Suzdak, Schwartz, et al., 1986) or potentiate $GABA_A$ receptor-mediated $36Cl^-$ uptake (Allan and Harris, 1986; Mehta and Ticku, 1988; Suzdak, Schwartz, and Paul, 1987; Suzdak, Schwartz, et al., 1986; Ticku, Lowrimore, and Lehoullier, 1986). Electrophysiological studies have confirmed that ethanol enhances $GABA_A$ receptor-mediated Cl-conductance, but only in specific brain regions (Celentano, Gibbs, and Farb, 1988; Givens and Breese, 1990a,b; Mereu and Gessa, 1985; Nestores, 1980) or cell populations (Aguayo, 1990; Reynolds and Prasad, 1991). The regional specificity of ethanol interactions with GABA was first observed by Givens and Breese (1990a,b), who demonstrated that ethanol enhances GABA responses in the medial septal nucleus, but not the lateral septal nucleus. Subsequent studies have defined several brain regions where electrophysiological responses to GABA are both sensitive and insensitive to ethanol (Criswell et al., 1993, 1995). Several researchers have suggested that the subunit composition of $GABA_A$ receptors determines the presence or absence of ethanol sensitivity (Breese et al., 1993; Criswell et al., 1993; Givens and Breese, 1990a; Morrow, Herbert, and Montpied, 1992; Wafford et al., 1990). This hypothesis has been supported by studies of mammalian brain regions in which ethanol sensitivity is highly correlated with the simultaneous presence of benzodiazepine type I ([3H]zolpidem) binding sites (Breese et al., 1993; Criswell et al., 1993, 1995) and $GABA_A$ receptor $\alpha 1$, $\beta 2$, and $\gamma 2$ subunits (Criswell et al., 1993; Duncan et al., 1995). It is not clear from these studies whether the $\gamma 2$ subunit splice variants influence ethanol sensitivity in the rat brain, as $\gamma 2L$ subunits were abundant in both ethanol-sensitive and ethanol-insensitive sites (Criswell et al., 1993; Duncan et al., 1995). However, it is clear that ethanol potentiation of $GABA_A$ receptors may be limited to very specific subtypes of $GABA_A$ receptors that have a unique regional distribution in the brain.

Additional evidence suggests that other $GABA_A$ receptor isoforms may exhibit ethanol sensitivity under certain circumstances. Several investigators have found that ethanol modulates GABA responses in cerebellar Purkinje cells if α-adrenergic receptors are coactivated (Knapp, Criswell, and Breese, 1995; Lin, Freund, and Palmer, 1991; Palmer et al., 1988). Cerebellar granule cells contain recognition sites for the benzodiazepine inverse agonist, Ro15-4513, which antagonizes the effects of ethanol on GABA-mediated responses such as the righting reflex. As this site is not sensitive to zolpidem, it is assumed that it identifies a distinct $GABA_A$ receptor isoform that responds to ethanol. The subunit composition of this receptor is likely to include $\alpha 6$ subunits as this subunit appears to contain the Ro15-4513 recognition site (Lüddens et al., 1990). In the cerebral cortex, Ro15-4513 appears to label a $GABA_A$ receptor comprised of $\alpha 4$ subunits (Wisden et al., 1991).

Chronic ethanol administration increases [3H]Ro15-4513 binding in the cortex and cerebellum (Mhatre, Mehta, and Ticku, 1988), as well as $\alpha4$ (Devaud, Morrow, et al., 1995) and ~6 subunits (Mhatre and Ticku, 1993; Morrow, Herbert, and Montpied, 1992), respectively. Therefore, these GABA$_A$ receptor isoforms probably exhibit ethanol sensitivity in vivo.

The question of whether ethanol enhancement of GABA responses is dependent on receptor subunit composition has been directly addressed in various recombinant expression systems. In frog oocytes, the expression of the human γ2L subunit has been reported to be required for ethanol potentiation of GABA responses (Wafford and Whiting, 1992; Wafford et al., 1991), but other studies have not confirmed this effect (Mihic et al., 1994; Sigel, Baur, and Malherbe, 1993). In mouse LTK cells, $\alpha1\beta1$ γ2L and $\alpha1\beta1$ γ2S recombinant receptors are sensitive to ethanol, though greater sensitivity was observed when the γ2L subunit was expressed (Ryan-Jastrow and Macdonald, 1993). Using the HEK293 expression system, the γ2 splice variant does not influence ethanol enhancement of GABA responses (Ryan-Jastrow and Macdonald, 1993). Conversely, stably transfected PA3 cells are only sensitive to ethanol when the γ2L variant is expressed with $\alpha1$ and $\beta1$ subunits (Harris, Proctor, et al., 1995). The lack of consistent results in recombinant expression systems suggests that factors other than subunit composition can influence ethanol interactions with GABA$_A$ receptors. These factors could include *differences* in membrane properties, intracellular messengers, and/or receptor assembly that may exist among recombinant expression systems and mammalian brains. The extent to which these factors modulate the functional properties of GABA$_A$ receptors is a question of considerable importance in the interpretation of structure-function studies in recombinant expression systems.

Ethanol's Effects on GABA$_A$ Receptors Mediated by Posttranslational Modifications

Recent studies in recombinant receptor systems, where subunit expression is controlled by a dexamethasone-sensitive promoter, exhibit changes in receptor function that cannot be attributed to alterations in subunit expression (Klein et al., 1995). A possible explanation for these changes in receptor function may involve posttranslational modification of GABA$_A$ receptors and secondary messenger systems. Tyrosine phosphorylation of GABA$_A$ receptors has been shown to enhance GABA$_A$ receptor-gated currents (Valenzuela et al., 1995). As noted previously, tyrosine phosphorylation of NMDA receptors has also been linked to the development of acute tolerance of NMDA receptors. PKC, protein kinase A (PKA), and calmodulin kinase II have been reported to phosphorylate and/or alter the function of NMDA or GABA$_A$ receptors. In addition, mouse mutants that lack a PKC isoform exhibit a loss of ethanol sensitivity both in vivo and at the cellular level (Harris, McQuilkin, et al., 1995). Thus, ethanol tolerance and dependence may also involve secondary messengers associated with GABA$_A$ receptors.

CHANGES IN NMDA AND GABA$_A$ RECEPTORS DURING CHRONIC ALCOHOL ABUSE AND WITHDRAWAL

Chronic Ethanol Alters NMDA Receptor Function and Expression

Hyperexcitability of the central nervous system (CNS) is a key component of ethanol withdrawal and a sign of alcohol dependence (Frye, McCown, and Breese, 1983a,b; Grant et al., 1990). Both a reduction in GABA-mediated inhibition (Frye, McCown, and Breese, 1983a,b) and a supersensitive NMDA response appear to be involved. One of the earliest findings suggesting glutamate involvement was the finding that [^{3}H]glutamate binding is increased in the hippocampus of alcoholics (Michaelis et al., 1990). Although the isoform of glutamate receptor involved is not known, this is consistent with increased glutamate receptor density. Several studies of neuronal cells in culture have indicated that a few days of chronic ethanol treatment leads to supersensitive NMDA-stimulated calcium flux (Ahern, Lustig, and Greenberg, 1994; Iorio et al., 1992), as well as NMDA-stimulated excitotoxicity (Ahern, Lustig, and Greenberg, 1994; Chandler et al., 1993; Crews and Chandler, 1993; Crews et al., 1993; Iorio, Tabakoff, and Hoffman, 1993) and NMDA-stimulated nitric oxide formation (Chandler, Sumners, and Crews, 1995). Although the mechanisms are not totally resolved, it is clear that chronic ethanol can induce NMDA supersensitivity and likely contributes to the hyperexcitability and seizures associated with ethanol withdrawal. It may also cause neurotoxicity. Supersensitivity could occur through a number of mechanisms including increased density of the NMDA receptors, changes in subunit composition, and increased release of glutamate.

Nitric oxide has been implicated in toxicity due to the formation of highly oxidative metabolites (Crews and Chandler, 1993). Although both nitric oxide and excitotoxicity show supersensitivity as indicated by left shifts in the dose response curves, the finding that nitric oxide production is maximal at the minimum threshold concentration for NMDA-stimulated excitotoxicity suggests that nitric oxide may contribute to excitotoxicity, but is not likely to be the only factor involved. Although supersensitivity was found in both nitric oxide and excitotoxicity, changes in the amount of NMDAR-1 immunoreactivity were not found, suggesting that changes in the NMDA receptor subunit composition, phosphorylation, or other posttranslational factors are most likely responsible for the super-sensitive NMDA response.

Ligand-binding studies support the hypothesis that changes in subunit composition are involved. Grant et al. (1990) reported that seven days of 7 percent ethanol diet increased [^{3}H]MK-801 binding in hippocampal membranes by approximately 16 percent. Another autoradiographic study also reported increased [^{3}H]MK-801 binding in the cortex, hippocampus, and striatum (Gulya et al., 1991). Well-controlled extensions of these experiments found changes in the hippocampus but not the cerebral cortex (Snell, Tabakoff, and Hoffman, 1993). These studies found that [^{3}H]MK-801 and NMDA-specific [^{3}H]glutamate binding slightly increased in the hippocampus during chronic ethanol treatment, but there were no changes in [^{3}H]glycine or [^{3}H]CGS19755, a competitive NMDA antagonist, in the hippocampus. No changes in ligand binding were found in the cerebral cortex (Snell, Tabakoff, and Hoffman, 1993). Reconstitution studies using NMDAR-1A and NMDAR-2A subunits found receptors containing both glutamate antagonist and channel-blocking antagonist binding sites (Lynch et al., 1994). Further studies combining NMDAR-1A and NMDAR-2B subunits resulted in different receptor properties, particularly in the modulation of the channel by polyamines and high-affinity ifenprodil binding. Thus, subunit composition changes and not an increased density of channels may cause the changes in NMDA ligand-binding sites seen in these experiments.

Further supporting this theory, Trevisan et al. (1994) found that 12 weeks of ethanol liquid diet in rats increased the levels of NMDAR-1 immunoreactivity in the hippocampus, but not the cortex, striatum, or nucleus accumbens. Of interest, studies of levels of NMDAR-1 mRNA have indicated that chronic ethanol does not change NMDAR-1 mRNA but increases NMDAR-2A and NMDAR-2B mRNA levels in the hippocampus and cortex (Follesa and Ticku, 1995). As Merck compound 801 (MK801) requires both an NMDAR-1 and NMDAR-2 subunit for binding, an increase in binding could be due to changes in receptor subunits without a concomitant increase in the density of channels. Other studies have not found increases in MK801 binding following chronic ethanol treatment of mice (Carter et al., 1995) or rats (Rudolph et al., 1997). These differences could be due to different ethanol treatment protocols or the responses of different animals. Long-term treatment of rats with ethanol (12 weeks) increased NMDAR-1 immunoreactivity in the ventral tegmental area, whereas one or six weeks of chronic 5 percent ethanol liquid diet did not (Ortiz et al., 1995). Another factor that may relate to differences in ethanol treatment is that stress and treatment with glucocorticoids have been shown to increase NMDA receptor binding in a manner similar to ethanol (Yoneda, Enomoto, and Kiyokazu, 1994). As ethanol increases glucocorticoids and is a stressor, it is possible that increased glucocorticoid levels play a role in ethanol-induced increases in NMDA receptor binding in the brain. However, the supersensitivity observed in vitro by several groups cannot be related to stress-induced changes in NMDA receptor binding. Although the exact molecular processes require additional experimentation, a number of studies support the hypothesis that chronic ethanol consumption results in supersensitive NMDA receptors.

Chronic ethanol consumption also affects the functioning of NMDA receptors by altering the levels of extracellular glutamate through changes in glutamate release. Although an acute dose of ethanol lowers extracellular glutamate levels in the CNS (Carboni et al., 1993; Moghaddam and Bolinao, 1994), ethanol-dependent rats show tolerance as their levels of extracellular glutamate return to normal levels. During withdrawal, however, levels of extracellular glutamate increased threefold, paralleling the time course of the withdrawal syndrome (Fadda and Rossetti, 1998; Gonzales et al., 1996; Rossetti and Carboni, 1995). It is therefore likely that the hyperexcitable state seen during ethanol withdrawal is not only caused by supersensitive NMDA receptor response, but also due to an increase in glutamate release.

Chronic Ethanol Consumption Alters GABA$_A$ Receptor Function and Receptor Subunit Assembly

Ethanol shares several pharmacologic actions with barbiturates and benzodiazepines including anxiolytic and sedative activity (Liljequist and Engel, 1984), cross-tolerance, and dependence (Boisse and Okamoto, 1980; Le et al., 1986). The similarities between the actions of ethanol, benzodiazepines, and barbiturates suggest that all three drugs share some mechanism(s) of action. Tolerance to the sedative and intoxicating effects of ethanol has been postulated to result from a compensatory decrease in GABA-mediated inhibition in the brain (Hunt, 1983). Other studies suggest that alterations in the function of GABA$_A$ receptor chloride channels also contribute to the signs and symptoms of ethanol withdrawal syndrome. Chronic exposure of rats to ethanol produces physical dependence and tolerance (Frye et al., 1981; Goldstein and Pal, 1971; Karanian et al., 1986; Morrow, Suzdak, and Paul, 1988; Morrow, Herbert, and Montpied, 1992), which are associated with a decreased sensitivity of the GABA$_A$ receptor in the cerebral cortex (Sanna et al., 1993), when blood ethanol levels were greater than 0.15 percent (Morrow, Suzdak, and Paul, 1988). In vitro studies have also shown that chronic ethanol decreases the sensitivity of GABA$_A$ receptors. Muscimol-stimulated ^{36}Cl$^-$ uptake was decreased by 26 percent and pentobarbital-stimulated ^{36}Cl$^-$ uptake was decreased by 25 percent following chronic ethanol treatment. Following chronic ethanol administration, the ability of ethanol (20 mM) to potentiate muscimol-stimulated ^{36}Cl$^-$ uptake was completely lost in rat cerebral cortical synaptoneurosomes (Morrow, Suzdak, and Paul, 1988) and in mouse cerebellar microsacs (Allan and Harris, 1987). Cross-tolerance was also demonstrated as benzodiazepine enhancement of muscimol-stimulated chloride flux was reduced in the cerebral cortex of mouse microsacs, while the functional efficacy of inverse agonists was enhanced (Buck and Harris, 1990). This cross-tolerance was also seen in behavioral responses to injections of muscimol into the substantia nigra (Gonzalez and Czachura, 1989) and to subcutaneous THIP (a GABA agonist) injections (Martz, Dietrich, and Harris, 1983) that were reduced following chronic ethanol administration. Following the completion of ethanol withdrawal, the decrease in muscimol-stimulated ^{36}Cl$^-$ uptake in rat cerebral cortical synaptoneurosomes (Morrow, Suzdak, and Paul, 1988) and flunitrazepam potentiation in mouse cortical microsacs (Buck and Harris, 1990) was completely reversed, as would be predicted if these neurochemical changes were related to the behavioral states of alcohol withdrawal.

Alterations in the density or affinity of brain GABA$_A$ receptors following chronic ethanol administration have yielded conflicting results and cannot explain the development of tolerance or withdrawal. For example, Ticku and Burch (1980), Ticku et al. (1986), and Unwin and Taberner (1980) have reported a decrease in the density of low-affinity [^{3}H]agonist binding sites in the brain following chronic ethanol exposure to rats or mice. de Vries et al. (1987) have reported a reduction in the ability of GABA to enhance [^{3}H]flunitrazepam binding in brain membranes prepared from ethanol-treated mice. However, others have failed to find alterations in the number or affinity of GABA$_A$ receptors (Volicer, 1980; Volicer and Biagioni, 1982b). Chronic ethanol administration does not alter the density of [^{3}H]flunitrazepam (Karobath, Rogers, and Bloom, 1980; Rastogi et al., 1986; Volicer and Biagioni, 1982a) or [^{35}S]t-butylbicyclophosphorothionate binding sites (Rastogi et al., 1986; Thyagarajan and Ticku, 1985) in brain. Mhatre, Mehta, and Ticku (1988) reported an increase in the density of specific binding sites for [^{3}H] Ro15-4513 in the rat cortex and cerebellum following chronic ethanol administration, as well as increased sensitivity to its behavioral effects (Mehta and Ticku, 1989). It has been proposed that the alterations in GABA$_A$ receptor function observed following chronic ethanol administration are the result of a change in the synthesis and expression of GABA$_A$ receptor isoforms. Chronic ethanol administration may have differential effects on the expression of individual GABA$_A$ receptor subunits, accounting for the diverse effects of ethanol on *different* radioligand binding sites. If ethanol alters the expression of specific populations of GABA$_A$ receptor isoforms, radioligands, which measure all GABA receptors, may lack the selectivity to detect changes in one or more receptor subunits or populations of GABA$_A$ receptor isoforms.

Chronic ethanol administration differentially alters the expression of GABA$_A$ receptor subunit mRNAs in the cerebral cortex (Devaud, Smith, et al., 1995; Montpied et al., 1991; Morrow et al., 1990) and cerebellum (Morrow, Herbert, and Montpied, 1992). The levels of GABA$_A$ receptor α1 subunit mRNAs are reduced while α4 subunit mRNAs are increased by approximately equal amounts in the cerebral cortex (Devaud, Smith, et al., 1995). Likewise in the cerebellum, decreases in GABA$_A$ receptor α1 subunit mRNAs and increases in α6 subunit mRNA levels are found (Mhatre and Ticku, 1992; Morrow, Herbert, and Montpied, 1992). These changes in mRNA levels suggest alterations in the expression of the corresponding proteins that could account for the alterations in receptor function and binding that have been observed. For example, the increases in α4 and α6 subunit expression probably explain the increases in [^{3}H] Ro-15-4513 (Mhatre, Mehta, and Ticku, 1988) and sensitivity (Buck and Harris, 1990; Mehta and Ticku, 1989) following chronic ethanol administration. The increased expression of α4 subunits may also underlie the reduced sensitivity to GABA (Morrow, Suzdak, and Paul, 1988) and benzodiazepine agonists (Buck and Harris, 1990), as recombinant GABA receptors with α4 β2γ2 subunits are less sensitive to GABA agonists and benzodiazepines than α1 β2γ2 receptors (Whittemore et al., 1995). Ethanol-dependent and withdrawn rats are also sensitized to the effects of the neurosteroid 3α,5αTHP (Devaud, Purdy, and Morrow, 1995; Devaud et al., 1996). This effect may be related to the increase in γ1 subunit mRNAs following chronic ethanol exposure (Devaud, Smith, et al., 1995; Devaud et al., 1996), as γ1 subunits convey greater neurosteroid sensitivity in recombinant expression studies (Puia et al., 1994).

As seen with chronic ethanol exposure, ethanol withdrawal is also associated with dynamic changes in GABA$_A$ receptor subunit mRNAs. During withdrawal, GABA$_A$ receptor α1 and α4 subunit mRNAs return to control levels, while β2 and β3 subunit mRNA levels increase compared with both control and dependent rats (Devaud et al., 1996). At this time, corresponding changes in protein expression are unlikely as the receptor turnover rate (t½) is estimated to be one to two days. Therefore, although GABA$_A$ receptor polypeptide expression during withdrawal is probably similar to that found in ethanol-dependent rats, profound changes in GABA$_A$ receptor expression may occur shortly after withdrawal.

The observation that ethanol tolerance is associated with changes in subunit composition also supports the hypothesis that subunit composition influences ethanol sensitivity. As previously discussed, ethanol potentiation of $GABA_A$ receptor function is abolished at the cellular level in rats that are ethanol tolerant and dependent. The changes in subunit expression resulting from chronic exposure to ethanol may contribute to this reduction in ethanol sensitivity (Devaud, Smith, et al., 1995; Morrow, Herbert, and Montpied, 1992).

Chronic Ethanol Alters Phosphorylation and Localization of NMDA and GABA_A Receptors

Whether the phosphorylation state of NMDA and $GABA_A$ receptors is altered by chronic ethanol exposure is not yet known. Chronic ethanol exposure can increase PKC levels and activity (Coe, Yao, et al., 1996; DePetrillo and Liou, 1993; Gordon et al., 1997; Messing, Petersen, and Henrich, 1991; Roivainen, McMahon, and Messing, 1993) and induce heterologous desensitization of cAMP signaling with decreased PKA activity (Coe, Dohrman, et al., 1996; Gordon, Collier, and Diamond, 1986; Rabin, Edelman, and Wagner, 1992). Some of these effects of ethanol could relate to changes in subcellular translocation and localization. Ethanol has been shown to stimulate translocation to the nucleus of the catalytic subunit of PKA where it remains sequestered for as long as ethanol is present (Dohrman, Diamond, and Gordon, 1996), and to stimulate translocation of PKC-δ and PKC-ε to new intracellular sites (Gordon et al., 1997). Translocation of PKC and PKA isozymes to subcellular anchoring proteins is thought to be important in targeting specific signaling events. Furthermore, PKA and calcineurin (protein phosphatase 2B) are concentrated in postsynaptic densities via a common A-kinase anchoring protein (AKAP79), putting them in a position to regulate phosphorylation and/or dephosphorylation of key postsynaptic proteins (Coghlan et al., 1995). Clearly, changes in PKA and/or PKC activity and subcellular targeting could play an important role in ethanol-induced changes in synaptic function, including modulation of NMDA and $GABA_A$ receptors.

Another potentially important process in NMDA and $GABA_A$ receptor adaptation during ethanol exposure is receptor-cytoskeletal interaction (Chandler, Harris, and Crews, 1998). NMDA receptors are required for ctivity-dependent synaptic remodeling during development, and studies in hippocampal cultures have shown that the subcellular distribution of NMDA receptors is modulated by receptor activity. Chronic treatment with an NMDA receptor antagonist leads to increased NMDA receptor clustering at synaptic sites and, conversely, spontaneous activity leads to decreased synaptic NMDA receptor clustering (Rao and Craig, 1997). As studies in primary neuronal cell cultures might more closely model developmental processes, an important question to be addressed is whether this activity-dependent redistribution of NMDA receptors also occurs in mature neurons. Furthermore, it is not known whether the functional property of the NMDA receptor itself is altered by clustering and redistribution (i.e., synaptic versus nonsynaptic). However, receptor redistribution could represent a novel form of activity-dependent synaptic modification (plasticity), and prolonged inhibition of the NMDA receptor during chronic ethanol exposure might also lead to an increase in NMDA receptor clustering at synaptic sites.

BRAIN DAMAGE IN ALCOHOLICS

Morphological Changes Caused by Chronic Alcohol Abuse

Alcohol-induced changes in brain structure have been studied in both humans and rodents. A variety of postmortem histological analyses, as well as supporting imaging analysis, suggest that chronic alcohol intoxication changes brain structure (Crews, 2000; Sullivan, Rosenbloom, and Pfefferbaum, 2000). Computerized tomography (CT) and magnetic resonance imaging (MRI) studies have repeatedly shown enlargement of the cerebral ventricles and sulci in most alcoholics. The enlargement of the ventricles and sulci reflect a shrinking of brain mass. This is consistent with studies on postmortem brain tissue, wherein alcoholics have a reduction in total brain weight. Particularly severe alcoholics also have reductions in global cerebral hemisphere and cerebellar brain weights compared to controls and moderate drinkers (Harper and Kril, 1993). Some of this loss of brain mass is likely due to loss of neurons (gray matter) and myelin sheaths (white matter). However, a portion of the loss in brain mass is also likely to be due to a reduction in the brain parenchyma, that is, the size of the cells and their processes, during chronic alcohol abuse. Recent studies have indicated that within one to five months of sustained abstinence, the size of the brain returns to normal levels. It is likely that this return involves an increase in neuronal cell size, arborization, and density of the neuronal processes that make up cellular brain mass, as well as increases in the number and size of glial cells (Franke et al., 1997). Although it is not exactly clear how alcoholism leads to a reduction in brain weight and volume, it is clear that this occurs during active alcohol abuse, and that some recovery of brain mass occurs during abstinence. More research is needed to clearly understand how chronic alcohol abuse leads to a reduction in brain mass and how recovery of brain mass occurs during abstinence.

The frontal lobes appear to be particularly affected in persons with chronic alcoholism as first observed in neuropathological studies (Courville, 1955) and confirmed more recently with neuropathological (Harper and Kril, 1990) and in vivo neuroradiological studies (Nicolas et al., 1997; Pfefferbaum et al., 1997; Ron et al., 1982). Quantitative morphometry suggests that the frontal lobes of the human brain show the greatest loss, and account for much of the associated ventricular enlargement (Jernigan et al., 1991). Studies have found that neuronal density in the superior frontal cortex is reduced by 22 percent in alcoholics compared to nonalcoholic controls, in contrast to other areas of the cortex, which were not different between the groups (Harper, Kril, and Daly, 1987). Further, the complexity of the basal dendritic arborization of layer III pyramidal cells in both superior frontal and motor cortices were significantly reduced in alcoholics compared to controls. Decreases in the amounts of *N*-acetyl aspartate in the frontal lobe, a measure of neuron levels, also illustrates frontal lobe degeneration in alcoholics (Jagannathan, Desai, and Raghunathan, 1996). One reason these frontal lobe changes are more evident is the greater proportion of white matter to cortical gray matter in the frontal regions.

Other brain regions are also affected by chronic alcohol abuse. A reduction in dendritic arborization of Purkinje cells in the anterior superior vermis of the cerebellum is also found in alcoholics. Temporal lobe shrinkage occurs particularly in individuals with alcohol-withdrawal seizure history (Sullivan et al., 1996). Taken together, the data demonstrate a selective neuronal loss, dendritic simplification, and reduction of synaptic complexity in specific brain regions of alcoholics.

In addition to the global shrinkage of brain regions, certain key neuronal nuclei that have broad-ranging functions on brain activity are selectively lost with chronic alcohol abuse. One important nucleus altered in alcoholism is the cholinergic basal forebrain nuclei, which is also lost in Alzheimer's disease, causing loss of memory formation. Arendt (1993) found a significant loss of neurons in this region in alcoholic Korsakoff psychosis patients. Cholinergic blockade has been shown to cause the anterograde amnesia seen in both Korsakoff and Alzheimer patients (Kopelman and Corn, 1988).

Additional brain nuclei such as the locus coeruleus and raphe nuclei appear to be particularly sensitive. These two nuclei contain many of the noradrenergic and serotonergic neurons within the brain, respectively. Although these nuclei are small in size, they are particularly important because their neuronal processes project throughout the brain and modulate global aspects of brain activity. Chemical studies have shown abnormally low levels of serotonergic metabolites in the cerebrospinal fluid of alcoholics with Wernicke-Korsakoff syndrome, and more recent morphological studies have found a 50 percent reduction in the number of serotonergic neurons from the raphe nuclei of all alcoholic cases studied compared to controls. Thus the serotonergic system appears to be disrupted in alcoholics, especially in severe alcoholics (Baker et al., 1996; Halliday, Baker, and Harper, 1995). Several studies have also reported significant noradrenergic cell loss in the locus coeruleus (Arango et al., 1996; Arendt et al., 1995; Lu et al., 1997), although not all studies have found this loss (Harper and Kril, 1993). Studies have also indicated that certain neurons that contain the peptide vasopressin may be sensitive to chronic ethanol-induced neurotoxicity in both rats and humans (Harding et al., 1996; Madeira et al., 1997). Damage to hypothalamic vasopressin and other peptide-containing neurons could disrupt a variety of hormone functions as well as daily rhythms that are important for healthy living. Thus, studies have suggested that cholinergic and biogenic amine brain nuclei appear particularly sensitive to ethanol neurotoxicity.

Although human alcoholic neuropathology is associated with years of alcohol abuse, studies have found that long-term ethanol intoxication is not necessary to cause brain damage. Just a few days of intoxication can lead to neuronal loss in several brain areas including temporal dentate gyrus, entorhinal, piriform, and perirhinal cortices, and in the olfactory bulb (Collins, Zou, and Neafsey, 1998; Crews et al., 2000). These structures are involved in integrating cortical inputs through the limbic system. These findings are consistent with recent human studies that report damage to the entorhinal cortex (Ibanez et al., 1995) and significant hippocampal shrinkage in alcoholics (Harding et al., 1997). Hippocampal damage during chronic ethanol treatment has been correlated with deficits in spatial learning and memory (Franke et al., 1997). Thus, cortical and hippocampal damage occur with chronic ethanol treatment and relatively short durations of alcohol abuse may cause some form of damage.

Cognitive Dysfunction Caused by Chronic Alcohol Abuse

Alcoholics who do not have Korsakoff's syndrome show decreased neuropsychological performance on tests of learning, memory, abstracting, problem solving, visuospatial and perceptual motor functioning, and information processing when compared with peer nonalcoholics (Parsons, 1993). Alcoholics are not only less accurate, they take considerably longer to complete tasks. Alcoholics are differentially vulnerable to these deficits. Further, many of the deficits appear to recover to age-appropriate levels of performance over a four- to five-year period of abstinence (Parsons, 1993). Although global cerebral atrophy rebounds to normal levels with extended abstinence, not all cognitive functions return. Some abstinent alcoholics appear to have permanent cognitive impairments, particularly in memory and visual-spatial-motor skills (Di Sclafani et al., 1995). Other studies support a loss of logical memory and paired association learning tasks in alcoholics that may be long lasting (Eckardt et al., 1996; see Chapter 3 for further discussion). Thus, various psychological tests suggest long-term changes in brain function following chronic alcohol abuse.

Exciting studies have begun to address the effects of gender on brain damage. Interestingly, alcoholic women appear to have an increased sensitivity for brain damage when compared with alcoholic men (Hommer et al., 1996). This appears to be true for liver disease as well. Although more men than women are diagnosed as alcoholic, the number of female alcoholics is increasing. The increased susceptibility of women to alcoholic pathology is an area that needs further investigation.

Mechanisms of Alcohol-Induced Brain Damage

Although the neurotoxicity of alcohol is well established, the mechanisms of alcohol-induced brain damage are not clear. Human studies indicate loss of both white matter and gray matter, for example, myelinated nerve track areas and primarily neuronal areas, respectively. It is generally thought that the loss of neurons leads to a loss of myelinated tracks. However, there is little or no evidence to support this hypothesis in humans. Although their methodologies are different, basic studies report neuronal toxicity with no clear loss of myelin or the oligodendroglia that form myelin. A number of mechanisms have been proposed for alcohol-induced brain damage with strong evidence for NMDA-mediated excitotoxicity and losses of trophic factors with less evidence for osmotic and oxidative stress mechanisms. These mechanisms, in combination with diet and other factors, such as genetics, cause alcohol-induced brain damage. Understanding the mechanisms of alcohol-induced brain damage will improve prevention, intervention, treatment, and recovery efforts as well as increase our understanding of neurodegeneration and neurobiological health.

Excitotoxicity

One of the leading theories that explains ethanol-induced neurotoxicity is excitotoxicity. Hyperexcitability of the central nervous system is a key component of ethanol withdrawal and a supersensitive NMDA response appears to be involved. Early research showing that [³H]glutamate binding was increased in the hippocampus of alcoholics (Michaelis et al., 1990) reinforced the hypothesis that a supersensitive NMDA response was responsible, either through an increase in NMDA receptor density or a change in subunit composition. NMDA receptors have a unique property, in that, excessive stimulation of these receptors triggers a process in neurons that leads to neuronal death. This process is referred to as excitotoxicity. Glutamate can be excitotoxic in vivo through NMDA in combination with kainate and other glutamate receptors. Excitotoxicity plays a key role in neurodegenerative diseases in general, as well as stroke, brain trauma, and other types of brain damage (Crews and Chandler, 1993).

In vitro studies of excitotoxicity have indicated that long-term exposure to ethanol is not necessary to induce NMDA excitotoxic supersensitivity. Several studies of isolated neuronal cells have indicated that only a few days of ethanol treatment leads to supersensitive NMDA-stimulated calcium flux (Ahern, Lustig, and Greenberg, 1994; Iorio et al., 1992), as well as NMDA-stimulated excitotoxicity (Crews and Chandler, 1993; Crews et al., 1993; Iorio, Tabakoff, and Hoffman, 1993). This led researchers to investigate the role of excitotoxicity in an in vivo rat binge model of ethanol exposure which found extensive mesocorticolimbic neuronal damage. Attempts to block binge ethanol-induced brain damage with NMDA antagonists were not successful (Table 5.1). Thus, general agreement exists among laboratories that chronic alcohol consumption leads to NMDA receptor supersensitivity. This finding predicts that NMDA antagonists would block alcohol withdrawal and alcohol-induced brain damage. Although alcohol withdrawal is blocked, brain damage is not.

Although thiamin deficiency is thought to play a key role in Wernicke's syndrome, the mechanism of the neurodegeneration in this model appears to involve excitotoxicity from glutamate (Langlais and Zhang, 1993). An animal model of Wernicke's syndrome that used pyrithiamine to create thiamine-deficient animals found extracellular concentrations of glutamate increased several fold during ethanol withdrawal seizures (Langlais and Zhang, 1993). Furthermore, MK-801, an NMDA antagonist, reduced experimental neurological symptoms and decreased neural lessening in models of thiamine deficiency in rats (Langlais and Mair, 1990). In any case, there is strong evidence that ethanol withdrawal hyperexcitability is related at least in part to NMDA supersensitivity and that this supersensitivity could underlie ethanol-induced brain damage.

Osmotic Changes and Increased Intracranial Pressure

Another possible mechanism of ethanol-induced brain damage involves osmotic changes and increases in intracranial pressure. Although difficult

TABLE 5.1. Drugs tested for effects on neurodegeneration caused by binge ethanol exposure.

Drug	Class	Hypothesis	Effect	References
Nimodipine	Voltage-gated Ca^{2+} channel blocker	Chronic EtoH increases Ca^{2+} channels in brain	Reduced damage in dentate gyrus Increased damage in piriform cortex	Corso et al., 1998
Nimodipine	L-type Ca^{2+} channel blocker	Chronic EtoH increases Ca^{2+} channels in brain	No neuroprotection	Hamelink, 1998, 2000
DNQX	AMPA antagonist NMDA antagonist at glycine site	High densities of AMPA receptors in the dentate gyrus, Ca fields, entorhinal cortex, piriform, frontal cortex	No effect	Corso et al., 1998
MK-801	NMDA antagonist	Chronic EtoH causes excitotoxicity	Increased damage in entorhinal cortex, orbital cortex, and periamygdala	Corso et al., 1998
MK-801	NMDA antagonist	Chronic EtoH causes excitotoxicity	No effect	Collins et al., 1998
MK-801	NMDA antagonist	Chronic EtoH causes excitotoxicity	No neuroprotection	Hamelink, 1998, 2000
Memantine	NMDA antagonist	Chronic EtoH causes excitotoxicity	No neuroprotection	Hamelink, 1998, 2000
Olfactory bulbectomies	Surgical procedure	Chronic EtoH causes excitotoxic cascade	No neuroprotection	Hamelink, 1998, 2000
L-NAME	Nitric oxide synthase inhibitor	Chronic EtoH increases NO production	No change/increased damage	Zou et al., 1996

Note: Table 5.1 sets out the results of experiments which tested hypotheses regarding mechanisms of alcohol-induced brain damage, particularly those regarding glutamate NMDA receptor supersensitivity to excitotoxicity (see Crews and Chandler, 1993). Each of the hypotheses has a basis in the basic brain studies that are referenced. Specific antagonists were used as tests. Binge treatment with ethanol differs slightly among studies, but in general involves very high alcohol consumption for several days. Although NMDA supersensitivity appears to be involved in ethanol dependence and withdrawal, it does not appear to be central to ethanol-induced neurotoxicity in these bingle-drinking models.

to test, some studies have hypothesized that cerebral edema occurs with moderate doses of ethanol (McQueen and Posey, 1975; Weiss and Craig, 1978) and that this may cause alcoholic brain damage (Lambie, 1985). Recent investigations have tested the edema mechanisms of binge-drinking-induced brain damage using furosemide, which could reduce vasogenic and cytotoxic edema, and mannitol, a commonly used agent to reduce intracerebral pressure. Mannitol is an inert molecule that increases the osmolarity of the blood and decreases water content and brain volume (Paczynski et al., 1997). No protective effects have been found with binge-drinking models (see Figure 5.1). However, Collins, Zou, and Neafsey (1998) treated rats once daily with ethanol, much less than binge-drinking models, for ten days and found that furosemide reduced brain hydration and neurodegeneration in the entorhinal cortex and dentate gyrus, though no attenuation of olfactory bulb degeneration was found. Neurodegeneration mechanisms may differ depending upon the extent and duration of alcohol consumption.

Oxidative Stress

Another possible mechanism of ethanol-induced brain damage involves increased oxidative stress on neurons. Cells use oxygen for energy metabolism and normally have mechanisms that protect against oxidative damage. Studies that have examined the effects of both acute and chronic ethanol administration upon cellular oxidation have primarily focused either on ethanol's effects upon intracellular antioxidant mechanisms such as α-tocopherol, ascorbate, glutathione, catalase, and superoxide dismutase (SOD) activity (Ledig, M'Paria, and Mandel, 1981; Montoliu et al., 1994; Nordmann, 1987; Rouach et al., 1987) or potential sources of oxidative radicals such as CYP2E1 (Montoliu et al., 1994, 1995). Chronic ethanol-induced increases in CYP2E1 and other oxidases have been related to increased lipid peroxidation and reactive oxygen radicals in the brain (Montoliu et al., 1994). As the brain is rich in polyunsaturated fatty acids, which are especially prone to reactive oxygen injury, it is particularly susceptible to lipid peroxidation. It has been demonstrated that a single dose of ethanol elevates lipid hydroperoxide levels and decreases glutathione levels in rat brain homogenates (Nordmann, Ribiere, and Rouach, 1990, 1992; Uysal et al., 1986, 1989). However, it is not clear how this increased oxidation translates to increased brain damage or whether it does at all. Oxidative stress has been implicated in a variety of conditions, particularly aging, Alzheimer's disease, Parkinson's disease, stroke, and other neurodegenerative diseases. More research is needed to completely understand how oxidation damages neurons, and how other brain cells respond to increased oxidative stress. Ethanol-

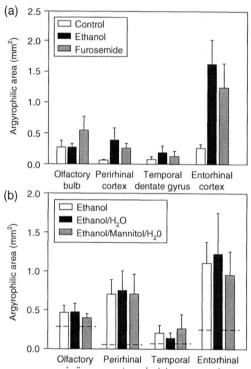

FIGURE 5.1. Edema and binge ethanol-induced brain damage. To determine whether cerebral edema was involved in binge ethanol-induced brain damage, furosemide (a loop diuretic) was concomitantly administered to binge ethanol-exposed rats (a). Sprague-Dawley rats were treated using a four-day binge ethanol episode, as previously described (Knapp and Crews, 1999). Furosemide, 6.7 mg/kg, was administered three times daily i.p. Immediately after the last dose of ethanol was administered, the rats were euthanized and their brains sectioned at 40 μm. Every eighth section was stained by the amino curpric silver method of de Olmos (1994). Shown is the mean total argyrophilia per rat SE. There was a main effect of drug treatment $(F(2,17) = 5.481; p < .05)$. To determine whether vasogenic edema or hydration state was involved in binge ethanol-induced brain damage, the experiment in panel B was performed. Mannitol is an inert molecule that increases the osmolarity of the blood and decreases brain water content (Paczynski et al., 1997). The rats were hydrated to 25.9 ml/kg water per day and/or 0.75 g/kg mannitol was administered three times daily. After the final dose of ethanol, the rats were euthanized and treated as in panel A. Shown is the mean total argyrophilia per rat SE. The broken lines represent the average level of argyrophilic area in control-treated animals. There was no significant effect of hydration or mannitol $(F(2,13) = .032; p > .05)$ on binge ethanol-induced brain damage as measured by argyrophilic area.

induced neurodegeneration may be related to an induction of oxidative enzymes, and alcohol research provides an opportunity to clearly address this aspect of neurodegeneration which could impact a broad range of mental diseases.

Hepatic Encephalopathy

Hepatic encephalopathy (HE) is caused by liver cirrhosis and other hepatotoxic syndromes that start with subtle personality changes and disturbances of sleep patterns and progress to muscle incoordination, flapping tremors, coma, and death. HE is caused by several factors, including increased levels of neurotoxic substances in the brain, in particular ammonia and manganese, and is often associated with alcohol cirrhosis (Hazell and Butterworth, 1999). HE causes severe alterations in astrocytes, including changes in expression of peripheral-type benzodiazepine receptors (Lavoie, Layrargues, and Butterworth, 1990), monoamine oxidase B (Rao et al., 1993) and glutamine synthetase (Lavoie et al., 1987), and the glutamate transporter GLT-1 (Knecht et al., 1997; Norenberg et al., 1997). These changes during acute liver failure cause accumulation of glutamine (an ammonia metabolite) in the brain and cytotoxic edema (Levin et al., 1989; Takahashi et al., 1991), and in chronic liver failure result in Alzheimer type II astrocytosis (Hazell and Butterworth, 1999). Neurotransmitter systems such as glutamate, serotonin, GABA, and opioids are also disturbed in HE, although the causes and effects of these alterations are not as well understood (Bergeron et al., 1989; Layrargues and Butterworth, 1992; Thornton and Losowsky, 1988; Young et al., 1975). This suggests that the neurodegeneration associated with chronic alcoholism may be caused in part by changes in hepatic function.

Brain Damage, Alcohol Dependence, and Recovery

Alcoholism is a progressive disease that begins with experimentation and progresses to addiction, usually over the course of 10 to 15 years (Vaillant, 1996). Progressive increases in abuse often develop into complete fixation on obtaining and consuming alcohol. Addiction involves the loss of control over the ability to abstain from alcohol or other drugs, even in the face of adverse consequences, and perseverative preoccupation with obtaining and using the drugs desired. Perseveration refers to continued repetitive behaviors of a previous appropriate or correct response, even though the repeated response has since become inappropriate and incorrect. Perseveration is associated with cortical damage. One hypothesis regarding the development of alcoholism is that an initial state of disinhibition/hyperexcitability, perhaps due to low frontal-cortical impulse inhibition, predisposes a person to developing alcoholism (Begleiter and Porjesz, 1999). Both clinical and experimental studies support frontal-cortical involvement in neuropsychological dysfunction in alcoholics, particularly those with Korsakoff's syndrome (Oscar-Berman and Hutner, 1993). Studies have found that the ventromedial prefrontal cortex mediates goal-oriented actions that are guided by motivational and emotional factors (Gallagher, McMahan, and Schoenbaum, 1999). Damage to this area results in a loss of the ability to associate incentive values with stimuli. Thus the effects of negative stimuli on behavior are blunted by ventromedial prefrontal damage and result in maladaptive behaviors (Bechara, Tranel, and Damasio, 2000; Gallagher, McMahan, and Schoenbaum, 1999). Humans with ventromedial prefrontal cortical lesions are insensitive to future consequences and are primarily guided by immediate prospects (Bechara, Tranel, and Damasio, 2000). As mentioned earlier, a variety of evidence has focused attention on the prefrontal cortex as an area of brain that is particularly sensitive to alcohol-induced brain damage. Various regions of the frontal and prefrontal cortex are involved in learned associations, emotional decision making, and executive cognitive functions. Executive cognitive function (ECF) is the ability to utilize higher mental abilities, such as attention, planning, organization, sequencing, and abstract reasoning, to adaptively modulate future behavior based on external and internal feedback (Foster, Eskes, and Stuss, 1994). ECF is disrupted in alcoholics and other patients who exhibit prefrontal damage (Boller et al., 1995), and this disruption has been implicated in aggression associated with alcohol and drug abuse (Hoaken, Giancola, and Pihl, 1998). ECF/prefrontal disruption is associated with decreased regulation of human social behavior, including disinhibition syndrome (characterized by impulsivity, socially inappropriate behavior, and aggression) (Giancola and Zeichner, 1995). These studies suggest that some of the greatest sociopathic problems of alcoholism, for example, violence and loss of control over the drug, may be directly related to the neurotoxic effects of ethanol on prefrontal cortical function. The prefrontal cortex is closely linked to the amygdala and temporal lobes which also show damage in cases of alcoholism. These structures are known to play a role in automatic or nonconscious decision making (Kubota et al., 2000). Emotional factors are often subconscious processes that are below the level of awareness. Addiction involves continued behaviors out of conscious control. The progression from experimentation with alcohol to alcohol addiction generally occurs over an extended period of many years with increased consumption of alcohol, increased neurotoxicity, increased distortions of thinking, and preoccupation with the drug. A hypothetical scheme of the progression to alcoholism is depicted in the "spiral of distress" (Figure 5.2; see Koob and Le Moal, 1997, for additional discussions). Figure 5.2 attempts to relate the neurochemical changes in the brain induced by alcohol to the progression to addiction. Addiction is presented as an end point reached when cortical damage results in perseverative drinking behavior without conscious recognition of the negative consequences, and the inability to consciously control behavior. Each of these characteristics occurs with frontal and temporal lobe cortical lesions suggesting that progressive neurotoxicity may underlie the progression to addiction. Future studies are needed to directly determine the relationship of prefrontal cortical function to alcohol-induced brain damage and addiction.

Treatment and Recovery for Alcoholism

The principal approach to treatment for alcoholism is abstinence from drinking alcohol. A variety of treatments including elements of supportive therapy, cognitive-behavioral therapy, and Alcoholics Anonymous and other group therapies and recovery programs in various forms and combinations have helped millions of people. In general, treatments are effective for many, but not all, individuals. During recovery, behavioral and neuroanatomical changes persist long after the end of the physical alcohol withdrawal syndrome, which typically lasts less than one week. Human studies have shown that within the first month of recovery alcoholics show a significant decrease in ventricular and sulci size (i.e., the brain mass actually increases and returns to normal values) (Pfefferbaum et al., 1995). Over the following months regrowth of brain mass continues. In abstinent alcoholics, a significant increase in brain volume occurs over a period of months. Relapsing alcoholics do not show increased gains in brain mass (Pfefferbaum et al., 1995). It is possible that changes in behavior essential for successful recovery from addiction require neurophysiological and perhaps anatomical changes in the brain to sustain the recovery. The findings that those who are successful at recovery have brain regrowth whereas those who relapse have no regrowth could be due to continued ethanol neurotoxicity in relapsing addicts (Pfefferbaum et al., 1998) or due to the need for brain regrowth and return of key brain functions to sustain abstinence. Those individuals without regrowth and return of functions (e.g., executive functions that include setting and maintaining goals) may be more prone to relapse. Behavioral counseling and other therapies may activate and train cortical regions, strengthen and stimulate neuronal function and neuronal regrowth. Thus, successful recovery may involve brain regrowth due to abstinence and the removal of ethanol neurotoxicity, as well as exercising the emotional-association cortical areas to regain functions needed for appropriate emotional

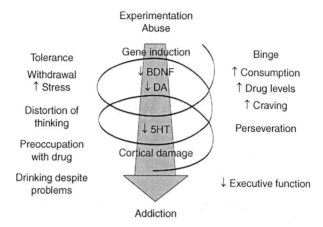

FIGURE 5.2. The spiral of distress. This model depicts the progression from experimentation to addiction. On the left are criteria for the diagnosis of alcohol dependence. Included are increasing tolerance; alcohol withdrawal due to physical dependence, which increases stress; increasing preoccupation with the drug; spending large amounts of time obtaining and consuming alcohol; and continued use despite negative consequences and problems associated with the use of alcohol. In the middle are known changes in the brain that occur during chronic alcohol use. Changes in gene expression are well documented as occurring during the development of dependence. Studies have shown changes in biogenic amines, particularly serotonin (5-hydroxytryptamine, 5HT) and dopamine, key neurotransmitters involved in dependence (see Crews et al., 1999, for more details). Cortical damage and shrinkage occur in alcoholics, particularly in frontal and temporal regions. Binge drinking, on the right, is indicative of the behavior most likely to induce tolerance, dependence, and changes in brain structure and function. Loss of biogenic amines could increase craving and drinking. Cortical damage can cause perseveration—the persistence of behavior once the reward is removed—and could be analogous to preoccupation with alcohol. Frontal cortical damage is associated with loss of executive functions and could be related to failure to associate negative consequences with drinking, inability to set goals, and inability to inhibit behaviors, ultimately leading to addiction. *Source:* Adapted from Koob and Le Moal, 1997.

decision making, executive function, and appropriate responses to environmental stimuli (Figure 5.3).

SUMMARY AND CONCLUSIONS

Alcohol dependence is one of the most common maladies in our society, touching most families and communities. At least part of the acute actions

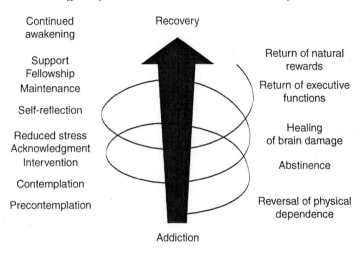

FIGURE 5.3. The path to recovery. This model illustrates the stages of change, including reversal of brain damage and return of executive function, involved in recovery from addiction (Prochasta and DiClemente, 1992). These stages begin with precontemplation, in which individuals are unaware of the problem, have no intention of changing, and possibly have difficulty associating negative consequences of drug taking due to cortical dysfuction. Contemplation refers to the point at which individuals are aware of the problem and interventions to make the patient aware help and motivate change. Abstinence allows the return of cortical functions and regrowth of the cortex. Self-reflection strengthens associations of negative consequences with drug taking, perhaps invigorating cortical regions involved in these associations. Return of executive functions, including impulse inhibition and goal setting, support the maintenance of abstinence. Increased fellowship with other abstainers reduces craving and helps with motivation, leading to continued awakening and return of natural rewards. Models of this type can be used to test associations between recovery and changes in brain function. *Source:* Adapted from Koob and LeMoal, 1997.

of alcohol are due to its effects at glutamate and GABA receptors. Glutamate NMDA receptors are abundant excitatory receptors in the brain and are among the most sensitive receptors to inhibition by ethanol. NMDA receptors are heterogeneous and the effects of alcohol on NMDA receptors *differ* among brain regions, likely due to differences in subunit composition, phosphorylation state, and other factors. Kainate and AMPA glutamate excitatory receptors are also inhibited in certain circumstances. In contrast, the major inhibitory receptor in the brain, the $GABA_A$ receptor, is potentiated by ethanol. $GABA_A$ receptor potentiation also varies across brain regions due to subunit composition, phosphorylation state, and other possible heterogeneous modulators. $GABA_A$ receptor potentiation is shared by ethanol with barbiturates and benzodiazepines as well as many sedative, anticonvulsant, and anxiolytic behavioral actions. Chronic ethanol abuse leads to adaptive changes in both NMDA glutamate and $GABA_A$ receptor responses. NMDA receptor supersensitivity likely contributes to the hyperexcitability of the ethanol withdrawal syndrome and may contribute to alcoholic brain damage, although other mechanisms appear to contribute as well. The mechanism of supersensitivity appears to be more complicated than a simple increased number of receptors and requires additional studies to elucidate the mechanisms of NMDA supersensitivity in alcohol dependence. $GABA_A$ receptor responses are altered during chronic ethanol consumption as well in a complex manner consistent with tolerance and dependence. It is clear that many of ethanol's acute and chronic pharmacological effects are due to actions at glutamate NMDA and $GABA_A$ receptors.

Alcohol abuse and dependence clearly result in neurodegeneration. Alcoholics have lesions in specific cholinergic, biogenic amine, and other brain nuclei as well as cortical shrinkage and ventricular enlargement. The frontal, prefrontal, associative, and temporal lobe cortexes appear to be particularly sensitive to alcohol neurotoxicity. The mechanisms of neurotoxicity appear to be multifaceted, including NMDA supersensitivity and other toxic factors that lead to neuronal loss and degeneration. The progressive nature of addiction may be related to a progressive loss of brain tissue associated with chronic alcohol abuse neurotoxicity. Recovery from alcoholism is associated with a return of cerebral mass that could play a role in the success of the recovery process. Additional studies are needed to understand fully the process of addiction and how it relates to the effects of chronic alcohol abuse on brain function.

REFERENCES

Aguayo, L.G. (1990). Ethanol potentiates the GABAA-activated Cl⁻ current in mouse hippocampal and cortical neurons. *Eur Pharmacol* 187:127-130.

Ahern, K.B.; Lustig, H.S.; Greenberg, D.A. (1994). Enhancement of NMDA toxicity and calcium responses by chronic exposure of cultured cortical neurons to ethanol. *Neurosci Lett* 165:211-214.

Allan, A.M.; Harris, R.A. (1986). Gamma-aminobutyric acid and alcohol actions: Neurochemical studies of long sleep and short sleep mice. *Life Sci* 39:2005-2015.

Allan, A.M.; Harris, R.A. (1987). Acute and chronic ethanol treatments alter GABA receptor-operated chloride channels. *Pharmacol Biochem Behav* 27:665-670.

Arango, V.; Underwood, M.D.; Pauler, D.K.; Kass, R.E.; Mann, J.J. (1996). Differential age-related loss of pigmented locus coeruleus neurons in suicides, alcoholics, and alcoholic suicides. *Alcohol Clin Exp Res* 20:1141-1147.

Arendt, T. (1993). The cholinergic differentiation of the cerebral cortex induced by chronic consumption of alcohol: Reversal by cholinergic drugs and transplantation. In Hunt, W.A.; Nixon, S.J. (Eds.), *Alcohol-Induced Brain Damage*, Vol. 22, pp. 431-460. Rockville, MD: NIAAA/NIH.

Arendt, T.; Bruckner, M.K.; Magliusi, S.; Krell, T. (1995). Degeneration of rat cholinergic basal forebrain neurons and reactive changes in nerve growth factor expression after chronic neurotoxic injury-I. Degeneration and plastic response of basal forebrain neurons. *Neuroscience* 65:633-645.

Baker, K.G.; Halliday, G.M.; Kril, J.J.; Harper, C.G. (1996). Chronic alcoholism in the absence of Wernicke-Korsakoff syndrome and cirrhosis does not result in the loss of serotonergic neurons from the median raphe nucleus. *Metab Brain Dis* 11:217-227.

Bechara, A.; Tranel, D.; Damasio, H. (2000). Characterization of the decision-making deficit of patients with ventromedial prefrontal cortex lesions. *Brain* 123:2189-2202.

Begleiter, H.; Porjesz, B. (1999). What is inherited in the predisposition toward alcoholism? A proposed model. *Alcohol Clin Exp Res* 23:1125-1135.

Bergeron, M.; Reader, T.A.; Layrargues, G.P.; Butterworth, R.F. (1989). Monoamines and metabolites in autopsied brain tissue from cirrhotic patients with hepatic encephalopathy. *Neurochem Res* 14:853-859.

Bettler, B.; Mulle, C. (1995). Neurotransmitter receptors II AMPA and kainate receptors. *Neuropharmacology* 34:123-139.

Boisse, N.N.; Okamoto, M. (1980). Ethanol as a sedative-hypnotic: Comparison with barbiturate and non-barbiturate sedative-hypnotics. In Rigter, H.; Crabbe, J.C. (Eds.), *Alcohol Tolerance and Dependence*, pp. 265-292. Amsterdam: Elsevier.

Boller, F.; Traykov, L.; Dao-Castellana, M.H.; Fontaine-Dabernard, A. (1995). Cognitive functioning in "diffuse pathology": Role of prefrontal and limbic structures. *Ann NY Acad Sci* 769:23-39.

Bowe, M.A.; Nadler, J.V. (1995). Polyamines antagonize N-methyl-D-aspartate evoked depolarizations, but reduce Mg^{2+} block. *Eur J Pharmacol* 278:55-65.

Breese, G.R.; Morrow, A.L.; Simson, P.E.; Criswell, H.E.; McCown, T.J.; Duncan, G.E.; Keir, W.J. (1993). The neuroanatomical specificity of ethanol action with ligand-gated ion channels: A hypothesis. *Alcohol and Alcoholism* Suppl 2:309-313.

Buck, K.J.; Harris, R.A. (1990). Benzodiazepine agonist and inverse agonist actions on GABAA receptor-operated chloride channels. II. Chronic effects of ethanol. *J Pharmacol Exp Ther* 253:713-719.

Buller, A.L.; Larson, H.C.; Morrisett, R.A.; Monaghan, D.T. (1995). Glycine modulates ethanol inhibition of heteromeric N-methyl-D-aspartate receptors expressed in Xenopus oocytes. *Mol Pharmacol* 48:717-723.

Buller, A.L.; Larson, H.C.; Schneider, B.E.; Beaton, J.A.; Morrisett, R.A.; Monoghan, D.T. (1994). The molecular basis of NMDA receptor subtypes:

Native receptor diversity is predicted by subunit composition. *J Neurosci* 14:5471-5484.

Butterworth, R.F. (1995). Pathophysiology of alcoholic brain damage: Synergistic effects of ethanol, thiamine deficiency and alcoholic liver disease. *Metab Brain Dis* 10:1-8.

Carboni, S.; Isola, R.; Gessa, G.L.; Rossetti, Z.L. (1993). Ethanol prevents the glutamate release induced by N-methyl-D-aspartate in the rat striatum. *Neurosci Lett* 152:133-136.

Carter, L.A.; Belknap, J.K.; Crabbe, J.C.; Janowsky, A. (1995). Allosteric regulation of the N-methyl-D-aspartate receptor-linked ion channel complex and effects of ethanol in ethanol-withdrawal seizure-prone and -resistant mice. *J Neurochem* 64:213-219.

Celentano, J.J.; Gibbs, T.T.; Farb, D.H. (1988). Ethanol potentiates GABA- and glycine-induced chloride currents in chick spinal cord neurons. *Brain Res* 455:377-380.

Chandler, L.J.; Harris, R.A.; Crews, F.T. (1998). Ethanol tolerance and synaptic plasticity. *Trends Pharmacol Sci* 19:491-495.

Chandler, L.J.; Sumners, C.; Crews, F.T. (1995). Chronic ethanol increases NMDA-stimulated NO formation but not MK-801 binding or NMDAR1 subunits in primary neuronal cultures. *Mol Pharmacol* 19:6A-14.

Chandler, L.J.; Newson, H.; Sumners, C.; Crews, F.T. (1993). Chronic ethanol exposure potentiates NMDA excitotoxicity in cerebral cortical neurons. *J Neurochem* 60:1578-1581.

Chandler, L.J.; Guzman, N.; Sumners, C.; Crews, F.T. (1994). Induction of nitric oxide synthase in brain glial cells: Possible interaction with ethanol in reactive neuronal injury. In Lancaster, F.E. (Ed.), *Alcohol and Glial Cells,* Vol. 27, pp. 195-214. Rockville, MD: NIAAA.

Chu, B.; Anantharam, V.; Treistman, S.N. (1995). Ethanol inhibition of recombinant heteromeric NMDA channels in the presence and absence of modulators. *J Neurochem* 65:140-148.

Coe, I.R.; Dohrman, D.P.; Constantinescu, A.; Diamond, I.; Gordon, A.S. (1996). Activation of cyclic AMP-dependent protein kinase reverses tolerance of a nucleoside transporter to ethanol. *J Pharmacol Exp Ther* 276:365-369.

Coe, I.R.; Yao, L.; Diamond, I.; Gordon, A.S. (1996). The role of protein kinase C in cellular tolerance to ethanol. *J Biol Chem* 271:29468-29472.

Coghlan, V.M.; Perrino, B.A.; Howard, M.; Langeberg, L.K.; Hicks, J.B.; Gallatin, W.M.; Scott, J.D. (1995). Association of protein kinase A and protein phosphatase 2B with a common anchoring protein. *Science* 267:108-111.

Collins, M.A.; Zou, J-Y.; Neafsey, E.J. (1998). Brain damage due to episodic alcohol exposure in vivo and in vitro: Furosemide neuroprotection implicates edema based mechanism. *FASEB J* 12:221-230.

Courville, C.B. (1955). *Effects of Alcohol on the Nervous System in Man.* Los Angeles: San Lucas Press.

Crews, F.T. (1999). Alcohol and neurodegeneration. *CNS Drug Reviews* 5:379-394.

Crews, F.T. (2000). Neurotoxicity of alcohol: Excitotoxicity, oxidative stress, neurotrophic factors, apoptosis, and cell adhesion molecules. In Noronha, M.; Eckardt, M.; Warren, K. (Eds.), *Review of NIAAA's Neuroscience and Behavioral Research Portfolio,* Monograph No. 34, pp. 189-206. Bethesda, MD: National Institutes of Health.

Crews, F.T.; Chandler, L.J. (1993). Excitotoxicity and the neuropathology of ethanol. In Hunt, W.A.; Nixon, S.J. (Eds.), *Alcohol-Induced Brain Damage,* Vol. 22, pp. 355-371. Rockville, MD: NIAAA Monograph.

Crews, F.T.; Newsom, H.; Gerber, M.; Sumners, C.; Chandler, L.J.; Freund, G. (1993). Molecular mechanisms of alcohol neurotoxicity. In Alling, C.; Sun, G. (Eds.), *Alcohol, Cell Membranes, and Signal Transduction in Brain,* pp. 123-138. Lund, Sweden: Plenum Press.

Crews, F.T.; Waage, H.G.; Wilkie, M.B.; Lauder, J.M. (1999). Ethanol pretreatment enhances NMDA excitotoxicity in biogenic amine neurons: Protection by brain derived neurotrophic factor. *Alcohol Clin Exp Res* 23:1834-1842.

Crews, F.T.; Braun, C.J.; Hoplight, B.; Switzer, R.C.; Knapp, D.J. (2000). Binge ethanol consumption causes differential brain damage in young-adolescent compared to adult rats. *Alcohol Clin Exp Res* 24:1712-1723.

Criswell, H.E.; Simson, P.E.; Duncan, G.E.; McCown, T.J.; Herbert, J.S.; Morrow, A.L.; Breese, G.R. (1993). Molecular basis for regionally specific action of ethanol on γ-aminobutyric acid A receptors: Generalization to other ligand-gated ion channels. *J Pharmacol Exp Ther* 267:522-537.

Criswell, H.E.; Simson, P.E.; Knapp, D.J.; Devaud, L.L.; McCown, T.J.; Duncan, G.E.; Morrow, A.L.; Breese, G.R. (1995). Effect of zolpidem on γ-aminobutyric acid (GABA)-induced inhibition predicts the interaction of ethanol with GABA on individual neurons in several rat brain regions. *J Pharmacol Exp Ther* 273:526-536.

Cutting, G.R.; Curristin, S.; Zoghbi, H.; O'Hara, B.; Seldin, M.F.; Uhl, G.R. (1992). Identification of a putative gamma-aminobutyric acid (GABA) receptor subunit rho2 cDNA and colocalization of the genes encoding rho2 (GABRR2) and rho1 (GABRR1) to human chromosome 6q14-q21 and mouse chromosome 4. *Genomics* 12:801-806.

Cutting, G.R.; Lu, L.; O'Hara, B.F.; Kasch, L.M.; Montrose-Rafizadeh, C.; Donovan, D.M.; Shimada, S. et al. (1991). Cloning of the gamma-aminobutyric acid (GABA) rho1 cDNA: A GABA receptor subunit highly expressed in the retina. *Proc Natl Acad Sci USA* 88:2673-2677.

Davies, J.; Francis, A.A.; Jones, A.W.; Watkins, J.C. (1981). 2-Amino-5-phosphonovalerate (2APV), a potent and selective antagonist of amino acid-induced and synaptic excitation. *Neurosci Lett* 21:77-81.

Davis, W.C.; Ticku, M.K. (1981). Ethanol enhances [3H]diazepan binding at the benzodiazepine-GABA receptor ionophore complex. *Mol Pharmacol* 20:287.

DePetrillo, P.B.; Liou, C.S. (1993). Ethanol exposure increases total protein kinase C activity in human lymphocytes. *Alcohol Clin Exp Res* 17:351-354.

Devaud, L.L.; Purdy, R.H.; Morrow, A.L. (1995). The neurosteroid 3α-hydroxy5α-pregnan-20-one protects against bicuculline-induced seizures during ethanol withdrawal in rats. *Alcohol Clin Exp Res* 19:350-355.

Devaud, L.L.; Morrow, A.L.; Criswell, H.E.; Breese, G.R.; Duncan, G.E. (1995). Regional differences in the effects of chronic ethanol administration on [3H]zolpidem binding in rat brain. *Alcohol Clin Exp Res* 19:910-914.

Devaud, L.L.; Purdy, R.H.; Finn, D.A.; Morrow, A.L. (1996). Sensitization of γ-aminobutyric acidA receptors to neuroactive steroids in rats during ethanol withdrawal. *J Pharmacol Exp Ther* 278:510-517.

Devaud, L.L.; Smith, F.D.; Grayson, D.R.; Morrow, A.L. (1995). Chronic ethanol consumption differentially alters the expression of g-aminobutyric acid A receptor subunit mRNAs in rat cerebral cortex: Competitive, quantitative reverse transcriptase-polymerase chain reaction analysis. *Mol Pharmacol* 48:861-868.

de Vries, D.J.; Johnston, G.A.R.; Ward, L.C.; Wilce, P.A.; Shanley, B.C. (1987). Effects of chronic ethanol inhalation on the enhancement of benzodiazepine binding to mouse brain membranes by GABA. *Neurochem Int* 10:231-235.

Di Sclafani, V.; Ezekiel, F.; Meyerhoff, D.J.; MacKay, S.; Dillon, W.P.; Weiner, M.W. (1995). Brain atrophy and cognitive function in older abstinent alcoholic men. *Alcohol Clin Exp Res* 19:1121-1126.

Dildy, J.E.; Leslie, S.W. (1989). Ethanol inhibits NMDA-induced increases in free intracellular Ca^{2+} in dissociated brain cells. *Brain Res* 499:383-387.

Dildy-Mayfield, J.E.; Harris, R.A. (1992a). Acute and chronic ethanol exposure alters the function of hippocampal kainate receptors expressed in Xenopus oocytes. *J Neurochem* 58:1569-1572.

Dildy-Mayfield, J.E.; Harris, R.A. (1992b). Comparison of ethanol sensitivity of rat brain kainate, DL-a-amino-3-hydroxy-5-methyl-4-isoxalone proprionic acid and N-methyl-D-aspartate receptors expressed in Xenopus oocytes. *J Pharmacol Exp Ther* 262:487-494.

Dildy-Mayfield, J.E.; Mihic, S.J.; Liu, Y.; Deitrich, R.A.; Harris, R.A. (1996). Actions of long chain alcohols on GABAA and glutamate receptors: Relation to in vivo effects. *Br J Pharmacol* 118:378-384.

Dohrman, D.P.; Diamond, I.; Gordon, A.S. (1996). Ethanol causes translocation of cAMP-dependent protein kinase catalytic subunit to the nucleus. *Proc Natl Acad Sci USA* 93:10217-10221.

Duncan, G.E.; Breese, G.R.; Criswell, H.E.; McCown, T.J.; Herbert, J.S.; Devaud, L.L.; Morrow, A.L. (1995). Distribution of [3H]zolpidem binding sites in relation to mRNA encoding the α1, β2 and γ2 subunits of GABAA receptors in rat brain. *Neuroscience* 64:1113-1128.

Durand, G.M.; Bennett, M.V.; Zukin, R.S. (1993). Splice variants of the N-methyl-D-aspartate receptor NR1 identify domains involved in regulation by polyamines and protein kinase C. *Proc Natl Acad Sci USA* 90:6731-6735.

Durand, G.M.; Gregor, P.; Zheng, X.; Bennett, M.L.V.; Uhl, G.R.; Zukin, R.S. (1992). Cloning of an apparent splice variant of the rat N-methyl-D-aspartate receptor NMDAR1 with altered sensitivity to polyamines and activators of protein kinase C. *Proc Natl Acad Sci USA* 89(19):9359-9363.

Eckardt, M.J.; Rohrbaugh, J.W.; Stapleton, J.M.; Davis, E.Z.; Martin, P.R.; Weingartner, H.J. (1996). Attention-related brain potential and cognition in alcoholism-associated organic brain disorders. *Biol Psychiatry* 39:143-146.

Fadda, F.; Rossetti, Z. (1998). Chronic ethanol consumption: From neuroadaptation to neurodegeneration. *Prog Neurobiol* 56:385-431.

Follesa, P.; Ticku, M. (1995). Chronic ethanol treatment differentially regulates NMDA receptor subunit mRNA expression in rat brain. *Mol Brain Res* 29:99-106.

Foster, J.; Eskes, G.; Stuss, D. (1994). The cognitive neuropsychology of attention: A frontal lobe perspective. *Cognitive Neuropsychology* 11:133-147.

Franke, H.; Kittner, H.; Berger, P.; Wirkner, K.; Schramek, J. (1997). The reaction of astrocytes and neurons in the hippocampus of adult rats during chronic ethanol treatment and correlations to behavioral impairments. *Alcohol* 14:445-454.

Frohlich, R.; Patzelt, C.; Illes, P. (1994). Inhibition by ethanol of excitatory amino acid receptors and nicotinic acetylcholine receptors at rat locus coeruleus neurons. *Naunyn Schmiedebergs Arch Pharmacol* 350(6):626-631.

Frye, G.D.; Breese, G.R. (1982). GABAergic modulation of ethanol-induced motor impairment. *J Pharmacol Exp Ther* 223:752-756.

Frye, G.; Chapin, R.; Vogel, R.; Mailman, R.; Kilts, C.; Mueller, R.; Breese, G. (1981). Effects of acute and chronic 1,3-butanediol treatment on central nervous system function: A comparison with ethanol. *J Pharmacol Exp Ther* 216:306-314.

Frye, G.D.; McCown, T.J.; Breese, G.R. (1983a). Characterization of susceptibility to audiogenic seizures in ethanol-dependent rats after microinjections of gammaaminobutyric acid (GABA) agonists into the inferior coliculus, substantia nigra or medial septum. *J Pharmacol Exp Ther* 227:663-670.

Frye, G.D.; McCown, T.J.; Breese, G.R. (1983b). Differential sensitivity of ethanol withdrawal signs in the rat to gamma-aminobutyric acid (GABA) mimetics: Blockade of audiogenic seizures but not forelimb tremors. *J Pharmacol Exp Ther* 226:720-725.

Gallagher, M.; McMahan, R.W.; Schoenbaum, G. (1999). Orbitofrontal cortex and representation of incentive value in associative learning. *J Neurosci* 19:6610-6614.

Giancola, P.R.; Zeichner, A. (1995). Alcohol-related aggression in males and females: Effects of blood alcohol concentration, subjective intoxication, personality, and provocation. *Alcohol Clin Exp Res* 19:130-134.

Givens, B.S.; Breese, G.R. (1990a). Electrophysiological evidence for an involvement of the medial septal area in the acute sedative effects of ethanol. *J Pharmacol Exp Ther* 253:95-103.

Givens, B.S.; Breese, G.R. (1990b). Site-specific enhancement of γ-aminobutyric acid-mediated inhibition of neural activity by ethanol in the rat medial septum. *J Pharmacol Exp Ther* 254:528-538.

Goldstein, D.B. (1973). Alcohol withdrawal reactions in mice: Effects of drugs that modify neurotransmission. *J Pharmacol Exp Ther* 186:1-9.

Goldstein, D.B.; Pal, N. (1971). Alcohol dependence produced in mice by inhalation of ethanol: Grading the withdrawal reaction. *Science* 172:288-290.

Gonzales, R.; Bungay, P.M.; Kiianmaa, K.; Samson, H.H.; Rossetti, Z.L. (1996). In vivo links between neurochemistry and behavioral effects of ethanol. *Alcohol Clin Exp Res* 20(suppl):203A-205A.

Gonzales, R.A. (1990). NMDA receptors excite alcohol research. *Trends Pharmacol Sci* 11:137-139.

Gonzalez, L.P.; Czachura, J.F. (1989). Reduced behavioral responses to intranigral muscimol following chronic ethanol. *Physiol Behav* 46:473-477.

Gordon, A.S.; Collier, K.; Diamond, I. (1986). Ethanol regulation of adenosine receptor-stimulated cAMP levels in a clonal neural cell line: An in vitro model of cellular tolerance to ethanol. *Proc Natl Acad Sci USA* 83:2105-2108.

Gordon, A.S.; Yao, L.; Wu, Z.L.; Coe, I.R.; Diamond, I. (1997). Ethanol alters the subcellular localization of delta- and epsilon protein kinase C in NG 108-15 cells. *Mol Pharmacol* 52:554-559.

Grant, B.F.; Dawson, D.A. (1997). Age of onset of alcohol use and its association with DSM-IV alcohol abuse and dependence: Results from the National Longitudinal Alcohol Epidemiologic Survey. *J Substance Abuse* 9:103-110.

Grant, K.A.; Colombo, G. (1993). Discriminative stimulus effects of ethanol: Effect of training dose on the substitution of N-methyl-D-aspartate antagonists. *J Pharmacol Exp Ther* 264:1261-1247.

Grant, K.A.; Knisely, J.S.; Tabakoff, B.; Barrett, J.E.; Balster, R.L. (1991). Ethanol like discriminative stimulus effects of noncompetitive N-methyl-D-aspartate antagonists. *Behavioral Pharmacology* 2:87-95.

Grant, K.A.; Valverius, P.; Hudspith, M.; Tabakoff, B. (1990). Ethanol withdrawal seizures and the NMDA receptor complex. *Eur J Pharmacol* 176:289-296.

Greenberg, D.A.; Cooper, E.C.; Gordon, A.; Diamond, I. (1984). Ethanol and the γ-aminobutyric acid receptor complex. *J Neurochem* 42:1062-1068.

Gulya, K.; Grant, K.A.; Valverius, P.; Hoffman, P.L.; Tabakoff, B. (1991). Brain regional specificity and time-course of changes in the NMDA receptor-ionophore complex during ethanol withdrawal. *Brain Res* 547:129-134.

Gyenes, M.; Farrant, M.; Farb, D.H. (1988). "Run-down" of γ-aminobutyric acid A receptor function during whole cell recording: A possible role for phosphorylation. *Mol Pharmacol* 34:719-723.

Halliday, G.; Baker, K.; Harper, C. (1995). Serotonin and alcohol-related brain damage. *Metab Brain Dis* 10:25-30.

Hamelink, C.R.; Carpenter-Hylana, E.P.; Meiri, N.; Ondo, J.G.; Castronguay, T.W.; Eskay, R.L. (1998). Short-term binge alcohol exposure lesions hippocampa-lentorhinal cortex and impairs spatial memory. *Society for Neuroscience Abstracts* 24:1239.

Harding, A.J.; Halliday, G.M.; Ng, J.L.; Harper, C.G.; Kril, J.J. (1996). Loss of vasopressin-immunoreactive neurons in alcoholics is dose-related and time-dependent. *Neuroscience* 72:699-708.

Harding, A.J.; Wong, A.; Svoboda, M.; Kril, J.J.; Halliday, G.M. (1997). Chronic alcohol consumption does not cause hippocampal neuron loss in humans. *Hippocampus* 7:78-87.

Harper, C.G.; Kril, J.J. (1990). Neuropathology of alcoholism. *Alcohol* 25:207-216.

Harper, C.G.; Kril, J.J. (1993). Neuropathological changes in alcoholics. In Hunt, W.A.; Nixon, S.J. (Eds.), *Alcohol-Induced Brain Damage,* Vol. 22, pp. 39-70. Rockville, MD: NIAAA/NIH.

Harper, C.G.; Kril, J.J.; Daly, J. (1987). Are we drinking our neurons away? *Br Med J* 294:534-536.

Harris, R.A.; McQuilkin, S.J.; Paylor, R.; Abeliovich, A.; Tonegawa, S.; Wehner, J.M. (1995). Mutant mice lacking the gamma isoform of protein kinase C show decreased behavioral actions of ethanol and altered function of gamma-aminobutyrate type A receptors. *Proc Natl Acad Sci USA* 92:3658-3662.

Harris, R.A.; Proctor, W.R.; McQuilkin, S.J.; Klein, R.L.; Mascia, M.P.; Whatley, V.; Whiting, P.J.; Dunwiddie, T.V. (1995). Ethanol increases GABAA responses in cells stably transfected with receptor subunits. *Alcohol Clin Exp Res* 19:226-232.

Hazell, A.S.; Butterworth, R.F. (1999). Hepatic encephalopathy: An update of pathophysiologic mechanisms. *Proc Soc Exp Biol Med* 222:99-112.

Heuschneider, G.; Schwartz, R.D. (1989). cAMP and forskolin decrease γ-aminobutyric acid-gated chloride flux in rat brain synaptoneurosomes. *Proc Natl Acad Sci USA* 86:2938-2942.

Hoaken, P.N.S.; Giancola, P.R.; Pihl, R.O. (1998). Executive cognitive functions as mediators of alcohol-related aggression. *Alcohol and Alcoholism* 33:47-54.

Hoffman, P.L.; Moses, F.; Tabakoff, B. (1989). Selective inhibition by ethanol of glutamate-stimulated cyclic GMP production in primary cultures of cerebellar granule cells. *Neuropharmacology* 28:1239-1243.

Hoffman, P.L.; Rabe, C.S.; Moses, F.; Tabakoff, B. (1989). N-methyl-D-aspartate receptors and ethanol: Inhibition of calcium flux and cyclic GMP production. *J Neurochem* 52:1937-1940.

Hollmann, M.; Boulter, J.; Maron, C.; Beasley, L.; Sullivan, J.; Pecht, G.; Heinemann, S. (1993). Zinc potentiates agonist-induced currents at certain splice variants of the NMDA receptor. *Neuron* 10:943-954.

Hollmann, M.; Heineman, S. (1994). Cloned glutamate receptors. *Annu Rev Neurosci* 17:31-108.

Hollmann, M.; O'shea-Greenfield, A.; Rogers, S.W.; Heinemann, S. (1989). Cloning by functional expression of a member of the glutamate receptor family. *Nature* 342:643-648.

Hommer, D.; Momenan, R.; Rawlings, R.; Ragan, P.; Williams, W.; Rio, D.; Eckardt, M. (1996). Decreased corpus callosum size among alcoholic women. *Arch Neurol* 53:359-363.

Huganir, R.L.; Greengard, P. (1990). Regulation of neurotransmitter receptor desensitization by protein phosphorylation. *Neuron* 5:555-567.

Hunt, W.A. (1983). The effect of ethanol on GABAergic transmission. *Neurosci Biobehav Rev* 7:87-95.

Ibanez, J.; Herrero, M.T.; Insausti, R.; Balzunegui, T.; Tunon, T.; Garcia-Bragado, F.; Gonzalo, L.M. (1995). Chronic alcoholism decreases neuronal nuclear size in the human entorhinal cortex. *Neurosci Lett* 183:71-74.

Igarashi, K.; Williams, K. (1995). Antagonist properties of polyamines and bis(ethyl)polyamines at N-methyl-D-aspartate receptors. *J Pharmacol Exp Ther* 272:1101-1109.

Iorio, K.R.; Reinlib, L.; Tabakoff, B.; Hoffman, P.L. (1992). Chronic exposure of cerebellar granule cells to ethanol results in increased N-methyl-D-aspartate receptor function. *Mol Pharmacol* 41:1142-1148.

Iorio, K.R.; Tabakoff, B.; Hoffman, P.L. (1993). Glutamate-induced neurotoxicity is increased in cerebellar granule cells exposed chronically to ethanol. *Eur J Pharmacol* 248:209-212.

Ishii, T.; Moriyoshi, K.; Sugihara, H.; Sakurada, K.; Kadotani, H.; Tokoi, M.; Akazawa, C. et al. (1993). Molecular characterization of the family of the NMDA receptor subunits. *J Biol Chem* 286:2636-2643.

Jagannathan, M.R.; Desai, M.G.; Raghunathan, P. (1996). Brain metabolite changes in alcoholism: An in vivo proton magnetic resonance spectroscopy. *Magn Reson Imaging* 14:553-557.

Jernigan, T.L.; Butters, N.; DiTraglia, G.; Schafer, K.; Smith, T.; Irwin, M.; Grant, I.; Schuckit, M.; Cermak, L.S. (1991). Reduced cerebral grey matter observed in alcoholics using magnetic resonance imaging. *Alcohol Clin Exp Res* 15:418-427.

Johnson, J.W.; Ascher, P. (1987). Glycine potentiates the NMDA response in cultured mouse brain neurons. *Nature* 325:529-531.

Karanian, J.W.; Yergey, J.; Lister, R.; D'souza, N.; Linnoila, M.; Salem, N. (1986). Characterization of an automated apparatus for precise control of inhalation chamber ethanol vapor and blood ethanol concentrations. *Alcohol Clin Exp Res* 10:443-447.

Karobath, M.; Rogers, J.; Bloom, F.E. (1980). Benzodiazepine receptors remain unchanged after chronic ethanol administration. *Neuropharmacology* 19:125-128.

Keinanen, K.; Wisden, W.; Sommer, B.; Werner, P.; Herb, A.; Verdoorn, T.A.; Sakmann, B.; Seeburg, P.H. (1990). A family of AMPA-selective glutamate receptors. *Science* 249:556-560.

Kleckner, N.W.; Dingledine, R. (1988). Requirement for glycine in activation of NMDA-receptors expressed in Xenopus oocytes. *Science* 241:835-837.

Klein, R.L.; Mascia, M.P.; Whiting, P.J.; Harris, R.A. (1995). GABAA receptor function and binding in stably transfected cells: Chronic ethanol treatment. *Alcohol Clin Exp Res* 19:1338-1344.

Knapp, D.J.; Criswell, H.E.; Breese, G.R. (1995). Regional effects of isoproterenol on ethanol enhancement of GABA responses in vivo. *Soc Neurosci Abstr* 21:354.

Knecht, K.; Michalak, A.; Rose, C.; Rothstein, J.D.; Butterworth, R.F. (1997). Decreased glutamate transporters (GLT-1) expression in frontal cortex of rats with acute liver failure. *Neurosci Lett* 229:201-203.

Koltchine, V.; Anantharam, V.; Wilson, A.; Bayley, H.; Treistman, S.N. (1993). Homomeric assemblies of NMDAR1 splice variants are sensitive to ethanol. *Neurosci Lett* 152:13-16.

Koob, G.F.; Le Moal, M. (1997). Drug abuse: Hedonic homeostatic dysregulation. *Science* 278:52-58.

Koob, G.F.; Percy, L.; Britton, K.T. (1989). The effects of Ro15-4513 on the behavioral actions of ethanol in an operant reaction time test and a conflict test. *Pharmacol Biochem Behav* 31:757-760.

Kopelman, M.D.; Corn, T.H. (1988). Cholinergic "blockade" as a model for cholinergic depletion. A comparison of the memory deficits with those of Alzheimer-type dementia and the alcoholic Korsakoff syndrome. *Brain* 111:1079-1110.

Kubota, Y.; Sato, W.; Murai, T.; Toichi, M.; Ikeda, A.; Sengoku, A. (2000). Emotional cognition without awareness after unilateral temporal lobectomy in humans. *J Neurosci* 20:1-5.

Kumar, K.N.; Tilakaratne, N.; Johnson, P.S.; Allen, A.E.; Michaelis, E.K. (1991). Cloning of cDNA for the glutamate-binding subunit of an NMDA receptor complex. *Nature* 354:70-73.

Kutsuwada, T.; Kashiwabuchi, N.; Mori, H.; Sakimura, K.; Kushiya, E.; Araki, K.; Meguro, H. et al. (1992). Molecular diversity of the NMDA receptor channel. *Nature* 358:36-41.

Lambie, D.G. (1985). Alcoholic brain damage and neurological symptoms of alcohol withdrawal—manifestations of overhydration. *Med Hypotheses* 16:377-388.

Langlais, P.J.; Mair, R.G. (1990). Protective effects of the glutamate antagonist MK-801 on pyrithiamine-induced lesions and amino acid changes in rat brain. *J Neurosci* 10:1664-1674.

Langlais, P.J.; Zhang, S.X. (1993). Extracellular glutamate is increased in thalamus during thiamine deficiency-induced lesions and is blocked by MK-801. *J Neurochem* 61:2175-2182.

Laurie, D.J.; Seeburg, P.H. (1994). Regional and developmental heterogeneity in splicing of the rat brain NMDAR1 mRNA. *J Neurosci* 14:335-345.

Lavoie, J.; Giguere, J.F.; Layrargues, G.P.; Butterworth, R.F. (1987). Activities of neuronal and astrocytic marker enzymes in autopsied brain tissue from patients with hepatic encephalopathy. *Metab Brain Dis* 2:283-290.

Lavoie, J.; Layrargues, G.P.; Butterworth, R.F. (1990). Increased densities of peripheral-type benzodiazepine receptors in brain autopsy samples from cirrhotic patients with hepatic encephalopathy. *Hepatology* 11:874-878.

Layrargues, G.P.; Butterworth, R.F. (1992). Efficacy of Ro15-1788 in cirrhotic patients with hepatic coma: Results of a randomized, double-blind placebocontrolled crossover trial. *Hepatology* 16:311-319.

Le, A.D.; Khanna, J.M.; Kalant, H.; Grossi, F. (1986). Tolerance to and crosstolerance among ethanol, pentobarbital and chlordiazepoxide. *Pharmacol Biochem Behav* 24:93-98.

Ledig, M.; M'Paria, J.; Mandel, P. (1981). Superoxide dismutase activity in rat brain during acute and chronic alcohol intoxication. *Neurochem Res* 6:385-390.

Leidenheimer, N.J.; Browning, M.D.; Dunwiddie, T.V.; Hahner, L.D.; Harris, R.A. (1990). Phosphorylation-independent effects of second messenger system modulators on gamma-aminobutyric acidA receptor complex function. *Mol Pharmacol* 38:823-828.

Levin, L.H.; Koehler, R.C.; Brusilow, S.W.; Jones, J.; Traystman, R.J. (1989). Elevated brain water during urease-induced hyperammonemia in dogs. In Hoff, J.T.; Betz, A.L. (Eds.), *Intracranial Pressure,* pp. 1032-1088. Berlin: SpringerVerlag.

Levitan, E.S.; Schofield, P.R.; Burt, D.R.; Rhee, L.M.; Wisden, W.; Kohler, M.; Fujita, N. et al. (1988). Structural and functional basis for GABAA receptor heterogeneity. *Nature* 335:76-79.

Lieberman, D.N.; Mody, I. (1994). Regulation of NMDA channel function by endogenous Ca^{2+}-dependent phosphatase. *Nature* 369:235-239.

Liljequist, S.; Engel, J.A. (1984). The effects of GABA and benzodiazepine receptor antagonists on the anti-conflict action of diazepam or ethanol. *Pharmacol Biochem Behav* 21:521-526.

Lima-Landman, M.T.; Albuquerque, E.X. (1989). Ethanol potentiates and blocks NMDA-activated single-channel currents in rat hippocampal pyramidal cells. *FEBS Lett* 247:61-67.

Lin, A.M-Y.; Freund, R.K.; Palmer, M.R. (1991). Ethanol potentiation of GABA-induced electrophysiological responses in cerebellum: Requirement for catecholamine modulation. *Neurosci Lett* 122:154-158.

Lister, R.G. (1988). Partial reversal of ethanol-induced reductions in exploration by two benzodiazepine antagonists (flumazenil and ZK 93426). *Brain Res Bull* 21:765-770.

Lovinger, D.M. (1993). High ethanol sensitivity of recombinant AMPA-type glutamate receptors expressed in mammalian cells. *Neurosci Lett* 159:83-87.

Lovinger, D.M. (1995). Developmental decrease in ethanol inhibition of N-methyl D-aspartate receptors in rat neocortical neurons: Relation to the actions of ifenprodil. *J Pharmacol Exp Ther* 274:164-172.

Lovinger, D.M.; White, G.; Weight, F.F. (1989). Ethanol inhibits NMDA-activated ion current in hippocampal neurons. *Science* 243:1721-1724.

Lovinger, D.M.; White, G.; Weight, F.F. (1990). NMDA receptor-mediated synaptic excitation selectively inhibited by ethanol in hippocampal slice from adult rat. *J Neurosci* 10:1372-1379.

Lu, W.; Jaatinen, P.; Rintala, J.; Sarviharju, M.; Kiianmaa, K.; Hervonen, A. (1997). Effects of life-long ethanol consumption on rat locus coeruleus. *Alcohol and Alcoholism* 32:463-470.

Lüddens, H.; Pritchett, D.B.; Kohler, M.; Killisch, I.; Keinanen, K.; Monyer, H.; Sprengel, R.; Seeburg, P.H. (1990). Cerebellar GABAA receptor selective for a behavioral alcohol antagonist. *Nature* 346:648-651.

Lynch, D.R.; Anegawa, N.J.; Verdoorn, T.; Pritchett, D.B. (1994). N-methyl-D-aspartate receptors: Different subunit requirements for binding of glutamate antagonists, glycine antagonists, and channel-blocking agents. *Mol Pharmacol* 45:540-545.

Lynch, D.R.; Lawrence, J.J.; Lenz, S.; Anegawa, N.J.; Dichter, M.; Pritchett, D.B. (1995). Pharmacological characterization of heterodimeric NMDA receptors composed of NR 1a and 2B subunits: Differences with receptors formed from NR 1a and 2A. *J Neurochem* 64:1462-1468.

Macdonald, R.L.; Olsen, R.W. (1994). GABA A receptor channels. *Annu Rev Neurosci* 17:569-602.

Madeira, M.D.; Andrade, J.P.; Lieberman, A.R.; Sousa, N.; Almeida, O.F.; Paula Barbosa, M.M. (1997). Chronic alcohol consumption and withdrawal do not induce cell death in the suprachiasmatic nucleus, but lead to irreversible depression of peptide immunoreactivity and mRNA levels. *J Neurosci* 17:1302-1319.

Martin, D.; Tayyeb, M.I.; Swartzwelder, H.S. (1995). Ethanol inhibition of AMPA and kainate receptor-mediated depolarizations of hippocampal area CA1. *Alcohol Clin Exp Res* 19:1312-1316.

Martin, P.R.; Adinoff, B.; Weingartner, H.; Mukherjee, A.B.; Edhardt, M.J. (1986). Alcoholic organic brain disease: Nosology and pathophysiologic mechanisms. *Prog Neuropsychopharmacol Biol Psychiatry* 10:147-164.

Martz, A.; Dietrich, R.A.; Harris, R.A. (1983). Behavioral evidence for the involvement of γ-aminobutyric acid in the actions of ethanol. *Eur J Pharmacol* 89:53-62.

Masood, K.; Wu, C.; Brauneis, U.; Weight, F.F. (1994). Differential ethanol sensitivity of recombinant N-methyl-D-aspartate receptor subunits. *Mol Pharmacol* 45:324-329.

Massey, J.T.; Moore, T.F.; Parsons, V.L.; Tadros, W. (1989). Design and estimation for the National Health Interview Survey, 1985-1994. *Vital and Health Statistics*, Vol 2(110), pp. 1-33. Hyattsville, MD: National Center for Health Statistics.

Matsumoto, I.; Leah, J.; Shanley, B.; Wilce, P. (1993). Immediate early gene expression in the rat brain during ethanol withdrawal. *Mol Cell Neurosci* 4:485-491.

Mayer, M.L.; Westbrook, G.L.; Guthrie, P.B. (1984). Voltage-dependent block by Mg^{2+} of NMDA responses in spinal cord neurons. *Nature* 309:261-263.

McQueen, J.D.; Posey, J.B. (1975). Changes in intracranial pressure and brain hydration during acute ethanolism. *Surgical Neurology* 4(4):375-379.

Meguro, H.H.; Mori, K.; Araki, E.; Kushiya, T.; Kutsuwada, M.; Yamazaki, T.; Kumanishi, M.; Arakawa, T.; Sakimura, S.; Mishina, M. (1992). Functional characterization of a heteromeric NMDA receptor channel expressed from cloned cDNAs. *Nature* 357:70-74.

Mehta, A.K.; Ticku, M.K. (1988). Ethanol potentiation of GABAergic transmission in cultured spinal cord neurons involves γ-aminobutyric acid-gated chloride channels. *J Pharmacol Exp Ther* 246:558-564.

Mehta, A.K.; Ticku, M.K. (1989). Chronic ethanol treatment alters the behavioral effects of Ro 15-4513, a partially negative ligand for benzodiazepine binding sites. *Brain Res* 489:93-100.

Mereu, G.; Gessa, G.L. (1985). Low doses of ethanol inhibit the firing of neurons in the substantia nigra pars reticulata: A GABAergic effect? *Brain Res* 360:325-330.

Messing, R.O.; Petersen, P.J.; Henrich, C.J. (1991). Chronic ethanol exposure increases levels of protein kinase C delta and epsilon and protein kinase C-mediated phosphorylation in cultured neural cells. *J Biol Chem* 266:23428-23432.

Mhatre, M.C.; Ticku, M.K. (1992). Chronic ethanol administration alters gamma aminobutyric acidA receptor gene expression. *Mol Pharmacol* 42:415-422.

Mhatre, M.C.; Ticku, M.K. (1993). Alcohol: Effects on GABAA receptor function and gene expression. *Alcohol and Alcoholism* Suppl 2:331-335.

Mhatre, M.; Mehta, A.K.; Ticku, M.K. (1988). Chronic ethanol administration increases the binding of the benzodiazepine inverse agonist and alcohol antagonist [3H]Ro15-4513 in rat brain. *Eur J Pharmacol* 153:141-145.

Michaelis, E.K.; Freed, W.J.; Galton, N.; Foye, J.; Michaelis, M.L.; Phillips, I.; Kleinmann, J.E. (1990). Glutamate receptor changes in brain synaptic membranes from human alcoholics. *Neurochemical Research* 15:1055-1063.

Mihic, S.J.; McQuilkin, S.J.; Eger, E.I. II; Ionescu, P.; Harris, R.A. (1994). Potentiation of gamma-aminobutyric acid type A receptor-mediated chloride currents by novel halogenated compounds correlates with their abilities to induce general anesthesia. *Mol Pharmacol* 46:851-857.

Mirshahi, T.; Woodward, J.J. (1995). Ethanol sensitivity of heteromeric NMDA receptors: Effects of subunit assembly, glycine and NMDAR1 Mg^{2+}-insensitive mutants. *Neuropharmacology* 34:347-355.

Moghaddam, B.; Bolinao, M.L. (1994). Biphasic effect of ethanol on extracellular accumulation of glutamate in the hippocampus and the nucleus accumbens. *Neurosci Lett* 178:99-102.

Molinoff, P.B.; Williams, K.; Pritchett, D.B.; Zhong, J. (1994). Molecular pharmacology of NMDA receptors: Modulatory role of NR2 subunits. *Prog Brain Res* 100:39-45.

Monaghan, D.T. (1991). Differential stimulation of [3H]-MK-801 binding to subpopulations of NMDA receptors. *Neurosci Lett* 122:21-24.

Montoliu, C.; Sancho-Tello, M.; Azorin, I.; Burgal, M.; Valles, S.; Renau-Piqueras, J.; Guerri, C. (1995). Ethanol increases cytochrome P4502E1 and induces oxidative stress in astrocytes. *J Neurochem* 65:2561-2570.

Montoliu, C.; Valles, S.; Renau-Piqueras, J.; Guerri, C. (1994). Ethanol-induced oxygen radical formation and lipid peroxidation in rat brain: Effect of chronic alcohol consumption. *J Neurochem* 63:1855-1862.

Montpied, P.; Morrow, A.L.; Karanian, J.W.; Ginns, E.I.; Martin, B.M.; Paul, S.M. (1991). Prolonged ethanol inhalation decreases gamma-aminobutyric acid A receptor alpha subunit mRNAs in the rat cerebral cortex. *Mol Pharmacol* 39:157-163.

Monyer, H.; Burnashev, N.; Laurie, D.J.; Sakmann, B.; Seeburg, P.H. (1994). Developmental and regional expression in rat brain and functional properties of four NMDA receptors. *Neuron* 12:529-540.

Monyer, H.; Sprengel, R.; Schoepfer, R.; Herb, A.; Higuchi, M.; Lomeli, H.; Burnashev, N.; Sakmann, B.; Seeburg, P.H. (1992). Heteromeric NMDA receptors: Molecular and functional distinction of subtypes. *Science* 258:597-603.

Moriyoshi, K.; Masu, M.; Ishii, T.; Shigemoto, R.; Mizuno, N.; Nakanishi, S. (1991). Molecular cloning and characterization of the rat NMDA receptor. *Nature* 354:31-37.

Morrow, A.L.; Herbert, J.S.; Montpied, P. (1992). Differential effects of chronic ethanol administration on GABAA receptor $\alpha 1$ and $\alpha 6$ subunit mRNA levels in rat cerebellum. *Mol Cell Neurosci* 3:251-258.

Morrow, A.L.; Pace, J.R.; Purdy, R.H.; Paul, S.M. (1990). Characterization of steroid interactions with gamma-aminobutyric acid receptor-gated chloride ion channels: Evidence for multiple steroid recognition sites. *Mol Pharmacol* 37: 263-270.

Morrow, A.L.; Suzdak, P.D.; Paul, S.M. (1988). Chronic ethanol administration alters GABA, pentobarbital and ethanol-mediated 36Cl- uptake in cerebral cortical synaptoneurosomes. *J Pharmacol Exp Ther* 246:158-164.

Nakanishi, N.; Axel, R.; Shneider, N.A. (1992). Alternative splicing generates functionally distinct N-methyl-D-aspartate receptors. *Proc Natl Acad Sci USA* 89: 8552-8556.

Nayeem, N.; Green, T.P.; Martin, I.L.; Barnard, E.A. (1994). Quarternary structure of the native GABAA receptor determined by electron microscopic image analysis. *J Neurochem* 62:815-818.

Nestores, J.N. (1980). Ethanol specifically potentiates GABA-mediated neurotransmission in the feline cerebral cortex. *Science* 209:708-710.

Nicolas, C.; Carter, C. (1994). Autoradiographic distribution and characteristics of high- and low-affinity polyamine-sensitive [3H]ifenprodil sites in the rat brain: Possible relationship to NMDAR2B receptors and calmodulin. *J Neurochem* 63:2248-2258.

Nicolas, J.M.; Estruch, R.; Salamero, M.; Orteu, N.; Fernandez-Sola, J.; Sacanella, E.; Urbano-Marquez, A. (1997). Brain impairment in well-nourished chronic alcoholics is related to ethanol intake. *Ann Neurol* 41:590-598.

Nordmann, R. (1987). Oxidative stress from alcohol in the brain. *Alcohol and Alcoholism* Suppl 1:75-82.

Nordmann, R.; Ribiere, C.; Rouach, H. (1990). Ethanol-induced lipid peroxidation and oxidative stress in extrahepatic tissues. *Alcohol and Alcoholism* 25:231-237.

Nordmann, R.; Ribiere, C.; Rouach, H. (1992). Implication of free radical mechanisms in ethanol induced cellular injury. *Free Radic Biol* 12:219-240.

Norenberg, M.D.; Huo, Z.; Neary, J.T.; Roig-Cantesano, A. (1997). The glial glutamate transporter in hyperammonemia and hepatic encephalopathy: Relation to energy metabolism and glutamatergic neurotransmission. *Glia* 21:124-133.

Nowak, L.; Bregestovski, P.; Ascher, A.; Herbert, A.; Prochiantz, A. (1984). Magnesium gates glutamate-activated channels in mouse central neurons. *Nature* 307:462-465.

Ortiz, J.; Fitzgerald, L.W.; Charlton, M.; Lane, S.; Trevisan, L.; Guitart, X.; Shoemaker, W.; Duman, R.S.; Nestler, E.J. (1995). Biochemical actions of chronic ethanol exposure in the mesolimbic dopamine system. *Synapse* 21:289-298.

Oscar-Berman, M.; Hutner, N. (1993). Frontal lobe changes after chronic alcohol ingestion. In Hunt, W.A.; Nixon, S.J. (Eds.), *Alcohol-Induced Brain Damage*, Vol. 22, pp. 121-156. Rockville, MA: NIAAA/NIH.

Paczynski, R.P.; He, Y.Y.; Diringer, M.N.; Hsu, C.Y. (1997). Multiple-dose mannitol reduces brain water content in a rat model of cortical infarction. *Stroke* 28:1437-1444.

Palmer, M.R.; van Horne, C.G.; Harlan, J.T.; Moore, E.A. (1988). Antagonism of ethanol effects on cerebellar Purkinje neurons by the benzodiazepine inverse agonists Ro15-4513 and FG 7142: Electrophysiological studies. *J Pharmacol Exp Ther* 247:1018-1024.

Parsons, O.A. (1993). Impaired neuropsychological cognitive functioning in sober alcoholics. In Hunt, W.A.; Nixon, S.J. (Eds.), *Alcohol-Induced Brain Damage,* Vol. 22, pp. 173-194. Rockville, MD: NIAAA/NIH.

Peoples, R.W.; Weight, F.F. (1992). Ethanol inhibition of N-methyl-D-aspartate activated ion current in rat hippocampal neurons is not competitive with glycine. *Brain Res* 571:342-344.

Peters, S.; Koh, J.; Choi, D.W. (1987). Zinc selectively blocks the action of N-methyl-D-aspartate on cortical neurons. *Science* 236:589-593.

Pfefferbaum, A.; Lim, K.O.; Desmond, J.E.; Sullivan, E.V. (1996). Thinning of the corpus callosum in older alcoholic men: A magnetic resonance imaging study. *Alcohol Clin Exp Res* 20:752-757.

Pfefferbaum, A.; Sullivan, E.V.; Mathalon, D.H.; Lim, K.O. (1997). Frontal lobe volume loss observed with magnetic resonance imaging in older chronic alcoholics. *Alcohol Clin Exp Res* 21:521-529.

Pfefferbaum, A.; Sullivan, E.V.; Mathalon, D.H.; Shear, P.K.; Rosenbloom, M.J.; Lim, K.O. (1995). Longitudinal changes in magnetic resonance imaging brain volumes in abstinent and relapsed alcoholics. *Alcohol Clin Exp Res* 19:1177-1191.

Pfefferbaum, A.; Sullivan, E.V.; Rosenbloom, M.J.; Mathalon, D.H.; Lim, K.O. (1998). A controlled study of cortical gray matter and ventricular changes in alcoholic men over a 5-year interval. *Arch Gen Psychiatry* 55:905-912.

Porter, N.M.; Twyman, R.E.; Uhler, M.D.; Macdonald, R.L. (1990). Cyclic AMP dependent protein kinase decreases GABAA receptor current in mouse spinal neurons. *Neuron* 5:789-796.

Pritchett, D.B.; Lüddens, H.; Seeburg, P.H. (1989). Type I and type II GABAA benzodiazepine receptors produced in transfected cells. *Science* 245:1389-1392.

Pritchett, D.B.; Sontheimer, H.; Shivers, B.D.; Ymer, S.; Kettenmann, H.; Schofield, P.R.; Seeburg, P.H. (1989). Importance of a novel GABAA receptor subunit for benzodiazepine pharmacology. *Nature* 338:582-585.

Prochasta, J.O.; DiClemente, C.D. (1992). Stages of change in the modification of problem behaviors. *Prog Behav Modif* 28:183-218.

Puia, G.; Ducic, I.; Vicini, S.; Costa, E. (1994). Does neurosteroid modulatory efficacy depend on GABAA receptor subunit composition? *Receptors Channels* 1:135-142.

Puia, G.; Vicini, S.; Seeburg, P.H.; Costa, E. (1991). Influence of recombinant gamma-aminobutyric acid-A receptor subunit composition on the action of allosteric modulators of gamma-aminobutyric acid-gated Cl⁻ currents. *Mol Pharmacol* 39:691-696.

Rabe, C.S.; Tabakoff, B. (1990). Glycine site-directed agonists reverse the actions of ethanol at the N-methyl-D-aspartate receptor. *Mol Pharmacol* 38:753-757.

Rabin, R.A.; Edelman, A.M.; Wagner, J.A. (1992). Activation of protein kinase A is necessary but not sufficient for ethanol-induced desensitization of cyclic AMP production. *J Pharmacol Exp Ther* 262:257-262.

Ransom, R.W.; Stec, N.L. (1988). Cooperative modulation of [3H]MK-801 binding to the N-methyl-D-aspartate receptor ion channel complex by L-glutamate, glycine, and polyamines. *J Neurochem* 51:830-836.

Rao, A.; Craig, A.M. (1997). Activity regulates the synaptic localization of the NMDA receptor in hippocampal neurons. *Neuron* 19:801-812.

Rao, V.L.; Giguere, J.F.; Layrargues, G.P.; Butterworth, R.F. (1993). Increased activities of MAOA and MAOB in autopsied brain tissue from cirrhotic patients with hepatic encephalopathy. *Brain Res* 621:349-352.

Rastogi, S.K.; Thyagarajan, R.; Clothier, J.; Ticku, M.K. (1986). Effect of chronic treatment of ethanol on benzodiazepine and picrotoxin sites on the GABA receptor complex in regions of the brain of the rat. *Neuropharmacology* 25:1179-1184.

Reynolds, I.J. (1990). Arcaine uncovers dual interactions of polyamines with the N-methyl-D-aspartate receptor. *J Pharmacol Exp Ther* 255:1001-1007.

Reynolds, I.J.; Miller, R.J. (1989). Ifenprodil is a novel type of N-methyl-D-aspartate receptor antagonist: Interaction with polyamines. *Mol Pharmacol* 36: 758-765.

Reynolds, I.J.; Murphy, S.N.; Miller, R.J. (1987). 3H-labeled MK-801 binding to the excitatory amino acid receptor complex from rat brain is enhanced by glycine. *Proc Natl Acad Sci USA* 84:7744-7748.

Reynolds, J.N.; Prasad, A. (1991). Ethanol enhances GABAA receptor-activated chloride currents in chick cerebral cortical neurons. *Brain Res* 564:138-142.

Rock, D.M.; Macdonald, R.L. (1995). Polyamine regulation of *N*-methyl-D-aspartate receptor channels. *Annu Rev Pharmacol Toxicol* 35:463-482.

Roivainen, R.; McMahon, T.; Messing, R.O. (1993). Protein kinase C isozymes that mediate enhancement of neurite outgrowth by ethanol and phorbol esters in PC12 cells. *Brain Res* 624:85-93.

Ron, M.A.; Acker, R.W.; Shaw, G.K.; Lishman, W.A. (1982). Computerized tomography of the brain in chronic alcoholism: A survey and follow-up study. *Brain* 105:497-514.

Rossetti, Z.L.; Carboni, S. (1995). Ethanol withdrawal is associated with increased extracellular glutamate in the rat striatum. *Eur J Pharmacol* 283:177-183.

Rouach, H.; Park, M.K.; Orfanelli, M.T.; Janvier, B.; Nordmann, R. (1987). Ethanol-induced oxidative stress in the rat cerebellum. *Alcohol and Alcoholism* 22:207-211.

Rudolph, J.G.; Walker, D.W.; Iimuro, Y.; Thurman, R.G.; Crews, F.T. (1997). NMDA receptor binding in adult rat brain after several chronic ethanol treatment protocols. *Alcohol Clin Exp Res* 21:1508-1519.

Ryan-Jastrow, T.; Macdonald, R.L. (1993). Ethanol sensitivity of recombinant α1β1γ2 GABAA receptors expressed in mammalian cells do not require the γ2L splice variant. *Soc Neurosci Abstr* 19:852.

Sanna, E.; Serra, M.; Cossu, A.; Colombo, G.; Follesa, P.; Cuccheddu, T.; Concas, A.; Biggio, G. (1993). Chronic ethanol intoxication induces differential effects on GABAA and NMDA receptor function in the rat brain. *Alcohol Clin Exp Res* 17:115-123.

Schofield, P.R. (1989). The GABAA receptor: Molecular biology reveals a complex picture. *Trends Pharmacol Sci* 10:476-478.

Schofield, P.R.; Darlison, M.G.; Fujita, N.; Burt, D.R.; Stephenson, F.A.; Rodriguez, H.; Rhee, L.M. et al. (1987). Sequence and functional expression of the GABAA receptor shows a ligand-gated super-family. *Nature* 328:221-227.

Seeburg, P.H.; Wisden, W.; Verdoorn, T.A.; Pritchett, D.B.; Werner, P.; Herb, A.; Lüddens, H.; Sprengel, R.; Sakmann, B. (1990). The GABAA receptor family: Molecular and functional diversity. *Cold Spring Harbor Sym Quant Biol* 55:29-38.

Sellers, E.M.; Kalant, H. (1976). Alcohol intoxication and withdrawal. *New Eng J Med* 294:757-762.

Sheng, M.; Cummings, J.; Roldan, L.A.; Jan, Y.N.; Jan, L.Y. (1994). Changing subunit composition of heteromeric NMDA receptors during development of rat cortex. *Nature* 368:144-147.

Sigel, E.; Baur, R.; Malherbe, P. (1993). Recombinant GABAA receptor function and ethanol. *FEBS Lett* 324:140-142.

Simson, P.E.; Criswell, H.E.; Breese, G.R. (1993). Inhibition of NMDA-evoked electrophysiological activity by ethanol in selected brain regions: Evidence for ethanol-sensitive and ethanol-insensitive NMDA responses. *Brain Res* 607:9-16.

Simson, P.E.; Criswell, H.E.; Johnson, K.B.; Breese, G.R. (1991). Ethanol inhibits NMDA-evoked electrophysiological activity in vivo. *J Pharmacol Exp Ther* 257:225-231.

Skolnick, P.; Paul, S.M. (1982). Molecular pharmacology of the benzodiazepines. *Int Rev Neurobiol* 23:103-140.

Snell, L.D.; Tabakoff, B.; Hoffman, P.L. (1993). Radioligand binding to the N-methyl D-aspartate receptor/ionophore complex: Alterations by ethanol in vitro and by chronic in vivo ethanol ingestion. *Brain Res* 602:91-98.

Snell, L.D.; Tabakoff, B.; Hoffman, P.L. (1994). Involvement of protein kinase C in ethanol-induced inhibition of NMDA receptor function in cerebellar granule cells. *Alcohol Clin Exp Res* 18:81-85.

Sommer, B.; Seeburg, P.H. (1992). Glutamate receptor channels: Novel properties and new clones. *Trends Pharmacol Sci* 13:291-296.

Sprengel, R.; Seeburg, P.H. (1993). The unique properties of glutamate receptor channels. *FEBS Lett* 325:90-94.

Standaert, D.G.; Testa, C.M.; Penney, J.B.; Young, A.B. (1993). Alternatively spliced isoforms of the NMDAR1 receptor subunit: Differential expression in the basal ganglia of the rat. *Neurosci Lett* 152:161-164.

Stelzer, A.; Kay, A.R.; Wong, R.K.S. (1988). GABAA receptor function in hippocampal cells is maintained by phosphorylation factors. *Science* 241:339-341.

Sugihara, H.; Moriyoshi, K.; Ishii, T.; Masu, M.; Nakanishi, S. (1992). Structures and properties of seven isoforms of the NMDA receptor generated by alternative splicing. *Biochem Biophys Res Commun* 185:826-832.

Sullivan, J.M.; Traynelis, S.F.; Hen, H-S.V.; Escobar, W.; Heinemann, S.F.; Lipton, S.A. (1994). Identification of two cystine residues that are required for redox modulation of NMDA subtype of glutamate receptor. *Neuron* 13:929-936.

Sullivan, E.V.; Marsh, L.; Mathalon, D.H.; Lim, K.O.; Pfefferbaum, A. (1996). Relationship between alcohol withdrawal seizures and temporal lobe white matter volume deficits. *Alcohol Clin Exp Res* 20:348-354.

Sullivan, E.V.; Rosenbloom, M.J.; Lim, K.O.; Pfefferbaum, A. (2000). Longitudinal changes in cognition, gait, and balance in abstinent and relapsed alcoholic men: Relationships to changes in brain structure. *Neuropsychology* 14:178-188.

Sullivan, E.V.; Rosenbloom, M.J.; Pfefferbaum, A. (2000). Pattern of motor and cognitive deficits in detoxified alcoholic men. *Alcohol Clin Exp Res* 24:611-621.

Suzdak, P.D.; Glowa, J.R.; Crawley, J.N.; Schwartz, R.D.; Skolnick, P.; Paul, S.M. (1986). A selective imidazobenzodiazepine antagonist of ethanol in the rat. *Science* 234:1243-1247.

Suzdak, P.D.; Glowa, J.R.; Crawley, J.N.; Skolnick, P.; Paul, S.M. (1988). Is ethanol antagonist Ro15-4513 selective for ethanol? Response to K.T. Britton et al. *Science* 239:649-650.

Suzdak, P.D.; Schwartz, R.D.; Paul, S.M. (1987). Alcohols stimulate GABA receptor-mediated chloride uptake in brain vesicles: Correlation with intoxication potency. *Brain Res* 444:340-344.

Suzdak, P.D.; Schwartz, R.D.; Skolnick, P.; Paul, S.M. (1986). Ethanol stimulates γ-aminobutyric acid receptor-mediated chloride transport in rat brain synaptoneurosomes. *Proc Natl Acad Sci USA* 83:4071-4075.

Tabakoff, B. (1995). Ethanol's action on the GABAA receptor: Is there a requirement for parsimony? *Alcohol Clin Exp Res* 24:810-821.

Takahashi, H.; Koehler, R.C.; Brusilow, S.W.; Traystman, R.J. (1991). Inhibition of brain glutamine accumulation prevents cerebral edema in hyperammonemia in rats. *Am J Physiol* 281:H826-H829.

Thornton, J.R.; Losowsky, M.S. (1988). Plasma methionine enkephalin concentration and prognosis in primary biliary cirrhosis. *Br Med J* 297:1241-1242.

Thyagarajan, R.; Ticku, M.K. (1985). The effect of in vitro and in vivo ethanol administration on [35S]t-butylbicyclophosphorothionate binding in C57 mice. *Brain Res Bull* 15:343-345.

Ticku, M.K.; Burch, T. (1980). Alterations in gamma-aminobutyric acid receptor sensitivity following acute and chronic ethanol treatments. *J Neurochem* 34:417-423.

Ticku, M.K.; Lowrimore, P.; Lehoullier, P. (1986). Ethanol enhances GABA induced 36Cl- influx in primary spinal cord cultured neurons. *Brain Res Bull* 17:123-126.

Trevisan, L.; Fitzgerald, L.W.; Brose, N.; Gasic, G.P.; Heinemann, S.F.; Duman, R.S.; Nestler, E.J. (1994). Chronic ingestion of ethanol up-regulates NMDAR1 receptor subunit immunoreactivity in rat hippocampus. *J Neurochem* 62:1635-1638.

Unwin, N. (1989). The structure of ion channels in membranes of excitable cells. *Neuron* 3:665-676.

Unwin, J.W.; Taberner, P.V. (1980). Sex and strain differences in GABA receptor binding after chronic ethanol drinking in mice. *Neuropharmacology* 19:1257-1259.

Uysal, M.; Keyer-Uysal, M.; Kocak-Toker, N.; Aykac, G. (1986). Effect of chronic ethanol ingestion on brain lipid peroxide and glutathione levels in rats. *Drug Alcohol Depend* 18:73-75.

Uysal, M.; Kutalp, G.; Ozdemirler, G.; Aykac, G. (1989). Ethanol-induced changes in lipid peroxidation and glutathione content in rat brain. *Drug Alcohol Depend* 23:227-230.

Vaillant, G.E. (1996). A long-term follow-up of male alcohol abuse. *Arch Gen Psychiatry* 53:243-249.

Valenzuela, C.F.; Cardoso, R.A.; Lickteig, R.; Browning, M.D.; Nixon, K.M. (1998). Acute effects of ethanol on recombinant kainate receptors: Lack of role of protein phosphorylation. *Alcohol Clin Exp Res* 22:1292-1299.

Valenzuela, C.F.; Machu, T.K.; McKernan, R.M.; Whiting, P.; VanRenterghem, B.B.; McManaman, J.L.; Brozowski, S.J.; Smith, G.B.; Olsen, R.W.; Harris, R.A. (1995). Tyrosine kinase phosphorylation of GABAA receptors. *Brain Res Mol Brain Res* 31:165-172.

Volicer, L. (1980). GABA levels and receptor binding after acute and chronic ethanol administration. *Brain Res Bull* 5:809-813.

Volicer, L.; Biagioni, T.M. (1982a). Effect of ethanol administration and withdrawal on benzodiazepine receptor binding in the rat brain. *Neuropharmacology* 21: 283-286.

Volicer, L.; Biagioni, T.M. (1982b). Effect of ethanol administration and withdrawal on GABA receptor binding in rat cerebral cortex. *Subst Alcohol Actions Misuse* 3:31-39.

Wafford, K.A.; Burnett, D.M.; Dunwiddie, T.V.; Harris, R.A. (1990). Genetic differences in the ethanol sensitivity of GABAA receptors expressed in Xenopus oocytes. *Science* 249:291-293.

Wafford, K.A.; Burnett, D.M.; Leidenheimer, N.J.; Burt, D.R.; Wang, J.B.; Kofuji, P.; Dunwiddie, T.V.; Harris, R.A.; Sikela, J.M. (1991). Ethanol sensitivity of the GABAA receptor expressed in Xenopus oocytes requires 8 amino acids contained in the gamma 2L subunit. *Neuron* 7:27-33.

Wafford, K.A.; Whiting, P.J. (1992). Ethanol potentiation of GABAA receptors requires phosphorylation of the alternatively spliced variant of the gamma2 subunit. *FEBS Lett* 313:113-117.

Wang, J.B.; Burt, D.R. (1991). Differential expression of two forms of GABAA receptor gamma2-subunit in mice. *Brain Res Bull* 27:731-735.

Watkins, J.C. (1962). The synthesis of some acidic amino acids possessing neuropharmacological activity. *J Med Pharm Chem* 5:1187-1199.

Weight, F.F. (1992). Cellular and molecular physiology of alcohol actions in the nervous system. *Int Rev of Neurobiol* 33:289-348.

Weight, F.F.; Peoples, R.W.; Wright, J.M.; Li, C.; Aguayo, L.G.; Lovinger, D.M.; White, G. (1993). Neurotransmitter-gated ion channels as molecular sites of alcohol action. In Alling, C. (Ed.), *Alcohol, Cell Membranes, and Signal Transduction in Brain,* pp. 107-122. New York: Plenum Press.

Weiner, J.L.; Dunwiddie, T.V.; Valenzuela, C.F. (1999). Ethanol inhibition of synaptically evoked kainate responses in rat hippocampal CA3 pyramidal neurons. *Mol Pharmacol* 56:85-90.

Weiss, M.H.; Craig, J.R. (1978). The influence of acute ethanol intoxication on intracranial physical dynamics. *Bull Los Angeles Neurol Soc* 43:1-5.

Westbrook, G.L.; Mayer, M.L. (1987). Micromolar concentration of Zn^{2+} antagonize NMDA and GABA responses of hippocampal neurons. *Nature* 328:640-643.

White, G.; Gurley, D.A. (1995). Primate-derived GABAA α1, α2, α3, α5 subunits in combination with either β1γ2L, β2g2L, form twelve pharmacologically distinct receptor subtypes in Xenopus oocytes. *Soc Neurosci Abstr* 21:850.

Whiting, P.; McKernan, R.M.; Iversen, L.L. (1990). Another mechanism for creating diversity in γ-aminobutyrate type A receptors: RNA splicing directs expression of two forms of gamma 2 phosphorylation site. *Proc Natl Acad Sci USA* 87:9966-9970.

Whittemore, E.R.; Yang, W.; Drewe, J.A.; Woodward, R.M. (1995). Functional and pharmacological characterization of the human GABAA receptor α4 subunit expressed in Xenopus oocytes. *Soc Neurosci Abstr* 21:850.

Williams, K.; Russel, S.L.; Shen, Y.M.; Molinoff, P.B. (1993). Developmental switch in the expression of NMDA receptors occurs in vivo and in vitro. *Neuron* 10:267-278.

Williams, K.; Zappia, A.M.; Pritchett, D.B.; Shen, Y.M.; Molinoff, P.B. (1994). Sensitivity of the N-methyl-D-aspartate receptor to polyamines is controlled by NR2 subunits. *Mol Pharmacol* 45:803-809.

Wilson, W.R.; Bosy, T.Z.; Ruth, J.A. (1990). NMDA agonists and antagonists alter the hypnotic response to ethanol in LS and SS mice. *Alcohol* 7:389-395.

Wisden, W.; Herb, A.; Wieland, H.; Keinänen, K.; Lüddens, H.; Seeburg, P.H. (1991). Cloning, pharmacological characteristics, and expression pattern of the rat GABAA receptor α4 subunit. *FEBS Lett* 289:227-230.

Wright, M.S.; Sefland, I.; Walaas, S.I. (1993). Cloning of the long intracellular loop of the AMPA-selective glutamate receptor for phosphorylation studies. *J Receptor Res* 13:653-665.

Yamazaki, M.; Araki, K.; Shibata, A.; Mishina, M. (1992). Molecular cloning of a cDNA encoding a novel member of the mouse glutamate receptor channel family. *Biochem Biophys Res Commun* 183:886-892.

Yang, X.; Criswell, H.E.; Simson, P.; Moy, S.S.; Breese, G.R. (1996). Evidence for a selective effect of ethanol on NMDA responses: Ethanol affects a subtype of the ifenprodil-sensitive NMDA receptor. *J Pharmacol Exp Ther* 278:782-786.

Ymer, S.; Schofield, P.R.; Draguhn, A.; Werner, P.; Kohler, M.; Seeburg, P.H. (1989). GABAA receptor ß subunit heterogeneity: Functional expression of cloned cDNAs. *EMBO J* 8:1665-1670.

Yoneda, Y.; Enomoto, R.; Kiyokazu, O. (1994). Supporting evidence for negative modulation by protons of an ion channel associated with the N-methyl-D-aspartate receptor complex in rat brain using ligand binding techniques. *Brain Res* 636:298-307.

Young, S.N.; Lal, S.; Feldmuller, F.; Aranoff, A.; Martin, J.B. (1975). Relationships between tryptophan in serum and CSF and -hydroxyindoleacetic acid in CSF of man: Effects of cirrhosis of the liver and probenecid administration. *J Neurol Neurosurg Psychiatry* 38:322-330.

Zhang, J-H.; Gong, Z.H.; Hellstrom-Lindahl, E.; Nordberg, A. (1995). Regulation of α4 and ß2 nicotinic acetylcholine receptors in M10 cells following treatment with nicotinic agents. *NeuroReport* 6:313-317.

Zhong, J.; Russell, S.L.; Pritchett, D.B.; Molinoff, P.B.; Williams, K. (1994). Expression of mRNAs encoding subunits of the N-methyl-D-aspartate receptor in cultured cortical neurons. *Mol Pharmacol* 45:846-853.

Chapter 6

Neuroanatomical and Neurobehavioral Effects of Heavy Prenatal Alcohol Exposure

Tara S. Wass

INTRODUCTION AND OVERVIEW

Suspicions about the harmful effects of prenatal alcohol exposure have surfaced throughout history (Streissguth, 1997). However, these suspicions were for the most part unsubstantiated until researchers in France (Lemoine et al., 1968) and the United States (Jones and Smith, 1973; Jones et al., 1973) identified a cluster of abnormalities in the children of female alcohol abusers, which came to be referred to as fetal alcohol syndrome (FAS). Three criteria provide the basis for the FAS diagnosis: a characteristic pattern of craniofacial anomalies (see Figure 6.1), growth retardation, and central nervous system (CNS) dysfunction (Jones et al., 1973). Although the diagnostic criteria for FAS have been scrutinized and even criticized because many children thought to be affected by prenatal alcohol exposure do not meet criteria for the diagnosis, FAS continues to be diagnosed on the basis of the triad of features delineated in those original articles (Institute of Medicine [IOM], 1996).

The effects of prenatal alcohol exposure may be viewed as a continuum with FAS and fetal death at the extreme end of the spectrum. At the opposite end of the spectrum, there may be no observable effect on the fetus follow-

Author's note: Original version of this chapter funded by grants AA10417 and AA07456 from NIAAA.

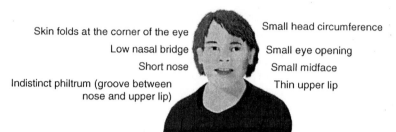

Skin folds at the corner of the eye
Low nasal bridge
Short nose
Indistinct philtrum (groove between nose and upper lip)

Small head circumference
Small eye opening
Small midface
Thin upper lip

FIGURE 6.1. Example of facial features associated with FAS. *Source:* Illustration available at http://www.niaaa.nih.gov/gallery/fetal/FASkids.htm and reprinted from Warren and Foudin (2001).

ing minimal exposure. A wide range of effects has been observed between these extremes, including attention deficits, learning disabilities, and physical birth defects (IOM, 1996). The term "fetal alcohol effects" (FAE) has been used to refer to alcohol-exposed children who do not meet the diagnostic criteria for FAS but exhibit one or more of these effects. However, this term has repeatedly been criticized because of its lack of diagnostic specificity (Aase, Jones, and Clarren, 1995; IOM, 1996). In response to these criticisms, the Institute of Medicine (1996) proposed several diagnostic categories for alcohol-exposed children who did not meet the criteria for an FAS diagnosis. Two of these diagnoses, alcohol-related neurodevelopmental disorder (ARND) and alcohol-related birth defects (ARBD), are particularly important because they enable the classification of alcohol-affected children who do not present with craniofacial anomalies characteristic of FAS. These children may be particularly at risk for the development of secondary disabilities because they are not identified early in life and frequently do not *qualify* for services. However, research suggests that these children display neurobehavioral deficits (Mattson et al., 1997; Mattson et al., 1999; Streissguth et al., 1997) and neuroanatomical changes (Bookstein, 2001; Bookstein, Streissguth et al., 2002) that are comparable to those observed in children with FAS.

Estimating the number of children affected by prenatal alcohol exposure can be difficult, in part due to the diagnostic issues just mentioned. Incidence estimates vary widely, to some extent due to different methods used to identify children with FAS (May and Gossage, 2001). Several studies estimated the incidence of FAS in the United States and around the world. In a recent review of studies, May and Gossage argued that the prevalence of FAS in the United States is between 0.5 and 2 cases per 1,000 live births. Estimates vary widely across populations within the United States, with the highest rates typically observed in African American and Native American communities. The high rate of poverty among minority communities, rather than race, is thought to be a major factor influencing the higher rates of FAS in these communities (Abel, 1995). The estimates in previous text only refer to children diagnosed with FAS. However, as already mentioned, many children are affected by prenatal alcohol exposure, but do not qualify for the FAS diagnosis. Sampson et al. (1997) estimated the combined prevalence rate of FAS and ARND to be at least 9.1 cases per 1,000 live births. Overall, these statistics suggest that alcohol may be a bigger public health threat than previously realized.

Since the identification of FAS, a multitude of animal and human studies have examined the impact of prenatal alcohol exposure on the developing organism. The most obvious and debilitating effects of heavy prenatal alcohol exposure are the persistent and pervasive neurobehavioral deficits, which may include reductions in IQ, deficits in learning and memory, attention deficits, and increased behavioral problems (Mattson et al., 1998). These neurobehavioral changes presumably reflect alcohol-induced changes in the structure and/or function of the brain. To date, numerous studies have begun to characterize the neuropathological changes present in the brains of children with FAS or heavy prenatal exposure to alcohol (PEA) as a means of understanding the neurological underpinnings of the disorder and providing direction for further refining the behavioral phenotype of FAS. The current chapter reviews findings from autopsy, structural imaging, and functional imaging studies on children with FAS and PEA. In addition, research on cognitive and psychosocial functioning is briefly reviewed.

AUTOPSY STUDIES

Evidence that prenatal alcohol exposure affects human brain development first came from autopsy studies. Clarren (1986) summarized the findings from the first 16 autopsy reports that were available for infants with FAS who died within a year of birth. Since that time, a total of 25 autopsies have been reported and reviewed (Mattson and Riley, 1996).

The first autopsy was conducted on a child of a chronic alcoholic mother (Jones and Smith, 1973). The child, who was delivered at 32-weeks gestation and died at five days of age, had an abnormally small brain (microcephaly). Further, the child's left cerebral hemisphere was covered by a leptomeningeal neuroglial heterotopia, an abnormal sheet of neural and glial tissue. Below the leptomeningeal neuroglial heterotopia there was evidence of extensive neuronal disorganization, which ranged from cortical thinning to an absence of the normative laminar structure of the cortex. Abnormalities were not localized solely in the cerebral cortex. Agenesis (absence) of the corpus callosum and the anterior commissure were noted, as were abnormalities in both the cerebellum and the brainstem. The cerebellum was small and poorly shaped, while the medulla was covered by another small leptomeningeal neuroglial heterotopia. Thus, in this first autopsy case, damage to the brain was extensive and widespread.

Later autopsies have similarly reported widespread damage to cortical and subcortical structures following heavy PEA. By far, the most consistent and common neuropathological change is a reduction in the size of the cranium, also referred to as microcephaly (see Figure 6.2). Samson (1986) reported that microcephaly is present in more than 80 percent of children with FAS. In a review of autopsies done on children with FAS who died within one year of birth, Clarren (1986) reported that 56 percent of cases had micro-cephaly. In a later review, Mattson and Riley (1996) found that 73 percent of the 22 autopsy or magnetic resonance imaging (MRI) cases had microce-phaly. Microcephaly could be caused by a variety of *different* mechanisms including disruptions in neuronal generation, neuronal differentiation, the

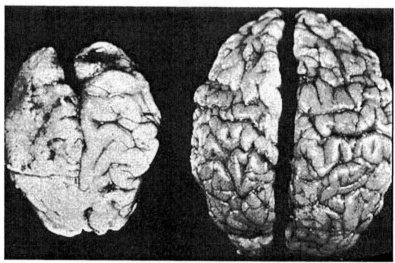

FIGURE 6.2. Pictures show the brains of two infants who died shortly after birth. The brain on the right represents normal development while the brain on the left is from an infant who was exposed to alcohol in utero. *Source:* From Research Society on Alcoholism Lecture Series (Riley, 2001) and reprinted from Clarren (1986). From *Alcohol and Brain Development,* edited by James R. West, copyright © 1986 by Oxford University Press, Inc. Used by permission of Oxford University Press, Inc.

establishment and maintenance of synaptic connections between neurons, and increased cell death. Many of these effects have been observed in animal models of FAS (Bonthius and West, 1990; Guerri, 1998; Miller, 1988).

Porencephaly and hydrocephaly have also been reported (Clarren et al., 1978; Peiffer et al., 1979). Hydrocephaly is characterized by an overabundance of cerebrospinal fluid (CSF), which results in enlargement of the ventricles. Enlargement of the ventricles causes the cerebral gray matter to be displaced and compressed, ultimately resulting in neuronal damage if the pressure is not released. In contrast, porencephaly is characterized by one or more fluid-filled cysts in the cerebral cortex, which are typically caused by a brain hemorrhage, trauma, or partial to complete occlusion of blood vessels.

Another neuropathological finding is holoprosencephaly (Coulter et al., 1993; Jellinger et al., 1981), a condition in which the forebrain fails to completely develop into two hemispheres. In the most severe cases, known as alobar holoprosencephaly, there is a complete fusion of all forebrain structures. Ronen and Andrews (1991) presented one case of alobar holoprosencephaly and two less-severe cases of semilobar holoprosencephaly. In all three cases, there was only a single "square-shaped ventricle" and midline fusion of the basal ganglia and thalamic nuclei (p. 152). Holoprosencephaly has been induced in nonhuman primate and mouse models of FAS (Siebert, Astley, and Clarren, 1991; Sulik and Johnston, 1982), further strengthening the suggestion that alcohol exposure is one possible cause of this disorder. Finally, it is interesting to note that infants with FAS or holoprosencephaly both exhibit midline facial anomalies (Ronen and Andrews, 1991), although the anomalies observed in the two disorders are not identical. In both disorders, the severity of these craniofacial anomalies may covary with the severity of the underlying neuropathological abnormalities (Swayze et al., 1997).

In addition to these macroscopic cortical anomalies, microscopic changes and abnormalities resulting from abnormal neuronal and glial cell migration have frequently been reported. These include ectopic neurons scattered throughout the cortex, nonspecific cerebral disorganization or dysgenesis, incompletely developed sulci, and polymicrogyria (Clarren et al., 1978; Coulter et al., 1993; Konovalov et al., 1997; Peiffer et al., 1979; Wisniewski et al., 1983).

Abnormalities are not limited to the cerebral cortex. Both cerebellar and brainstem anomalies have been documented. For example, brainstem abnormalities have included absence of the pons and medulla, leptomeningeal neuroglial heterotopias, and brainstem dysgenesis (Clarren et al., 1978; Peiffer et al., 1979). Cerebellar abnormalities have been more widely reported and include underdevelopment of the cerebellum or the cerebellar vermis, hyperplastic folds of the cerebellum, and agenesis of the cerebellar vermis

(Clarren et al., 1978; Konovalov et al., 1997; Peiffer et al.,1979; Wisniewski et al., 1983). In all, 10 of the 16 autopsy cases reviewed by Clarren (1986) displayed evidence of cerebellar abnormalities.

Agenesis of the corpus callosum and the anterior commissure was noted in Clarren et al.'s (1978) original autopsy case (Jones and Smith, 1973). Two additional autopsy cases presented with agenesis of the corpus callosum and one also presented with agenesis of the anterior commissure (Peiffer et al., 1979; Wisniewski et al., 1983). When the corpus callosum is present, significant thinning has been reported (Clarren et al., 1978; Coulter et al., 1993).

A variety of other abnormalities have been found in numerous autopsy cases. These include fusion of the thalami or basal ganglia nuclei, absence of the olfactory bulbs, and hypoplasia of the optic nerves and hippocampus (Coulter et al., 1993; Peiffer et al., 1979; Wisniewski et al., 1983).

Even a cursory examination of the autopsy findings suggests that the damage caused by PEA is widespread. On the basis of these autopsy findings, Clarren (1986) argued that due to the variability in the neuropathological findings in children with FAS, future research would be unable to document a pattern of behavioral or neuropsychological deficits that is representative of all children with FAS. Though others have agreed with this position (Peiffer et al., 1979), it may be premature to presume that no commonalities in the neurological underpinnings or phenotypic expression of FAS will emerge across children. The cases evaluated in the autopsy studies represent the extreme for children with FAS. Primate studies suggest that prenatal alcohol exposure may not be lethal in the majority of cases. Two nonhuman primate studies demonstrated that although exposure does decrease viability, 68 to 70 percent of exposed cases were live born (Clarren and Astley, 1992; Clarren, Bowden, and Astley, 1987). Furthermore, only 6 percent (3 out of 47) of the live-born alcohol-exposed infants died within the first six months of life. Thus, in the vast majority of cases, prenatal alcohol exposure is not lethal, which suggests that the cases reviewed in the autopsy studies may be more severely affected than the average child with FAS. Consequently, it is possible that an examination of the brains of children with FAS who have survived will yield a more consistent pattern of neuropathological findings. Rapid advances in structural and functional imaging techniques have enabled researchers to examine living children with FAS or PEA and a much more consistent pattern of neuropathological findings is beginning to emerge.

MAGNETIC RESONANCE IMAGING STUDIES

Brain imaging techniques such as MRI have become increasingly popular tools for documenting structural changes in the brain associated with various developmental disorders. These techniques have the potential to advance our understanding of the neuroanatomical changes associated with disorders such as FAS. Some MRI studies have provided clinical assessments and descriptions of MRI scans, indicating whether the images are normal or abnormal, while others have assessed the size of structures. Clinical assessments of MRI data are sensitive to gross structural malformations of the brain that can be detected by the human eye. However, subtle changes such as small reductions in volume may not be observable. Furthermore, clinical assessments negate the possibility of controlling for alcohol's global effect on the brain when examining individual brain structures. As we already know that prenatal alcohol exposure frequently results in a reduction in overall brain size, it may be more informative to determine whether this reduction is uniform across the brain or whether specific structures appear to be more susceptible to alcohol's teratogenic effects.

The most recent studies utilized new advances in computer software and statistical techniques to examine variation in the shape and location of key brain structures (Bookstein, Sampson, et al., 2002), as well as localization of white and gray matter alterations in the cortex (Sowell et al., 2001). With the combination of these techniques, a clearer picture of the neuroanatomical damage caused by prenatal alcohol exposure is emerging that suggests that while alcohol-induced damage can be widespread, discrete regions of the brain including the corpus callosum, cerebellum, and portions of the parietal and temporal lobes may be particularly vulnerable to alcohol's effects. Understanding the impact of these structural changes on brain function should lead to a better understanding of the neurobehavioral deficits observed in these children.

Cerebral Cortex

The most consistent and common neuropathological change associated with heavy prenatal alcohol exposure is a reduction in overall head or brain size (Roebuck, Mattson, and Riley, 1998). A series of structural MRI studies documented significant reduction in cranial vault volume of children with FAS or PEA (Archibald et al., 2001; Mattson et al., 1992; Mattson et al., 1994; Mattson, Riley, Sowell, et al., 1996). In one study, these reductions were accompanied by increases in cortical and subcortical fluid, which is further suggestive of brain atrophy (Mattson et al., 1992). Studies from other laboratories noted cortical atrophy, enlargement of the lateral ventricles, and enlargement of the subarachnoid space, which are consistent with brain atrophy and reductions in overall brain size (Goldstein and Arulanantham, 1978; Johnson et al., 1996; Riikonen et al., 1999; Robin and Zachai, 1994;

Swayze et al., 1997). In addition to microcephaly, imaging studies documented other changes to the cortex, including a large infarct in the left hemisphere, delayed myelination, multifocal encephalopathy, and an abnormal configuration of the occipital lobes (Clark et al., 2000; Gabrielli et al., 1990; Riikonen et al., 1999).

In an attempt to move beyond global effects on the brain, Archibald et al. (2001) used morphometric MRI analyses to examine whether the proportional cortical volume comprised by the frontal, parietal, temporal, and occipital lobes differed between children with FAS and normally developing children. After adjusting for overall brain size, only the parietal lobe was disproportionately reduced in children with FAS, indicating that all areas of the cortex were not equally affected. These findings are consistent with later studies examining regional differences in cortical white and gray matter density, hemispheric asymmetry, and brain shape (Sowell, Thompson, Mattson, et al., 2002; Sowell, Thompson, Peterson, et al., 2002).

Two studies examined the effect of prenatal alcohol exposure on cerebral white and gray matter (Archibald et al., 2001; Sowell et al., 2001). Using the same pool of participants researchers examined the relative density and volume of these tissue types. Both studies revealed that prenatal alcohol exposure was related to disproportionate reductions in cerebral white matter with relative sparing of cerebral gray matter. When overall microcephaly is taken into account, it appears that the parietal region is particularly affected, with marked white matter volume reductions occurring along with reductions in white matter density and increases in gray matter density.

In a later study, Sowell, Thompson, Peterson, et al. (2002) hypothesized that alcohol-related alternations in white and gray matter density might be associated with a reduction in hemispheric asymmetries typically observed in the brains of normally developing individuals. Normative studies demonstrated hemispheric asymmetry in the perisylvian region (Sowell, Thompson, Rex, et al., 2002; Steinmetz et al., 1991, 1995), an area where alcohol related abnormalities were previously documented (Sowell et al., 2001). For example, the sylvian fissure tends to be longer in the left hemisphere than in the right hemisphere and the right Sylvian fissure tends to have a greater slope. Another common asymmetry is observed in the temporal lobes where the planum temporale is larger in the left hemisphere than in the right hemisphere.

Sowell, Thompson, Peterson, et al. (2002) compared the distances between analogous points in the left and right hemispheres after matching them using cortical landmarks. Both nonexposed and exposed individuals exhibited hemispheric asymmetries. Focusing on anterior-posterior displacement, the data indicated that across the frontal, parietal, temporal, and occipital lobes, the left hemisphere tended to be located more posterior than the right hemisphere. The perisylvian region had the greatest asymmetry in all groups. Thus, the data suggest that hemispheric asymmetries along the anterior-posterior dimension are not disrupted by prenatal alcohol exposure.

In contrast to the displacement analyses, an alteration of cortical gray matter asymmetry was observed in the temporal cortex. In the control groups, cortical density was greater in the right temporal cortex than in the left temporal cortex. This asymmetry was not significant in the alcohol exposed (ALC) group. Within the temporal cortex the difference in asymmetry between the ALC and control groups was only significant in the posterior inferior portion (Sowell, Thompson, Peterson, et al., 2002), primarily where Brodmann's areas 21, 22, and 37 join together. Volumetric analyses also confirmed this difference in gray matter asymmetry.

In a related study, Sowell, Thompson, Mattson, et al. (2002) examined abnormalities in regional brain shape by computing the distance between a center point, defined as the midline decussation of the anterior commissure, and individual points on the brain surface (Sowell, Thompson, Mattson, et al., 2002). An average distance from center (DFC) for surface points within each cortical lobe and various regions of interest was computed. Significant differences in DFC were observed in the anterior and orbital frontal cortex, most prominently in the left hemisphere, and bilaterally in the inferior parietal/perisylvian cortical region. The reductions in the inferior parietal/perisylvian cortical region remained significant even after controlling for the overall reduction in brain size suggesting that the brain is narrower than expected in this region. Interestingly, gray matter density analyses indicated a greater density in the inferior parietal/perisylvian cortical regions in the ALC group compared to controls.

Cerebellum

Historically, studies of the cerebellum have focused on its role in the control of motor functions. This focus was driven in part by the knowledge that the cerebellum has reciprocal connections with multiple motor areas of the CNS including the spinal cord, the vestibular system, and the motor cortex, among others. Furthermore, a number of studies have detailed the performance of individuals with cerebellar lesions on motor tasks. From the accumulated data, it is clear that the cerebellum is involved in a variety of motor skills, including postural control, gait, balance, and the coordination of bilateral movements (Diener et al., 1993).

Although largely overlooked, the idea that the cerebellum also plays a role in cognition is not new. For example, classical conditioning of the eyeblink response is known to be dependent upon the cerebellum and research on this phenomenon dates as far back as the early part of the twentieth century (Woodruff-Pak, 1997). There has been a surge of interest in the nonmotor functions of the cerebellum with researchers focusing on the role that the cerebellum plays in learning and memory (Ivry and Baldo, 1992; Schmahmann, 1997). The idea that the cerebellum could play a role in cognition is reinforced by neuroanatomical research that has demonstrated afferents from the association areas of the cortex via the pontine nucleus and efferents to the cortex via the thalamus (Schmahmann and Pandya, 1997). Current theories suggest that in addition to influencing motor control, the cerebellum influences attention (Townsend et al., 1999), planning (Hallett and Grafman, 1997), and temporal computation and perception (Ackermann et al., 1999; Keele and Ivry, 1990). Interestingly, deficits in attention and planning have been reported in children with FAS (Kodituwakku et al., 1995; Kopera-Frye, Carmichael-Olson, and Streissguth, 1997; Mattson et al., 1999).

Cerebellar abnormalities associated with heavy PEA have received extensive attention in the animal and human literature. Both autopsy studies and animal studies suggest that the cerebellum is one of several neural structures sensitive to prenatal alcohol exposure. For example, animal studies demonstrated that prenatal alcohol exposure causes a reduction in the number of cerebellar neurons resulting in a reduction in overall cerebellar volume (Bonthius and West, 1990; Cragg and Phillips, 1985; Pierce, Goodlett, and West, 1989).

MRI studies also revealed changes in the cerebellum in children with FAS or PEA. In a series of three MRI studies, significant reductions in the volume of the cerebellar vault of children with FAS were documented (Mattson et al., 1992; Mattson, Riley, Sowell, et al., 1996), along with marginally significant volume reductions in children with PEA (Mattson et al., 1994). Overall, 80 percent of the children with FAS or PEA who received MRI scans in these studies had a cerebellar vault volume below the range observed in normal controls. In a recent study, the earlier finding of significant reductions in the cerebellar vault of children with FAS was confirmed, along with marginal reductions in the cerebellar vault of children with PEA (Archibald et al., 2001).

Archibald et al. (2001) also examined the proportion of the cerebellar cortex composed of white and gray matter, but failed to find a significant difference. Thus, in contrast to the cerebral cortex data presented previously, white and gray matter appeared to be similarly affected in the cerebellum. This appeared to be due to relatively more severe effects on cerebellar gray matter, as cerebellar hypoplasia overall was more severe than was cerebral hypoplasia.

A global analysis of the cerebellum may not be sufficient to understand the relationship between cerebellar changes and behavior in this population.

Animal studies have demonstrated regional differences in sensitivity to prenatal alcohol exposure within the cerebellum. For example, animal research indicated that earlier maturing regions of the cerebellar vermis (lobules I-V, IX, and X) were more susceptible to the effects of alcohol than later maturing regions (lobules VI and VII) (Goodlett, Marcussen, and West, 1990). Using MRI analyses in humans, the cerebellar vermis was divided into the anterior vermis (lobules I-V), the posterior vermis (lobules VI and VII), and the remaining vermal area (lobules VIII-X) to examine whether reductions in volume were widespread or limited to the anterior regions and remaining vermal area, as would be predicted from the animal studies (Sowell et al., 1996). Results indicated there was a significant reduction in the anterior vermis of children with FAS or PEA. In contrast, neither the posterior vermis nor the remaining vermal area differed from controls.

These results are particularly interesting for two reasons. First, they are consistent with the animal literature. Second, these findings are inconsistent with cerebellar abnormalities observed in other developmental disorders. Specifically, studies of attention-deficit/hyperactivity disorder (ADHD) reported reductions in the posterior vermis with sparing of the anterior vermis (Berquin et al., 1998; Mostofsky et al., 1998). Studies of autism (Bauman, Filipek, and Kemper 1997; Courchesne, Townsend, and Saitoh, 1994; Townsend et al., 1999) reported subtypes of autism patients who display either hyperplasia or hypoplasia in the posterior vermis with sparing of the anterior vermis. This pattern is opposite to what was observed in children with FAS or PEA, suggesting that although cerebellar abnormalities are not solely caused by alcohol, the pattern of damage caused by prenatal alcohol exposure differs. This raises the possibility that specific patterns of strengths and weaknesses reflective of cerebellum function and dysfunction could be observed across these disorders. This pattern, in conjunction with other neuropathological findings, could increase the specificity of the behavioral phenotype observed in children with FAS or PEA, thereby improving the accuracy of the diagnosis.

Corpus Callosum

The corpus callosum is a large bundle of axonal fibers that connects the left and right hemispheres of the brain and allows for the efficient transfer of information between them. It is comprised of about 300 million fibers (Heimer, 1995) and can be separated into four sections: the rostrum, genu, body, and splenium (Kolb and Whishaw, 1996). Autopsy studies initially documented corpus callosum abnormalities. In fact, as mentioned previously, the first autopsied brain of an infant with FAS displayed agenesis (absence) of the corpus callosum (Clarren et al., 1978; Jones and Smith, 1973).

Agenesis of the corpus callosum is estimated to occur in 0.3 percent of the general population and in 2.3 percent of the developmentally disabled population (Jeret et al., 1986). In a sample of children in San Diego with FAS or PEA, the estimated incidence of complete agenesis of the corpus callosum was 6.8 percent (3 out of 44 children) (Riley et al., 1995). In addition to complete agenesis of the corpus callosum, other abnormalities such as partial agenesis or hypoplasia of the corpus callosum have been observed (Clark et al., 2000; Riikonen et al., 1999; Swayze et al., 1997) (see Figure 6.3). Corpus callosum abnormalities, even complete agenesis, are not unique to FAS, but rather have been observed in multiple developmental and genetic disorders including ADHD (Hynd et al., 1991), mental retardation (Schaefer et al., 1991), and Down's syndrome (Wang et al., 1992).

Riley et al. (1995) conducted quantitative analyses of the corpus callosum in children with FAS or PEA. During an MRI analyses, the corpus

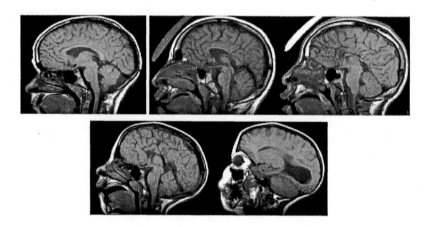

FIGURE 6.3. The top left picture shows the brain of a normally developing child; the remaining images are of children with FAS. The FAS images show varying levels of corpus callosum damage. In the top middle image, the corpus callosum is substantially thinned. In the top right and bottom left pictures, the corpus callosum is essentially absent. The bottom right image shows a fluid-filled sac where gray matter should be located, a condition known as coprocephaly. *Source:* From Research Society on Alcoholism Lecture Series (Riley, 2001) and reprinted from Mattson et al. (1994), Mattson and Riley (1995), and Riley et al. (1995). From *Alcohol and Brain Development,* edited by James R. West, copyright © 1986 by Oxford University Press, Inc. Used by permission of Oxford University Press, Inc.

callosum was divided into five equiangular regions, with region 1 corresponding to the genu, region 5 corresponding to the splenium, and regions 2 to 4 corresponding to the body of the corpus callosum. In addition, the area of the midsagittal section was computed in order to control for reductions in overall brain size when examining group differences. The midsagittal area was reduced by 14 percent in alcohol-exposed children. In addition, there were significant reductions in areas 1, 3, 4, and 5 of the corpus callosum. Even after controlling for the reduction in the midsagittal area, areas 1, 4, and 5 were still significantly reduced in the corpus callosum of children with FAS or PEA. Thus, it was the most anterior and posterior regions of the corpus callosum that were affected by prenatal exposure. The selective pattern of reductions can provide information regarding the types of deficits one would expect to observe in children with FAS. For example, the anterior region of the corpus callosum contains fibers for the prefrontal cortex, while the posterior region contains fibers for the visual cortex, as well as the superior and inferior temporal cortexes.

A recent series of studies shifted the emphasis from volumetric reductions to variability in the shape of the corpus callosum (Bookstein et al., 2001; Bookstein, Sampson, et al., 2002; Bookstein, Streissguth, et al., 2002). In the first study (Bookstein et al., 2001), the authors identified 33, primarily subcortical, landmarks in the brains of male and female adults categorized as PEA, FAS, or control. They also identified 40 semi-landmarks placed along the curvature of the corpus callosum to represent its shape (Bookstein et al., 2001). The data indicated that the location of landmarks between the brainstem and diencephalon was much more variable within the ALC group than the control group. The ALC group also displayed more variability in the location of the semi-landmark locations that defined the curvature of the corpus callosum, although the excess variability was isolated and varied by sex. In male participants exposed to alcohol, excess variance tended to be localized to the underside of the isthmus. In contrast, the excess variance tended to be localized in the arch of the corpus callosum in exposed female participants.

In a second study, with an expanded sample that included adolescents, Bookstein, Sampson, et al. (2002) again documented excess variability in the shape of the corpus callosum. Within the entire sample, they argued that they could successfully differentiate exposed and nonexposed individuals using four landmarks and two scores that characterized the shape of the corpus callosum. The four landmarks included the genu, interior genu, head of the caudate and the rostrum. Plotting the location of the interior genu and the caudate relative to a line drawn between the genu and the rostrum enabled them to identify an area that contained most of the nonexposed individuals and excluded most of the exposed. The first callosal shape variable represented the thickness of the front relative to the thickness of the back. The second callosal shape variable represented either a compression of the area around the genu with a relative thickening of the rest of the arch or an expansion of the genu area with a relative thinning of the rest of the arch. Plotting these two shape scores against one another also provided good differentiation of exposed from nonexposed individuals. The combination of the landmark and shape analyses enabled the authors to correctly identify 87 percent of the exposed individuals while maintaining a high level of specificity (82 percent).

Findings from a follow-up study suggested that the neurobehavioral deficits in alcohol exposed individuals may vary with corpus callosum shape (Bookstein, Streissguth et al., 2002). The first significant shape reflected variation in the anterior-posterior length and the height of the arch, which correlated strongly with a cluster of neuropsychological tests that primarily tapped intellectual functioning. Lower performance on this cluster of tests was associated with a corpus callosum that was shortened in the anterior-posterior dimension coupled with a relatively high arch. The second significant shape reflected the relative thickness of the corpus callosum. Excessive thinning of the corpus callosum was associated with poor performance on a battery of tests that assessed motor skills including balance, coordination, and spatial learning. At the other extreme, excessive thickness of the corpus callosum was associated with poor performance on tests of verbal memory and executive functioning.

Overall, data from numerous studies with several independent samples suggests that the corpus callosum is particularly sensitive to the effects of prenatal alcohol exposure. While early studies focused on reductions in size and demonstrated that the anterior and posterior regions tended to be most affected, recent studies suggest that alcohol-related variation in shape may be at least as important as variation in size. The ability to utilize shape variability to differentiate different neuropsychological profiles within an exposed sample suggests a promising avenue for future research. If future studies replicate these findings using independent samples and variability in shape can also differentiate alcohol exposed individuals from individuals with other disabilities, these findings could substantially change the way that alcohol-related disorders are diagnosed potentially leading to earlier diagnosis and treatment.

Basal Ganglia

The basal ganglia are a group of subcortical nuclei that can be subdivided into the caudate and lenticular nuclei. The lenticular nuclei can be further subdivided into the globus pallidus and the putamen (Heimer, 1995). The basal ganglia have traditionally been thought to participate in motor activity for several reasons. First, the basal ganglia are part of a corticostriatal loop in which information is projected from the somatosensory and motor cortices to basal ganglia and eventually back to the motor and premotor cortices. This motor loop enables the basal ganglia to participate in both the initiation and modulation of motor activity (Kolb and Whishaw, 1996). Further, two diseases with known pathology in the basal ganglia, Huntington's and Parkinson's diseases, result in prominent motor dysfunction such as akinesia and hyperkinesia.

Current perspectives suggest that the basal ganglia play a role not only in motor activity, but also in cognitive functioning (Middleton and Strick, 1994, 2000; Rao et al., 1997). Cognitive deficits have been observed in patients with either Huntington's disease or Parkinson's disease and the degree of cognitive deficits has in some cases been linked to the degree of basal ganglial pathology (Bäckman et al., 1997; Watkins et al., 2000). Further, there is a second corticostriatal loop (cognitive loop) in which frontal, parietal, and temporal cortical association areas send projections to the caudate nucleus of the basal ganglia, which in turn sends projections back to the cortex, providing a means for the basal ganglia to influence cognition (Heimer, 1995).

A series of MRI studies examined the basal ganglia in alcohol-exposed children and a remarkable consistency emerged. A clinical examination of the MRI scans taken by these studies revealed no abnormalities in the basal ganglia of children with FAS compared with normally developing children or children with Down's syndrome (Mattson et al., 1992). However, *differences* were revealed when morphometric analyses were conducted. The volume of the basal ganglia in the alcohol-exposed children was reduced beyond what would be expected given their overall brain size. In contrast, the children with Down's syndrome had proportionally larger basal ganglia than would be expected. Subsequently, two children with PEA were evaluated. In these less affected children, the volume of the basal ganglia was still significantly reduced even after controlling for the overall reduction in head size. Thus, analyses indicated that the basal ganglia were disproportionately reduced in the children with FAS or PEA and that mental retardation, degree of dysmorphology, and overall reductions in head size were not sufficient to explain the finding.

In a later study, six children with FAS were compared with seven age-appropriate, normally developing control children (Mattson, Riley, Sowell, et al., 1996). The morphometric analysis differentiated the caudate nucleus from the lenticular nuclei, as the caudate nucleus is more involved in the "cognitive loop," whereas the lenticular nuclei are more involved in the "motor loop." Analyses revealed that the caudate nucleus and lenticular nuclei were reduced in children with FAS relative to control children. However, only the caudate nucleus displayed a disproportionate reduction in volume after controlling for brain size. A recent study which incorporated a larger sample of FAS ($N = 14$), PEA ($N = 12$), and normally developing control children ($N = 14$) replicated this finding (Archibald et al., 2001). On the basis of their intellectual functioning (range of intelligence scores: 40 to 103), this new sample was also more representative of the FAS and PEA populations on the whole. Archibald et al. (2001) found that the caudate nucleus, but not the lenticular nuclei, was disproportionately reduced in FAS children. There was a trend for a similar reduction in children with PEA; however, this was not significant, suggesting that either the magnitude or the consistency of basal ganglial damage is diminished in children who do not manifest the full FAS phenotype.

OTHER STUDIES

Electroencephalogram (EEG) and Event-Related Potential (ERP) Studies

The earliest studies examining brain activity in children utilized EEG and event-related potential (ERP) methodologies. Numerous case studies have appeared throughout the literature. These reports indicated abnormal brain-wave activity, which included reduced voltage in the left temporal lobe (Goldstein and Arulanantham, 1978), markedly abnormal brain stem-auditory-evoked-response potentials (Johnson et al., 1996), theta-wave activity (Riikonen et al., 1999), and occasional delta-wave activity in the posterior cortex (Mattson et al., 1992).

Two studies systematically utilized EEG or ERP methodologies to evaluate neural activity in children with FAS. Kaneko, Phillips, et al. (1996) compared brain-wave activity in normally developing children with children who had either FAS or Down's syndrome. The EEG records for the children with FAS were distinguishable from both the normally developing children and those with Down's syndrome. Brain activity in the children with Down's syndrome was characterized by a generalized slowing and a predominance of delta and theta waves. In contrast, the FAS children did not present with a generalized slowing of neural activity. However, alpha-frequency activity was significantly affected. Specifically, FAS children had significantly lower mean power in the alpha-frequency range in the left fronto-central and left parietal-occipital leads. They also displayed lower peak frequencies in the alpha frequency. These findings suggest immaturity of the cerebral cortex, particularly in the left hemisphere.

In a second study, Kaneko, Ehlers, et al. (1996) examined the same group of children using an oddball-plus-noise paradigm and ERP technology. Again, children with FAS were distinguishable from normally developing controls or children with Down's syndrome. Both children with Down's syndrome and FAS displayed longer P300 latencies. However, this finding was widespread in the Down's syndrome children and occurred in the presence of both the noise burst and infrequent tones. In the FAS children, the longer P300 latencies were isolated to the parietal cortex and only occurred in response to the noise burst.

Positron Emission Tomography (PET) and Single-Photon Emission Computerized Tomography (SPECT) Studies

While EEG provides information about the pattern of neuronal activity, its specificity is limited as it is typically difficult to accurately localize the source of the activity. Recently two new studies utilized newer neuroimaging techniques to examine brain function in children with FAS.

Riikonen et al. (1999) utilized SPECT to examine the changes in the brain structure and activity of 11 children with FAS. SPECT is a variant of the better known PET methodology, which enables researchers to examine the amount of glucose utilized by different brain regions. Glucose utilization reflects the activity level of the brain with greater utilization indicating greater activity. Results indicated an absence of the hemispheric asymmetry characteristic of normally developing brains. Specifically, in normally developing children there is greater glucose utilization and cerebral blood flow in the left hemisphere. This hemispheric difference was absent in FAS children. Further, this finding was most pronounced in the frontal and parietooccipital regions.

In a similar study, Clark et al. (2000) utilized PET to examine brain activity in high-functioning children with FAS. Rather than focus on cerebral asymmetry, Clark et al. (2000) examined the glucose metabolism of various cortical and subcortical structures relative to age-appropriate controls. Standardized glucose metabolism in the thalamus, head of the caudate, and the caudate/putamen was significantly lower in individuals with FAS than in controls. There was a bilateral reduction in glucose metabolism in each structure, with the exception of the caudate/putamen where the reduction was limited to the right side.

These newer studies complement the findings from the structural imaging studies. First, Riikonen, et al. (1999) demonstrated a disruption of the normal hemispheric asymmetry, which was predominantly localized to the frontal and parietooccipital regions. Likewise, Riley et al. (1995) found that corpus callosum abnormalities were predominantly located in the anterior and posterior portions, which carry fibers from the frontal and occipital cortical regions and allow for the efficient transfer of information across the hemispheres. Second, Clark et al. (2000) demonstrated decreased rates of glucose metabolism in the thalamus, caudate, and caudate/putamen. These data are consistent with the findings of a disproportionate reduction in the size of the caudate nucleus of the basal ganglia. Thus, it appears that both the structure and activity of the basal ganglia are impaired.

NEUROBEHAVIORAL EFFECTS

Intelligence

The effect of prenatal alcohol exposure on intelligence has received considerable attention, perhaps because prenatal alcohol exposure is the most frequent and preventable cause of mental retardation (Pulsifer, 1996). However, not all children with FAS or PEA are mentally retarded. In fact, it is estimated that only 25 percent of children with FAS have IQ scores that fall within the mental retardation range (IQ < 70) (Streissguth, 1997).

IQ scores vary widely in children with FAS or PEA. For example, IQ scores ranging from a low of 20 (Streissguth, Randels, and Smith, 1991) to a high of at least 120 have been reported (Olson et al., 1998). Mean IQ for children with FAS is estimated to be between 65 and 72 (Mattson and Riley, 1997). At least during childhood, IQ scores tend to be correlated with dysmorphology (Steinhausen, Willms, and Spohr, 1994). Children with more dysmorphic features tend to have lower IQ scores than children with fewer dysmorphic features. Consequently, IQ scores tend to be higher in children classified as PEA than in those with FAS (Streissguth et al., 1997; Streissguth, Randels, and Smith, 1991). However, it should be noted that children with PEA have significantly lower IQ scores than normally developing, alcohol-exposed children (Mattson et al., 1997). Thus, they tend to be less impaired in overall intellectual functioning than children with FAS, but are impaired when compared with non-alcohol-exposed peers.

Research indicates that the IQ scores of children with FAS derived from standardized intelligence tests such as the Wechsler Intelligence Scale for Children (WISC) (Wechsler, 1991) are very stable over time (Steinhausen and Spohr, 1998; Steinhausen, Willms, and Spohr, 1993). For example, Streissguth, Randels, and Smith (1991) found that test-retest correlations over an average eight-year interval ranged from 0.78 to 0.88 for FAS and PEA children, respectively, indicating a high degree of stability in intellectual functioning across time.

Language

Delays in language development have been reported in a variety of studies. For example, Iosub et al. (1981) reported that in a sample of 63 patients with FAS, 84 percent of patients displayed some evidence of delayed or disordered speech or language development. Shaywitz, Caparulo, and Hodgson (1981) described two preschool-aged children who had expressive and receptive language skills that were delayed by at least two years. Further, they noted that these children failed to use language as a tool for initiating social interactions. Thus, early reports suggested that language impairments were widespread within this population.

Several systematic studies examined language functioning in this population using standardized measures. Carney and Chermak (1991) tested 10 children with FAS and 17 normally developing children using the Test of Language Development. They found widespread impairments in language functioning, which included impairments in vocabulary and sentence imitation, grammatical understanding, and word discrimination. Impairments were noted in both expressive and receptive language. However, impairments appeared to be more extensive in the younger children. Older children were primarily impaired in their understanding and use of syntax. Although this study did not use a longitudinal design, it does suggest that language development may be delayed but not deviant.

This possibility was addressed in a study by Becker, Warr-Leeper, and Leeper (1990). Children with FAS were compared with chronological age (CA) and mental age (MA) control groups. A deficit in comparison to the CA group would suggest that language development was delayed. In contrast, a deficit in comparison with the MA group would suggest a qualitative shift in language development that is not easily accounted for by general cognitive functioning. This study utilized tests of grammar, semantics, and short-term memory. Significant differences were found between the children with FAS and the CA control group on a variety of measures including grammar, semantics, and memory. Thus, the data suggested that language development was delayed. However, the FAS group never differed significantly from the MA control group, indicating that while language development is delayed, the observed language skills are consistent with the general intellectual functioning of the FAS group.

Overall, the data strongly indicate that language development is delayed, although consistent with general intellectual functioning. A variety of issues are likely to impede language development in this population. For example, Church et al. (1997) found that while 82 percent of their patients had receptive language delays, almost all of them also had a hearing disorder. In addition, both Church et al. (1997) and Becker, Warr-Leeper, and Leeper (1990) reported abnormalities in the structure and function of the speech apparatus including cleft palate, high or narrow arches, and functional movements of the tongue and larynx, among other things. Both hearing disorders and abnormalities in the structure and function of the speech apparatus are likely to hinder age-appropriate language development.

Learning and Memory

Both verbal and nonverbal learning has been assessed in children with FAS and appears to be impaired. Mattson, Riley, Delis, et al. (1996) examined verbal learning and memory in children with FAS in relation to chronological- and mental-age-matched controls using the California Verbal Learning Test–Children's Version (CVLT-C). Across five learning trials, children learn a 15-word list, which must be recalled following each presentation as well as after a 20-minute delay. Results indicated that children with FAS learned fewer words across the five learning trials relative to chronological, but not mental age-matched controls.

Other studies have replicated these deficits using the verbal learning subscale of the Wide Range Assessment of Memory and Learning (WRAML). The WRAML verbal learning subscale and the CVLT-C are similar with two major exceptions. The CVLT-C offers one more learning trial and the words on the CVLT can be semantically clustered whereas words on the WRAML are unrelated. In studies with two different samples (Kaemingk and Halverson, 2000; Kaemingk, Mulvaney, and Halverson, 2003; Mattson and Roebuck, 2002; Roebuck-Spencer and Mattson, 2004), children with FAS learned significantly fewer words than normally developing children did.

Roebuck-Spencer and Mattson (2004) noticed that the learning pattern differed across the CVLT-C and the WRAML. Although children with FAS benefited from exposure to the words over multiple trials in both tasks, performance on the CVLT-C reached a plateau before the end of the task, while performance on the WRAML continued to improve across all trials. They argued that the learning on the CVLT-C may be facilitated by the ability to cluster words semantically. Analyses indicated that children with FAS utilized semantic clustering as much as control children early in the task. However, the last two trials, nonexposed, but not FAS, children increased their use of this strategy. The use of semantic clustering, was significantly correlated with the amount of information learned in the CVLT-C. Thus, the data suggest that although verbal memory may be impaired, performance can be improved with repetition and the use of learning strategies such as semantic clustering.

Learning of nonverbal material also appears to be impaired in children with FAS. The Biber Figure Learning Test (BFLT) and the visual subscale of the WRAML are two tests in which children learn nonverbal information over multiple trials. In the BFLT, children view multiple stimuli which they are expected to draw after the last stimulus is presented. In the WRAML, children learn the spatial location of multiple stimuli that are individually presented in a 4 × 4 grid. Data from two independent samples demonstrated that learning spatial and the object information was impaired (Kaemingk and Halverson, 2000; Kaemingk, Mulvaney, and Halverson, 2003; Mattson and Roebuck, 2002).

Children with FAS were also impaired on a virtual analog of the Morris water task, which assesses place learning. In this task, children start at various places within a virtual pool and must navigate to a platform that is hidden in the water. The platform is always in the same location and markers along the pool can be used to determine where they are in the pool. With the exception of the first trial, children with FAS took significantly longer paths to the platform. On a probe trial after the learning phase, children with FAS spent less time in the quadrant where the platform had been located, took a longer path to that quadrant, and spent less time searching for the platform in the appropriate quadrant. Interestingly, after the task, the children with FAS said that they thought the platform appeared in different locations throughout the training, even though they were initially told it would always appear in the same location.

Given that children with FAS tend to learn less material even with repeated trials, any assessment of memory deficits should take into account initial learning as memory deficits could occur due to disruptions in various cognitive processes including encoding, storage, and retrieval. Studies using the CVLT-C have documented memory impairments (Mattson, Riley, Delis, et al., 1996; Mattson and Roebuck, 2002; Roebuck-Spencer and Mattson, 2004). Mattson, Riley, Delis, et al. found that after a 20-minute delay, children with FAS exhibited significantly poorer recall for the list of words relative to their chronological, but not mental, age-matched controls. It is interesting that, when the number of words recalled after the 20-minute delay was compared with the number of words learned by the fifth learning trial, the groups did not differ in the percentage of learned words that were retained across the delay period. Thus, information that was learned tended to be equally retained by all groups. Some differences emerged between children with FAS and the mental-age-matched controls. Specifically, children with FAS had more difficulty discriminating the list words from distracters during a yes/no recognition test, resulting in more false positive errors. In addition, they tended to make more perseverative errors during free- and cued-recall conditions.

A later study expanded these findings by comparing implicit and explicit memory in children with FAS. Mattson and Riley (1999) used a word-stem completion task to assess priming, a type of implicit memory, and used free recall and recognition memory tasks to assess explicit memory. Results indicated that the children with FAS performed comparably to normally developing control children and better than children with Down's syndrome on the priming task, strongly suggesting that implicit memory is spared following. In contrast, children with FAS were significantly impaired in their ability to recall a list of words relative to normal controls. Further, they tended to make more perseveration errors when recalling the list of words. Thus, these studies suggest that although memory is impaired, it is not globally impaired. Both recognition and implicit (priming) memory appear to be spared while free recall is impaired.

A similar disassociation occurs when one examines memory for objects and spatial location (Uecker and Nadel, 1996, 1998). In two related studies, children with FAS exhibited deficits in spatial memory, but not object memory. Specifically, children were instructed to remember the identity and spatial location of various objects they either estimated the price of or named. Children with FAS recalled a comparable number of objects during an immediate delay condition, but were significantly worse at accurately determining the original location of the object. After a 24-hour delay, children with FAS were still impaired in their ability to remember where the objects were originally located. On the whole, the data suggested that spatial memory was impaired while object memory was spared.

The observed memory dissociations have implications for the types of neuroanatomical changes one would expect to find in alcohol-exposed children. For example, Mattson and Riley (1999) argued that the pattern of spared implicit memory and impaired explicit memory is comparable to that observed in patients with Huntington's disease. As mentioned previously, Huntington's disease is associated with pathological changes in the basal ganglia, an area that is reduced in children with FAS. Thus, the emerging neurobehavioral data converge with the existing neuroanatomical data. The dissociation between object and spatial memory provides us with a new avenue for exploration. The deficit in spatial memory suggests damage to the right hemisphere, particularly the temporal lobe and hippocampus (Smith and Milner, 1981) as well as damage to the basal ganglia (Lawrence et al., 2000). Damage to the hippocampus has been repeatedly observed in animal models of FAS (Berman and Hannigan, 2000). However, Riikonen et al. (1999) found that the right hippocampus was significantly larger than the left in children with FAS. Archibald et al. (2001) also found that the hippocampus was larger than expected in children with FAS given the size of other subcortical structures. As more sensitive neuroimaging techniques become available, further research should examine whether neuroanatomical differences in the hippocampus and temporal cortex emerge.

Attention and Activity

Attention and activity levels have received considerable focus. The inattentiveness and hyperactive behavioral patterns of children with FAS are frequently compared to those of children with ADHD. High levels of ADHD-like symptoms in this population would not be particularly surprising, as the prevalence of ADHD in special education classrooms is conservatively estimated to be between 9 and 33 percent (Pearson et al., 2000).

Steinhausen et al. (Steinhausen and Spohr, 1998; Steinhausen, Willms, and Spohr, 1993, 1994) examined rates of psychopathology in a sample of children with FAS and found that 63 percent displayed one or more psychiatric disorders, with hyperkinetic disorders (e.g., ADHD) predominant within the sample. The prevalence of hyperkinetic disorders ranged from approximately 42 to 63 percent depending upon the time of the assessment and the subsample evaluated. Further, while the presence of many other disorders, such as enuresis and language disorders, appeared to be age related, hyperkinetic disorders were present from an early age and persisted through adolescence in the majority of affected cases. The prevalence of hyperactivity in this sample is higher than the estimates for special education populations, suggesting that prenatal alcohol exposure may be one of many potential etiologies for hyperactivity.

A number of studies utilized neuropsychological measures of attention to determine whether children with FAS exhibit deficits in attention, but provide conflicting data about whether sustained attention is globally impaired. Kerns et al. (1997) reported that adults with FAS performed within normal limits on tests of simple auditory attention. However, complex sustained and alternating auditory attention were impaired. In a similar study, Connor et al. (1999) compared the visual and auditory attention abilities of adults with FAS or PEA to nonexposed adults. The adults with FAS/PEA performed more poorly than controls on most measures in both modalities and the results suggested that adults with FAS/PEA have difficulty focusing, sustaining, and shifting auditory attention, as well as focusing and sustaining visual attention. Overall, auditory attention appeared to be more affected than visual attention.

Coles et al. (2002) reported conflicting findings. When collapsed across modality, they found no evidence of attention deficits among alcohol exposed adolescents using a continuous performance task. Group differences only emerged when the visual and auditory data were analyzed separately. The performance of alcohol-exposed adolescents who had dysmorphic features was significantly worse than that of nonexposed adolescents, or that of those who were exposed, but had no dysmorphic features. However, this difference was only observed on the visual task, not the auditory task.

The source of the discrepancy between these studies is unclear but is probably due to differences in samples and methodology. For example, Kerns et al. (1997) did not utilize a control group, but rather compared performance with test norms. In contrast, Coles et al. (2002) compared the performance of the alcohol affected children to a sample of adolescents from special education classrooms, and adolescents drawn from the same low socioeconomic neighborhoods in terms of level of intellectual impairment and socioeconomic status. Developmental changes may also influence these differences (Coles et al., 2002). Further research examining the development of attention across the life span and across modalities should help clarify whether the pattern of attention deficits observed in alcohol-exposed individuals is unique and could be used to identify exposed children as has been suggested (Lee, Mattson, and Riley, 2004).

Although children with FAS are frequently compared to children with ADHD, it is unclear whether the behavioral phenotype expressed by children with FAS is identical to that expressed by children with ADHD. Two studies explicitly compared the performance of children with ADHD or FAS. Nanson and Hiscock (1990) used parental reports and laboratory measures of attention to compare the performance of children with FAS or PEA to children with ADHD or normally developing children. The parental reports for children with FAS/PEA or ADHD were indistinguishable, suggesting that the presence and severity of hyperactive and inattentive symptoms was perceived to be significant in both groups. Likewise, children with ADHD or FAS exhibited increased rates of impulsive errors on a delayed reaction time task. Although children with ADHD appeared to make a speed accuracy trade-off, children with FAS/PEA responded slowly and made many errors, indicating an increased difficulty with the task as well as possible impulsive responding. The slower responses exhibited by the FAS/ PEA children on delayed reaction time task and vigilance tasks were likely attributable in part to the *differences* in IQ observed between the FAS/PEA children and other groups.

In a similar study, Coles et al. (1997) used parental reports and an attention battery to examine the profile of FAS/PEA children and ADHD children on four components of attention: focus, sustain, encode, and shift. Unlike the previous study, Coles et al. (1997) found that parents rated children with FAS/PEA differently from children with ADHD. Ratings for children with ADHD indicated that they displayed significantly more behaviors associated with the disorder than either children with FAS/PEA or control children. Likewise, the profile of children with FAS/PEA tended to differ from that of children with ADHD on the attention battery. Both groups had difficulty focusing attention as measured by the WISC-Revised coding subtest. In addition, children with FAS/PEA had some difficulty encoding information and shifting attention. The performance of children with ADHD was significantly worse on measures of sustained attention. However, more than 50 percent of children with FAS/PEA or ADHD were unable to complete the sustained attention tasks, so the findings are difficult to interpret. Overall, Coles et al. (1997) found that although children with FAS/PEA exhibit attention deficits, the profile of deficits varies from that observed in children with ADHD. These phenotypic differences suggest that prenatal alcohol exposure may not cause classic ADHD symptoms, but rather a variant, which potentially could require different pharmacological and behavioral treatment protocols from those employed with nonexposed children with ADHD.

Executive Functioning

Executive functioning (EF) is a complex psychological construct that has been broadly defined as "the ability to maintain an appropriate problem solving set for the attainment of a goal" (Welsh and Pennington, 1988, p. 201). A variety of cognitive domains are subsumed under this general definition including inhibition, set shifting and set maintenance, planning, working memory, and the ability to integrate information across time and space (Pennington and Ozonoff, 1996). EF plays a big role in our day-to-day functioning, as it is utilized in such diverse activities as interpersonal relations, organizing and conducting a search for missing keys, or organizing the tools and skills necessary to achieve a job or school assignment. Although EF is typically associated with the frontal cortex, damage to subcortical or cortical regions that send projections to the frontal cortex could also disrupt EF. Thus, deficits in EF would be consistent with MRI studies that documented a reduction in the size of the basal ganglia. Studies of Parkinson's disease and Huntington's disease have documented impaired performance on EF tasks in association with the pathology of the basal ganglia (Bäckman et al., 1997; Watkins et al., 2000).

The first systematic study of executive functioning in children with FAS investigated deficits in the self-regulation of action (Kodituwakku et al., 1995). Specifically, they measured three constructs: planning, the regulation of behavior, and the ability to utilize feedback to adapt behavior. Children with FAS or PEA were compared to normally developing children. The FAS/PEA children performed significantly worse on the Standard Progressive Matrices, a measure of fluid intelligence, indicating that overall they were more impaired than the control children. Results from the EF battery were mixed. Children with FAS/PEA performed significantly worse on the Progressive Planning Test that was used to measure planning but also has a strong inhibitory component (Goel and Grafman, 1995). However, there were no group differences on two of the three tests of behavioral regulation. Finally, the FAS/PEA group performed significantly worse on one utilization of feedback test, the Wisconsin Card Sorting Test (WCST), but not on the go/no-go task. Children with FAS/PEA made significantly more perseverative responses and consequently did not complete as many categories as did control children in the WCST. These data are consistent with those reported by Olson et al. (1998), although Coles et al. (1997) found no significant *difference* between children with FAS and normally developing children on this measure. Thus, although there were some deficits in EF, they were not as consistent as might have been expected, particularly as the two groups differed significantly on fluid intelligence.

Another systematic examination of EF in this population was recently published by Mattson et al. (1999). This study utilized the new Delis Kaplan Executive Function System (D-KEFS) battery (Delis et al., 2001) to assess four domains of EF: cognitive flexibility, response inhibition, planning, and concept formation and reasoning. FAS/PEA children had significantly lower IQ scores than the normally developing control children and group *differences* emerged across all four domains.

Cognitive flexibility and response inhibition were assessed with the California Trail Making Test and California Stroop Test, respectively. Both tests incorporate control conditions, although no group *differences* emerged across any control tasks. In the California Trail Making Test, the critical test requires children to connect a series of letters and numbers, alternating between the two categories (e.g., 1-A-2-B). FAS/PEA children performed significantly worse on this test. The California Stroop Test contains two critical tests: interference and set shifting. During the interference condition, children see a color name printed in a different color of ink and are supposed to name the ink's color. During the set-shifting condition, children were presented with the same stimuli but were directed to read the word or name the ink color depending on a cue. The FAS/PEA children were significantly impaired on the interference condition. Only children with FAS differed from control children on the set-shifting condition. Thus, the data suggest that both cognitive flexibility and response inhibition may be impaired in children with FAS/PEA.

Schonfeld et al. (2001) later demonstrated verbal and nonverbal fluency deficits in this same sample. Fluency tests provide an estimate of mental flexibility. In the verbal fluency task, the participant names as many unique words that fit a designated category as possible in a short period. For example, they may be asked to name words that begin with the letter F (phonetic) or animals (semantic). The D-KEFS (Delis et al., 2001) nonverbal fluency tasks requires participants to create unique designs by connecting dots on a page. The simplest version involves connecting black dots with no other symbols or distractors present. In contrast, the set shifting version involves alternately connecting black dots and open circles to form unique designs. Children with FAS/PEA performed worse than nonexposed children did on both the verbal and nonverbal fluency tasks. These findings support their earlier contention that cognitive flexibility is impaired following heavy prenatal alcohol exposure.

Planning was assessed using the Tower of California Test, a variant of the progressive planning test used by Kodituwakku et al. (1995), while concept formation and reasoning was assessed with the California Word Context Test. Consistent with Kodituwakku et al. (1995), the FAS/PEA children violated more rules and passed fewer items on the Tower of California Test, suggesting that planning was impaired. In the California Word Context Test, children must guess a target word on the basis of a series of five sequentially presented sentences that provide clues about the target word. Likewise, children with FAS/PEA required significantly more sentence cues to guess the target word than normally developing children.

Although the earlier data suggested EF impairments in this population, none of these studies adequately controlled for overall intellectual functioning that is known to covary with EF (Denckla, 1996). This is particularly problematic because each of these studies utilized control groups that scored on average 15-30 points higher on tests of overall cognitive functioning. Connor et al. (2000) argued that while alcohol could have a direct impact on EF, the impact of alcohol exposure on EF could also be mediated through the well-documented reduction in overall intellectual functioning. Using a battery of EF tasks that overlapped substantially with those described previously, they examined EF in clinically referred adults with FAS or PEA and compared them with over 400 control participants drawn from two previous studies.

Utilizing data from the control sample, they estimated the difference between the FAS/PEA participants' actual performance on each EF task and their expected performance given their measured intelligence (Connor et al., 2000). Performance was not uniformly poor as might be expected. Adults with FAS or PEA performed worse than expected given their IQ on measures of set shifting and perseveration, nonverbal fluency, response inhibition and one (out of three) measure of working memory. In contrast, performance on measures of verbal fluency, cognitive estimation, working memory, and error scores on multiple tasks was consistent with their level of overall intellectual functioning. Thus, it appears that some of the deficits in EF may be indirectly influenced by alcohol's effect on intelligence while other EF skills may be directly affected.

Further research on EF in alcohol-exposed individuals is clearly needed to resolve remaining inconsistencies and to integrate the neuroanatomical and behavioral data. For example, Connor et al.'s (2000) data suggest that all, or at least the majority, of the adults with FAS or PEA exhibited EF deficits. However, in a later study, which included this sample, examining the relationship between variability in corpus callosum shape and neuropsychological functioning (Bookstein, Streissguth et al., 2002), two distinct groups emerged: individuals with EF deficits but spared motor skills and individuals with spared EF skills but impaired motor skills. These two profiles should be validated in a larger sample. Given the emphasis placed on EF deficits underlying observed deficits in psychosocial functioning (see following section), it will be important to examine whether the individuals with spared EF skills exhibited better adaptive functioning than individuals meeting the other profile.

Psychosocial Functioning

The majority of the research on the neurobehavioral consequences of heavy prenatal alcohol exposure focused on cognitive skills and capabilities. However, the behavioral consequences of prenatal alcohol exposure are not limited to the cognitive arena as emphasized by a study on secondary disabilities across the life span in individuals with FAS and PEA (Streissguth et al., 1997). Secondary disabilities are those problems that are not directly caused by alcohol, but emerge after birth, and presumably could be prevented or ameliorated with intervention efforts. This initial study provided some alarming statistics. For example, 90 percent of 415 patients sought help for or experienced a mental health problem. Further, more than half of the individuals with FAS experienced trouble with the law, and either dropped out of school, or had been suspended or expelled (Streissguth et al., 1997). These data indicate that individuals with FAS have significant and pervasive adaptive functioning deficits that persist into adulthood.

Early studies examining adaptive behaviors, problem behaviors, or social skills demonstrated a spectrum of attention and social problems among children with FAS. However, the implications of these studies was unclear (Streissguth, Randels, and Smith, 1991; Steinhausen and Spohr, 1998; Steinhausen, Willms, and Spohr, 1993) because these studies typically compared children with FAS to normally developing children or national norms. As behavioral and social problems are not uncommon in developmentally disabled populations, it was not clear whether the problems documented are similar to those in other disabled populations or whether the difficulties exhibited by children with FAS are in some way unique.

Several new studies provide data on the issue. Whaley, O'Connor, and Gunderson (2001) compared children with FAS or PEA to a sample of children previously referred to a mental health clinic. The groups were matched on age, sex, and IQ. Parents reported that both the exposed and clinical control groups were significantly impaired in communication skills, daily living skills, and socialization using the Vineland Adaptive Behavior Scales (VABS). Both groups had overall adaptive functioning scores that were approximately two standard deviations below the mean for their age and did not differ significantly from each other. Adaptive functioning standardized scores declined with age for both groups, although the decline was significantly steeper for the alcohol exposed children. Thus, in a preadolescent sample, children with FAS did not differ in adaptive functioning skills from a clinical control group. Given the age-related steep decline in adaptive functioning skills, it will be important to follow these children to determine whether group differences emerge during adolescence.

On the surface, this study contradicts an earlier study that found that children with FAS had significant deficits in social skills, using the same index of socialization as Whaley, O'Connor, and Gunderson (2001). In this earlier study (Thomas et al., 1998) children with FAS were impaired on the socialization subscale of the VABS. Specifically, they were significantly impaired in their interpersonal relationships and their ability to make appropriate use of their play and leisure time, even when compared with children with similar verbal IQ scores.

The difference in findings is likely attributable to sample ages and supports the suggestion that the discrepancy in social skills between children with FAS and normally developing or cognitively impaired children increases with age. The Whaley, O'Connor, and Gunderson's FAS sample had a mean age of 6 and included children between the ages of 20 months and 10.5 years. The Thomas et al. (1998) FAS sample included children between the ages of 5 and 12.92 years, but only included one child less than eight years old. Whaley, O'Connor, and Gunderson demonstrated that standardized socialization scores declined substantially as a function of age. By age ten, the FAS sample had standardized socialization scores around 60, which is similar to the mean scores reported by Thomas et al. for their FAS sample which had a mean age of 10.3 years. Thomas et al. calculated age-equivalent scores and found that the socialization scores of children with FAS tended to plateau around the four to six year level. Thus, the increasing discrepancy in social skills appears to occur because the social skills of the children with FAS remain stable after they reach the four to six year old level, while the skills of normally developing children, clinically referred children, and children with modest reductions in intellectual ability continue to increase, at varying rates, with age.

Behavioral and emotional disturbances have been reported in a variety of studies. One study compared parental reports of behavioral and emotional disturbances in children with FAS or mild FAS/PEA to a group of children with unspecified intellectual impairment who were matched to the FAS group on age, sex, and IQ (Steinhausen et al., 2003). Both alcohol-exposed groups scored higher than the control group on disruptive behavior, self-absorbed behavior, communication disturbances, anxiety, and antisocial behavior. These differences cannot be accounted for solely by intelligence. Both the FAS and the control groups had mean intelligence scores more than two standard deviations below the mean, while the mild FAS/PEA group had a mean intelligence score that was only one standard deviation below the mean. The two exposed groups were remarkably similar across all subscales despite the large intelligence difference and they both differed significantly from the control group. These data suggest that behavioral disturbances often reported in this population emerge early in development and that parents of alcohol-exposed children report higher rates of behavioral disturbance than parents of children with comparable or worse intellectual impairments that are unrelated to alcohol-exposure.

FAS children also display more problematic behaviors than children with comparable IQ scores (Mattson and Riley, 2000). Parents reported that children with FAS engaged in more externalizing behaviors and had more social, thought, and attention problems. Further, according to their parents, FAS children engaged in more aggressive and delinquent behavior. These problems were not limited to the most severely affected children. Children with PEA displayed the same pattern of social and behavioral problems as children with FAS, indicating that overall intellectual functioning and dysmorphology were not sufficient to explain the pattern of maladaptive behaviors.

A related study used the Personality Inventory for Children (PIC) to further examine the behavioral and psychological problems present in this population (Roebuck, Mattson, and Riley, 1999). As expected, FAS and PEA children scored poorly on the three subtests that measured intelligence, cognitive development, and achievement. In addition, they were in the clinical range for the subscales measuring delinquency and psychosis, with PEA children showing a level of impairment comparable to the FAS children.

Across multiple studies it is becoming clear that alcohol-exposed children display a wide variety of maladaptive behaviors and have significant difficulties in their social interactions. These maladaptive behaviors tend to be directed toward others rather than themselves and do not appear to be commensurate with their level of cognitive disability. FAS and PEA children are more likely to engage in externalizing and delinquent behaviors and to disregard or fail to comprehend the rights and feelings of others. These findings are consistent with the secondary disabilities documented by Streissguth et al. (1997).

These studies have not determined why these children engage in these behaviors. Are children with FAS deliberately misbehaving or do their misdeeds reflect an inability to understand the consequences of their behaviors and the potential effect of their behaviors on others? Currently, many believe the latter to be the case. As mentioned previously, some have suggested that children with FAS/PEA have deficits in EF (Kodituwakku et al., 1995; Mattson et al., 1999). Although this hypothesis needs to be validated further, EF deficits could be expressed as an inability to plan and foresee the consequences of actions as well as the inability to inhibit actions that may be inappropriate. Thus, although children with FAS may be engaging in risky and aversive behaviors, these behaviors may not be intentionally mischievous or antisocial. Rather they may reflect core deficits in foresight, planning, and the ability to read and understand social cues. Further research needs to be directed at determining the cause of social deficits and increased behavioral problems in children with FAS.

SUMMARY AND CONCLUSIONS

In summary, understanding of the neuroanatomical and neurobehavioral consequences of prenatal alcohol exposure is increasing rapidly. Although autopsy studies have suggested that heavy prenatal exposure to alcohol resulted in a diffuse, nonspecific pattern of neuropathological abnormalities, newer neuroimaging techniques are revealing a consistent pattern of anomalies across alcohol-affected children. Microcephaly is still the most common outcome following heavy exposure. However, it is now clear that the entire brain is not equally sensitive to the teratogenic effects of alcohol. The basal ganglia, corpus callosum, cerebellum, and perisylvian cortex appear to have a heightened susceptibility relative to other brain structures. Further research on the neuroanatomical effects of prenatal alcohol exposure is still needed. Most notably, there is a need for more studies that use developmentally disabled, rather than normally developing, children as controls in order to determine whether the observed neuropathology is in any way unique from that observed in a variety of other developmental disorders. Bookstein, Streissguth, et al. (2002) offer the possibility that utilizing multiple pieces of information about alterations, shape, and relative location of neuroanatomical landmarks may aid in the diagnosis of alcohol-affected individuals and in the identification of subgroups of alcohol-affected individuals whose core deficits vary. If further research supports their findings, it could substantially change the way the field diagnoses and provides treatment for alcohol-affected individuals.

Intellectual deficits have received considerable attention and this is not surprising as prenatal alcohol exposure remains the leading preventable cause of mental retardation and results in significant impairments in academic functioning. A number of other cognitive domains have also been examined including attention, learning and memory, executive functioning, and language. Questions remain unanswered in each of these domains. Most pressing is the need to determine the extent to which deficits in cognitive domains are consistent general declines in intellectual functioning. New research clearly indicates that deficits are not isolated to the cognitive domain. Children with FAS exhibit a high level of problem behaviors as well as impairments in their interpersonal relationships. It is critical that more research be directed toward exploring and alleviating these problems at a very young age in order to prevent secondary disabilities such as the observed problems in psychosocial adjustment, juvenile delinquency, and mental health.

REFERENCES

Aase, J.M.; Jones, K.L.; and Clarren, S.K. (1995). Do we need the term "FAE"? *Pediatrics,* 95, 428-430.

Abel, E.L. (1995). An update on incidence of FAS: FAS is not an equal opportunity birth defect. *Neurotoxicology and Teratology,* 17, 437-443.

Ackermann, H.; Graber, S.; Hertrich, I.; and Daum, I. (1999). Cerebellar contributions to the perception of temporal cues within the speech and nonspeech domain. *Brain and Language, 67*, 228-241.

Archibald, S.L.; Fennema-Notestine, C.; Gamst, A.; Riley, E.P.; Mattson, S.N.; and Jernigan, T.L. (2001). Brain dysmorphology in individuals with severe prenatal alcohol exposure. *Developmental Medicine and Child Neurology, 43*, 148-154.

Bäckman, L.; Robins-Wahlin, T.B.; Lundin, A.; Ginovart, N.; and Farde, L. (1997). Cognitive deficits in Huntington's disease are predicted by dopaminergic PET markers and brain volumes. *Brain, 120*, 2207-2217.

Bauman, M.L.; Filipek, P.A.; and Kemper, T.L. (1997). Early infantile autism. In: J.D. Schmahmann (Ed.), *International Review of Neurobiology*, Vol. 4: *The Cerebellum and Cognition* (pp. 367-386). San Diego, CA: Academic Press.

Becker, M.; Warr-Leeper, G.A.; and Leeper, H.A., Jr. (1990). Fetal alcohol syndrome: A description of oral motor, articulatory, short-term memory, grammatical, and semantic abilities. *Journal of Communication Disorders, 23*, 97-124.

Berman, R.F. and Hannigan, J.H. (2000). Effects of prenatal alcohol exposure on the hippocampus: Spatial behavior, electrophysiology, and neuroanatomy. *Hippocampus, 10*, 94-110.

Berquin, P.C.; Giedd, J.N.; Jacobsen, L.K.; Hamburger, S.D.; Krain, A.L.; Rapoport, J.L.; and Castellanos, F.X. (1998). Cerebellum in attention-deficit hyperactivity disorder: A morphometric MRI study. *Neurology, 50*, 1087-1093.

Bonthius, D.J. and West, J.R. (1990). Alcohol-induced neuronal loss in developing rats: Increased brain damage with binge exposure. *Alcoholism: Clinical and Experimental Research, 14*, 107-118.

Bookstein, F.L.; Sampson, P.D.; Connor, P.D.; and Streissguth, A.P. (2002). Midline corpus callosum is a neuroanatomical focus of fetal alcohol damage. *The Anatomical Record, 269*, 162-174.

Bookstein, F.L.; Sampson, P.D.; Streissguth, A.P.; and Conner, P.D. (2001). Geometric morphometrics of corpus callosum and subcortical structures in the fetal-alcohol-affected brain. *Teratology, 64*, 4-32.

Bookstein, F.L.; Streissguth, A.P.; Sampson, P.D.; Conner, P.D.; and Barr, H.M. (2002). Corpus callosum shape and neuropsychological deficits in adult males with heavy fetal alcohol exposure. *NeuroImage, 15*, 233-251.

Carney, L.J. and Chermak, G.D. (1991). Performance of American Indian children with fetal alcohol syndrome on the test of language development. *Journal of Communication Disorders, 24*, 123-134.

Church, M.W.; Eldis, F.; Blakley, B.W.; and Bawle, E.V. (1997). Hearing, language, speech, vestibular, and dentofacial disorders in fetal alcohol syndrome. *Alcoholism: Clinical and Experimental Research, 21*, 227-237.

Clark, C.M.; Li, D.; Conry, J.; Conry, R.; and Loock, C. (2000). Structural and functional brain integrity of fetal alcohol syndrome in nonretarded cases. *Pediatrics, 105*, 1096-1099.

Clarren, S.K. (1986). Neuropathology in fetal alcohol syndrome. In: J.R. West (Ed.), *Alcohol and Brain Development* (pp. 158-166). New York: Oxford University Press.

Clarren, S.K.; Alvord, E.C.; Sumi, S.M.; Streissguth, A.P.; and Smith, D.W. (1978). Brain malformations related to prenatal exposure to ethanol. *Journal of Pediatrics,* 92, 64-67.

Clarren, S.K. and Astley, S.J. (1992). Pregnancy outcomes after weekly oral administration of ethanol during gestation in the pig-tailed macaque: Comparing early gestational exposure to full gestational exposure. *Teratology,* 45, 1-9.

Clarren, S.K.; Bowden, D.M.; and Astley, S.J. (1987). Pregnancy outcomes after weekly oral administration of ethanol during gestation in the pig-tailed macaque *(Macaca nemestrina). Teratology,* 35, 345-354.

Coles, C.D.; Platzman, K.A.; Lynch, M.E.; and Freides, D. (2002). Auditory and visual sustained attention in adolescents prenatally exposed to alcohol. *Alcoholism: Clinical and Experimental Research,* 26, 263-271.

Coles, C.D.; Platzman, K.A.; Raskind-Hood, C.L.; Brown, R.T.; Falek, A.; and Smith, I.E. (1997). A comparison of children affected by prenatal alcohol exposure and attention deficit, hyperactivity disorder. *Alcoholism: Clinical and Experimental Research,* 21, 150-161.

Connor, P.D.; Sampson, P.D.; Bookstein, F.L.; Barr, H.M.; and Streissguth, A.P. (2000). Direct and indirect effects of prenatal alcohol damage on executive function. *Developmental Neuropsychology,* 18, 331-354.

Connor, P.D.; Streissguth, A.P.; Sampson, P.D.; Bookstein, F.L.; and Barr, H.M. (1999). Individual differences in auditory and visual attention among fetal alcohol-affected adults. *Alcoholism: Clinical and Experimental Research,* 23, 1395-1402.

Coulter, C.L.; Leech, R.W.; Schaefer, B.; Scheithauer, B.W.; and Brumbak, R.A. (1993). Midline cerebral dysgenesis, dysfunction of the hypothalamic-pituitary axis, and fetal alcohol effects. *Archives of Neurology,* 50, 771-775.

Courchesne, E.; Townsend, J.; and Saitoh, O. (1994). The brain in infantile autism: Posterior fossa structures are abnormal. *Neurology,* 44, 214-223.

Cragg, B. and Phillips, S. (1985). Natural loss of Purkinje cells during development and increased loss with alcohol. *Brain Research,* 325, 151-160.

Delis, D.C.; Kaplan, E.; Kramer, J.H.; and Ober, B.A. (2001). *Delis-Kaplan Executive Function Scale.* San Antonio, TX: Harcourt Assessment.

Denckla, M.B. (1996). A theory and model of executive function: A neuropsychological perspective. In: G.R. Lyon and N.A. Krasnegor (Eds.), *Attention, Memory, and Executive Function* (pp. 263-278). Baltimore: Brookes.

Diener, H.C.; Hore, J.; Ivry, R.; and Dichgans, J. (1993). Cerebellar dysfunction of movement and perception. *The Canadian Journal of Neurological Sciences,* 20, S62-S69.

Gabrielli, O.; Salvolini, U.; Coppa, G.V.; Catassi, C.; Rossi, R.; Manca, A.; Lanza, R.; and Giorgi, P.L. (1990). Magnetic resonance imaging in the malformative syndromes with mental retardation. *Pediatric Radiology,* 21, 16-19.

Goel, V. and Grafman, J. (1995). Are the frontal lobes implicated in "planning" functions? Interpreting data from the tower of Hanoi. *Neuropsychologia,* 33, 623-642.

Goldstein, G. and Arulanantham, K. (1978). Neural tube defect and renal anomalies in a child with fetal alcohol syndrome. *Journal of Pediatrics,* 93, 636-637.

Goodlett, C.R.; Marcussen, B.L.; and West, J.R. (1990). A single day of alcohol exposure during the brain growth spurt induces brain weight restriction and cerebellar Purkinje cell loss. *Alcohol,* 7, 107-114.

Guerri, C. (1998). Neuroanatomical and neurophysiological mechanisms involved in central nervous system dysfunctions induced by prenatal alcohol exposure. *Alcoholism: Clinical and Experimental Research,* 22, 304-312.

Hallett, M. and Grafman, J. (1997). Executive function and motor skill learning. In: J.D. Schmahmann (Ed.), *International Review of Neurobiology,* Vol. 4: *The Cerebellum and Cognition* (pp. 297-323). San Diego, CA: Academic Press.

Heimer, L. (1995). *The Human Brain and Spinal Cord: Functional Neuroanatomy and Dissection Guide* (3rd ed.). New York: Springer-Verlag.

Hynd, G.W.; Semrud-Clikeman, M.; Lorys, A.R.; Novey, E.S.; Eliopulos, D.; and Lyytinen, H. (1991). Corpus callosum morphology in attention deficit-hyperactivity disorder: Morphometric analysis of MRI. *Journal of Learning Disabilities,* 24, 141-146.

Institute of Medicine (1996). *Fetal Alcohol Syndrome: Diagnosis, Epidemiology, Prevention, and Treatment.* Washington, DC: National Academy Press.

Iosub, S.; Fuchs, M.; Bingol, N.; and Gromisch, D.S. (1981). Fetal alcohol syndrome revisited. *Pediatrics,* 68, 475-479.

Ivry, R.B. and Baldo, J.V. (1992). Is the cerebellum involved in learning and cognition? *Current Opinion in Neurobiology,* 2, 212-216.

Jellinger, K.; Gross, H.; Kaltenback, E.; and Grisold, W. (1981). Holoprosencephaly and agenesis of the corpus callosum: Frequency of associated malformations. *Acta Neuropathology,* 55, 1-10.

Jeret, J.S.; Serur, D.; Wisniewski, K.; and Fisch, C. (1986). Frequency of agenesis of the corpus callosum in the developmentally disabled population as determined by computerized tomography. *Pediatric Neuroscience,* 12, 101-103.

Johnson, V.P.; Swayze, V.W.; Sato, Y.; and Andreasen, N.C. (1996). Fetal alcohol syndrome: Craniofacial and central nervous system manifestations. *American Journal of Medical Genetics,* 61, 329-339.

Jones, K.L. and Smith, D.W. (1973). Recognition of the fetal alcohol syndrome in early infancy. *Lancet,* 2, 999-1001.

Jones, K.L.; Smith, D.W.; Ulleland, C.N.; and Streissguth, A.P. (1973). Pattern of malformation in offspring of chronic alcoholic mothers. *Lancet,* 1, 1267-1271.

Kaemingk, K.L. and Halverson, P.T. (2000). Spatial memory following prenatal alcohol exposure: More than a material specific memory deficit. *Child Neuropsychology,* 6, 115-128.

Kaemingk, K.L.; Mulvaney, S.; and Halverson, P.T. (2003). Learning following prenatal alcohol exposure: Performance on verbal and visual multitrial tasks. *Archives of Clinical Neuropsychology,* 18, 33-47.

Kaneko, W.M.; Ehlers, C.L.; Phillips, E.L.; and Riley, E.P. (1996). Auditory event related potentials in fetal alcohol syndrome and Down's syndrome children. *Alcoholism: Clinical and Experimental Research,* 20, 35-42.

Kaneko, W.M.; Phillips, E.L.; Riley, E.P.; and Ehlers, C.L. (1996). EEG findings in fetal alcohol syndrome and Down's syndrome children. *Electroencephalography and Clinical Neurophysiology,* 98, 20-28.

Keele, S.W. and Ivry, R. (1990). Does the cerebellum provide a common computation for diverse tasks? In: A. Diamond (Ed.), *The Development and Neural Bases of Higher Cognitive Functions,* Vol. 608 (pp. 179-211). New York: New York Academy of Sciences.

Kerns, K.A.; Don, A.; Mateer, C.A.; and Streissguth, A.P. (1997). Cognitive deficits in nonretarded adults with fetal alcohol syndrome. *Journal of Learning Disabilities,* 30, 685-693.

Kodituwakku, P.W.; Handmaker, N.S.; Cutler, S.K.; Weathersby, E.K.; and Handmaker, S.D. (1995). Specific impairments in self-regulation in children exposed to alcohol prenatally. *Alcohol: Clinical and Experimental Research,* 19, 1558-1564.

Kolb, B. and Whishaw, I.Q. (1996). *Fundamentals of Human Neuropsychology* (4th ed.). New York: W. H. Freeman and Company.

Konovalov, H.V.; Kovetsky, N.S.; Bobryshev, Y.V.; and Ashwell, K.W.S. (1997). Disorders of brain development in the progeny of mothers who used alcohol during pregnancy. *Early Human Development,* 48, 153-166.

Kopera-Frye, K.; Carmichael-Olson, H.; and Streissguth, A.P. (1997). Teratogenic effects of alcohol on attention. In: J.A. Burack and J.T. Enns (Eds.), *Attention, Development, and Psychopathology* (pp. 171-204). New York: The Guilford Press.

Lawrence, A.D.; Watkins, L.H.A.; Sahakian, B.J.; Hodges, J.R.; and Robbins, T.W. (2000). Visual object and visuospatial cognition in Huntington's disease: Implications for information processing in corticostriatal circuits. *Brain,* 123, 1349-1364.

Lee, K.T.; Mattson, S.N.; and Riley, E.P. (2004). Classifying children with heavy prenatal alcohol exposure using measures of attention. *Journal of the International Neuropsychological Society,* 10, 271-277.

Lemoine, P.; Harousseau, H.; Borteryu, J.P.; and Menuet, J.C. (1968). Les enfants des parents alcooliques: Anomalies observees. A proposos de 127 cas [Children of alcoholic parents: Abnormalities observed in 127 cases]. *Ouest-médical,* 21, 476-482.

Mattson, S.N.; Goodman, A.M.; Caine, C.; Delis, D.C.; and Riley, E.P. (1999). Executive functioning in children with heavy prenatal alcohol exposure. *Alcoholism: Clinical and Experimental Research,* 23, 1808-1815.

Mattson, S.N.; Jernigan, T.L.; and Riley, E.P. (1994). MRI and prenatal alcohol exposure. *Alcohol Health & Research World,* 18, 49-52.

Mattson, S.N. and Riley, E.P. (1995). Prenatal exposure to alcohol: What the images reveal. *Alcohol Health & Research World,* 19, 273-277.

Mattson, S.N. and Riley, E.P. (1996). Brain anomalies in fetal alcohol syndrome. In: E.L. Abel (Ed.), *Fetal Alcohol Syndrome: From Mechanism to Prevention* (pp. 51-68). Boca Raton, FL: CRC Press.

Mattson, S.N. and Riley, E.P. (1997). Neurobehavioral and neuroanatomical effects of heavy prenatal exposure to alcohol. In: A. Streissguth and J. Kanter (Eds.),

The Challenge of Fetal Alcohol Syndrome: Overcoming Secondary Disabilities. Seattle, WA: University of Washington Press.

Mattson, S.N. and Riley, E.P. (1999). Implicit and explicit memory functioning in children with heavy prenatal alcohol exposure. *Journal of International Neuropsychological Society,* 5, 462-471.

Mattson, S.N. and Riley, E.P. (2000). Parent ratings of behavior in children with heavy prenatal alcohol exposure and IQ-matched controls. *Alcoholism, Clinical and Experimental Research,* 24, 226-231.

Mattson, S.N.; Riley, E.P.; Delis, D.C.; Stern, C.; and Jones, K.L. (1996). Verbal learning and memory in children with fetal alcohol syndrome. *Alcoholism: Clinical and Experimental Research,* 20, 810-816.

Mattson, S.N.; Riley, E.P.; Gramling, L.; Delis, D.C.; and Jones, K.L. (1997). Heavy prenatal alcohol exposure with or without physical features of fetal alcohol syndrome leads to IQ deficits. *Journal of Pediatrics,* 131, 718-721.

Mattson, S.N.; Riley, E.P.; Gramling, L.; Delis, D.C.; and Jones, K.L. (1998). Neuropsychological comparison of children with or without physical features of fetal alcohol syndrome. *Neuropsychology,* 12, 146-153.

Mattson, S.N.; Riley, E.P.; Jernigan, T.L.; Ehlers, C.L.; Delis, D.C.; Jones, K.L.; Stern, C.; Johnson, K.A.; Hesselink, J.R.; and Bellugi, U. (1992). Fetal alcohol syndrome: A case report of neuropsychological, MRI, and EEG assessment of two children. *Alcoholism: Clinical and Experimental Research,* 16, 1001-1003.

Mattson, S.N.; Riley, E.P.; Jernigan, T.L.; Garcia, A.; Kaneko, W.M.; Ehlers, C.L.; and Jones, K.L. (1994). A decrease in the size of the basal ganglia following prenatal alcohol exposure: A preliminary report. *Neurotoxicology and Teratology,* 16, 283-289.

Mattson, S.N.; Riley, E.P.; Sowell, E.R.; Jernigan, T.L.; Sobel, D.F.; and Jones, K.L. (1996). A decrease in the size of the basal ganglia in children with fetal alcohol syndrome. *Alcoholism: Clinical and Experimental Research,* 20, 1088-1093.

Mattson, S.N. and Roebuck, T.M. (2002). Acquisition and retention of verbal and nonverbal information in children with heavy prenatal alcohol exposure. *Alcoholism: Clinical and Experimental Research,* 26, 875-882.

May, P.A. and Gossage, J.P. (2001). Estimating the prevalence of fetal alcohol syndrome: A summary. *Alcohol Research & Health,* 25, 159-167.

Middleton, F.A. and Strick, P.L. (1994). Anatomical evidence for cerebellar and basal ganglia involvement in higher cognitive function. *Science,* 266, 458-461.

Middleton, F.A. and Strick, P.L. (2000). Basal ganglia and cerebellar loops: Motor and cognitive circuits. *Brain Research Reviews,* 31, 236-250.

Miller, M.W. (1988). Effect of prenatal exposure to ethanol on the development of cerebral cortex: I. Neuronal generation. *Alcoholism: Clinical and Experimental Research,* 12, 440-449.

Mostofsky, S.H.; Reiss, A.L.; Lockhart, P.; and Denckla, M.B. (1998). Evaluation of cerebellar size in attention-deficit hyperactivity disorder. *Journal of Child Neurology,* 13, 434-439.

Nanson, J.L. and Hiscock, M. (1990). Attention deficits in children exposed to alcohol prenatally. *Alcoholism: Clinical and Experimental Research,* 14, 656-661.

National Institute on Alcohol Abuse and Alcoholism (2005). *Graphics gallery, 2005.* Available at: http://www.niaaa.nih.gov.

Olson, H.C.; Feldman, J.J.; Streissguth, A.P.; Sampson, P.D.; and Bookstein, F.L. (1998). Neuropsychological deficits in adolescents with fetal alcohol syndrome: Clinical findings. *Alcoholism: Clinical and Experimental Research,* 22, 1998-2012.

Pearson, D.A.; Lachar, D.; Loveland, K.A.; Santos, C.W.; Faria, L.P.; Azzam, P.N.; Hentges, B.A.; and Cleveland, L.A. (2000). Patterns of behavior adjustment and maladjustment in mental retardation: Comparison of children with and without ADHD. *American Journal on Mental Retardation,* 105, 236-251.

Peiffer, J.; Majewski, F.; Fischbach, H.; Bierich, J.R.; and Volk, B. (1979). Alcohol embryo- and fetopathy. *Journal of the Neurological Sciences,* 41, 125-137.

Pennington, B.F. and Ozonoff, S. (1996). Executive functions and developmental psychopathology. *Journal of Child Psychology and Psychiatry,* 37, 51-87.

Pierce, D.R.; Goodlett, C.R.; and West, J.R. (1989). Differential neuronal loss following early postnatal alcohol exposure. *Teratology,* 40, 113-126.

Pulsifer, M.B. (1996). The neuropsychology of mental retardation. *Journal of the International Neuropsychological Society,* 2, 159-176.

Rao, S.M.; Bobholz, J.A.; Hammeke, T.A.; Rosen, A.C.; Woodley, S.J.; Cunningham, J. M.; Cox, R.W.; Stein, E.A.; and Binder, J.R. (1997). Functional MRI evidence for subcortical participation in conceptual reasoning skills. *Neuroreport,* 8, 1987-1993.

Riikonen, R.; Salonen, I.; Partanen, K.; and Verho, S. (1999). Brain perfusion SPECT and MRI in foetal alcohol syndrome. *Developmental Medicine and Child Neurology,* 41, 652-659.

Riley, E.P. (2001). Fetal alcohol syndrome and fetal alcohol effects. In: D. Gruol and Y. Israel (Eds.), *The Research Society on Alcoholism Lecture Series* [CD-ROM]. Austin, TX: Research Society on Alcoholism.

Riley, E.P.; Mattson, S.N.; Sowell, E.R.; Jernigan, T.L.; Sobel, D.F.; and Jones, K.L. (1995). Abnormalities of the corpus callosum in children prenatally exposed to alcohol. *Alcoholism: Clinical and Experimental Research,* 19, 1198-1202.

Robin, N.H. and Zachai, E.H. (1994). Unusual craniofacial dysmorphia due to prenatal alcohol and cocaine exposure. *Teratology,* 50, 160-164.

Roebuck, T.M.; Mattson, S.N.; and Riley, E.P. (1998). A review of the neuroanatomical findings in children with fetal alcohol syndrome or prenatal exposure to alcohol. *Alcoholism: Clinical and Experimental Research,* 22, 339-344.

Roebuck, T.M.; Mattson, S.N.; and Riley, E.P. (1999). Behavioral and psychosocial profiles of alcohol-exposed children. *Alcoholism: Clinical and Experimental Research,* 23, 1070-1076.

Roebuck-Spencer, T.M. and Mattson, S.N. (2004). Implicit strategy affects learning in children with heavy prenatal alcohol exposure. *Alcoholism: Clinical and Experimental Research,* 28, 1424-1431.

Ronen, G.M. and Andrews, W.L. (1991). Holoprosencephaly as a possible embryonic alcohol effect. *American Journal of Medical Genetics,* 40, 151-154.

Sampson, P.D.; Streissguth, A.P.; Bookstein, F.L.; Little, R.E.; Clarren, S.K.; Dehaene, P.; Hanson, J.W.; and Graham, J.M., Jr. (1997). Incidence of fetal alcohol syndrome and prevalence of alcohol-related neurodevelopmental disorder. *Teratology*, 56, 317-326.

Samson, H.H. (1986). Microcephaly and fetal alcohol syndrome: Human and animal studies. In: J.R. West (Ed.), *Alcohol and Brain Development* (pp. 167-183). New York: Oxford University Press.

Schaefer, G.B.; Bodensteiner, J.B.; Thompson, J.N.; and Wilson, D.A. (1991). Clinical and morphometric analysis of the hypoplastic corpus callosum. *Archives of Neurology*, 48, 933-936.

Schmahmann, J.D. (1997). *International Review of Neurobiology*, Vol. 4: *The Cerebellum and Cognition*. San Diego, CA: Academic Press.

Schmahmann, J.D. and Pandya, D.N. (1997). The cerebrocerebellar system. In: J.D. Schmahmann (Ed.), *International Review of Neurobiology*, Vol. 4: *The Cerebellum and Cognition* (pp. 31-60). San Diego, CA: Academic Press.

Schonfeld, A.M.; Mattson, S.N.; Lang, A.R.; Delis, D.C.; and Riley, E.P. (2001). Verbal and nonverbal fluency in children with heavy prenatal alcohol exposure. *Journal of Studies on Alcohol,* 62, 239-246.

Shaywitz, S.E.; Caparulo, B.K.; and Hodgson, E.S. (1981). Developmental language disability as a consequence of prenatal exposure to ethanol. *Pediatrics,* 68, 850-855.

Siebert, J.R.; Astley, S.J.; and Clarren, S.K. (1991). Holoprosencephaly in a fetal macaque *(Macaca nemestrina)* following weekly exposure to ethanol. *Teratology,* 44, 29-36.

Smith, M.L. and Milner, B. (1981). The role of the right hippocampus in the recall of spatial location. *Neuropsychologia,* 27, 781-793.

Sowell, E.R.; Jernigan, T.L.; Mattson, S.N.; Riley, E.P.; Sobel, D.F.; and Jones, K.L. (1996). Abnormal development of the cerebellar vermis in children prenatally exposed to alcohol: Size reduction in lobules I-V. *Alcoholism: Clinical and Experimental Research,* 20, 31-34.

Sowell, E.R.; Thompson, P.M.; Mattson, S.N.; Tessner, K.D.; Jernigan, T.L.; Riley, E.P.; and Toga, A.W. (2001). Voxel-based morphometric analyses of the brain in children and adolescents prenatally exposed to alcohol. *Neuroreport,* 12, 515-523.

Sowell, E.R.; Thompson, P.M.; Mattson, S.N.; Tessner, K.D.; Jernigan, T.L.; Riley, E.P.; and Toga, A.W. (2002). Regional brain shape abnormalities persist into adolescence after heavy prenatal alcohol exposure. *Cerebral Cortex,* 12, 856-865.

Sowell, E.R.; Thompson, P.M.; Peterson, B.S.; Mattson, S.N.; Welcome, S.E.; Henkenius, A.L.; Riley, E.P.; Jernigan, T.L.; and Toga, A.W. (2002). Mapping cortical gray matter asymmetry patterns in adolescents with heavy prenatal alcohol exposure. *NeuroImage,* 17, 1807-1819.

Sowell, E.R.; Thompson, P.M.; Rex, D.; Kornsand, D.; Tessner, K.D.; Jernigan, T.L.; and Toga, A.W. (2002). Mapping sulcal pattern asymmetry and local cortical surface gray matter distribution in vivo: Maturation in perisylvian cortices. *Cerebral Cortex,* 12, 17-26.

Steinhausen, H.C. and Spohr, H.L. (1998). Long-term outcome of children with fetal alcohol syndrome: Psychopathology, behavior, and intelligence. *Alcoholism: Clinical and Experimental Research,* 22, 334-338.

Steinhausen, H.C.; Wilms, J.; Metzke, C.W.; and Spohr, H.L. (2003). Behavioural phenotype in foetal alcohol syndrome and foetal alcohol effects. *Developmental Medicine & Child Neurology,* 45, 179-182,

Steinhausen, H.C.; Willms, J.; and Spohr, H.L. (1993). Long-term psychopathological and cognitive outcome of children with fetal alcohol syndrome. *Journal of the American Academy of Child and Adolescent Psychiatry,* 32, 990-994.

Steinhausen, H.C.; Willms, J.; and Spohr, H.L. (1994). Correlates of psychopathology and intelligence in children with fetal alcohol syndrome. *Journal of Child Psychology and Psychiatry,* 35, 323-331.

Steinmetz, H.; Herzog, A.; Schlaug, G.; Huang, Y.; and Jancke, L. (1995). Brain (A) symmetry in monozygotic twins. *Cerebral Cortex,* 5, 296-300.

Steinmetz, H.; Volkmann, J.; Jancke, L.; and Freund, H.J. (1991). Anatomical left-right asymmetry of language-related temporal cortex is different in left- and right-handers. *Annals of Neurology,* 29, 315-319.

Streissguth, A. (1997). *Fetal Alcohol Syndrome: A Guide for Families and Communities.* Baltimore, MD: Paul H. Brooks Publishing.

Streissguth, A.; Barr, H.; Kogan, J.; and Bookstein, F. (1997). Primary and secondary disabilities in fetal alcohol syndrome. In: A. Streissguth and J. Kanter (Eds.), *The Challenge of Fetal Alcohol Syndrome: Overcoming Secondary Disabilities* (pp. 25-39). Seattle, WA: University of Washington Press.

Streissguth, A.P.; Randels, S.P.; and Smith, D.F. (1991). A test-retest study of intelligence in patients with fetal alcohol syndrome: Implications for care. *Journal of the American Academy of Child and Adolescent Psychiatry,* 30, 584-587.

Sulik, K.K. and Johnston, M.C. (1982). Embryonic origin of holoprosencephaly: Interrelationship of the developing brain and face. *Scanning Electron Microscopy,* 1, 309-322.

Swayze, V.W., II.; Johnson, V.P.; Hanson, J.W.; Piven, J.; Sato, Y.; Giedd, J.N.; Mosnik, D.; and Andreasen, N.C. (1997). Magnetic resonance imaging of brain anomalies in fetal alcohol syndrome. *Pediatrics,* 99, 232-240.

Thomas, S.E.; Kelly, S.J.; Mattson, S.N.; and Riley, E.P. (1998). Comparison of social abilities of children with fetal alcohol syndrome to those of children with similar IQ scores and normal controls. *Alcoholism: Clinical and Experimental Research,* 22, 528-533.

Townsend, J.; Courchesne, E.; Covington, J.; Westerfield, M.; Harris, N.S.; Lyden, P.; Lowry, T.P.; and Press, G.A. (1999). Spatial attention deficits in patients with acquired or developmental cerebellar abnormality. *The Journal of Neuroscience,* 19, 5632-5643.

Uecker, A. and Nadel, L. (1996). Spatial locations gone awry: Object and spatial memory deficits in children with fetal alcohol syndrome. *Neuropsychologia,* 34, 209-223.

Uecker, A. and Nadel, L. (1998). Spatial but not object memory impairments in children with fetal alcohol syndrome. *American Journal on Mental Retardation,* 103, 12-18.

Wang, P.P.; Doherty, S.; Hesselink, J.R.; and Bellugi, U. (1992). Callosal morphology concurs with neurobehavioral and neuropathological findings in two neurodevelopmental disorders. *Archives of Neurology,* 49, 407-411.

Warren, K.R. and Foudin, L.L. (2001). Alcohol-related birth defects: The past, present, and future. *Alcohol Research & Health,* 25, 153-158.

Watkins, L.H.A.; Rogers, R.D.; Lawrence, A.D.; Sahakian, B.J.; Rosser, A.E.; and Robbins, T.W. (2000). Impaired planning but intact decision making in early Huntington's disease: Implications for specific fronto-striatal pathology. *Neuropsychologia,* 38, 1112-1125.

Wechsler, D. (1991). *WISC-III Manual: Wechsler Intelligence Scale for Children* (3rd ed.). New York: The Psychological Corporation.

Welsh, M.C. and Pennington, B.F. (1988). Assessing frontal lobe functioning in children: Views from developmental psychology. *Developmental Neuropsychology,* 4, 199-230.

Whaley, S.E.; O'Connor, M.J.; and Gunderson, B. (2001). Comparison of the adaptive functioning of children exposed to alcohol to a nonexposed clinical sample. *Alcoholism: Clinical and Experimental Research,* 25, 1018-1024.

Wisniewski, K.; Dambska, M.; Sher, J.H.; and Qazi, Q. (1983). A clinical neuropathological study of the fetal alcohol syndrome. *Neuropediatrics,* 14, 197-201.

Woodruff-Pak, D.S. (1997). Classical conditioning. In: J.D. Schmahmann (Ed.), *International Review of Neurobiology,* Vol. 4: *The Cerebellum and Cognition* (pp. 342-366). San Diego, CA: Academic Press.

Chapter 7

The Medical and Developmental Consequences of Prenatal Drug Exposure

Karen K. Howell
Claire D. Coles
Julie A. Kable

INTRODUCTION AND OVERVIEW

This chapter addresses the medical and developmental consequences of prenatal exposure to commonly used drugs during pregnancy, such as nicotine, cocaine, and marijuana. The impact of opiate use during pregnancy is also discussed. Both the direct impact of the teratogenic agent as well as the social and environmental factors which influence the expression of these agents are presented. When available, the effects of these substances on the growth, cognition, behavior, and social-emotional development of the prenatally exposed child are addressed.

PRINCIPLES OF TERATOLOGY AND BEHAVIORAL TERATOLOGY

The concepts of teratogen exposure and the factors that influence the expression of the teratogen on offspring are important variables in any discussion of the medical and developmental consequences of prenatal drug exposure. A teratogen is defined as a substance that causes fetal malformations. The teratogenic theory on the effects of prenatal exposure to drugs explains the negative consequences of prenatal exposure in terms of direct damage to the fetus caused by exposure during gestation (Coles, 1995). The

Handbook of the Medical Consequences of Alcohol and Drug Abuse
© 2008 by The Haworth Press, Taylor & Francis Group. All rights reserved.
doi:10.1300/6039_07

general principles and mechanisms of teratogenic response were outlined by Wilson (1977), who described six generalizations. These generalizations or principles outline important concepts regarding prenatal exposure to potential teratogens, such as the interaction between the genotype of the fetus and environmental factors; the issue of critical periods for exposure and its expression; the specificity of teratogenic agents; the final manifestations of teratogenic response; the access and nature of the teratogenic agent; and the dose-response relationship of teratogenic agents (Wilson, 1977). More recently, a parallel set of generalizations has been posited for behavioral teratogenic responses, or the postnatal effects on behavior of prenatal exposure to teratogenic agents such as drugs (Vorhees, 1986). Finally, recent advances in research on prenatal and postnatal drug exposure has focused on how contextual factors, such as parental psychopathology, may act as mediating and moderating variables to influence and interact with the impact of parental substance abuse on developmental outcome (Jacobson and Jacobson, 2001).

MATERNAL SUBSTANCE USE AND DEVELOPMENTAL IMPACT: TOBACCO

Epidemiology of Tobacco Use in Pregnancy

According to the latest estimates, approximately 21 percent of women of childbearing age are smokers (Cnattingus, 2004). Although increasing pressure is being placed on those who smoke to cease during pregnancy, the majority of expecting mothers fail to do so. The Centers for Disease Control (CDC) reports that 20 to 25 percent of expectant mothers continue tobacco use during gestation (Ebrahim et al., 2000). In the National Health Interview Survey, only 27 percent of women were able to immediately quit use when told that they were pregnant and an additional 12 percent were able to quit by the third trimester of pregnancy (Fingerhut, Kleinman, and Kendrick, 1990). Ershoff, Ashford, and Goldenberg (2004) reported that it was rare for cessation programs for women smokers who are pregnant to achieve quit rates above 20 percent.

Growth Effects

Tobacco use by pregnant women raises concerns about potential teratogenic effects. Nicotine and its by-product, cotinine, are found in fetal serum and amniotic fluid at 15 percent higher concentrations than in maternal blood and last for 15 to 20 hours (Slotkin, 1998). Large amounts of nicotine and cotinine can be ingested by nursing infants of women who smoke (Polifka, 1998). It has been well documented for many years that tobacco exposure affects fetal growth even after controlling for pertinent demographic and confounding variables (Abel, 1984; Werler, Pober, and Holmes, 1985). The earliest reported study on human infants who were prenatally exposed to tobacco smoke was done by Simpson (1957). She found that the incidence of low birth weight (<2,599 g) among infants whose mothers smoked was twice as high as the incidence rate among mothers who did not smoke. The incidence of low birth weight in this study was dose-related to the quantity of cigarettes smoked per day. Subsequent numerous studies have investigated the relationship between cigarette smoking and birth weight. In reviews of the effects of maternal smoking during pregnancy, authors all agree that there is overwhelming evidence to support the original finding that low birth weight is associated with maternal cigarette smoking (Abel, 1984; Landesman-Dwyer and Emanuel, 1979; Werler, Pober, and Holmes, 1985; Witter and King, 1980). In addition, this dose-response relationship is found when controlling for factors such as age, parity, maternal weight gain, pre-pregnancy weight/height ratio, gestational age, socioeconomic status, and race (Abel, 1984; Werler, Pober, and Holmes, 1985). The risk of having a small-for-gestational age (SGA) infant is two to four times higher for smokers, with smokers' neonates weighing an average of 200 to 300 g less than nonsmokers' infants (Kearney, 1999). This effect was not found, however, among smokers who quit during their pregnancy. Hebel, Fox, and Sexton (1988) report no effect on birth weight among women who quit before week 30 of gestation. Rantakallio (1978) also reported no differences in birth weight between infants whose mothers quit smoking by the third trimester and infants whose mothers did not smoke during pregnancy.

Although newborns have a weight deficit, the most recent evidence suggests that older children who were exposed prenatally to tobacco smoke may have a reversal of this trend as they age. Kries et al. (2002) report a 1.43 greater incidence of being overweight and a 2.06 increase in meeting criteria for obesity among five-to-six-year-old offspring of women who smoke. In another study, six-year-olds whose mothers smoked during pregnancy had increased skinfold thickness (Cornelius et al., 2002) in comparison to controls after controlling for a host of potential confounds.

Additional physical and medical outcomes that have been linked to tobacco smoke exposure after controlling for pertinent demographic and confounding variables include decreased gestational length (Landesman-Dwyer and Emanuel, 1979), increased risk of spontaneous abortion (Himmelberger, Brown, and Cohen, 1978; Kline et al., 1983), increased risk for cleft palate

(Little, Cardy, and Munger, 2004), and of sudden infant death syndrome (Haglund and Cnattingus, 1990).

Respiration Effects

Among the respiratory effects of maternal smoking, increased incidence rates of bronchitis and pneumonia have been found (Colley, Holland, and Corkhill, 1974; Harlap and Davies, 1974). Increased incidences of asthma (e.g., Jaakkola and Gissler, 2004; Kershaw, 1987) and increased severity of asthmatic symptoms (Evans et al., 1987) have also been associated with maternal smoking. Sawnani et al. (2004) found that infants whose mothers smoked during pregnancy were more at risk for obstructive apnea while sleeping.

Cognitive and Learning Effects

Evidence for a general cognitive deficit during infancy and early childhood is mixed. General cognitive deficits have been found on some studies (e.g., Fried and Watkinson, 1990; Mortensen et al., 2005; Sexton, Fox, and Hebel, 1990) but not on others (e.g., Makin, Fried, and Watkinson, 1991; Streissguth et al., 1989). Deficits in learning and achievement have also been posited as being associated with maternal smoking. Data from the National Collaborative Perinatal Project (NCPP) has shown that children of smokers have deficiencies in achievement, particularly in the areas of reading and spelling (Hardy and Mellits, 1972; Naeye and Peters, 1984). Reduced scores on tests of spelling and arithmetic were found in a large cohort from Netherlands (Batstra, Hadders-Algra, and Neeleman, 2003). No difference in achievement has been found in other studies comparing children of smokers and nonsmokers (Fergusson and Lloyd, 1991; Makin, Fried, and Watkinson, 1991).

Language Effects

Investigations into verbal ability have yielded mixed results as well. Fried and Watkinson (1990) found a difference between the receptive verbal abilities of children of smokers and nonsmokers, although not the expressive abilities of these two groups. This finding was later replicated, with a significant difference between the receptive language skills of children who were prenatally exposed to nicotine and the children of nonsmokers (Makin, Fried, and Watkinson, 1991). Although these deficits in verbal processing have been found, these skills are known to be highly correlated with general cognitive ability. As such, it is difficult to determine the relative contribution of a general cognitive deficit from a specific deficit in verbal processing.

Auditory Processing Effects

Although there are few studies in this area, the evidence for a negative impact on the early auditory development of the children of women who smoked during pregnancy has been more consistent than that for most other neurodevelopmental outcomes (Fried, 1998). Poorer auditory habituation on standardized infant assessment has been found repeatedly (Fried and Makin, 1987; Jacobson et al., 1985; Picone et al., 1982; Saxton, 1978). In polygraphic studies of sleep, Franco et al. (1999) reported that infants of smokers, both newborns and 12-week-olds, showed decreased arousal to auditory stimuli compared to infants of nonsmokers. The evidence in older infants and children is more limited but consistent (e.g., Fried and Watkinson, 1988; Kristjansson, Fried, and Watkinson, 1989). These findings suggest that there may be an underlying auditory processing deficit associated with prenatal exposure to tobacco smoke that manifests in delays in early language development and specific aspects of reading development.

Behavioral Regulation Difficulties

The role which early tobacco exposure plays in producing behavioral regulation difficulties has been explored by a number of researchers. Results of these studies suggest that children who were exposed to tobacco during early development may have subtle deficits in their ability to control and regulate their behavior to meet environmental demands. Naeye and Peters (1984) examined behavioral ratings of children of mothers who smoked during their pregnancy, and found that these children were rated as having lower attention spans and greater motor activity. Streissguth et al. (1984) found that maternal cigarette use was significantly related to poorer attention and orientation to a vigilance task in children. Kristjansson, Fried, and Watkinson (1989) also found deficits in auditory and visual vigilance and greater levels of motor activity among children of smokers.

More recently, a growing number of studies have reported associations between maternal smoking during pregnancy and externalizing behavioral problems during childhood and adolescence (Fergusson, Horwood, and Lynskey, 1993; Fergusson, Woodward, and Horwood, 1998; Linnet et al., 2003; Wakschlag et al., 1997; Weitzman, Gortmaker, and Sobol, 1992). Several studies using diverse samples throughout the world have related maternal smoking to an increased prevalence of ADHD symptoms (Batstra,

Hadders-Algra, and Neeleman, 2003; Kotimaa et al., 2003; Mick et al., 2002; Rodriguez and Bohlin, 2005; Thapar et al., 2003), oppositional or conduct problems (Day et al., 2000; Silberg et al., 2003; Wakschlag and Hans, 2002), and an increased use of substances in adolescence (Porath and Fried, 2005). It remains to be seen whether this possible causal relationship may be the result of uncontrolled confounding variables, including characteristics of the mother that influence the child's environment, differences in parenting practices, and/or inherited characteristics.

Social and Environmental Considerations

There is some evidence that the relationship between early tobacco smoke exposure and behavioral outcomes may be the consequence of a different psychosocial environment created by a parent who chooses to smoke. Differences have been found in the manner in which parents who are smokers relate to their children when compared to parents who are nonsmokers. Fried and Watkinson (1988) found that nicotine use was negatively related to maternal involvement with the child, opportunities for variety in daily routines, emotional/verbal responsivity to the mother, avoidance of restriction and punishment, organization of the physical and temporal environment, and provision of appropriate play materials. Furthermore, researchers have hypothesized that there may be important personality characteristics, behaviors, and lifestyle variables that differentiate smokers and nonsmokers. Smokers have been found to differ from nonsmokers on measures of anxiety, extroversion, nurturance, and deference. They report more symptoms of psychopathology, have more hospitalizations, lower status occupations, and more job changes than nonsmokers (Eysenck, 1980; Eysenck, 1991; Eysenck et al., 1960; Krogh, 1991; Lilienfeld, 1959; Matarazzo and Saslow, 1960; Maughan et al., 2004; McManus and Weeks, 1982; Reiter, 1970; Schneider and Houston, 1970). It remains to be seen whether any of these characteristics that exist between smokers and nonsmokers may be capable of mediating the relationship found between tobacco smoke exposure and teratogenic outcome variables.

Summary

Maternal smoking during pregnancy has not been consistently associated with major structural anomalies but has been linked to several physical outcomes, including disruption of growth, alterations in fetal cardiorespiratory status, sudden infant death syndrome (Behnke and Eyler, 1993), and poor outcomes on measures of neurodevelopmental functioning. Although the evidence is mixed on outcomes related to general intellectual functioning and academic achievement, consistent deficits have been found in auditory processing and poorer behavioral regulation skills among children prenatally exposed to tobacco smoke.

ILLICIT DRUG USE: COCAINE

Epidemiology of Cocaine Use in Pregnancy

Although the epidemic of cocaine and crack use that began in the 1980s has waned to some extent, the problem of prenatal exposure to cocaine persists. According to the National Institute on Drug Abuse (NIDA, 1996), approximately 2.3 percent of women of childbearing age have used cocaine in the past year and many of these women continue to use cocaine when pregnant. This figure may be higher in certain population subgroups and lower in others. In 1994, when blood drawn from a cohort of neonates was analyzed, about 0.1 percent of all births were reported to have been exposed to cocaine (Brantley et al., 1996), with a higher incidence among older women, those delivering without prenatal care, and inner-city populations. Most women reporting cocaine use also used tobacco, and alcohol, and some combined the use of cocaine or crack with heroin (Day, Cottreau, and Richardson, 1993).

Owing to concerns raised during the "crack baby" period (Coles, 1993), extensive examination of the teratogenic potential of this drug in both animal models and clinical studies was carried out. Although in 1993, one could conclude that inadequate data existed to support conclusions about the effects of this drug (e.g., Coles and Platzman, 1993), during the latter half of the 1990s many studies were published that provide considerable insight into this area, at least during infancy and the preschool period (see Eyler and Behnke, 1999; Frank et al., 2001; Tronick and Beeghly, 1999, for reviews).

Growth and Other Health Effects

Cocaine exposure has been associated with lower gestational age and reduced growth parameters at birth in a number of studies (Chouteau, Namerow, and Leppert, 1988; Kliegman et al., 1994). As cocaine users have many other characteristics that may be associated with such outcomes, interpretation of these effects can be difficult (Holtzman and Paneth, 1994). However, Kliegman et al. (1994) found that cocaine exposure was associated with preterm birth as well as lower birth weight even when associated factors were controlled for statistically. Richardson et al. (1999) controlled for the effects of prenatal care by comparing the effects of cocaine use for both those who had prenatal care and those who did not. They found that cocaine had a significant impact on both gestational age and birth weight in each group even when the effects of alcohol, marijuana, and tobacco were controlled. Even when growth effects are observed, interpreting the relationship may not be straightforward. While examining the relationship between gestational age and cocaine exposure in neonates, Brown et al. (1998) found that lower birth weight was characteristic only of full-term cocaine-exposed infants, suggesting that such effects occurred in the third trimester. In contrast, Richardson et al. (1999) found that growth effects in their sample were attributable to exposure during the first and second trimesters. Finally, even when statistically significant effects are found during the neonatal period, cocaine-exposed children do not have "clinically significant" growth failure and often appear to have a postnatal "catch-up" in growth. For instance, while comparing preterm and full-term cocaine-exposed infants to socioeconomic status (SES)–matched contrast groups, Coles et al. (2000) found that growth differences could no longer be observed by eight weeks of age and there were no differences in growth rate over 24 months for weight, length, or ponderal index. In the same sample, at eight years postpartum, there were no effects of prenatal exposure on growth, including height, weight, and head circumference (Coles et al., 2004).

Motor Development

Early studies of cocaine effects identified reflexive behavior and motor development as areas of concern. Schneider and Chasnoff (1992) compared 30 full-term four-month-old infants exposed to cocaine (and other drugs) to 50 unexposed infants using the Movement Assessment of Infants (MAI). Exposed infants were found to have higher risk scores on motor tone, primitive reflexes, and volitional movements. Swanson et al. (1999) found poorer mean scores on the volitional movements subscale of the MAI as well as the total risk score among four-month-old exposed infants compared to controls. Fetters and Tronick (1996) followed 28 cocaine-exposed and 22 control infants for 15 months and found a negative drug effect on motor performance at this age. The authors note, however, that both cocaine-exposed and contrast groups of children performed more poorly than would be expected from the age norms. In contrast, in a study published in 2004, the same research group (Tronick et al., 2004) reported that experimental studies of kinematic reaching parameters in infants at 7 and 15 months revealed no decrements in performance associated with either drug exposure or with

SES. This study had been undertaken with the assumption that lack of significant differences in motor development reported by other studies might be attributable to lack of precision in methodology. However, this experimental procedure did not reveal any deficiencies in motor development associated with drug exposure.

Arendt et al. (1999) used the Psychomotor Index of the Bayley Scales of Infant Development (BSID) (Bayley, 1993) and the MAI as well as other measures of sensorimotor development in a sample of inner-city children exposed to cocaine. They found small but significant effects of cocaine and other drug exposure on a variety of motor indicators both early in infancy and at 12 months. At 24 months, children from this sample were reassessed using the Peabody Developmental Motor Scales with the cocaine-exposed group performing significantly lower on both fine and gross motor development indices. The effects appeared to be more significant in the fine motor rather than the gross motor area. However, in a subsequent study, the same research group reported that, while cocaine-related decrements were observed in cognitive development, no problems were noted in psychomotor development until 24 months, when a small but significant correlation was noted (Singer et al., 2002).

Later in infancy (e.g., Chasnoff et al., 1992; Jacobson et al., 1996), motor differences are not described by most investigators. This discrepancy may be the result of differences in the measurement tools used. Those studies reporting effects often used the MAI, while those that did not used the BSID. As more longitudinal data is published, it will be possible to evaluate the implications of observed differences in motor function for later development.

Behavioral Effects

Initially, severe consequences were anticipated in this area of development (Coles, 1993), although the evidence to support such effects was not strong. Studies of newborns provided conflicting information about the immediate impact of maternal cocaine use during gestation. In a meta analysis, Held, Riggs, and Dorman (1999) critically reviewed Brazelton Neurobehavioral Assessment Scale (BNBAS) studies of infants (Brazelton, 1984; Brazelton and Nugent, 1995). It was concluded that while effects could be found reliably on motor performance, abnormal reflexes, orientation, and autonomic regulation, the effect size was small and tended to diminish over the first month of life. As well-controlled studies of later development are reported, evidence of direct teratogenic effects on cognition have been limited (Hurt et al., 1997; Tronick and Beeghly, 1999), although children born to drug-using mothers in low SES populations continue to be at risk for nonoptimal development in many domains (e.g., Brown et al., 2004; Frank et al., 2002). For instance, in a follow-up study that examined outcomes at four to six years, Chasnoff et al. (1998) reported that differences in developmental functioning in their clinical samples can be accounted for by environmental factors, principally, caregiver behavior. Singer et al. (1997) reported that prenatal cocaine and alcohol exposure as well as maternal postpartum psychological distress directly impacted the BSID Mental Development Index (MDI) while Psychomotor Index (PI) scores were affected only by cocaine. Kilbride et al. (2000) reported that at 36 months, no effects on cognition, psychomotor skills, or language were observed in exposed children who had received case management services, compared with those who did not receive services, and a nonexposed contrast group. Kilbride et al. (2000) also found that exposed children who remained with their mothers and did not receive services had lower verbal scores on intelligence tests and measures of language development. Similarly, in a follow-up study examining outcomes at four to six years, Chasnoff et al. (1998) reported that differences in developmental functioning in their clinical samples could be accounted for by environmental factors, principally, caregiver behavior. In contrast, Mayes et al. (2003) reported that cocaine exposed children showed "delayed developmental indices" (p. 323) relative to controls than children exposed to other drugs but that their developmental trajectories from 3 to 36 months are parallel to those of other groups. Examination of mean scores suggests that none of the groups tested can be defined as "delayed" although by 36 months all groups are scoring about one standard deviation below the mean on the MDI of the Bayley Scales, a phenomenon commonly associated with environmental deprivation. The cocaine group's scores are 2 points lower than those of the unexposed controls. Similarly, Richardson (1998) found that in three-year-olds, cocaine exposure was associated with lower scores on some of the subtests of the Stanford-Binet Intelligence Scales, Fourth Edition), including composite IQ scores and short term memory scores, although all children scored within the typical range of development. A previous study of a different cohort of children by the same author (Richardson, Conroy, and Day, 1996) did not show effects on cognition, demonstrating the extent to which these outcomes are dependent on sampling and other methodological considerations.

Language Development

A number of studies have identified deficiencies in the early language development of children born to cocaine-using women. Bland-Stewart et al. (1998) compared semantic content category in a small sample of low-SES infants exposed to cocaine with a contrast group matched for social class and ethnicity and found some restriction in the development of semantic representations (meaning) in the children of cocaine users. No effect was observed in the structural features of language, that is, mean length of utterance (MLU) and utterance type, or for general language and cognitive functioning. Bandstra et al. (2004) and Morrow et al. (2003) report subtle effects on language development in children during the first seven years when controlling for growth and environmental lead exposure. The effects were stronger in males than for females. In contrast, Hurt et al. (1997) found no differences in language functioning at two-and-a-half years when cocaine-exposed and contrast children from the same SES group were compared using the Preschool Language Scale (PLS), a standardized measure of early language development. In reviewing the literature in this area, Mentis (1998) suggested that there is insufficient evidence for definitive statements about the language development of this group of children. Although language development may be disrupted, the factors affecting such development are numerous and their interaction is complex. She also suggested that deficits may be specific to certain areas of language function and are only evident under stressful conditions.

Play Behavior

Play behavior is often assessed as an indicator of children's functional status that does not require standardized testing. Play behavior has been examined in a number of studies of cocaine- and polydrug-exposed children that followed an initial study by Rodning, Beckwith, and Howard (1989) which reported alterations in the usual play patterns. Subsequent studies have been inconsistent in reported outcomes. Metosky and Vondra (1995) reported differences in play analogous to Rodning, Beckwith, and Howard (1989), while several other investigators have not found evidence of differences in the play of toddlers that can be attributed to the direct effects of cocaine (e.g., Beeghly et al., 1995; Hagan and Myers, 1997; Hurt et al., 1996) when associated factors are controlled. These outcomes suggest that such behavioral observations may be accounted for by environmental factors or group differences.

Behavior Problems

An increased incidence of behavior problems has been reported in children of drug-using mothers and it is not surprising that it should also be the case for children with prenatal cocaine exposure (e.g., Delaney-Black et al.,

1998). Bendersky, Bennet, and Lewis (2006) found that cocaine was associated with more aggressive behavior in five-year-old boys from high-risk environments and Coles et al. (2004) reported that eight-year-olds with cocaine and other drug exposure had significantly higher scores on many of the indices on the Child Behavior Checklist (CBCL) (Achenbach, 1991). However, as with other aspects of this literature, there is a good deal of inconsistency in reported outcomes. Accornero et al. (2002) examined child behavior at age five in the children in the Maternal Lifestyles study using the CBCL. Using structural equation modeling to evaluate both prenatal exposure and environmental factors on child behavior in the preschool period, these authors found that cocaine exposure was unrelated to outcome while maternal psychological functioning did account for child behavior. Overall, it seems likely that children of users of cocaine and other drugs will show more behavior problems but whether this is the result of prenatal exposure or related factors is not yet clear.

Arousal Regulation and Attention

The most persuasive evidence for a behavioral effect of cocaine concerns the impact on physiological arousal (e.g., heart rate, respiration) in early infancy and, by extension, on temperament and social/emotional development. Mayes (1999) provides an animal model of this phenomenon that suggests that dopamine regulation has been impacted, a view supported by a recent review of the literature in this area (Harvey, 2004). Several investigators have identified increased irritability (Brown et al., 1998; DiPietro et al., 1994; Bada et al., 2002) in young infants and alterations in psychophysiology, including heart rate and respiration (Mehta et al., 2002). As such effects appear to be the result of polydrug exposure and might be related to the acute effects of maternal use, it is important to examine whether these effects persist beyond the neonatal period. A few investigators have examined this question. At eight weeks, Bard et al. (2000) identified cocaine-related alterations in baseline heart rate and respiration as well as differences in response to moderate stress that appeared to be drug-related. Karmel and Gardner (1996) and Karmel, Gardner, and Freedland (1996) identified cocaine-related differences in attention and arousal modulation in newborns that persisted through four months of age. At four months, Bendersky and Lewis (1998) found that exposed infants were less able to modulate arousal. Other systems, such as sleep (Coles et al., 2000), appear to be impacted during the toddler period. Studies of older children are limited. Bendersky et al. (2003) report that cocaine exposed five-year-olds have more difficulty with inhibition of motor responses (an "executive function"). However, a significant difference from controls was observed only among boys living in "low risk" caregiving situations. Those in "high risk" situations did not differ nor did females in any groups. In a longitudinal study of eight-year-olds prenatally exposed to cocaine and other drugs, Coles et al. (2004) found that drug-exposed children responded to acute environmental and cognitive stressors with alterations in psychophysiology (e.g., HR, galvanic skin response) in a way that is more similar to that of children with behavior disorders than to normal controls.

That cognition may also be affected in some manner is suggested by reported effects on early attention. Mayes et al. (1995) reported that cocaine exposure affected three-month-old children's ability to complete a procedure measuring attention. Coles et al. (1999) found differences in attentional response associated with prenatal cocaine, but not other drug exposure at eight weeks. However, as these authors note, the caregiving instability associated with maternal drug use independently accounted for more variance in attentional response than did the direct effect of cocaine. In an older sample, Savage et al. (2005) report "subtle" effects on errors of commission and task efficiency on a vigilance task in prenatally exposed ten-year-olds who were otherwise not different from controls on a number of behavioral measures. These findings raise concerns about the vulnerability of exposed children. In addition to physiological dysregulation associated with prenatal exposure to cocaine and other drugs, exposed children are clearly also at environmental risk to an increased incidence of developmental psychopathology.

Medical, Social, and Environmental Considerations

Cocaine use in pregnancy is clearly a marker for a host of other factors that may affect subsequent child development, either directly or as part of a constellation of factors (see Figure 7.1). For that reason, most investigations have included medical, social, and caregiving factors as part of the research design. A review of the literature indicates that a number of these factors either account for the observed effects of cocaine or contribute to (moderate) these effects when children are made more vulnerable by drug exposure. A clear example is birth weight (see Behnke et al., 2006; Frank et al., 2002; Lester et al., 2002; Morrow et al., 2003), whether because of growth retardation or prematurity in the high risk samples that have been used to study the effects of this drug. Gender differences in development have been noted by Brown et al. (2004), Bendersky, Bennet, and Lewis (2006), Bendersky et al. (2003), and Delaney-Black et al. (2004), with males appearing to be more vulnerable than females to prenatal exposure and to

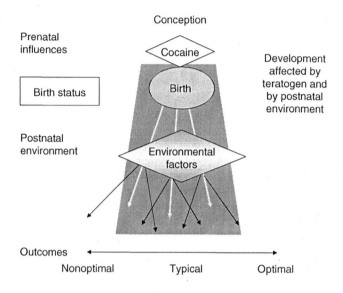

FIGURE 7.1. Developmental outcomes.

associated environmental effects. Environmental factors affecting health also interact with the effects of cocaine exposure. For instance, Nelson et al. (2004) report that iron deficiency, anemia, and lead exposure account for differences in cognition at two and four years in their cocaine-exposed sample. Maternal psychological state or psychopathology has been found to account for many of the behavioral and developmental effects observed in children of drug users (e.g., Accornero et al., 2002). Finally, caregiving status—that is, whether the child remains with their drug-using mother, their extended family, or goes into foster or adoptive care—can determine whether effects of cocaine are observed (see Brown et al., 2004; Frank et al., 2002).

Summary

Prenatal cocaine exposure is a marker for a number of risk factors that appear to have negative consequences for the infant and developing child. No specific "cocaine syndrome" has yet emerged and many of the problems previously anticipated have not manifested. However, the weight of the evidence suggests that cocaine exposure may produce an increased vulnerability to certain environmental stressors. The interactions of these factors may have long-term negative consequences for children.

MARIJUANA

Epidemiology of Marijuana Use in Pregnancy

In a recent NIDA survey (1996) of the prevalence and patterns of substance use among pregnant women, 2.8 percent reported marijuana use during their first trimester of pregnancy. This indicates that marijuana is the most commonly used illicit drug and, after alcohol and tobacco, the most commonly used drug during pregnancy (Goldschmidt, Day, and Richardson, 2000). As Fried observed (1996), this makes the paucity of objective information on the relationship between marijuana use during pregnancy and the impact of such use upon the development of the child all the more striking.

Growth Effects

Of the longitudinal studies of marijuana use during pregnancy, most find few significant effects on growth parameters. Cornelius et al. (2002) found that exposure to any prenatal marijuana in the second trimester was significantly associated with shorter stature in a sample of six-year olds. Day et al. (1991) obtained neonatal outcome data on more than 500 infants born prenatally exposed to varying amounts of marijuana in utero. There were few significant effects of marijuana use during pregnancy on birth weight, head or chest circumference, gestational age, or growth retardation. There was a small but significant negative effect of marijuana use during the first two months of pregnancy on birth length and a positive effect of marijuana use during the third trimester on birth weight. In a study of growth from birth to early adolescence in offspring prenatally exposed to marijuana, this exposure was not significantly related to any growth measure (Fried, Watkinson, and Gray, 1999), nor was there any impact on growth or timing of pubertal milestones in the same children when they were assessed in later adolescence (Fried, James, and Watkinson, 2001).

Cognitive Effects

Most research results regarding the impact of in utero marijuana exposure report no significant impact on composite measures representing general or overall intelligence (Fried, 2002). However, particular aspects of cognition at different ages have been negatively associated with prenatal marijuana exposure. Although some observations of a neurobehavioral effect of prenatal marijuana exposure on verbal ability of four-year-old subjects was noted by Fried, Watkinson, and Gray (1999), this relationship did not persist at ages two, three, five, or six years after statistically adjusting for other important variables such as ratings of the home environment. In another study, exposure to one or more marijuana joints per day during the first trimester predicted deficits in academic achievement areas such as reading and spelling, while second trimester marijuana use was significantly associated with reading comprehension and underachievement at age ten (Goldschmidt et al., 2004). In his review of two longitudinal investigations of prenatal marijuana exposure, Fried (2002) concludes that in utero exposure to marijuana does not impact cognitive abilities as measured by most standardized measures of intelligence.

Behavioral Effects

Much of the existing information concerning the behavioral effects of prenatal exposure to marijuana comes from reports of the Ottawa Prenatal Prospective Study (OPPS) (Fried, 1996) and the work of Day et al. (1991). The first report from the Ottawa study examined four-day-old infants born to regular marijuana users and found that prenatal exposure to marijuana was associated with decreased rates of visual habituation and increased tremors. Similar observations were also noted at nine and 30 days of age (Fried and Makin, 1987). When these same children were examined at one year of age, no adverse effects of prenatal marijuana exposure were noted on behavioral outcomes (Fried and Watkinson, 1988). Fried, Watkinson, and Gray (1992) noted the difficulty in unraveling the long-term consequences of in utero marijuana exposure.

Arousal Regulation and Attention

A few research findings indicate that prenatal marijuana exposure has an effect on child behavior problems at preschool and school age. In a prospective study of the effects of prenatal marijuana exposure on child behavior problems at age ten, prenatal marijuana exposure in the first and third trimesters predicted significantly increased hyperactivity, inattention, and impulsivity symptoms (Goldschmidt, Day, and Richardson, 2000). These results are consistent with the work of O'Connell and Fried (1991) who found a significant tendency for mothers who used marijuana heavily during pregnancy to rate their children as being more impulsive or hyperactive. The authors note, however, that it remains to be seen whether these results indicate a true behavioral difference in the attention-related domain or a lowered parental tolerance. More recent work by Fried and Watkinson (2001) found that prenatal marijuana exposure was associated with a factor they describe as stability of attention over time in their sample of 13- to 16-year-olds. The authors also note the inconsistency of findings across studies of marijuana's impact on attention, due to the multifaceted nature of attention. Results from Richardson et al. (2002) indicate that prenatal marijuana exposure had an effect on learning and memory, as well as impulsivity. In his review of two longitudinal investigations of prenatal marijuana exposure, Fried (2002) concludes that in utero exposure to marijuana does not impact cognitive abilities as measured by most standardized measures of intelligence but does impact attentional behavior and visual analysis/hypothesis testing. Kalant's review (2004) of the adverse effects of marijuana on health concludes that there is a small but growing body of evidence that indicates subtle but important effects on memory, information processing, and executive functions in children prenatally exposed to marijuana. Currently, research regarding prenatal marijuana exposure is focused on aspects of executive functioning such as attention, memory, and organization.

Social and Environmental Considerations

According to Goldschmidt, Day, and Richardson (2000), it is difficult to isolate the effects of marijuana exposure from its correlates and from environmental risk factors. Variables such as socioeconomic status, access to medical and social services, and the presence or absence of a male figure in the household have a significant influence on child development. Chatterji and Markowitz (2001) found, for example, that current maternal marijuana use within the household was associated with increases in child behavior problems. Maternal mental health, social support networks, stressful life events such as exposure to violence or domestic abuse, are also important variables that impact long-term developmental outcomes. The poor quality of caregiving due to maternal substance abuse may certainly result in a number of social and emotional challenges:

- Attachment disorders
- Aggression
- Conduct disorders
- ADHD
- Depression
- Parentification
- Anxiety
- School failure
- Substance abuse

Many environmental risk factors are directly associated with maternal marijuana use, making it difficult to identify the impact of prenatal exposure in isolation.

Summary

After statistically controlling for maternal personality and home environment conditions, many of the neurobehavioral consequences of prenatal exposure to marijuana do not remain significant. According to Fried (1996), the only definitive statement regarding prenatal exposure to marijuana would be that, if there are long-term consequences of prenatal exposure to marijuana, such effects are very subtle. At this point there are few human studies on the effects of marijuana use during pregnancy and no precise mechanism of action has been substantiated (Behnke and Eyler, 1993).

OPIATES

Epidemiology of Opiate Use in Pregnancy

The literature on developmental outcomes for infants prenatally exposed to opiates is relatively sparse and was primarily generated in the 1970s and early 1980s. The literature is also made more problematic by the issue of polysubstance abuse, as research investigating prenatal opiate exposure includes exposure to heroin, methadone, or both, and may also include exposure to amphetamines, barbiturates, benzodiazepines, cocaine, alcohol, and nicotine (Kaltenbach, 1996). Recent studies report prevalence for opiate use during pregnancy to range from less than 1 to 2 percent to as high as 21 percent (Chasnoff, Landress, and Barrett, 1990; McCalla et al., 1991; Ostrea et al., 1992).

Growth/Physiological Effects

There is no consistent pattern of congenital anomalies associated with prenatal exposure to heroin and heroin is not considered to be a teratogenic agent (Chasnoff, 1988; Eyler and Behnke, 1999). The most consistently reported effect of prenatal opiate exposure is associated with fetal growth retardation and neonatal abstinence syndrome (Behnke and Eyler, 1993). Within one to three days of birth, most infants born to opiate-addicted women show clear clinical signs of narcotic abstinence, or withdrawal (Kandall, 1998). Neonatal abstinence is described by Kaltenbach and Finnegan (1986) as a generalized disorder characterized by the signs and symptoms of central nervous system hyperirritability, gastrointestinal dysfunction, respiratory distress, and vague autonomic symptoms that include yawning, sneezing, mottling, and fever. These early neurobehavioral outcomes do not persist, however (Finnegan, 1979; Householder et al., 1982).

Within the past decade, methadone maintenance has become accepted as the standard of care for opiate addiction during pregnancy (Kandall et al., 1999). Methadone treatment stabilizes maternal drug levels and reduces the amount of polydrug use and associated complications (Kearney, 1997). According to Kandall et al. (1999), no study has yet reported either a higher rate of malformations compared with control populations or an increase in any specific dysmorphic syndrome which could be related to maternal methadone use during pregnancy. Methadone treatment during pregnancy is associated with increased fetal growth and higher birth weights in offspring compared with heroin-exposed infants (Connaughton et al., 1975; Ludlow, Evans, and Hulse, 2004; Zelson, 1973), although these findings have not been consistent across all studies (Householder et al., 1982; Zuckerman and Bresnahan, 1991).

Cognitive Effects

Studies on the early development of methadone-exposed offspring indicate relatively normal development, at least during infancy (de Cubas and Field, 1993). In studies by Hans (1989) and Hans and Marcus (1983), no differences in mental development were found at 4, 12, and 24 months of age when comparing opiate-exposed and nonexposed children (Hans, 1989; Hans and Marcus, 1983). Kaltenbach and Finnegan (1986) found no differences in mental development scores at 6, 12, and 24 months when the two groups were compared. Between three and six years of age, heroin-exposed children performed more poorly than their peers on a cognitive index in one study, but the same on behavior and skills in another study (Kearney, 1999). In the largest at-risk sample observed longitudinally to date (Messinger et al., 2004), infant prenatal exposure to opiates was not associated with mental, motor, or behavioral deficits after controlling for birth weight and environmental risks. Kaltenbach (1996) concludes her review of the effects of prenatal opiate exposure by stating that opiate-exposed infants through two years of age function well within the normal range of development and children between two and five years of age do not differ in cognitive function from other high-risk populations. According to Hans and Jeremy (2001), it appears that much of the effect of maternal opioid drug use on mental development of infant offspring is attributable to the experience of more social-environmental risk factors by children in substance-abusing families.

Social and Environmental Considerations

Illicit drug use is associated with late and inadequate prenatal care, poverty, poor nutrition, domestic and stranger violence, and other severe threats to maternal and infant health (Frohna, Lantz, and Pollack, 1999). It is especially difficult to identify the impact of a specific illicit substance such as heroin due to the issue of polysubstance abuse. As with cocaine exposure, outcomes of heroin and methadone exposure are more strongly related to home and parenting environment variables than to direct drug effects (Hans, 1996; Kaltenbach, 1996; Ornoy, 2003; Ornoy et al., 2001).

SUMMARY AND CONCLUSIONS

Children of mothers who abuse drugs during pregnancy are affected by a range of biological and environmental factors. At the present , it is clear that there are negative effects of substance abuse on fetal development and family function and that these consequences must be addressed. The physical and behavioral problems seen in children with prenatal exposure to drugs are the result of many related factors such as poverty, exposure to violence, parental psychopathology, and lack of access to medical and social services. These factors likely interact with the initial prenatal drug exposure to negatively impact long-term developmental outcomes for the child.

REFERENCES

Abel, E.L. (1984). Smoking and pregnancy. *Journal of Psychoactive Drugs,* 16, 327-338.

Accornero, V.H.; Morrow, C.E.; Bandstra, E.S.; Johnson, A.L.; Anthony, J.C. (2002). Behavioral outcome of preschoolers exposed prenatally to cocaine: Role of maternal behavioral health. *Journal of Pediatric Psychology,* 27(3), 259-269.

Achenbach, T.M. (1991). *Manual for the Child Behavior Checklist/4-18 and 1991 Profile.* Burlington, VT: University of Vermont.

Arendt, R.; Angelopoulos, J.; Salvator, A.; Singer, L. (1999). Motor development of cocaine-exposed children at age two years. *Pediatrics,* 103, 86-92.

Bada, H.S.; Bauer, C.R.; Shankaran, S.; Lester, B; Wright, L.L.; Das, A.; Poole, K.; Smeriglio, V.L.; Finnegan, L.P.; Maza, P.L. (2002). Central and autonomic system signs with in utero drug exposure. *Archives of Disease in Childhood Fetal and Neonatal Edition,* 87, F106-F112.

Bandstra, E.S.; Vogel, A.L.; Morrow, C.E.; Xue, L.; Anthony, J.C. (2004). Severity of prenatal cocaine exposure and child language functioning through age seven years: A longitudinal latent growth curve analysis. *Substance Use and Misuse,* 39, 25-50.

Bard, K.A.; Coles, C.D.; Platzman, K.A.; Lynch, M.A. (2000). The effects of prenatal drug exposure, term status, and caregiving on arousal and arousal modulation in 8-week-old infants. *Developmental Psychobiology,* 36, 194-212.

Batstra, L.; Hadders-Algra, M.; Neeleman, J. (2003). Effect of antenatal exposure to maternal smoking on behavioral problems and academic achievement in childhood: Prospective evidence from a Dutch birth cohort. *Early Human Development,* 75, 21-33.

Bayley, N. (1993). *Bayley Scales of Infant Development.* San Antonio, TX: Psychological Corporation.

Beeghly, M.; Tronick, E.; Brilliant, G.; High, A.; Flaherty, C.; Cabral, H.; Frank, D. (1995). Object play and affect of in-utero cocaine exposed and nonexposed infants at 1 year: Characteristics and context effects (abstract). Presented at the biennial meeting of the Society for Research on Child Development. Providence, RI, April.

Behnke, M.; Eyler, F.D. (1993). The consequences of prenatal substance use for the developing fetus, newborn, and young child. *The International Journal of the Addictions,* 28(13), 1341-1391.

Behnke, M.; Eyler, F.D.; Warner, T.D.; Garvan, C.W.; Hou, W.; Wobie, K. (2006). Outcome from a prospective longitudinal study of prenatal cocaine use: Preschool development at 3 years of age. *Journal of Pediatric Psychology,* 31(1), 41-49.

Bendersky, M.; Bennet, D.; Lewis, M. (2006). Aggression at age 5 as a function of prenatal exposure to cocaine, gender, and environmental risk. *Journal of Pediatric Psychology,* 31(1), 71-84.

Bendersky, M.; Gambini, G; Lastella, A; Bennett, D.S.; Lewis, M. (2003). Inhibitory motor control at five years as a function of prenatal cocaine exposure. *Developmental and Behavioral Pediatrics,* 24(5), 345-351.

Bendersky, M.; Lewis, M. (1998). Arousal modulation in cocaine-exposed infants. *Developmental Psychology,* 34, 555-564.

Bland-Stewart, L.M.; Seymour, H.N.; Beeghly, M.; Frank, D.A. (1998). Semantic development of African-American children prenatally exposed to cocaine. *Seminars in Speech and Language,* 19, 167-187.

Brantley, M.; Rochat, R.; Floyd, V.; Norris, D.; Franko, E.; Blake, P.; Toomey, K.; Mayer, L.; Ziegler, B.; Fernhoff, P.M. (1996). Population-based prevalence of perinatal exposure to cocaine—Georgia, 1994. *Morbidity and Mortality Weekly Report,* 41, 887-891.

Brazelton, T.B. (1984). *Neonatal Behavioral Assessment Scale* (Second Edition). *Clinics in Developmental Medicine,* Volume 88. London: Spastics International Medical Publication.

Brazelton, T.B.; Nugent, J.K. (1995). *Neonatal Behavioral Assessment Scale* (Third Edition). *Clinics in Developmental Medicine,* Volume 137. Cambridge: McKeith Press.

Brown, J.V.; Bakeman, R.; Coles, C.D.; Platzman, K.A.; Lynch, M.E. (2004). Prenatal cocaine exposure: A comparison of 2-year-old children in parental and nonparental care. *Child Development,* 75, 1282-1295.

Brown, J.V.; Bakeman, R.; Coles, C.D.; Sexson, W.R.; Demi, A. (1998). Maternal drug use, fetal growth, and newborn behavior: Are preterms and fullterms affected differently? *Developmental Psychology,* 34(3), 540-554.

Chasnoff, I.J. (1988). Drug use in pregnancy. *Pediatric Clinics of North America,* 35, 1403-1412.

Chasnoff, I.J.; Anson, A.; Hatcher, R.; Stenson, H.; Iaukea, K.; Randolph, L.A. (1998). Prenatal exposure to cocaine and other drugs: Outcome at four to six years. *Annals of the New York Academy of Sciences,* 846, 314-328.

Chasnoff, I.J.; Griffith, D.R.; Freier, C.; Murray, J. (1992). Cocaine/polydrug use in pregnancy: Two year follow-up. *Pediatrics,* 89(2), 284-289.

Chasnoff, I.J.; Landress, H.J.; Barrett, M.E. (1990). The prevalence of illicit-drug or alcohol use during pregnancy and discrepancies in mandatory reporting in Pinellas County, Florida. *New England Journal of Medicine,* 322, 1202-1206.

Chatterji, P.; Markowitz, S. (2001). The impact of maternal alcohol and illicit drug use on children's behavior problems: Evidence from the children of the national longitudinal survey of youth. *Journal of Health Economics,* 20, 703-731.

Chouteau, M.; Namerow, P.B.; Leppert, P. (1988). The effect of cocaine abuse on birth weight and gestational age. *Obstetrics and Gynecology,* 72, 351-354.

Cnattingus, S. (2004). The epidemiology of smoking during pregnancy: Smoking prevalence, maternal characteristics, and pregnancy outcomes. *Nicotine and Tobacco Research,* 6, S125-S140.

Coles, C.D. (1993). Saying "goodbye" to the "crack baby." *Neurotoxicology and Teratology,* 5, 290-292.

Coles, C.D. (1995). Children of parents who abuse drugs and alcohol. In: Smith, G.H.; Coles, C.D.; Poulsen, M.K.; Cole, C.K. (Eds.), *Children, Families, and Substance Abuse: Challenges for Changing Educational and Social Outcomes* (pp. 3-23). Baltimore: Paul H. Brookes.

Coles, C.D.; Bard, K.A.; Bakeman, R.; Platzman, K.A.; Lynch, M.E.; Moretto, S. (2000). Neurodevelopment and growth in drug-exposed and preterm infants. Poster presented at the International Conference on Infancy Studies. Brighton, UK, July.

Coles, C.D.; Bard, K.A.; Platzman, K.A.; Lynch, M.E. (1999). Attentional response at 8 weeks in prenatally drug-exposed and preterm infants. *Neurotoxicology and Teratology,* 21(5), 527-537.

Coles, C.D.; Kable, J.A.; Lynch, M.E.; Platzman, K.A. (2004). Prenatal cocaine exposure: 8-year-olds' arousal to social and cognitive challenges. Paper presented at the College on Problems of Drug Dependence Annual Meeting. San Juan, Puerto Rico, June.

Coles, C.D.; Platzman, K.A. (1993). Behavioral development in children prenatally exposed to drugs and alcohol. *The International Journal of the Addictions,* 28, 1393-1433.

Colley, J.R.; Holland, W.W.; Corkhill, R.T. (1974). Influence of passive smoking and parental phlegm on pneumonia and bronchitis in early childhood. *Lancet,* 2, 1031-1034.

Connaughton, J.F.; Finnegan, L.P.; Schut, J.; Emich, J.P. (1975). Current concepts in the management of the pregnant opiate addict. *Addictive Diseases,* 2, 21-35.

Cornelius, M.D.; Goldschmidt, L.; Day, N.L.; Larkby, C. (2002). Alcohol, tobacco and marijuana use among pregnant teenagers: 6-year follow-up of offspring growth effects. *Neurotoxicology and Teratology,* 24, 703-710.

Day, N.; Sambamoorthi, U.; Taylor, P.; Richardson, G.; Robles, N.; Jhon, Y.; Scher, M.; Stoffer, D.; Cornelius, M.; Jasperse, D. (1991). Prenatal marijuana use and neonatal outcome. *Neurotoxicology and Teratology,* 13, 329-334.

Day, N.L.; Cottreau, C.M.; Richardson, G.A. (1993). The epidemiology of alcohol, marijuana, and cocaine use among women of child-bearing age and pregnant women. *Clinical Obstetrics and Gynecology,* 36, 232-245.

Day, N.L.; Richardson, G.A.; Goldschmidt, L.; Cornelius, M.D. (2000). Effects of prenatal tobacco exposure on preschooler's behavior. *Journal of Developmental & Behavioral Pediatrics,* 21, 180-188.

de Cubas, M.M.; Field, T. (1993). Children of methadone-dependent women: Developmental outcomes. *American Journal of Orthopsychiatry,* 63(2), 266-276.

Delaney-Black, V.; Covington, C.; Nordstrom, B.; Ager, J.; Janisse, J.; Hannigan, J.H.; Chiodo, L.; Sokol, R.J. (2004). Prenatal cocaine: Quantity of exposure and gender moderation. *Journal of Developmental & Behavioral Pediatrics,* 25(4), 254-263.

Delaney-Black, V.; Covington, C.; Templin, T.; Ager, J.W.; Martier, S.S.; Sokol, R.J. (1998). Prenatal cocaine exposure and child behavior. *Pediatrics,* 102, 945-950.

DiPietro, J.A.; Caughy, M.O.; Cusson, R.; Fox, N.A. (1994). Cardiorespiratory functioning of preterm infants: Stability and risk associations for measures of heart rate variability and oxygen saturation. *Developmental Psychobiology,* 27, 137-152.

Ebrahim, S.H.; Floyd, R.L.; Merritt, R.K.; Decoufle, P.; Holtzman, D. (2000). Trends in pregnancy-related smoking rates in the United States, 1987-1996. *Journal of the American Medical Association,* 283(3), 361-366.

Ershoff, D.H.; Ashford, T.H.; Goldenberg, R.L. (2004). Helping pregnant women quit smoking: An overview. *Nicotine and Tobacco Research,* 6, S101-S105.

Evans, D.; Levison, M.J.; Feldman, C.H.; Clark, N.M.; Wasilewski, Y.; Levin, B.; Mellins, R.B. (1987). The impact of passive smoking on emergency room visits of urban children with asthma. *American Journal of Respiratory Disease,* 135, 567-572.

Eyler, F.D.; Behnke, M. (1999). Early development of infants exposed to drugs prenatally. *Clinics in Perinatology,* 26(1), 107-150.

Eysenck, H.J. (1980). *The Causes and Effects of Smoking.* London: Maurice Temple Smith.

Eysenck, H.J. (1991). *Smoking, Personality, and Stress: Psychosocial Factors in the Prevention of Cancer and Coronary Heart Disease*. New York: Springer-Verlag.

Eysenck, H.J.; Tarrant, M.; Woolf, M.; England, L. (1960). Smoking and personality. *British Medical Journal*, 1, 1456-1460.

Fergusson, D.M.; Horwood, L.J.; Lynskey, M.T. (1993). Maternal smoking before and after pregnancy: Effects on behavioral outcomes in middle childhood. *Pediatrics*, 92, 815-822.

Fergusson, D.M.; Lloyd, M. (1991). Smoking during pregnancy and its effects on child cognitive ability from the ages of 8 to 12 years. *Pediatric and Perinatal Epidemiology*, 5, 189-200.

Fergusson, D.M.; Woodward, L.J.; Horwood, L.J. (1998). Maternal smoking during pregnancy and psychiatric adjustment in late adolescence. *Archives of General Psychiatry*, 55(8), 721-727.

Fetters, L.; Tronick, E.Z. (1996). Neuromotor development of cocaine-exposed and control infants from birth through 15 months: Poor and poorer performance. *Pediatrics*, 98, 938-943.

Fingerhut, L.A.; Kleinman, J.C.; Kendrick, J.S. (1990). Smoking before, during, and after pregnancy. *American Journal of Pharmacy*, 80, 541-544.

Finnegan, L.P. (1979). Pathophysiological and behavioral effects of the transplacental transfer of narcotic drugs to the fetuses and neonates of narcotic dependent mothers. *Bulletin of Narcotics*, 31(3), 1-58.

Franco, P.; Groswasser, J.; Hassid, S.; Lanquart, J.P.; Scaillet, S.; Kahn, A. (1999). Prenatal exposure to cigarette smoking is associated with a decrease in arousal in infants. *Journal of Pediatrics*, 135, 34-38.

Frank, D.A.; Augustyn, M.; Knight, W.G.; Pell, T.; Zuckerman, B. (2001). Growth, development, and behavior in early childhood following prenatal cocaine exposure: A systematic review. *Journal of the American Medical Association*, 285, 1613-1625.

Frank, D.A.; Jacobs, R.R.; Beeghly, M.; Augustyn, M.; Bellinger, D.; Cabral, H. (2002). Level of prenatal cocaine exposure and scores on the Bayley Scales of Infant Development: Modifying effects of caregiver, early intervention, and birth weight. *Pediatrics*, 110, 1143-1152.

Fried, P.A. (1996). Behavioral outcomes in preschool and school-age children exposed prenatally to marijuana: A review and speculative interpretation. In: Wetherington, C.L.; Smeriglio, V.L.; Finnegan, L.P. (Eds.), *Behavioral Studies of Drug-Exposed Offspring: Methodological Issues in Human and Animal Research* (pp. 242-260). Rockville, MD: NIDA.

Fried, P.A. (1998). Cigarette smoke exposure and hearing loss. *Journal of the American Medical Association*, 280, 963.

Fried, P.A. (2002). Conceptual issues in behavioral teratology and their application in determining long-term sequelae of prenatal marihuana exposure. *Journal of Child Psychology and Psychiatry*, 43(1), 81-102.

Fried, P.A.; James, D.S.; Watkinson, B. (2001). Growth and pubertal milestones during adolescence in offspring prenatally exposed to cigarettes and marijuana. *Neurotoxicology and Teratology*, 23, 431-436.

Fried, P.A.; Makin, J.E. (1987). Neonatal behavioral correlates of prenatal exposure to marijuana, cigarettes, and alcohol in a low risk population. *Neurotoxicology and Teratology*, 9, 1-7.

Fried, P.A.; Watkinson, B. (1988). Twelve- and twenty-four-month neurobehavioral follow-up of children prenatally exposed to marijuana, cigarettes, and alcohol. *Neurotoxicology and Teratology*, 10, 305-313.

Fried, P.A.; Watkinson, B. (1990). Thirty-six- and forty-eight-month neurobehavioral follow-up of children prenatally exposed to marijuana, cigarettes, and alcohol. *Journal of Developmental & Behavioral Pediatrics*, 11, 49-58.

Fried, P.A.; Watkinson, B. (2001). Differential effects on facets of attention in adolescents prenatally exposed to cigarettes and marijuana. *Neurotoxicology and Teratology*, 23, 421-430.

Fried, P.A.; Watkinson, B.; Gray, R. (1992). A follow-up study of attentional behavior in 6-year-old children exposed prenatally to marijuana, cigarettes, and alcohol. *Neurotoxicology and Teratology*, 14, 299-311.

Fried, P.A.; Watkinson, B.; Gray, R. (1999). Growth from birth to early adolescence in offspring prenatally exposed to cigarettes and marijuana. *Neurotoxicology and Teratology*, 21(5), 513-525.

Frohna, J.G.; Lantz, P.M.; Pollack, H. (1999). Maternal substance abuse and infant health: Policy options across the life course. *The Milbank Quarterly*, 77(4), 531-570.

Goldschmidt, L.; Day, N.L.; Richardson, G.A. (2000). Effects of prenatal marijuana exposure on child behavior problems at age 10. *Neurotoxicology and Teratology*, 22, 325-336.

Goldschmidt, L.; Richardson, G.A.; Cornelius, M.D.; Day, N.L. (2004). Prenatal marijuana and alcohol exposure and academic achievement at age 10. *Neurotoxicology and Teratology*, 26, 521-532.

Hagan, J.C.; Myers, B.J. (1997). Mother-toddler play interaction: A contrast of substance exposed and nonexposed children. *Infant Mental Health Journal*, 18(1), 40-57.

Haglund, B.; Cnattingus, S. (1990). Cigarette smoking as a risk factor for sudden infancy death syndrome: A population-based study. *American Journal of Health*, 80, 29-32.

Hans, S.L. (1989). Developmental consequences of prenatal exposure to methadone. *Annals of the New York Academy of Science*, 562, 195-207.

Hans, S.L. (1996). Prenatal drug exposure: Behavioral functioning in late childhood and adolescence. In: Wetherington, C.L.; Smeriglio, V.L.; Finnegan, L.P. (Eds.), *Behavioral Studies of Drug-Exposed Offspring: Methodological Issues in Human and Animal Research* (pp. 261-276). Rockville, MD: NIDA.

Hans, S.L.; Jeremy, R.J. (2001). Postneonatal mental and motor development of infants exposed in utero to opioid drugs. *Infant Mental Health Journal*, 22(3), 300-315.

Hans, S.L.; Marcus, J. (1983). Motor and attentional behavior in infants of methadone maintained women. In: Harris, L. (Ed.), *Problems of Drug Dependence*. Rockville, MD: NIDA.

Hardy, J.B.; Mellits, E.D. (1972). Does maternal smoking during pregnancy have a long-term effect on the child? *Lancet,* 1, 1332-1336.

Harlap, S.; Davies, A.M. (1974). Infant admissions to hospital and maternal smoking. *Lancet,* 2, 529-532.

Harvey, J.A. (2004). Cocaine effects on the developing brain: Current status. *Neuroscience and Biobehavioral Reviews,* 27, 751-764.

Hebel, J.R.; Fox, N.L.; Sexton, M. (1988). Dose-response of birth weight to various measures of maternal smoking during pregnancy. *Journal of Clinical Epidemiology,* 41, 483-489.

Held, J.R.; Riggs, M.L.; Dorman, C. (1999). The effect of prenatal cocaine exposure on neonatal outcome. *Neurotoxicology and Teratology,* 21, 619-625.

Himmelberger, D.U.; Brown, B.W.; Cohen, E.N. (1978). Cigarette smoking during pregnancy and the occurrence of spontaneous abortion and congenital abnormality. *American Journal of Epidemiology,* 108, 470-479.

Holtzman, C.; Paneth, N. (1994). Maternal cocaine use during pregnancy and perinatal outcomes. *Epidemiological Review,* 16, 315-320.

Householder, J.; Hatcher, R.; Burns, W.; Chasnoff, I. (1982). Infants born to narcotic-addicted mothers. *Psychological Bulletin,* 92, 453-468.

Hurt, H.; Brodsky, N.L.; Betancourt, L.; Bratman, L.E.; Belsky, J.; Giannetta, J. (1996). Play behavior in toddlers with in utero cocaine exposure: A prospective, masked, controlled study. *Journal of Developmental Behavioral Pediatrics,* 17(6), 373-379.

Hurt, H.; Malmud, E.; Betancourt, L.; Braitman, L.E.; Brodsky, N.L.; Giannetta, J. (1997). Children with in utero cocaine exposure do not differ from control subjects on intelligence testing. *Archives of Pediatric and Adolescent Medicine,* 151, 1237-1241.

Jaakkola, J.J.; Gissler, M. (2004). Maternal smoking in pregnancy, fetal development, and childhood asthma. *American Journal of Public Health,* 94, 136-140.

Jacobson, J.L.; Jacobson, S.W.; Sokol, R.J.; Martier, S.S.; Chiodo, L.M. (1996). New evidence for neurobehavioral effects of in utero cocaine exposure. *Journal of Pediatrics,* 129(4), 581-590.

Jacobson, S.W.; Fein, G.G.; Jacobson, J.L.; Schwartz, P.M.; Dowler, J.K. (1985). The effect of PCB exposure on visual recognition memory. *Child Development,* 56, 853-860.

Jacobson, S.W.; Jacobson, J.L. (2001). Alcohol and drug-related effects on development: A new emphasis on contextual factors. *Infant Mental Health Journal,* 22(3), 416-430.

Kalant, H. (2004). Adverse effects of cannabis on health: An update of the literature since 1996. *Progress in Neuro-psychopharmacology & Biological Psychiatry,* 28, 849-863.

Kaltenbach, K.A. (1996). Exposure to opiates: Behavioral outcomes in preschool and school-age children. In: Wetherington, C.L.; Smeriglio, V.L.; Finnegan, L.P. (Eds.), *Behavioral Studies of Drug-Exposed Offspring: Methodological Issues in Human and Animal Research* (pp. 230-241). Rockville, MD: NIDA.

Kaltenbach, K.A.; Finnegan, L.P. (1986). Neonatal abstinence syndrome: Pharmacotherapy and developmental outcome. *Neurobehavioral Toxicology and Teratology,* 8, 353-355.

Kandall, S.R. (1998). Treatment options for drug-exposed neonates. In: Graham A.W.; Schultz T.K. (Eds.), *Principles of Addiction Medicine* (Second Edition, pp. 1211-1222). Chevy Chase, MD: American Society of Addiction Medicine, Inc.

Kandall, S.R.; Doberczak, T.M.; Jantunen, M.; Stein, J. (1999). The methadone-maintained pregnancy. *Clinics in Perinatology,* 26(1), 173-183.

Karmel, B.Z.; Gardner, J.M. (1996). Prenatal cocaine exposure effects on arousal-modulated attention during the neonatal period. *Developmental Psychobiology,* 29, 463-480.

Karmel, B.Z.; Gardner, J.M.; Freedland, R.L. (1996). Arousal-modulated attention at four months as a function of intrauterine cocaine exposure and central nervous system injury. *Journal of Pediatric Psychology,* 21, 821-832.

Kearney, M.H. (1997). Drug treatment for women: Traditional models and new directions. *Journal of Obstetric, Gynecologic, and Neonatal Nursing,* 26, 449-458.

Kearney, M.H. (1999). *Perinatal Impact of Alcohol, Tobacco, and other Drugs.* White Plains, NY: March of Dimes Publishing.

Kershaw, C.R. (1987). Passive smoking, potential atopy, and asthma in the first five years. *Journal of the Royal Society of Medicine,* 80, 683-688.

Kilbride, H.; Castor, C.; Hoffman, E.; Fuger, K.L. (2000). Thirty-six-month outcome of prenatal cocaine exposure for term or near-term infants: Impact of early case management. *Journal of Developmental & Behavioral Pediatrics,* 21, 19-26.

Kliegman, R.M.; Madura, D.; Kiwi, R.; Eisenberg, I.; Yamashita, T. (1994). Relation of maternal cocaine use to the risks of prematurity and low birth weight. *Journal of Pediatrics,* 124, 751-756.

Kline, J.; Levin, B.; Shrout, P.; Stein, Z.; Susser, M.; Warburton, D. (1983). Maternal smoking and trisomy among spontaneously aborted conceptions. *American Journal of Human Genetics,* 35, 421-431.

Kotimaa, A.J.; Moilanen, I.; Taanila, A.; Ebeling, H.; Smalley, S.L.; McGough, J.J.; Hartikainen, A.L.; Jarvelin, M.R. (2003). Maternal smoking and hyperactivity in 8-year-old children. *Journal of the American Academy of Child and Adolescent Psychiatry,* 42, 826-833.

Kries, R.; Toschke, A.M.; Koletzko, B.; Slikker, W. (2002). Maternal smoking during pregnancy and childhood obesity. *American Journal of Epidemiology,* 156, 954-961.

Kristjansson, E.A.; Fried, P.A.; Watkinson, B. (1989). Maternal smoking during pregnancy affects children's vigilance performance. *Drug and Alcohol Dependence,* 24, 11-19.

Krogh, D. (1991). *Smoking: The Artificial Passion.* New York: Freeman.

Landesman-Dwyer, S.; Emanuel, I. (1979). Smoking during pregnancy. *Teratology,* 19, 119-126.

Lester, B.; Tronick, E.Z.; LaGasse, L.; Seifer, R.; Bauer, C.R.; Shankaran, S.; Bada, H.S. et al. (2002). The maternal lifestyle study: Effects of substance exposure during pregnancy on neurodevelopmental outcome in 1-month-old infants. *Pediatrics,* 110, 1182-1192.

Lilienfeld, A.M. (1959). Emotional and other selected characteristics of cigarette smokers and nonsmokers as related to epidemiological studies of lung cancer and other diseases. *Journal of the National Cancer Institute,* 22, 259-282.

Linnet, K.M.; Dalsgaard, S.; Obel, C.; Wisborg, K.; Henriksen, T.B.; Rodriguez, A.; Kotimaa, A. et al. (2003). Maternal lifestyle factors in pregnancy risk of Attention Deficit Hyperactivity Disorder and associated behaviors: Review of the current evidence. *American Journal of Psychiatry,* 160, 1028-1040.

Little, J.; Cardy, A.; Munger, R.G. (2004). Tobacco smoking and oral clefts: A meta-analysis. *Bulletin of the World Health Organization,* 82(3), 213-218.

Ludlow, J.P.; Evans, S.F.; Hulse, G. (2004). Obstetric and perinatal outcomes in pregnancies associated with illicit substance abuse. *Australian and New Zealand Journal of Obstetrics and Gynecology,* 44, 302-306.

Makin, J.; Fried, P.A.; Watkinson, B. (1991). A comparison of active and passive smoking during pregnancy: Long-term effects. *Neurotoxicology and Teratology,* 13, 5-12.

Matarazzo, J.D.; Saslow, G. (1960). Psychological and related characteristics of smokers and nonsmokers. *Psychological Bulletin,* 57, 493-513.

Maughan, B.; Taylor, A.; Caspi, A.; Moffitt, T.E. (2004). Prenatal smoking and early childhood conduct problems: Testing genetic and environmental explanations of the association. *Archives of General Psychiatry,* 61, 836-843.

Mayes, L.C. (1999). Developing brain and in utero cocaine exposure: Effects on neural ontogeny. *Development and Psychopathology,* 11, 685-714.

Mayes, L.C.; Bornstein, M.H.; Chawarska, K.; Granger, R.H. (1995). Information processing and developmental assessments in three-month-olds exposed prenatally to cocaine. *Pediatrics,* 95, 539-545.

Mayes, L.C.; Cicchetti, D.; Acharyya, S.; Zhang, H. (2003). Developmental trajectories of cocaine and other-drug-exposed and non cocaine-exposed children. *Journal of Developmental & Behavioral Pediatrics,* 24, 323-335.

McCalla, S.; Minkoff, H.L.; Feldman, J.; Delke, I.; Salwin, M.; Valencia, G.; Glass, L. (1991). The biologic and social consequences of perinatal cocaine use in an inner-city population: Results of an anonymous cross-sectional study. *American Journal of Obstetrics and Gynecology,* 164, 625-630.

McManus, I.C.; Weeks, S.J. (1982). Smoking, personality, and reasons for smoking. *Psychological Medicine,* 12, 349-356.

Mehta, S.K.; Super, D.M.; Connuck, D.; Kirchner, L.; Salvator, A.; Singer, L.; Fradley, L.G.; Kaufman, E.S. (2002). Autonomic alterations in cocaine-exposed infants. *American Heart Journal,* 144, 1109-1115.

Mentis, M. (1998). In utero cocaine exposure and language development. *Seminars in Speech and Language,* 19, 147-165.

Messinger, D.S.; Bauer, C.R.; Das, A.; Seifer, R.; Lester, B.M.; Lagasse, L.L.; Wright, L.L. et al. (2004). The maternal lifestyle study: Cognitive, motor, and behavioral outcomes of cocaine-exposed and opiate-exposed infants through three years of age. *Pediatrics,* 113(6), 1677-1685.

Metosky, P.; Vondra, J. (1995). Prenatal drug exposure and coping in toddlers: A comparison study. *Infant Behavior and Development*, 18(1), 15-25.

Mick, E.; Biederman, J.; Faraone, S.V.; Sayer, J.; Kleinman, S. (2002). Case-control study of Attention-Deficit Hyperactivity Disorder and maternal smoking, alcohol use, and drug use during pregnancy. *Journal of the American Academy of Child and Adolescent Psychiatry*, 41, 378-385.

Morrow, C.E.; Bandstra, E.S.; Anthony, J.C.; Ofir, A.Y.; Xue, L.; Reyes, M.B. (2003). Influence of prenatal cocaine exposure on early language development: Longitudinal findings from four months to three years of age. *Journal of Developmental Medicine & Behavioral Pediatrics*, 24, 39-50.

Mortensen, E.L.; Michaelsen, K.F.; Sanders, S.A.; Reinisch, J.M. (2005). A dose-response relationship between maternal smoking during late pregnancy and adult intelligence in male offspring. *Paediatric and Perinatal Epidemiology*, 19, 4-11.

Naeye, R.L.; Peters, E.C. (1984). Mental development of children whose mothers smoked during pregnancy. *Obstetrics and Gynecology*, 64, 601-607.

National Institute on Drug Abuse (1996). *National Pregnancy and Health Survey*. Rockville, MD: NIDA.

Nelson, S.; Lerner, E.; Needlman, R.; Salvator, A.; Singer, L.T. (2004). Cocaine, anemia, and neurodevelopmental outcomes in children: A longitudinal study. *Journal of Developmental & Behavioral Pediatrics*, 25(1), 1-9.

O'Connell, C.M.; Fried, P.A. (1991). Prenatal exposure to cannabis: A preliminary report of postnatal consequences in school-age children. *Neurotoxicology and Teratology*, 13, 631-639.

Ornoy, A. (2003). The impact of intrauterine exposure versus postnatal environment in neurodevelopmental toxicity: Long-term neurobehavioral studies in children at risk for developmental disorders. *Toxicology Letters*, 140-141; 171-181.

Ornoy, A.; Segal, J.; Bar-Hamburger, R.; Greenbaum, C. (2001). Developmental outcome of school-age children born to mothers with heroin dependency: Importance of environmental factors. *Developmental Medicine & Child Neurology*, 43, 668-675.

Ostrea, E.M.; Brady, M.; Gause, S.; Raymondo, A.L.; Stevens, M. (1992). Drug screening of newborns by meconium analysis: A large-scale, prospective, epidemiologic study. *Pediatrics*, 89, 107-113.

Picone, T.A.; Allen, L.H.; Olsen, P.N.; Ferris, M.E. (1982). Pregnancy outcome in North American women: II. Effects of diet, cigarette smoking, stress, and weight gain on placentas, and on neonatal physical and behavioral characteristics. *The American Journal of Clinical Nutrition*, 36, 1214-1224.

Polifka, J.E. (1998). Drugs and chemicals in breast milk. In: Slikker, W.; Chang, L.W. (Eds.), *Handbook of Developmental Neurotoxicology* (pp. 383-400). San Diego: Academic Press.

Porath, A.J.; Fried, P.A. (2005). Effects of prenatal cigarette and marijuana exposure on drug use among offspring. *Neurotoxicology and Teratology*, 27, 267-277.

Rantakallio, P. (1978). Relationship of maternal smoking to morbidity and mortality of the child up to age of five. *Acta Paediatric Scandinavia*, 67, 621-631.

Richardson, G.A. (1998). Prenatal cocaine exposure: A longitudinal study of development. *Annals of the New York Academy of Science,* 846, 144-152.

Richardson, G.A.; Conroy, M.L.; Day, N.L. (1996). Prenatal cocaine exposure: Effects on the development of school-age children. *Neurotoxicology and Teratology,* 18, 627-634.

Richardson, G.A.; Hamel, S.C.; Goldschmidt, L.; Day, N.L. (1999). Growth of infants prenatally exposed to cocaine/crack: Comparison of a prenatal care and a no prenatal care sample. *Pediatrics,* 104, 1-10.

Richardson, G.A.; Ryan, C.; Willford, J.; Day, N.L.; Goldschmidt, L. (2002). Prenatal alcohol and marijuana exposure: Effects on neuropsychological outcomes at 10 years. *Neurotoxicology and Teratology,* 24, 309-320.

Rodning, C.; Beckwith, L.; Howard, J. (1989). Characteristics of attachment organization and play organization in prenatally drug exposed toddlers. *Development and Psychopathology,* 1, 277-287.

Rodriguez, A.; Bohlin, G. (2005). Are maternal smoking and stress during pregnancy related to ADHD symptoms in children? *Journal of Child Psychology and Psychiatry and Allied Disciplines,* 46, 246-254.

Savage, J.; Brodsky, N.L.; Malmud, E.; Giannetta, J.M.; Hurt, H. (2005). Attentional functioning and impulse control in cocaine-exposed and control children at age ten years. *Journal of Developmental & Behavioral Pediatrics,* 26, 42-47.

Sawnani, H.; Jackson, T.; Murphy, T.; Beckerman, R.; Simakajornboon, N. (2004). The effect of maternal smoking on respiratory and arousal patterns of preterm infants during sleep. *American Journal of Respiratory Care Medicine,* 169, 733-738.

Saxton, D.W. (1978). The behavior of infants whose mothers smoke in pregnancy. *Early Human Development,* 2, 363-369.

Schneider, J.W.; Chasnoff, I.J. (1992). Motor assessment of cocaine/polydrug exposed infants at 4 months. *Neurotoxicology and Teratology,* 14, 91-101.

Schneider, N.G.; Houston, J.P. (1970). Smoking and anxiety. *Psychological Reports,* 26, 941-942.

Sexton, M.; Fox, N.L.; Hebel, J.R. (1990). Prenatal exposure to tobacco: II. Effects on cognitive functioning at age three. *International Journal of Epidemiology,* 19, 72-77.

Silberg, J.L.; Parr, T.; Neale, M.C.; Rutter, M.; Angold, A.; Eaves, L.J. (2003). Maternal smoking during pregnancy and risk to boys' conduct disturbance: An examination of the causal hypothesis. *Biological Psychiatry,* 53, 130-135.

Simpson, K.J. (1957). A preliminary report of cigarettes and the incidence of prematurity. *American Journal of Obstetric Gynecology,* 73, 808.

Singer, L.; Arendt, R.; Farkas, K.; Minnes, S.; Huang, J.; Yamashita, T. (1997). Relationship of prenatal cocaine exposure and maternal postpartum psychological distress to child developmental outcome. *Development and Psychopathology,* 9(3), 473-489.

Singer, L.; Arendt, R.; Minnes, S.; Farkas, K.; Salvator, A.; Kirchner, H.L.; Kliegman, R. (2002). Cognitive and motor outcomes of cocaine-exposed infants. *Journal of the American Medical Association,* 287, 1952-1960.

Slotkin, T. (1998). Fetal nicotine or cocaine exposure: Which one is worse? *Journal of Pharmacology and Experimental Therapeutics,* 285, 931-945.

Streissguth, A.P.; Barr, H.M.; Sampson, P.D.; Darby, B.L.; Martin, D.C. (1989). IQ at age 4 in relation to maternal alcohol use and smoking during pregnancy. *Developmental Psychology,* 25, 3-11.

Streissguth, A.P.; Martin, D.C.; Barr, H.M.; Sandman, B.M. (1984). Intrauterine alcohol and nicotine exposure: Attention and reaction time in 4-year-old children. *Developmental Psychology,* 20, 533-541.

Swanson, M.W.; Streissguth, A.P.; Sampson, P.D.; Carmichael-Olsen, H. (1999). Prenatal cocaine and neuromotor outcome at four months: Effect of duration of exposure. *Journal of Developmental & Behavioral Pediatrics,* 20, 325-334.

Thapar, A.; Fowler, T.; Rice, F.; Scourfield, J.; van den Bree, M.; Thomas, H.; Harold, G.; Hay, D. (2003). Maternal smoking during pregnancy and Attention Deficit Hyperactivity Disorder symptoms in offspring. *American Journal of Psychiatry,* 160, 1985-1989.

Tronick, E.Z.; Beeghly, M. (1999). Prenatal cocaine exposure, child development, and the compromising effects of cumulative risk. *Clinics in Perinatology,* 26, 151-171.

Tronick, E.Z.; Fetters, L.; Olson, K.L.; Chen, Y. (2004). Similar and functionally typical kinematic reaching parameters in 7- and 15-month-old in utero cocaine-exposed and unexposed infants. *Developmental Psychobiology,* 44, 168-175.

Vorhees, C.V. (1986). Principles of behavioral teratology. In: Riley, E.P.; Vorhees, C.V. (Eds.), *Handbook of Behavioral Teratology* (pp. 23-48). New York: Plenum Press.

Wakschlag, L.S.; Hans, S.L. (2002). Maternal smoking during pregnancy and conduct problems in high-risk youth: A developmental framework. *Development and Psychopathology,* 14, 351-369.

Wakschlag, L.S.; Lahey, B.B.; Loeber, R.; Green, S.M.; Gordon, R.A.; Leventhal, B.L. (1997). Maternal smoking during pregnancy and the risk of conduct disorders in boys. *Archives of General Psychiatry,* 54, 670-676.

Weitzman, M.; Gortmaker, S.; Sobol, A. (1992). Maternal smoking and behavior problems in children. *Pediatrics,* 90, 342-349.

Werler, M.M.; Pober, B.R.; Holmes, L.B. (1985). Smoking and pregnancy. *Teratology,* 32, 473-481.

Wilson, J.G. (1977). Current status of teratology: General principles and mechanisms derived from animal studies. In: Wilson, J.G.; Fraser, F.C. (Eds.), *Handbook of Teratology General Principles and Etiology,* Volume 1 (pp. 49-60). New York: Plenum Press.

Witter, F.; King, T.M. (1980). Cigarettes and pregnancy. *Progress in Clinical and Biological Research,* 36, 83-92.

Zelson, C. (1973). Infant of the addicted mother. *New England Journal of Medicine,* 288, 1391-1395.

Zuckerman, B.; Bresnahan, K. (1991). Developmental and behavioral consequences of prenatal drug and alcohol exposure. *Pediatric Clinics of North America,* 38, 1387-1406.

Chapter 8

Health Consequences
of Marijuana Use

Alan J. Budney
Brent A. Moore
Ryan Vandrey

INTRODUCTION AND OVERVIEW

Marijuana smoking remains the most prevalent form of illicit drug use in the United States, Canada, Australia, New Zealand, and some European countries, and rates of heavy marijuana smoking are high in other countries where accurate epidemiological data are not available (Black and Casswell, 1993; Hall, Johnston, and Donnelly, 1999; Substance Abuse and Mental Health Services Administration [SAMHSA], 2005a,b). In the United States, conservative estimates indicate that more than 14 million people smoked marijuana during the last month, and approximately 25 percent of these smoke almost daily (SAMHSA, 2005a,b). The types of problems associated with regular marijuana use have been well documented. Heavy use has been linked to impairment in memory, concentration, motivation, health, interpersonal relationships, and employment, as well as decreased participation in conventional roles of adulthood, history of psychiatric symptoms and hospitalizations, and participation in deviant activities (Haas and Hendin, 1987; Halikas et al., 1983; Jones, 1980; Kandel, 1984; Rainone et al., 1987; Roffman and Barnhart, 1987). Given the large cohort of frequent marijuana users, it is vital that we have clear, scientific information available concerning the risks and consequences of acute and chronic use of marijuana and other forms of cannabis.

Author's note: Preparation of this chapter was supported, in part, by grants DA12471 and DA12157 from the National Institute on Drug Abuse.

Handbook of the Medical Consequences of Alcohol and Drug Abuse
doi:10.1300/6039_08

Cannabis is the generic name for the psychoactive substance(s) derived from the plant *Cannabis sativa*. Marijuana and hashish are the common forms of cannabis used to obtain psychoactive effects. Cannabis contains numerous chemical substances, but the one usually of primary interest is delta-9-tetrahydrocannabinol (THC). THC has been identified as the predominant substance in marijuana that produces the subjective "high" associated with smoking the plant. Some debate exists regarding whether other compounds in cannabis have direct psychoactive effects or whether they interact with THC to produce other physical or psychological effects. This distinction is important, as "pure" forms of THC that are used orally in medical settings (dronabinol, Marinol) may not have identical effects to smoked or orally ingested cannabis. Moreover, because the most common method of using cannabinoids is smoking (marijuana or hashish), the other substances present in the smoke (e.g., carcinogens, tar) are relevant to a discussion of the health consequences of marijuana use (see following sections on the respiratory, immune, and cardiovascular systems in this chapter).

Cannabis was used in the Western Hemisphere both medically and recreationally as early as the eighteenth century. Yet, it was not until the 1930s that scientific investigation began in response to concern over its nonmedical use. Two reports on the health consequences of marijuana use appeared in the mid-1900s (Mayor's Committee on Marijuana [MCM], 1944; Walton, 1938), and the Marijuana Tax Act of 1937 functionally served to prohibit the recreational use of marijuana in the United States. Subsequent to these reports, scientific efforts were limited until the 1960s and 1970s when the prevalence of marijuana use and abuse increased in Western cultures.

Cannabis use in the United States and other countries has long been a topic of controversy. Groups such as NORML (National Organization for the Reform of Marijuana Laws) have led an ongoing effort to decriminalize and legalize marijuana use, and a number of respected medical professionals have argued for legitimizing the medical use of marijuana (Grinspoon and Bakalar, 1997; Hollister, 2000). Marijuana supporters argue that cannabis (1) has many positive effects and benefits, (2) has few and minor adverse consequences, and (3) is less harmful than other legalized drugs such as alcohol. They further argue that government obstructionism and propaganda have misled the public regarding the adverse effects of cannabis.

Such controversy can bias the evaluation and interpretation of scientific findings regarding the health effects of cannabis use, creating general misperceptions and confusion about the current state of knowledge. Conflicting and inconclusive scientific findings have fueled the controversy. As this chapter will indicate, there is much that is still unknown about the effects of cannabis on human psychological and physical health. Epidemiological and experimental studies have provided clear evidence that many people experience problems related to cannabis use and that ingestion of cannabis is associated with multiple adverse effects. However, demonstrating causal relationships between cannabis use and many of these effects has proven difficult due to methodological challenges. The magnitude of risk and the functional significance of such effects also remains elusive.

This chapter summarizes the scientific literature on the effects of cannabis on physical health, cognitive and behavioral functioning, and mental/behavioral health. Data relevant to the addictive potential of cannabis use are also presented. We focus on areas with a substantial research base that have provided some indication of definitive findings. The space provided to each topic corresponds somewhat to the scope of the literature in that area. We comment on the strength and quality of data supporting the connection between cannabis use and specific effects, but, generally, detailed critical analyses of individual studies or purported causal mechanisms are not provided. Rather, the reader is referred to original sources and previous reviews. In particular, detailed reviews and recent updates on each topic area are available in Kalant (1999; 2004).

RESPIRATORY SYSTEM

Perhaps the most significant health effects of cannabis are those that effect the respiratory system. Smoking is the primary method for use of cannabis, and almost all chronic users smoke either marijuana cigarettes ("joints") or use pipes to smoke marijuana or hashish. Chronic cannabis smoking has the potential for significant respiratory health consequences comparable to tobacco cigarette smoking. The smoke of marijuana and tobacco have similar levels of tar and respiratory toxic chemicals. Marijuana smoke contains up to 50 percent more carcinogens and results in substantially greater tar deposits in the lungs than filtered tobacco cigarettes. Such increased effects likely occur because marijuana users smoke unfiltered material, inhale the smoke more deeply, and hold the smoke longer in their lungs than tobacco smokers (Hoffman et al., 1975; Institute of Medicine, 1982; Roth et al., 1998; Tashkin et al., 1987, 1991; Wu et al., 1988). However, marijuana smokers tend to smoke significantly less material per day than tobacco smokers, which serves to counter its impact on the lungs.

Acute Effects

The most significant acute effect of smoking marijuana is its action as a bronchodilator, which increases vulnerability to the smoke by decreasing airway resistance and increasing specific airway conductance (Tashkin, Shapiro, and Frank, 1973; Vachon et al., 1973). Marijuana-induced bronchodilation has been demonstrated with healthy control participants and asthmatics, and under conditions of experimentally induced asthma (Tashkin et al., 1975). Placebo-controlled studies suggest that bronchodilation is due to the THC content in marijuana (Tashkin et al., 1975). Of note, marijuana's effect, which is brochodilation, distinguishes it from tobacco smoking, which produces bronchoconstriction.

Marijuana smoking also increases absorption of carbon monoxide, resulting in elevated levels of blood carboxyhemoglobin (COHb) (Tilles et al., 1986; Wu et al., 1988). Although smoking tobacco also boosts COHb, the increase found with smoking marijuana is as much as four times greater than with tobacco. These elevated levels of COHb lead to reduced oxygen in the blood and impairment in oxygen release from hemoglobin. Reduced blood oxygen levels can stress a number of organs including the heart (see section on cardiovascular effects this chapter). In placebo-controlled studies, examinations of other short-term aspects of respiration such as breathing rate, breath depth, CO_2 production, respiratory exchange ratio, and arterial blood gases have revealed no significant effects of marijuana smoking (Shapiro et al., 1976).

Chronic Effects

The impact of chronic marijuana smoking on respiratory health has many similarities to that of tobacco smoking (Tashkin, 1999; VanHoozen and Cross, 1997). Compared with nonsmokers, chronic marijuana smokers show increased likelihood of outpatient visits due to respiratory illness and exhibit respiratory symptoms of bronchitis at comparable rates to tobacco smokers (Bloom et al., 1987; Moore et al., 2005; Polen et al., 1993; Tashkin et al., 1987; Taylor et al., 2000). Chronic bronchitis can be moderately debilitating and increases the risk of additional infections. As THC appears to suppress immune system function, recurrent bronchitis may further increase the risk of opportunistic respiratory infections such as pneumonia and aspergillosis (see the following section on immune systems effects). This is of concern particularly for those individuals with already compromised immune functions such as cancer and AIDS patients.

Airway obstruction and symptoms of chronic cough, sputum production, shortness of breath, and wheezing characterize chronic bronchitis. These symptoms are the result of airway inflammation and tissue damage caused by marijuana smoke that results in increased fluid production, cellular abnormalities, and reduced alveolar permeability (Gil et al., 1995; Tashkin et al., 1987). This damage begins long before overt symptoms such as cough or wheezing are evident (Roth et al., 1998). Cellular abnormalities include reductions in ciliating surface cells of the lungs that function to clear fluid from the lungs to the mouth and throat. As a result, marijuana smokers have substantially higher bronchitis index scores than nonsmokers, and comparable scores to tobacco smokers, even at young ages with only short histories of marijuana use (Taylor et al., 2000, 2002).

Investigations of chronic obstructive pulmonary disease (COPD) in chronic marijuana smokers have been inconclusive. A common severe consequence of tobacco smoking, COPD includes chronic *obstructive* bronchitis or emphysema, and is characterized by impairment in small airway function rather than large airways. Marijuana smokers exhibit almost identical degrees of histopathologic and molecular abnormalities associated with progression to COPD in tobacco smokers (Barsky et al., 1998; Fligiel et al., 1991, 1997; Mao and Oh, 1998) and several case reports have been identified. However, two large-scale studies of COPD in chronic marijuana users have been inconclusive. Bloom et al. (1987) reported some indication of reduced small airway function suggestive of COPD, while Tashkin et al. (1987) found no evidence of small airway obstruction or other indicators of COPD.

Chronic cannabis smoking is likely associated with respiratory cancer, although this link is not definitive (see section on immune system effects). Cannabis smoking is clearly associated with similar processes and patterns of disease that lead to aerodigestive cancers among tobacco smokers (Hall, Christie, and Currow, 2005; MacPhee, 1999; Mao and Oh, 1998). As noted previously, marijuana smoke contains more carcinogens than cigarette smoke (Hoffman et al., 1975). Marijuana interferes with normal cell function, including synthesis and functions of DNA and RNA (Sherman et al., 1995; Tahir and Zimmerman, 1991), and appears to activate an enzyme that converts inactive carcinogens found in marijuana smoke into active carcinogens (Marques-Magallanes et al., 1997). Chronic marijuana smokers also show substantial cellular mutation associated with tumor progression (Barsky et al., 1998; Fligiel et al., 1997; Gong et al., 1987; Sherman et al., 1995). Marijuana also reduces the ability of pulmonary alveolar macrophages to kill pathogens, including tumor cells, allowing tumors to grow more rapidly (Baldwin et al., 1997; Roth et al., 2004; Shay et al., 2003; Zhu et al., 2000).

Clinical reports of aerodigestive cancers in individuals who had a history of marijuana smoking with limited or no tobacco exposure have provided suggestive evidence of a link between marijuana use and cancer (Caplan and Brigham, 1990; Donald, 1991; Fung, Gallagher, and Machtay, 1999; Sridhar et al., 1995; Taylor, 1988). In addition, Zhang et al. (1999) found increased risk for squamous-cell carcinoma of the head and neck for marijuana smokers compared with nonsmokers when tobacco smoking was statistically controlled. Similarly in a case-controlled hospital study in Casablanca, Morocco, Sasco et al. (2002) found that the use of hashish was independently predictive of lung cancer. The only epidemiological study that directly examined the risk of aerodigestive cancer in marijuana users reported no significant risk associated with cannabis (Sidney et al., 1997). This study, however, included a relatively young cohort comprised of primarily experimental and light marijuana users rather than chronic heavy users. Individuals who began smoking marijuana in the late 1960s are now approaching ages that are more likely to be associated with aerodigestive cancer, hence, future epidemiological studies should clarify better the risk of cancer associated with chronic cannabis use.

Smoking both cannabis and tobacco warrants mention as this combination most likely produces an additive adverse effect on the respiratory system (Barsky et al., 1998; Roth et al., 1998). Tobacco smoking is common among cannabis users, as almost half of daily marijuana users also smoke tobacco (Moore and Budney, 2001; SAMHSA, 2005a,b). This subgroup of marijuana smokers merits careful study as they may be at particularly high risk for respiratory disease.

IMMUNE SYSTEM

Chronic use of cannabis appears to compromise the immune system, particularly the immune defense systems of the lungs (Baldwin et al., 1997; Klein, 1999; Roth, Baldwin, and Tashkin, 2002; Sherman et al., 1991). This suppressive effect occurs in a variety of immune cells including killer cells, T cells, and macrophages (Klein, Friedman, and Specter, 1998; Kusher et al., 1994; Newton, Klein, and Friedman, 1994). Most research has focused on pulmonary alveolar macrophages (PAMs) which are the killer cells that destroy infectious microorganisms in the lungs (Huber, First, and Grubner, 1991; Sherman et al., 1991). Compared with tobacco smokers and nonsmokers, PAMs of chronic cannabis smokers exhibit a reduced ability to kill tumor cells and many microorganisms, including fungi and bacteria (Baldwin et al., 1997; Roth et al., 2004; Shay et al., 2003; Sherman et al., 1991; Zhu et al., 2000). As with tobacco, cannabis smoking produces an inflammatory response in the lungs which increases growth in the number and concentration of PAMs. However, their efficacy for destroying microorganisms is compromised (Barbers et al., 1991; Wallace et al., 1994). Cannabis smoking also appears to impair phagocytosis and cytokine function of the PAMs (Baldwin et al., 1997). Recent studies have begun to explore the mechanisms that may be involved in the inhibitory responses associated with chronic cannabis smoking (Roth et al., 2004; Shay et al., 2003; Zhu et al., 2000).

The functional consequences of cannabis's effect on the suppression of the immune system in humans is poorly understood. Nonetheless, clinical findings suggest that such effects warrant some concern. Chronic cannabis smoking is associated with increased bronchitis and other respiratory illnesses. Chronic use may also increase risk of exposure to infectious organisms, as cannabis and tobacco plants are often contaminated with a variety of fungi and molds including aspergillus (Verweij et al., 2000). Lung illnesses in marijuana smokers have been attributed to fungal infection (Caiaffa et al., 1994; Marks et al., 1996; Verweij et al., 2000). Decreased immune system response could increase the vulnerability and risk of developing these respiratory illnesses and lung diseases. More research is needed to determine whether chronic marijuana use is directly responsible for an increased incidence of disease via its effects on immune system function.

It is worth noting that the medical use of marijuana has now been legalized in ten U.S. states and legislation is pending in others. Many of the patients deemed appropriate candidates for medical marijuana have illnesses that involve already compromised immune systems such as AIDS wasting syndrome and chronic pain from various types of cancer (Grinspoon and Bakalar, 1997; Hollister, 2000; Joy, Watson, and Benson, 1999). A better understanding of the functional significance of marijuana's effects on the immune system is imperative as attempts are made to develop safe and effective models for the medical use of marijuana.

CARDIOVASCULAR SYSTEM

Relatively little research has been conducted on the long-term cardiovascular effects of chronic cannabis use. Most studies have focused on acute changes and suggest a limited cardiovascular health impact associated with cannabis use. The primary acute effect of smoked marijuana or oral THC is tachycardia (Beaconsfield, Ginsburg, and Rainsbury, 1972; Perez-Reyes et al., 1973). The increase in heart rate appears dose dependent, is observed with nonusers and chronic users, and is reduced as tolerance develops (Benowitz and Jones, 1975; Jones and Benowitz, 1976).

Cannabis or oral THC can produce small increases in supine blood pressure and impair vascular reflexes (Jones and Benowitz, 1976; Maddock et al.,

1979; Perez-Reyes et al., 1991). Smoking marijuana also results in increased inhalation of carbon monoxide and subsequent COHb, which in combination with tachycardia, increases the work required of the heart. Cannabis use also may reduce exercise tolerance, which is likely due to the combination of tachycardia, reduced thermoregulation caused by decreased vascular reflexes, and the increase in carbon monoxide (Renaud and Cormier, 1986).

Although these findings show clear changes in cardiovascular functioning due to marijuana or THC use, the effects have not been associated with short-term or long-term cardiovascular or cerebrovascular injury or disease. Case reports suggest that regular cannabis smoking may increase risk for some serious disorders such as arteritis and transient ischemic attacks (Goldschmidt, Day, and Richardson, 2000; Mouzak et al., 2000), but no controlled studies support these reports. For most healthy young marijuana smokers, the stress to the heart produced by marijuana use does not appear clinically detrimental (Institute of Medicine, 1982). However, for individuals with cardiovascular or cerebrovascular disease, the additional cardiac stress may increase the risk for chest pain, heart attack, or stroke. Additional research is needed to further elucidate the effects of chronic cannabis use on cardiovascular health, including interactions with other risk factors.

REPRODUCTIVE FUNCTION

Hormones and Fertility

Research examining the effects of cannabis use on reproductive function in women or men has been sparse. In women, marijuana smoking can affect some reproductive hormones (e.g., luteinizing hormone, prolactin), but this effect may occur only when they smoke during specific phases of the menstrual cycle (Block, Farinpour, and Schelchtem, 1991; Mendelson et al., 1985, 1986). Chronic cannabis use appears to alter male reproductive hormones, but these effects are not conclusive. Some studies have demonstrated marijuana-related decreased levels of gonadotropin, testosterone, prolactin, and luteinizing hormones in men, while others have reported negative findings (Murphy, 1999). For both men and women, the functional significance of these findings remains elusive. Although one might suspect that these purported effects on the reproductive system would adversely influence fertility, this has not been carefully studied in humans.

Perinatal Effects

Pregnant women who use cannabis expose the fetus to its effects, as THC is known to cross the placenta (Howell, Coles, and Kable address the prenatal effects of cannabis use in Chapter 7 of this book). Here we provide an overview of the perinatal effects of cannabis use, focused primarily on cognitive functioning. It is estimated that 10 to 20 percent of women use marijuana during pregnancy (Chasnoff, 1990; Fried, Barnes, and Drake, 1985; Zuckerman et al., 1989). Thus, understanding the effects on fetal development is vital. Studying cannabis use during pregnancy in humans has proven difficult, as pregnant users generally have many additional risk factors for adverse effects such as tobacco smoking, alcohol use, other illicit drug use, poorer nutrition, and lower socioeconomic status SES. Moreover, multiple factors deterring self-disclosure in this population raise concern regarding the validity of self-reports of cannabis use.

A number of studies have made efforts to control for these influences other than cannabis that impact perinatal outcomes, hence, certain tentative conclusions appear justified. Risk of major congenital anomalies is not increased due to cannabis use in pregnant women (Tennes et al., 1985; Zuckerman et al., 1989). However, some reports suggest that risk of developing minor anomalies, particularly related to the visual system, may be related to heavy cannabis use, but these data are not robust (Hingson et al., 1982; O'Connell and Fried, 1984). Cannabis use during pregnancy may be related to reduced birth weight and length, and possibly shortened length of gestation, although studies have reported conflicting findings (Day and Richardson, 1991; Gibson, Baghurst, and Colley, 1983; Hatch and Bracken, 1986; Witter and Niebyl, 1990; Zuckerman et al., 1989). Overall, these perinatal effects, if valid, are clearly not as severe as those observed with tobacco smokers.

The cognitive and behavioral effects of prenatal exposure to cannabis are perhaps best addressed in one study, the Ottawa Prenatal Prospective Study (OPPS) (Fried, 1980). This study collected birth data on 700 women and has periodically assessed the children of a subsample of 150 to 200. Adverse effects of prenatal cannabis use were observed in testing the neonate during the first month. Possible indicators of an impact on the nervous system included increased tremors, decreased visual habituation, exaggerated startle, and increased hand-to-mouth behavior. However, at one and two years of age, no cannabis-related effects were observed when children were assessed using the Bayley Scales (Fried and Watkinson, 1988). No cannabis-related effects were observed at three years on tests of language expression, comprehension, and other general cognitive abilities, after controlling for confounding variables (Fried and Watkinson, 1990).

Age four assessments of OPPS children revealed cannabis-related performance decrements on verbal and memory tasks (Fried and Watkinson, 1990). These deficits were similar in type to another study of three-year-olds whose mothers smoked marijuana while pregnant (Day et al., 1994). One hypothesis for why impairment was not observed until age four is the possibility that such deficits may not be detectable until individuals reach a developmental age that allows for testing of more subtle effects on complex processes (Hutchings and Fried, 1999). However, similar testing at five and six years of age did not reveal any cannabis-related deficits. The authors suggested that environmental exposure to positive influences on cognitive abilities (e.g., school) might have obviated the subtle effects observed a year earlier. Thus, the researchers initiated additional testing of six-year-olds to assess other more general aspects of cognitive performance such as sustained attention and impulse control. Evidence of a deficit in sustained attention was observed in children whose mothers used marijuana heavily during pregnancy (O'Connell and Fried, 1991).

Testing at nine and twelve years of age showed marijuana-related deficits in measures of higher order or executive functioning that the investigators characterized as involving visual analysis, problem solving, hypothesis testing, and impulse control (Fried and Watkinson, 2000; Hutchings and Fried, 1999). Of note, these types of complex functioning deficits are similar to those observed in some studies of chronic adolescent and adult marijuana users (reviewed later in this chapter). Replication of these types of deficits has been reported in another sample in the United States (Goldschmidt, Day, and Richardson, 2000; Richardson et al., 2002). In this study, adverse effects of prenatal marijuana use in ten-year-olds were observed that included increased hyperactivity, impulsivity, inattention, and delinquency. A recent follow-up of the Ottawa sample showed continued effects of prenatal cannabis exposure on 14- to 16-year-olds on tests of visual memory, analysis, and integration (Fried, Watkinson, and Gray, 2003).

The observed effects of prenatal cannabis use on cognitive functioning appear subtle, and determining causality is difficult since genetic predispositions and multiple environmental factors after birth may interact with prenatal effects specific to cannabis use. The functional significance of these subtle deficits is also unclear; however, the types of impairment observed in the OPPS study could potentially affect general behavioral and cognitive performance abilities. Although these data are far from conclusive, they do raise concern regarding prenatal cannabis use and its effects on human offspring. As such, recommendations that pregnant women abstain from marijuana use appear warranted.

PSYCHOLOGICAL CONSEQUENCES

Acute Effects

A number of behavioral and emotional symptoms are associated with the intoxicating effects of cannabis. Generally, cannabis users experience mild euphoria, relaxation, and perceive an overall positive change of sensation and experience (food, music, and interpersonal). Mild problems in thought and speech (loss of train of thought, loose associations, distortion in time perception) commonly occur, but these are not deemed aversive by most users; rather, they are perceived as a positive aspect of the "high."

Cannabis intoxication appears to influence several aspects of social behavior, although relatively little research has been conducted in this area. The most consistent finding is some degree of introverted behavior (decreased verbal interactions), an effect that is uncommon among most drugs of abuse (Foltin and Fischman, 1988; Higgins and Stitzer, 1986; Kelly et al., 1990, 1994). In laboratory studies, cannabis intoxication generally does not change the amount of time individuals spend engaging in social activities (Heishman, Stitzer, and Yingling, 1989; Kelly et al., 1990, 1994). Rather, subjects tend to choose activities that do not require verbal communication (e.g., watching a movie with others). Cannabis intoxication may also increase the distance subjects maintain from each other in social situations (Rachlinski, Foltin, and Fischman, 1989). These social effects of cannabis intoxication might be considered consistent with the increased anxiety and mild paranoia reported by some users. In addition, such effects among frequent users could potentially impact adolescent peer development and the quality of adult social relationships.

The most common adverse psychological reactions to acute intoxication include anxiety attacks, mild paranoia, and increased general anxiety (Schuckit, 1990; Thomas, 1996). Little data on prevalence exist regarding these acute reactions, but they appear to occur in less experienced users, or in experienced users who ingest unusually high doses or use in a novel environment. These symptoms are typically of short duration and subside within hours of their onset. Most of the time they do not result in help-seeking, although they may be associated with marijuana-related emergency room visits. Such effects are typically managed with education, empathic support, and reassurance. With much less frequency, cannabis ingestion has been associated with more severe psychotic reactions, such as hallucinations and delusions (see the following section on psychosis for further information).

Mental Health/Nonpsychotic Disorders

Cross-sectional and longitudinal studies have reported a clear association between chronic cannabis use and impaired psychological functioning (Brooks, Balka, and Whiteman, 1999; Chen, Wagner, and Anthony, 2002; Deykin, Levy, and Wells, 1986; Fergusson and Horwood, 1997; Kandel, 1984; Kandel et al., 1986; McGee et al., 2000; Miller-Johnson et al., 1998; Patton et al., 2002). In particular, cannabis use has been associated with poorer life satisfaction, increased mental health treatment and hospitalization, higher rates of depression, anxiety disorders, suicide attempts, and conduct disorder.

Whether cannabis use contributes to or causes these mental health problems, or the converse, remains equivocal. Controlling for risk factors common to both problems appears to reduce but not eliminate the positive association (Ferguson and Horwood, 1997; Fergusson, Horwood, and Swain-Campbell, 2002; Kandel et al., 1986; McGee et al., 2000). The direction of influence may depend on the age of onset of cannabis use (Degenhardt, Hall, and Lynskey, 2003; Fergusson, Horwood, and Swain-Campbell, 2002; Green and Ritter, 2000; McGee et al., 2000). Early onset of cannabis use is a strong predictor of later mental health problems, but such early onset may be predicted from prior mental health problems. Of note, the types of mental health problems that remain associated with cannabis use, once common etiological factors are adequately controlled in longitudinal studies, are typically externalizing problems such as conduct/antisocial disorder or drug dependence disorders.

Cannabis use can be considered a risk factor for mental health problems and, as such, a target for prevention and intervention. Mental health problems and early cannabis use appear to share a pathway predicted by socioeconomic disadvantage and child behavior problems (McGee et al., 2000), however, cannabis use may also contribute directly to poor psychosocial outcomes (Fergusson, Horwood, and Swain-Campbell, 2002). More data on the causal nature of this relationship is needed.

Psychosis

Whether or not marijuana use can induce psychosis (hallucinations, delusions, thought disorder, and impaired reality testing) or psychotic disorders (e.g., schizophrenia) remains controversial, although data supporting such a causal relationship are emerging. Here we discuss data addressing the relationship between acute psychosis and cannabis, followed by a more extensive discussion of the relationship between cannabis and schizophrenia.

Acute Psychosis

Clinical case reports frequent the literature with examples of patients with psychotic symptoms whose onset closely follows ingestion of cannabis and whose symptoms remit within days or, at most, a few weeks of abstinence from cannabis (Schuckit, 1990). Typical symptoms include hallucinations, delusions, confusion, amnesia, paranoia, hypomania, and labile mood, although case reports vary regarding which and how many of these symptoms are observed across patients. Prevalence data on this phenomenon are limited and range from it being very rare to occurring in over 15 percent of cannabis users (Degenhardt and Hall, 2001; Johns, 2001; Thomas, 1996). Varying operational definitions of "acute psychosis" likely contribute to the wide range of prevalence estimates.

Suggestive evidence for a causal relationship between cannabis use and acute psychosis is of three types. First, in most case reports, the psychosis appears to involve large doses of cannabis. Large doses of THC have been shown to produce hallucinations in human and nonhuman laboratory studies (Georgotas and Zeidenberg, 1979; Kaymakcalan, 1973). Second, many cases of purported cannabis-induced psychosis involve patients without previous psychiatric histories. Third, the psychotic symptoms usually remit within days. Nonetheless, the literature linking cannabis use and acute psychosis includes only uncontrolled studies, thus other causes for the psychosis cannot be ruled out. One could reasonably conclude that high doses of cannabis can precipitate psychosis in some individuals, but whether or not a predisposition to psychotic illness or some other baseline factor is necessary for psychosis to occur is unknown.

Some researchers have attempted to differentiate acute toxic psychosis (due to direct intoxicating effects) from acute functional psychosis that is precipitated by chronic cannabis use but not necessarily due to its intoxicating effects (Thacore and Shukla, 1976). This distinction is difficult to operationalize since acute psychotic effects described across studies typically continue well after (days to weeks) the known duration of the direct effects of cannabis (hours). Hence, discriminating between "functional" or "toxic" effects presents a most difficult methodological challenge. Although studies have attempted to do so by examining differences in cannabis use patterns, responses to medication, and patterns of psychotic symptoms, results remain inconclusive (Thornicroft, 1990).

Schizophrenia

A number of research studies indicate that cannabis use has some relation to the development and course of schizophrenia, however, the causal nature of this association is difficult to study and remains unfounded. The argument for cannabis use precipitating schizophrenia is primarily supported by research showing that drug-abusing schizophrenics have an earlier onset of the disorder and drug use usually precedes reports of psychotic symptoms, show fewer negative symptoms, and show better response to medications than those schizophrenics who do not abuse drugs (Andreasson, Allebeck, and Rydberg, 1989; Mueser et al., 1990). The most well-cited study on this topic is a 15-year prospective study conducted in Sweden (Andreasson et al., 1987). Researchers found that cannabis use at age 18 significantly increased risk for development of schizophrenia after controlling for other premorbid characteristics related to risk of schizophrenia, and the more frequent the cannabis use, the greater the risk. A follow-up to that study with additional subjects confirmed these findings (Zammit et al., 2002).

Even this prospective study has methodological weaknesses that preclude drawing conclusions regarding the causal influence of cannabis. This literature has been critically reviewed in detail elsewhere (Channabasavanna, Paes, and Hall, 1999), thus, here we offer just a few limitations inherent to this research. First, cannabis use may be initiated due to a prodromal syndrome of schizophrenia, or conversely, as might be the case in the Swedish study, good premorbid adjustment of future schizophrenics might increase the likelihood of contact with peers who use illicit drugs. Second, use of other drugs that can produce acute psychosis, such as amphetamines, has typically not been accounted for in most studies. Third, some studies do a poor job of differentiating schizophrenia from acute psychotic episodes which results in the inclusion of acute, cannabis-associated psychoses when documenting cases of schizophrenia.

Course of Illness

How ongoing cannabis use affects the course of schizophrenia has important implications for the treatment and management of schizophrenia, as the rate of cannabis use among schizophrenics exceeds that of the general population and those with other types of psychiatric disorders (Negrete and Gill, 1999). The direct effects of cannabis intoxication, such as distorted time perception, cognitive impairment, and increased paranoia, along with reports of high doses causing hallucinations, delusions, and hypomania, would suggest that regular marijuana use may exacerbate psychiatric problems, particularly in those with major mental illnesses such as schizophrenia. Significant associations between drug use and increased use of treatment resources (hospitalizations and emergency room visits) and poor treatment compliance have been reported in psychiatric patients in general (Bartels et al., 1993; Leon et al., 1998; Richardson, Craig, and Haugland, 1985). The role of cannabis in most studies, however, has not been isolated from the use of other types of drugs. Marijuana use has been associated with increased rates of recurrent psychiatric symptomatology and relapse among schizophrenics (Jablensky et al., 1991; Linszen, Dingemans, and Lenior, 1994; Linszen et al., 1997; Martinez-Arevalo, Calcedo-Ordonez, and Varo-Prieto, 1994; Negrete, 1989; Soni and Brownlee, 1991), but, again, effects of other drug use cannot be completely ruled out in these studies. It must be noted that heavy cannabis use may also result in a misdiagnosis of cannabis-related psychosis resulting in a concomitant delay of a diagnosis and treatment of schizophrenia (Mathers et al., 1991). Recently, a three-year prospective study bolstered the evidence suggesting that cannabis use may adversely impact the course of psychosis (van Os et al., 2002). Cannabis use was associated with the more severe adverse effects among those showing psychosis prior to the study than those without psychotic symptoms. Also, those using cannabis at the start of the study were more likely to show severe symptoms at the follow-up.

As in the general population, cannabis use among psychiatric patients is associated with poorer psychosocial adjustment, criminal behavior, homelessness, and suicidality, but the causal direction of this association is unclear. These factors may contribute to the poor psychiatric outcome observed in schizophrenic cannabis users. As with the data on cannabis use and the development of psychotic disorders, a relatively strong association exists between cannabis use and a negative outcome in schizophrenics. Thus, cannabis use can be considered a risk factor for schizophrenia and a predictor of poor outcome in schizophrenic patients, but its role as an etiological factor remains uncertain.

COGNITIVE EFFECTS

Marijuana has long been thought to affect cognitive function. Early reviews, however, concluded that the scientific evidence for long-term deficits was inconclusive (Wert and Raulin, 1986a,b). This conclusion remains appropriate if one is referring to gross deficits with severe impairment of functioning. More recent findings from well-controlled studies indicate that cannabis use can lead to subtle, selective cognitive impairment (Solowij, 1999), although the functional significance of these deficits remains unclear. Specifically, tasks requiring "higher cognitive function" show significant deficits associated with chronic and frequent use of cannabis. The ability to organize and integrate complex information appears compromised, most likely due to an effect of cannabis on memory and attentional processes. A considerable research literature in this area has accumulated. Here, we provide a summary of the types of deficits associated with marijuana use in more recent studies and comment on the possible mechanisms involved.

Psychomotor Performance

Psychomotor performance measures provide a means of evaluating basic cognitive functions such as slowdown of response. We begin with a summary of this literature because general deficits in this area can affect performance on most of the other cognitive tasks. The Digit Symbol Substitution Task (DSST) (Lezak, 1995) has been the most commonly used measure of psychomotor performance in cannabis studies. Marijuana- or oral-THC-produced decrements in DSST response speed and accuracy have been observed in some studies, but not in others (Azorlosa et al., 1992; Foltin et al., 1993; Heishman, Arasteh, and Stitzer, 1997; Heishman, Stitzer, and Bigelow, 1988; Kamien et al., 1994; Kelly, Foltin, and Fischman, 1993; Kelly et al., 1990; Pickworth, Rohrer, and Fant, 1997). Marijuana's effects on other psychomotor tasks have also proved inconclusive. Performance decreases on circular lights, standing steadiness, and pursuit rotor tracking tasks have been reported in some studies (Chesher et al., 1990; Cone et al., 1986), while others have found no significant effects on circular light, tracking, card sorting, or reaction time tasks (Heishman, Arasteh, and Stitzer, 1997; Heishman, Stitzer, and Bigelow, 1988; Pickworth, Rohrer, and Fant, 1997).

With some exceptions, dose appears to partially account for study *differences*. Significant adverse effects are typically observed with higher doses, and dose-response effects have been observed in some studies that used multiple-dosing procedures. In summary, there appears to be moderately strong evidence that marijuana or THC used at higher doses can impair performance on some psychomotor tasks. This literature does not indicate a pervasive response slowing, such as decrements on simple reaction time tasks. Rather, tasks that are affected appear to depend more heavily on attention and motivation. As discussed later, cannabis intoxication may reduce the steady state of motivation. As performance on most cognitive tests is influenced by the degree of attention and motivation directed toward the specific task, determining how cannabis affects these processes is necessary for a better understanding of its influence on cognitive processing.

Attention and Memory

Acute Effects

Laboratory research on the acute effects of cannabis use on memory has generally shown subtle effects that appear linked to dose and an associated attention or learning deficit. Research on immediate word recall, digit span, and digit recognition tasks has produced equivocal results. Some studies show evidence of impaired performance on short-term memory tasks following marijuana intoxication (Block, Farinpour, and Braverman, 1992; Chait, Corwin, and Johanson, 1988; Galanter et al., 1973; Heishman, Stitzer, and Yingling, 1989), while others have not (Casswell and Marks, 1973; Heishman, Arasteh, and Stitzer, 1997; Hooker and Jones, 1987). Dose-related effects can explain some but not all of these conflicting outcomes, as impairment was evident primarily in studies that examined higher doses.

Cannabis intoxication also affects the subjective perception of time. Time estimates are shorter and time productions are longer in subjects after smoking marijuana compared with placebo or no drug use (Cappell and Pliner, 1973; Chait, 1990; Jones and Stone, 1970). Cannabis intoxication does not appear to affect the ability to reproduce a time interval that has been modeled (Dornbush, Fink, and Freedman, 1971; Heishman, Arasteh, and Stitzer, 1997). The mechanism for this temporal processing impairment is not clear, but deficits in attention warrant consideration.

The effects of marijuana on longer-term memory tasks (retrieval of information following a significant lapse in time) have proven more reliable across studies. Smoked marijuana has produced deficits in the recall of word lists and of prose material presented to subjects in placebo-controlled studies (Block, Farinpour, and Braverman, 1992; Heishman, Arasteh, and Stitzer, 1997; Hooker and Jones, 1987; Perez-Reyes et al., 1991; Wetzel, Janowsky, and Clopton, 1982; Zacny and Chait, 1989). Interestingly, when retrieval cues are used, the impairment of marijuana on these memory tasks may be obviated (Block and Wittenborn, 1984a, b; Hooker and Jones, 1987). Such findings suggest that effects on attentional or learning processes may be primary mechanisms for memory performance deficits associated with cannabis use. Indeed, marijuana has been shown to disrupt the ability to learn novel tasks (Kamien et al., 1994). Moreover, marijuana or THC-related deficits have generally been observed on divided attention tasks in which subjects must monitor multiple stimuli concurrently and make responses based on their observations (Azorlosa et al., 1992; Burns and Moskowitz, 1981; Chait, Corwin, and Johanson, 1988; Heishman, Stitzer, and Yingling, 1989; Kamien et al., 1994; Marks and MacAvoy, 1989; Perez-Reyes et al., 1988).

Methodological differences across studies make it difficult to interpret findings on cannabis and memory. Nonetheless, this literature indicates that the acute effects of cannabis on memory are moderate at most, and are likely dose dependent. The mechanism for these effects remains unclear, but deficits in attention and learning appear involved. How motivational factors impact these findings is also not clear. Interestingly, one early study reported that subjects performed better on memory tasks when they knew that the effects of marijuana on memory were being tested (Mendelson, Rossi, and Meyer, 1974).

Chronic Effects

Studies of the chronic effects of cannabis on cognitive processes have tried to examine the effects of chronic use while controlling for acute intoxication effects. A series of studies by Solowij (1999) examined the long-term effects of cannabis use on attentional processes. Regular cannabis users' performance on an auditory selective-attention task was measured after at least 24 hours of abstinence from cannabis use. Cannabis users' performances were significantly worse than that of matched controls, suggesting an inability to filter out complex irrelevant information. These findings were replicated in a second study that also demonstrated an association between years of marijuana use and the severity of attentional focus and information integration deficits. Moreover, a reduction in event-related potentials (P300 amplitude), a purported marker of cognitive processing, coincided with observed cognitive deficits.

Solowij et al. (1997) also reported significant deficits in a study of long-term, heavy cannabis users interested in quitting marijuana use. Increased perseveration on the Wisconsin Card Sorting Test and decreased memory on a verbal learning task were observed, and the severity of impairment was found to increase with the duration of regular marijuana use. Similarly, Leavitt et al. (1993) reported that the duration of chronic cannabis use was related to deficits on tasks of verbal learning, complex reaction time, complex reasoning, and short-term memory. Pope and Yurgelun-Todd (1996) reported similar deficits in a study of heavy versus light marijuana-using college students with shorter histories of cannabis use. Again, a 24-hour abstinence period was required prior to testing. Heavy marijuana users made significantly more perseverative errors on the Wisconsin Card Sorting Test, had poorer recall on a verbal learning task, and showed other deficits on specific tasks compared with light users. The authors characterized their findings as deficits of the attentional/executive system involving mental flexibility, learning, and sustained attention. Solowij et al. (2002) compared the neurocognitive functioning of longer-term cannabis users with shorter-term cannabis users seeking treatment for cannabis dependence and reported that the former faired worse following a short period of abstinence.

Two controlled studies of adolescent marijuana abusers reported deficits in specific types of memory and learning tasks, further extending the potential impact of cannabis use to a younger sample (Millsaps, Azrin, and Mittenberg, 1994; Schwartz et al., 1989). In addition, early onset of chronic cannabis use has recently been associated with impaired reaction time in visual scanning tasks but this relationship was not observed in late-onset users (Ehrenreich et al., 1999). This finding suggests the possibility of a specific vulnerability for development of an attentional impairment during early adolescence, and raises further concern about the impact of regular cannabis use on cognitive development and school performance.

The first study to examine whether cognitive impairment related to chronic cannabis use recovers following cessation of use compared ex-users (last use ranging from three months to six years), current long- and short-term users, and nonusers on a selective attention task and event-related potentials (Solowij et al., 1995). Findings suggested that ex-cannabis smokers continued to show impairment in their ability to filter out irrelevant information, although some evidence of partial recovery was noted. More recently, Bolla et al. (2002) examined heavy cannabis users following 28 days of abstinence and found continued impairment on multiple measures that increased in proportion to the severity of their cannabis use. In contrast, Pope et al. (2001) reported that heavy cannabis users showed signs of impairment for a least seven days post abstinence, but observed no cannabis associated deficits by day 28 of abstinence.

Historically, interpretation of findings on the chronic effects of cannabis use has been limited by multiple confounding variables such as possible acute marijuana intoxication effects, variable marijuana use histories, unknown cognitive abilities prior to marijuana exposure, concurrent use of other drugs, demographic influences, and comorbidity with other mental or physical illnesses. Recent studies have made strong effort to control for many of these variables, however, important confounds remain. For example, some studies have required a brief period of abstinence prior to testing to control for the acute intoxicating effects of cannabis. However, this procedure introduces another potential confound, that is, whether acute withdrawal effects impact performance testing (Budney et al., 2004). Moreover, as in studies of the acute effects of cannabis on cognitive performance tests, adverse effects on motivation may contribute to the deficits observed in studies of chronic cannabis use and performance. That is, chronic users may not expend as much effort toward testing as those in control groups. Much of this literature is summarized and discussed in a recent literature review (Grant et al., 2003).

Notwithstanding the methodological issues inherent to this research, the literature strongly suggests that chronic marijuana use can impair performance on various types of cognitive tests, specifically those thought to involve complex cognitive processes. These deficits may increase in form and severity in relation to the duration of exposure to cannabis. Future research is needed to better elucidate the processes that cause performance deficits and to determine their functional significance.

Academic Performance

Cannabis use has been linked to low grade-point averages, decreased academic satisfaction, negative attitudes toward school, poor overall performance in school, and absence from school (Lynskey and Hall, 2000). Early cannabis use (prior to age 16) is associated with dropping out of school before graduating high school and failure to complete college (Brooks, Balka, and Whiteman, 1999; Fergusson and Horwood, 1997; Fergusson, Horwood, and Beautrais, 2003; Fergusson, Lynskey, and Horwood, 1996). However, causality between cannabis use and poor academic achievement has not been established. Cannabis use also correlates significantly with delinquency, other drug problems, poor mental health, family dysfunction, and relationships with deviant peers, each of which is a likely contributor to academic problems. Studies that have statistically controlled to these factors have reported mixed results regarding the impact of cannabis use and academic performance (Ellickson et al., 1998; Fergusson, Horwood, and Beautrais, 2003; Krohn, Lizotte, and Perez, 1997; Tanner, Davies, and O'Grady, 1999).

Although one might expect that the adverse effects of cannabis use on attentional and complex cognitive processing would have some direct influence on optimal academic performance, the extent of this influence, if any, is unknown. Similarly, if cannabis use adversely affects motivation, one would expect a subsequent negative impact on academic performance through a decreased effort directed toward school work. The aforementioned other psychosocial problems associated with frequent cannabis use and concomitant effects on motivation to achieve in school would likely have a greater impact on a youth's academic performance than the subtle cannabis-related deficits in complex processing observed in laboratory studies. Whether marijuana use is a primary cause of academic problems or the converse, educational and behavioral problems lead to marijuana use, remains at issue.

Driving Performance

The effects of cannabis intoxication on driving have been examined using driving simulators and road tests during which lane position, emergency decisions (braking latency), and risk-taking behavior (speed, passing attempts, and headway distance) are assessed. Studies on lane position have produced mixed results (Casswell, 1977; Hansteen, Miller, and Lonero, 1976; Klonoff, 1974; Peck et al., 1986; Ramaekers, Robbe, and O'Hanlon, 2000; Robbe and O'Hanlon, 1999; Smiley, Moskowitz, and Zeidman, 1981; Stein et al., 1983). Cannabis intoxication has been shown to adversely affect performance in emergency situations (Dott, 1972; Liguori, Gatto, and Robinson, 1998; Smiley, Moskowitz, and Zeidman, 1981). When no warnings are provided, performance in emergency situations declines and brake latency increases. Cannabis has also been shown to adversely affect one's ability to attend to extraneous stimuli while driving, which may contribute to poor performance in emergency situations (Casswell, 1977; Smiley, Moskowitz, and Zeidman, 1981).

Cannabis use appears to decrease risk-taking behavior in driving situations. An association between cannabis intoxication and a reduction in speed has been observed across studies. In addition, subjects appear more hesitant to perform passing maneuvers and maintain a greater distance from other vehicles when under the influence of cannabis (Dott, 1972; Ellingstad, McFarling, and Struckman, 1973; Robbe and O'Hanlon, 1999; Smiley, Moskowitz, and Zeidman, 1981; Smiley, Noy, and Tostowaryk, 1986).

Adverse effects on driving performance appear most evident when assessed in close temporal proximity to cannabis ingestion and appear to be dose dependent. Performance decrements have not been shown to persist beyond three hours after ingestion. Negative results have typically been observed in studies that use smaller doses of marijuana, less-complicated driving tests, or less-sensitive assessment techniques. Overall, experimental data suggest that cannabis intoxication can decrease control of automobiles as evidenced by variability in lane position and poor performance in emergency situations. However, drivers may partially compensate for these deficits by engaging in low-risk driving behaviors.

Controlled studies have recently examined the effects of the combination of alcohol and cannabis on driving (Liguori, Gatto, and Jarrett, 2001; Ramaekers, Robbe, and O'Hanlon, 2000). Such studies are important as the majority of motor vehicle accidents in which the driver was known to have recently used cannabis, also show that alcohol was used by the same driver. One study of driving performance in real-world conditions reported clear synergistic effects of low doses of cannabis and alcohol on road tracking, time out of appropriate lane position, and increased variability in headway distance (Ramaekers, Robbe, and O'Hanlon, 2000). Performance in a driving simulator study, however, did not report such clear combination effects, as adverse performance effects observed with either substance alone were not exacerbated by the addition of the other (Liguori, Gatto, and Jarrett, 2001). Such conflicting results are difficult to interpret, and indicate the need for additional studies in this area.

Epidemiological studies have been conducted in the United States and Australia in an attempt to define the role of marijuana in major automobile accidents. A review of archival studies using police and laboratory reports assessed the relationship among marijuana use, alcohol use, combined use, and motor vehicle accidents in which serious injuries or fatalities occurred (Bates and Blakely, 1999). The authors concluded that use of marijuana alone was associated with reduced risk of a fatal accident relative to drug-free and alcohol-intoxication-related cases. Alcohol alone and in combination with marijuana was found to be a significant risk factor, with the combination showing slightly higher risk than alcohol alone. Studies of nonfatal injuries provided mixed results regarding the relative risk of marijuana use. A most recent study examined only plasma levels of THC and suggested that the probability of culpability for a specific accident increased with greater plasma levels of THC (Ramaekers et al., 2004).

These epidemiological studies have several important limitations. First, it is difficult to determine whether the obtained cannabinoid metabolite levels relate to acute intoxication at the time of the accident. Second, cases in which traces of cannabis and another illicit substance are found are typically excluded from these studies. As the combination of marijuana and other substances, including alcohol, is the most common finding in accident reviews, the relative contribution of marijuana to these accidents cannot be determined. Third, these studies rarely consider the base rates of cannabis use in comparable populations (young adults) and the concomitant accident rates in that population. More sophisticated methods of detecting marijuana intoxication, well-controlled studies, and inclusion of less severe accidents are needed to more fully understand the role of cannabis use in motor vehicle accidents.

Motivation

Marijuana use has long been associated with an "amotivational syndrome" characterized by lethargy, inactivity, loss of motivation, and decreased goal-directed behavior in heavy marijuana smokers (McGlothlin and West, 1968). Evidence for such amotivational effects comes primarily from case studies and clinical reports. Some chronic cannabis users attribute impaired vocational or academic performance and loss of ambition to their marijuana use (Hendin et al., 1987). Moreover, procrastination and impaired motivation are commonly reported as the consequences of using marijuana and as reasons for stopping use among heavy users and those seeking treatment (Jones, 1984; Schwartz, 1987; Stephens et al., 1993).

Controlled field studies have failed to provide clear evidence of an amotivational syndrome. However, these studies have many methodological limitations relating to sample selection and operational definitions of motivation (Carter, Coggins, and Doughty, 1977; Cohen, 1982; Halikas et al., 1982; Rubin and Comitas, 1976; Stefanis, Dornbush, and Fink, 1977). An Australian study of chronic users reported findings that typify this literature (Didcott et al., 1997). Many users appeared to be underemployed based on their education and abilities but were well integrated into family and community activities. Participants tended to attribute these circumstances to a lifestyle choice rather than an adverse effect of cannabis use. Family members provided mixed reports, as some noted amotivational effects in users, and others cited only positive effects.

Laboratory studies suggest that the motivational effects of cannabis intoxication on operant behavior are dependent on environmental context and contingencies. Miles et al. (1974) showed increased efficiency and no performance decrements when working for monetary reward while under the influence of marijuana. Pihl and Sigal (1978) found that they could reverse performance decrements induced by marijuana intoxication by providing monetary rewards. Other studies have failed to show adverse effects of marijuana on work output. However, the tasks and conditions of these studies may have been insensitive to cannabis effects as participants tended to show maximal performance across conditions (Foltin et al., 1990; Mendelson, Rossi, and Meyer, 1974).

Cherek et al., cited in Budney et al. (1997), used a more sensitive operant measure of motivation in a laboratory study of cannabis intoxication. Subjects could choose to spend time working on a high-demand task that earned monetary reinforcement, or switch to a no-demand task that earned a lower level of reinforcement. With this choice available, subjects spent less time working on the high-demand task when under the influence of marijuana than with placebo, suggesting an amotivational effect. This effect appeared dose dependent and was partially reversed by increasing the magnitude of the reinforcement in the high-demand task. This suggests that the amotivational effects of cannabis intoxication may occur by impacting the effects of reinforcement on various types of operant behavior (e.g., change sensitivity). The interaction among cannabis's behavioral effects and environmental variables needs further study to better understand the association between cannabis use and motivation.

There remains little scientific evidence that chronic cannabis use leads to an amotivational syndrome that could not be accounted for by chronic intoxication (Hall, Solowij, and Lemon, 1994). Laboratory studies that compare chronic users with nonusers on performance of operant tasks, while controlling for acute intoxication effects, may provide more important information and address the validity of a chronic effect of cannabis on motivation. It should be noted that the acute motivational effects on operant performance observed in the laboratory indicate that motivation should be considered when interpreting studies that examine the effects of cannabis on any cognitive or behavioral performance task.

Cannabis Dependence

Whether cannabis use can lead to dependence has been a controversial topic in both the lay and scientific communities. Personal experiences may bias many people toward the perception that cannabis is not addictive. More than one-third of the U.S. population has smoked marijuana in their lifetime. Most have not become addicted and have stopped using without difficulty. Moreover, unlike alcohol, cocaine, heroin, or nicotine dependence, most people are not familiar with personal acquaintances who have had problems with marijuana dependence, nor are sensational accounts of problems associated with marijuana common in the popular media.

The scientific community has also been reluctant to acknowledge the dependence potential of cannabis. Unlike most other drugs that humans abuse, animals do not readily self-administer THC in the laboratory. As drug-dependence research has a productive history of using animal models to explicate drug dependence, this methodological issue raised serious questions about the abuse potential of cannabis. Further quandries arose when early studies of THC withdrawal did not reveal a syndrome that included substantial physical symptoms such as those observed during classic opioid, barbiturate, or alcohol withdrawal. Until recently, the neurobiology of cannabis was poorly understood, leading to further uncertainty regarding this drug's addictive potential.

In contrast, the past 15 years of basic and clinical research has produced strong evidence for concluding that cannabis can and does produce dependence (see Budney and Moore, 2002, for a review). Here we review data addressing two facets of the dependence phenomenon: functional (behavioral) dependence and biological (physiological) dependence. Although this distinction can be considered artificial, it appears a logical way to organize new information in this area.

Functional (Behavioral) Dependence

Both the *Diagnostic and Statistical Manual of Mental Disorders,* Fourth Edition (DSM-IV) (American Psychiatric Association, 1994), and the *International Statistical Classification of Diseases and Related Health Problems,* Tenth Revision (ICD-10) (WHO, 1992), consider cannabis dependence a reliable and valid diagnostic category of mental disorder suggesting that individuals in the general population experience cannabis dependence in much the same way as they experience other substance dependence disorders (Budney et al., 2006). By definition, a diagnosis of dependence indicates that an individual although experiencing a cluster of cognitive, behavioral, or physiological symptoms associated with substance use continues to use the substance regularly. Two epidemiological studies conducted in the United States and another in New Zealand indicate that the lifetime prevalence of marijuana dependence approximates 4 to 5 percent of the population, the highest of any illicit drug (Anthony and Helzer, 1991; Anthony, Warner, and Kessler, 1994; Hall, Johnston, and Donnelly, 1999; Wells et al., 1992).

Such high prevalence of cannabis dependence in comparison with other illicit drugs is clearly due to the greater overall prevalence of cannabis use. The estimated conditional dependence rate for cannabis dependence is lower than most other drugs of abuse, but is certainly significant. That is, the risk of developing marijuana dependence among those who have used marijuana is approximately 9 percent compared with 12 percent for stimulants, 15 percent for alcohol, 17 percent for cocaine, 23 percent for heroin, and 32 percent for tobacco (Anthony, Warner, and Kessler, 1994). More frequent cannabis use results in greater risk of dependence. For example, rates of dependence are estimated at 20 to 30 percent among those who have used cannabis at least five times, and even higher (35 to 40 percent) estimates are reported among those who report near daily use (Hall, Solowij, and Lemon, 1994; Kandel and Davis, 1992).

Clinical studies indicate that the majority of individuals who seek treatment for marijuana-related problems clearly meet DSM dependence criteria (Budney et al., 2000, 2006; Stephens, Roffman, and Curtin, 2000; MTRPG, 2004). These individuals exhibit substantial psychosocial impairment and psychiatric distress, report multiple adverse consequences, report repeated unsuccessful attempts to stop using marijuana, and perceive themselves as unable to quit (Budney et al., 1998; Roffman and Barnhart, 1987;

Stephens, Roffman, and Simpson, 1993). A report comparing marijuana-dependent outpatients with cocaine-dependent outpatients found that the marijuana patients reported substance-use histories and psychosocial impairment comparable to the cocaine group, but showed less-severe dependence symptoms. The marijuana group was also more ambivalent and less confident about stopping their marijuana use than the cocaine group was about their cocaine use. Although marijuana-dependent outpatients typically do not experience the acute crises or severe consequences that many times drive alcohol-, cocaine-, or heroin-dependent individuals into treatment, they clearly show impairment that warrants clinical attention.

The number of individuals who enroll for treatment of marijuana-related problems is not small. Seeking treatment for marijuana abuse or dependence increased twofold between 1993 and 2005, such that the percentage of illicit-drug-abuse-treatment admissions in U.S. state-approved agencies for marijuana was 16 percent, was approximately 14 percent, for cocaine, and 14 percent for heroin (SAMHSA, 2005a,b). The response to treatment and relapse rates observed among marijuana-dependent outpatients appeared similar to those observed with other substances of abuse (Budney et al., 2006; Moore and Budney, 2003; Stephens, Roffman, and Curtin, 2000; Stephens, Roffman, and Simpson, 1994). In summary, clinical evidence for a cannabis dependence disorder is strong and indicative of a disorder of substantial severity.

Biological (Physiological) Dependence

Physiological dependence has typically been determined by evidence of tolerance or withdrawal. Tolerance to the physiological, cognitive, and social effects of marijuana or cannabinoids has been well documented. Controlled human laboratory studies have clearly shown that tolerance develops to the subjective high, heart rate increases, social interaction deficits, and some of the cognitive and psychomotor performance deficits associated with THC ingestion (Compton, Dewey, and Martin, 1990). In contrast, many regular marijuana users report a lack of tolerance to the subjective effects of marijuana use, with some reporting a sensitization effect (less of the drug is needed to produce the desired effect). Sensitization has not been demonstrated in controlled studies, and some have suggested that this phenomenon may be related to learning how to smoke more efficiently or to better identify the effects of cannabis (Stephens, 1999).

Withdrawal has generally been deemed a more robust indicator of dependence than tolerance. Early nonhuman studies of cessation of THC administration provided evidence of a withdrawal response, but the effects were mild and inconsistent (Beardsley, Balster, and Harris, 1986; Kaymakcalan, 1973).

Early studies with humans in residential laboratories also found evidence of withdrawal (Georgotas and Zeidenberg, 1979; Jones and Benowitz, 1976; Mendelson et al., 1984; Nowlan and Cohen, 1977). Common symptoms included decreased appetite, irritability, restlessness, sleep difficulties, and uncooperativeness. These effects were characterized as mild, transient, and without serious medical complications, and thus considered clinically insignificant when compared with the dramatic medical and physiological symptoms associated with severe opiate or alcohol withdrawal.

The discovery of a cannabinoid receptor (Devane et al., 1988) and the synthesis of a cannabinoid antagonist renewed scientific interest in cannabis dependence and withdrawal. Antagonist-challenge studies demonstrated a marked, precipitated withdrawal syndrome in rats and dogs (Aceto et al., 1996; Lichtman et al., 1998). Two placebo-controlled inpatient studies with humans, using moderate doses of oral THC and smoked marijuana, demonstrated withdrawal effects that included anxiety, decreased contentment and food intake, depressed mood, irritability, restlessness, sleep difficulty, and stomach pain (Haney, Comer, et al., 1999; Haney, Ward, et al., 1999). Controlled outpatient studies have now begun to demonstrate the reliability and validity of these withdrawal effects and examine their timecourse (Budney et al., 2001, 2003; Kouri and Pope, 2000).

Clinical studies indicate that the majority of persons seeking treatment for cannabis dependence, including adolescents, report histories of cannabis withdrawal (Budney et al., 2004; Vandrey, Budney, Kamon, et al., 2005). For example, in our research clinic the majority (57 percent) of marijuana-dependent outpatients reported experiencing >6 symptoms of at least moderate severity during previous abstinence attempts. Severity was associated with more frequent marijuana use (Budney, Novy, and Hughes, 1999).

Cannabis withdrawal is not currently recognized in the DSM-IV, which concludes that the clinical significance of the syndrome is yet to be established. We expect that findings from recent research will result in its inclusion in the next revision of the DSM (see Budney et al., 2004 for a review). Cannabis withdrawal syndrome resembles that observed during nicotine withdrawal (Vandrey, Budney, Moore, et al., 2005; Vandrey, Budney, Hughes, in press). It appears common among treatment seekers and may warrant attention in clinical settings. Additional research is needed to better determine its prevalent clinical significance.

Other recent neurobiological findings further support the conclusion that cannabis can produce dependence. The documentation of an endogenous cannabinoid system with identified cannabinoid receptors (CB1 and CB2) and an endogenous cannabinoid-like substance (anandamide) established that the actions of cannabinoids in the brain occur in a manner similar to that of other drugs with well-recognized addictive potential such as opiates or benzodiazepines. The aforementioned precipitated-withdrawal studies demonstrated that withdrawal from cannabinoids likely occurs via a process similar to that of other abused drugs. Studies that have examined neurochemical responses in animals following exposure to and withdrawal from cannabinoids have observed reductions in mesolimbic dopamine transmission and elevations in extracellular-releasing-factor concentrations in the limbic system that closely resemble the responses seen with other major drugs of abuse (deFonseca et al., 1997; Diana et al., 1998). The behavioral consequences of these neurobiological changes are consistent with the type of negative affective symptoms reported by patients withdrawing from marijuana and other substances, and may be primary contributing factors to the development and maintenance of drug dependence (Koob et al., 1997). In summary, research findings from the 1990s indicate that the biological risk factors for cannabis dependence appear more similar to other well-recognized addictive drugs than was previously believed.

MEDICAL MARIJUANA

In addition to the adverse consequences on health previously discussed, cannabis may also have beneficial effects for a number of medical conditions. Oral THC (dronabinol) has been approved by the U.S. Food and Drug Administration for use as an appetite- and food-intake stimulant in patients with AIDS wasting syndrome and as an antinausea and antivomiting agent in cancer patients receiving chemotherapy. In 1999, the Institute of Medicine and the National Institutes of Health acknowledged the importance of initiating additional scientific study of the risks and benefits of cannabis use and, in particular, the use of smoked marijuana for specific medical conditions. The interest in the benefits of smoked marijuana in contrast to oral THC arises primarily from *differences* in the pharmacokinetics of these two routes of administration. Through the oral route, THC absorption is slow and variable, and therefore clinical effects have a slower onset and longer duration than smoked marijuana. In addition, smoked marijuana not only delivers delta-9-THC, but other compounds (e.g., delta-8-THC and cannabidiol) are absorbed that may have direct or interactive effects of therapeutic interest.

Illnesses Involving Appetite, Food Intake, and Nausea Problems

Acute cannabis use can increase appetite and food intake. Single- and multiple-dose studies with marijuana and oral THC consistently show increases in food intake and food choice, as cannabis intoxication appears to result in frequent snacking and increased choice of sweet solid foods (Abel, 1971; Foltin, Brady, and Fischman, 1986; Greenburg et al., 1976; Haney, Comer, et al., 1999; Haney, Ward, et al., 1999; Hollister, 1971; Kelly et al., 1990). Interestingly, recent studies also show that abrupt discontinuation of oral THC or marijuana can result in decreased appetite and food intake, as well as concomitant weight loss during the first few days of withdrawal (Budney et al., 2001; Haney, Comer, et al., 1999; Haney,Ward, et al., 1999).

Cannabis's ability to facilitate appetite and food consumption prompted consideration of use of oral THC and smoked marijuana in clinical populations such as patients with AIDS wasting syndrome. Controlled case studies suggest some benefit from cannabis and THC for increasing appetite and weight gain in patients with AIDS wasting syndrome, but mixed results best characterize this literature (Beal et al., 1995, 1997; Plasse et al., 1991; Timpone et al., 1997).

Cancer patients' reports of the efficacy of smoked marijuana for relief from the nausea and vomiting associated with chemotherapy have stimulated study of such effects using oral THC and smoked marijuana (Grinspoon and Bakalar, 1997; Hollister, 2000). Placebo-controlled studies demonstrated the efficacy of dronabinol for this purpose, although other antiemetic drugs may work as well and are accompanied by fewer side effects (Gralla et al., 1984; Grunberg and Hesketh, 1993; Sallan, Zinberg, and Freii, 1975; Sallan et al., 1980; Schwartz and Beveridge, 1994). The efficacy of smoked marijuana in this clinical population has received little systematic study. Case reports commonly indicate the benefits of smoked marijuana, but the only controlled study conducted thus far did not demonstrate it to be superior to dronabinol (Grinspoon and Bakalar, 1997; Levitt et al., 1984).

As mentioned earlier, the problem with absorption of THC when taken orally in contrast to the efficiency of THC delivery with smoked marijuana has triggered the call for the more systematic study of smoked marijuana as an optimal method for achieving antiemetic and appetite effects in these clinical populations. However, the potential adverse effects of smoked marijuana on immune system function (reviewed previously) must be carefully considered as a contraindication for the use of smoked marijuana with immune-compromised clinical populations. Controlled research comparing the efficacy of oral THC and smoked marijuana is needed to determine whether cannabis should be considered a treatment of choice for severe problems with nausea and appetite in chronically ill populations. A most recent controlled study with HIV-positive individuals indicates comparable positive effects with oral THC and smoked marijuana (Haney et al., in press).

Analgesia

The discovery of the endogenous cannabinoid system has rekindled interest in the use of cannabis for the treatment of pain. Elevated levels of cannabinoid receptors are located in areas of the brain that modulate nociception and can also be found in peripheral tissue. Recent research in nonhumans using animal models of pain indicate that cannabinoid agonists clearly exert analgesic effects in both the central nervous system (CNS) and the periphery. The mechanisms for these analgesic effects differ from that of the opioids; hence, the potential use of cannabinoids as an adjunct or alternative treatment for acute or chronic pain has received increased attention.

The evidence for the analgesic effects of cannabis in humans is less clear. Historically, the few studies of the effects of cannabis, THC, or other cannabinoid analogues on acute pain (i.e., laboratory induced or surgical) have not produced impressive results (Clark et al., 1981; Hill et al., 1974; Jain et al., 1981; Libman and Stern, 1985; Raft et al., 1977). Greenwald and Stitzer (2000) reported significant dose-dependent antinociceptive effects of smoked marijuana using a radiant-heat pain stimulus. However, the effects on pain reduction were not clinically robust and lasted less than one hour. Unfortunately, most of the research in this area has not been methodologically strong, making interpretation of findings difficult.

Early research on chronic pain demonstrated that oral THC and a nitrogen analog produced analgesia similar to codeine, but side effects (sedation and depersonalization) were significant (Noyes, Brunk, Avery, et al., 1975; Noyes, Brunk, Baram, et al., 1975; Staquet, Gantt, and Machin, 1978). To date, most of the evidence for the efficacy of smoked marijuana in pain reduction in clinical populations experiencing chronic pain comes from case reports and survey studies. Patients have reported relief from cancer-related chronic pain, pain related to neurological disease, muscle spasticity, and headaches as well as phantom limb pain (Consroe et al., 1997; Dunn and Davis, 1974; Grinspoon and Bakalar, 1997). Many of these patients cite the superiority of smoked marijuana when compared with other treatments they have tried. Marijuana's positive effects on nausea and appetite make it particularly attractive for chronic-pain patients who also experience problems in these areas (e.g., cancer chemotherapy or AIDS patients). Moreover, the "positive" effect of cannabis on mood may further add to its desirability among patients with these types of chronic debilitating illnesses.

Again, the potential differences in the effects of delivering THC and the other compounds found in cannabis through smoking compared with oral administration are reason enough to pursue additional study of smoked marijuana as an analgesic agent. Controlled studies are needed to (1) compare smoked cannabis with dronabinol, (2) compare cannabis with other analgesics, and (3) examine the effects of combinations of cannabis and other analgesics (e.g., opioids). However, there is reason to hope that additional basic research on the analgesic effects of cannabinoids might result in the development of efficacious agents that do not produce the other problematic effects of THC such as sedation, memory problems, and intoxication.

Other Medical Indications

Spasticity Associated with Movement Disorders

Case studies have suggested that cannabis might help alleviate tremors, spasms, or loss of coordination associated with multiple sclerosis or other neurological disorders such as spinal cord injury (Clifford, 1983; Consroe, Sandyk, and Snider,1986; Consroe et al., 1997; Malec, Harvey, and Cayner, 1982; Meinck, Schonle, and Conrad, 1989; Ungerleider et al., 1987). Controlled studies have not been conducted. Uncontrolled trials of oral THC have produced some evidence for a reduction in spasticity in patients with multiple sclerosis and spinal cord injury, but the effect has not been uniform and multiple side effects including loss of impaired posture and balance have been reported (Clifford, 1983; Greenberg et al., 1994; Malec, Harvey, and Cayner, 1982; Petro and Ellenberger, 1981; Ungerleider et al., 1987). Conclusions regarding the efficacy of cannabis and other cannabinoids for the treatment of muscle spasticity await data from controlled studies.

Glaucoma

Both smoked marijuana and dronabinol can reduce intraocular pressure that contributes to glaucoma and its progression (Joy, Watson, and Benson, 1999). Nonetheless, cannabis use is no longer a good choice for treatment of this disease. THC clearly reduces intraocular pressure, but this effect is transient and thus requires chronic high doses, multiple times a day to achieve the desired therapeutic response. Although not the case 10 to 20 years ago, alternative local treatments are now available which require less frequent dosing and have fewer adverse side effects than cannabis. Hence, cannabis should no longer be considered a treatment of choice for glaucoma.

The current literature on medical indications for cannabis includes primarily uncontrolled case studies or open clinical trials with only a handful of controlled studies of dronabinol conducted, mostly in the 1970s. Nonetheless, a number of medical indications appear to have enough support to warrant additional investigation. Much more data on the efficacy of smoked marijuana and oral THC for various medical conditions will soon become available, as the NIH and other funding sources (e.g., Center for Medicinal Cannabis Research, UCSD, San Diego, CA) have initiated focused efforts to stimulate research in this area.

SUMMARY AND CONCLUSIONS

Cannabis use engenders health risks across many areas of functioning. The magnitude of such effects and their clinical significance remains difficult to discern in many domains. The probability of experiencing many of the adverse health effects mentioned in this chapter is also not clear. We know that dose, frequency, and duration of cannabis use increase risk, but this relationship has not been well quantified. We also remain uncertain regarding the etiologic role of cannabis use in the occurrence of many of the negative effects reported in the literature. Heavy cannabis users typically have numerous other characteristics that are known risk factors for health and behavior problems. Continued investigation directed toward a better understanding of the interaction between these factors and cannabis use is necessary to understand more fully the impact of cannabis use on human functioning and health.

Despite these caveats, the scientific evidence for substantial cannabis related adverse effects appears strong enough for individuals who use or who are considering using cannabis to be made aware of these potential negative outcomes. Overall, such outcomes appear less severe than those associated with alcohol, tobacco, heroin, or cocaine abuse (Hall, Room, and Bondy, 1999). However, that does not mean they should be ignored. As with other substances of abuse, many individuals use cannabis without significant consequence, but others misuse, abuse, or become dependent and experience adverse outcomes. Moreover, cannabis use may have positive effects and even legitimate medical benefits for persons with specific types of illnesses, yet this could also be said of the many other substances that are abused. The ongoing controversy and legalization debate over marijuana has spawned distrust in scientific data. If we stop treating cannabis as a special case, and consider it as we would other psychoactive substances, a reasonable assumption is that some level of use (i.e., misuse) will result in harmful effects (Hall, 1999). We still have much to learn about the parameters of cannabis use that result in adverse consequences, but a wealth of new knowledge has accumulated during the past decade of research. Our understanding of its potential for harm has increased and these new findings warrant our attention and additional study.

REFERENCES

Abel, E.L. (1971). Effects of marijuana on the solution of anagrams, memory, and appetite. *Nature,* 231:260-261.

Aceto, M.; Scates, S.; Lowe, J.; Martin, B. (1996). Dependence on delta-9 tetrahydrocannabinol: Studies on precipitated and abrupt withdrawal. *J Pharmacol Exp Ther,* 278:1290-1295.

American Psychiatric Association (1994). *Diagnostic and Statistical Manual of Mental Disorders,* Fourth Edition. Washington, DC: American Psychiatric Association.

Andreasson, S.; Allebeck, P.; Engstrom, A.; Rydberg, U. (1987). Cannabis and schizophrenia: A longitudinal study of Swedish conscripts. *Lancet,* 2:1483-1486.

Andreasson, S.; Allebeck, P.; Rydberg, U. (1989). Schizophrenia in users and nonusers of cannabis. A longitudinal study in Stockholm County. *Acta Psychiatr Scand,* 79:505-510.

Anthony, J.C.; Helzer, J.E. (1991). Syndromes of drug abuse and dependence. In: Robins, L.N.; Regier, D.A. (eds.), *Psychiatric Disorders in America* (pp. 116-154). New York: Free Press.

Anthony, J.; Warner, L.; Kessler, R. (1994). Comparative epidemiology of dependence on tobacco, alcohol, controlled substances, and inhalants: Basic findings from the National Comorbidity Survey. *Exp Clin Psychopharmacol,* 2:244-268.

Azorlosa, J.L.; Heishman, S.J.; Stitzer, M.L.; Mahaffey, J.M. (1992). Marijuana smoking: Effect of varying delta-9-tetrahydrocannabinol content and number of puffs. *J Pharmacol Exp Ther,* 261:114-122.

Baldwin, G.C.; Tashkin, D.P.; Buckley, D.M.; Park, A.N.; Dubinett, S.M.; Roth, M.D. (1997). Marijuana and cocaine impair alveolar macrophage function and cytokine production. *Am J Respir Crit Care Med,* 156:1606-1613.

Barbers, R.G.; Evans, M.J.; Gong, H.; Tashkin, D.P. (1991). Enhanced alveolar monocytic phagocyte (macrophage) proliferation in tobacco and marijuana smokers. *Am Rev Respir Dis,* 143:1092-1095.

Barsky, S.F.; Roth, M.D.; Kleerup, E.C.; Simmons, M.; Tashkin, D.P. (1998). Histopathologic and molecular alterations in bronchial epithelium in habitual smokers of marijuana, cocaine, and/or tobacco. *J Natl Cancer Inst,* 90:1198-1205.

Bartels, S.J.; Teague, G.B.; Drake, R.E.; Clark, R.E.; Bush, P.W.; Noordsy, D.L. (1993). Substance abuse in schizophrenia: Service utilization and costs. *J Nerv Ment Dis,* 181:227-232.

Bates, M.N.; Blakely, T.A. (1999). Role of cannabis in motor vehicle crashes. *Epidemiol Rev,* 21:222-232.

Beaconsfield, P.; Ginsburg, J.; Rainsbury, R. (1972). Marijuana smoking: Cardiovascular effects in man and possible mechanisms. *N Engl J Med,* 287:209-212.

Beal, J.F.; Olson, R.; Laubenstein, L.; Morales, J.O.; Bellman, P.; Yango, B.; Lefkowitz, L.; Plasse, T.F.; Shepard, K.V. (1995). Dronabinol as a treatment for anorexia associated with weight loss in patients with AIDS. *J Pain Symptom Manage,* 10:89-97.

Beal, J.F.; Olson, R.; Lefkowitz, L.; Laubenstein, L.; Bellman, P.; Yango, B.; Morales, J.O. et al. (1997). Long-term efficacy and safety of dronabinol for anorexia. *J Pain Symptom Manage*, 14:7-14.

Beardsley, P.M.; Balster, R.L.; Harris, L.S. (1986). Dependence on tetrahydrocannabinol in rhesus monkeys. *J Pharmacol Exp Ther*, 239:311-319.

Benowitz, N.L.; Jones, R.T. (1975). Cardiovascular effects of prolonged delta-9-tetrahydrocannabinol ingestion. *Clin Pharmacol Ther*, 18:287-297.

Black, S.; Casswell, S. (1993). *Drugs in New Zealand: A Survey in 1990*. Auckland, New Zealand: University of Auckland, Alcohol and Public Health Research Unit.

Block, R.I.; Farinpour, R.; Braverman, K. (1992). Acute effects of marijuana on cognition: Relationships to chronic effects and smoking techniques. *Pharmacol Biochem Behav*, 43:907-917.

Block, R.I.; Farinpour, R.; Schelchtem, J.A. (1991). Effects of chronic marijuana use on testosterone, luteinizing hormone, follicle stimulating hormone, prolactin and cortisol in men and women. *Drug Alcohol Depend*, 28:121-128.

Block, R.I.; Wittenborn, J.R. (1984a). Marijuana effects on semantic memory: Verification of common and uncommon category members. *Psychol Rep*, 55:503-512.

Block, R.I.; Wittenborn, J.R. (1984b). Marijuana effects on visual imagery in a paired-associate task. *Percept Mot Skills*, 58:759-766.

Bloom, J.W.; Kaltenborn, W.T.; Paoletti, P.; Camilli, A.; Lebowitz, M.D. (1987). Respiratory effects of non-tobacco cigarettes. *Br Med J*, 295:1516-1518.

Bolla, K.I.; Brown, K.; Eldreth, D.; Tate, K.; Cadet, J.L. (2002). Dose-related neurocognitive effects of marijuana use. *Neurology*, 59:1337-1343.

Brooks, J.S.; Balka, E.B.; Whiteman, M. (1999). The risks for late adolescence of early adolescent marijuana use. *Am J Public Health*, 89(10):1549-1554.

Budney, A.J.; Higgins, S.T.; Radonovich, K.J.; Novy, P.L. (2000). Adding voucher based incentives to coping-skills and motivational enhancement improves outcomes during treatment for marijuana dependence. *J Consult Clin Psychol*, 68:1051-1061.

Budney, A.J.; Hughes, J.R. (2006). The cannabis withdrawal syndrome. *Curr Opin Psychiatry*, 19:233-238.

Budney, A.J.; Hughes, J.R.; Moore, B.A.; Novy, P.L. (2001). Marijuana abstinence effects in marijuana smokers maintained in their home environment. *Arch Gen Psychiatry*, 58:917-924.

Budney, A.J.; Hughes, J.R.; Moore, B.A.; Vandrey, R.A. (2004). A Review of the validity and significance of the cannabis withdrawal syndrome. *Am J Psychiatry*, 161:1967-1977.

Budney, A.J.; Kandel, D.; Cherek, D.R.; Martin, B.R.; Stephens, R.S.; Roffman, R. (1997). Marijuana use and dependence: College on problems of drug dependence annual meeting, Puerto Rico (June, 1996). *Drug Alcohol Depend*, 45:1-11.

Budney, A.J.; Moore, B.A. (2002). Development and consequences of cannabis dependence. *J Clin Pharmacol*, 42(11 Suppl):28S-33S.

Budney, A.J.; Moore, B.A.; Higgins, S.T.; Rocha, H.L. (2006). Clinical trial of abstinence-based vouchers and cognitive-behavioral therapy for cannabis dependence. *J Consul Clin Psychol*, 74:307-316.

Budney, A.J.; Moore, B.A.; Vandrey, R.; Hughes, J.R. (2003). The time course and significance of cannabis withdrawal. *J Abnorm Psychol,* 112(3): 393-402.

Budney, A.J.; Novy, P.; Hughes, J.R. (1999). Marijuana withdrawal among adults seeking treatment for marijuana dependence. *Addiction,* 94(9):1311-1322.

Budney, A.J.; Radonovich, K.J.; Higgins, S.T.; Wong, C.J. (1998). Adults seeking treatment for marijuana dependence: A comparison to cocaine-dependent treatment seekers. *Exp Clin Psychopharmacol,* 6:419-426.

Burns, M.; Moskowitz, H. (1981). Alcohol, marijuana, and skills performance. In: Goldburg, L. (ed.), *Alcohol, Drugs and Traffic Safety* (pp. 954-968). Stockholm: Almqvist and Wiksell International.

Caiaffa, W.T.; Vlahov, D.; Graham, N.M.; Astemborski, J.; Solomon, L.; Nelson, K.E.; Munoz, A. (1994). Drug smoking, pneumocystis carinii pneumonia and immunosuppression increase risk of bacterial pneumonia in human immunodeficiency virus-seropositive injection drug users. *Am J Respir Crit Care Med,* 150:1493-1498.

Caplan, G.A.; Brigham, B.A. (1990). Marijuana smoking and carcinoma of the tongue: Is there an association? *Cancer,* 66:1005-1006.

Cappell, H.D.; Pliner, P.L. (1973). Volitional control of marijuana intoxication: A study of the ability to come down on command. *J Abnorm Psychol,* 1:428-434.

Carter, W.E.; Coggins, W.; Doughty, P.L. (1977). *Cannabis in Costa Rica: A Study of Chronic Marijuana Use.* Philadelphia: Institute for the Study of Human Issues.

Casswell, S. (1977). Cannabis and alcohol: Effects on closed course driving behaviour. In: Johnson, I. (ed.), *Seventh International Conference on Alcohol, Drugs, and Traffic Safety* (pp. 238-246). Melbourne, Australia.

Casswell, S.; Marks, D.F. (1973). Cannabis and temporal disintegration in experienced and naive subjects. *Science,* 179:803-805.

Chait, L.D. (1990). Subjective and behavioral effects of marijuana the morning after smoking. *Psychopharmacology (Berl),* 100:328-333.

Chait, L.D.; Corwin, R.L.; Johanson, C.E. (1988). A cumulative dosing procedure for administering marijuana smoke to humans. *Pharmacol Biochem Beh,* 29: 553-557.

Channabasavanna, S.M.; Paes, M.; Hall, W. (1999). Mental and behavioral disorders due to cannabis. In: Kalant, H.; Corrigall, W.A.; Hall, W.; Smart, R.G. (eds.), *The Health Effects of Cannabis* (pp. 267-290). Toronto: Centre for Addictions and Mental Health.

Chasnoff, I.J. (1990). Cocaine use in pregnancy: Effect on infant neurobehavioural functioning. Paper presented at the American Society for Pharmacology and Experimental Therapeutics, Washington, DC.

Chen, C.Y.; Wagner, F.A.; Anthony, J.C. (2002). Marijuana use and the risk of major depressive episode. Epidemiological evidence from the United States National Comorbidity Survey. *Soc Psychiatry Psychiatr Epidemiol,* 37:199-206.

Chesher, G.B.; Bird, K.D.; Jackson, D.M.; Perrignon, A.; Starmer, G.A. (1990). The effects of orally administered delta-9-tetrahydrocannabinol in man on mood and performance measures: A dose-response study. *Pharmacol Biochem Behav,* 35:861-864.

Clark, W.C.; Janal, M.N.; Zeidenberg, P.; Nahas, G.G. (1981). Effects of moderate and high doses of marihuana on thermal pain: A sensory decision theory analysis. *J Clin Pharmacol*, 21:S299-S310.

Clifford, D.B. (1983). Tetrahydrocannabinol for tremor in multiple sclerosis. *Ann Neurol*, 13:669-671.

Cohen, S. (1982). Cannabis effects upon adolescent motivation. *Marijuana and Youth: Clinical Observations on Motivation and Learning* (pp. 2-10). Rockville, MD: National Institute on Drug Abuse.

Compton, D.R.; Dewey, W.L.; Martin, B.R. (1990). Cannabis dependence and tolerance production. *Adv Alcohol Subst Abuse*, 9:129-147.

Cone, E.J.; Johnson, R.E.; Moore, J.D.; Roache, J.D. (1986). Acute effects of smoking marijuana on hormones subjective effects and performance in male human subjects. *Pharmacol Biochem Behav*, 24:1749-1754.

Consroe, P.; Musty, R.; Rein, J.; Tillery, W.; Pertwee, R. (1997). The perceived effects of smoked cannabis on patients with multiple sclerosis. *Eur Neurol*, 38:44-48.

Consroe, P.; Sandyk, R.; Snider, S.R. (1986). Open label evaluation of cannabidiol in dystonic movement disorders. *Int J Neurosci*, 30:277-282.

Crowley, T.J.; MacDonald, M.J.; Whitmore, E.A.; Mikulich, S.K. (1998). Cannabis dependence, withdrawal, and reinforcing effects among adolescents with conduct disorder symptoms and substance use disorders. *Drug Alcohol Depend*, 50:27-37.

Day, N.; Richardson, G.A. (1991). Prenatal marijuana use: Epidemiology, methodological issues and infant outcome. In: Chasnoff, I. (ed.), *Clinics in Perinatology* (pp. 77-92). Philadelphia: W.B. Saunders.

Day, N.; Richardson, G.A.; Goldschmidt, L.; Robles, N.; Taylor, P.M.; Stoffer, D.S.; Cornelius, M.D.; Geva, D. (1994). The effect of prenatal exposure on the cognitive development of offspring at age three. *Neurotoxicol Teratol*, 16:169-176.

deFonseca, F.R.; Carrera, M.R.A.; Navarro, M.; Koob, G.F.; Weiss, F. (1997). Activation of corticotropin-releasing factor in the limbic system during cannabinoid withdrawal. *Science*, 276:2050-2054.

Degenhardt, L.; Hall, W.; Lynskey, M. (2001). Alcohol, cannabis and tobacco use among Australians: A comparison of their associations with other drug use and use disorders, affective and anxiety disorders, and psychosis. *Addiction*, 96:1603-1614.

Degenhardt, L.; Hall, W.; Lynskey, M. (2003). Exploring the association between cannabis use and depression. *Addiction*, 98:1493-1504.

Devane, W.A.; Dysarz, F.A.; Johnson, M.R.; Melvin, L.S.; Howlett, A.C. (1988). Determination and characterization of a cannabinoid receptor in rat brain. *Mol Pharmacol*, 34:605-613.

Deykin, E.Y.; Levy, J.C.; Wells, V. (1986). Adolescent depression, alcohol, and drug abuse. *Am J Public Health*, 76:178-182.

Diana, M.; Melis, M.; Muntoni, A.L.; Gessa, G.L. (1998). Mesolimbic dopaminergic decline after cannabinoid withdrawal. *Proc Natl Acad Sci USA*, 95:10269-10273.

Didcott, P.; Reilly, D.; Swift, W.; Hall, W. (1997). *Long Term Cannabis Users on the New South Wales North Coast.* Sydney: National Drug and Alcohol Research Centre.

Donald, P.J. (1991). Advanced malignancy in the young marijuana smoker. *Adv Exp Med Biol,* 288:33-46.

Dornbush, R.L.; Fink, M.; Freedman, A.M. (1971). Marijuana memory and perception. *Am J Psychiatry,* 128:194-197.

Dott, A.B. (1972). *Effect of Marijuana on Risk Acceptance in a Simulated Passing Task.* Washington, DC: U.S. Government Printing Office.

Dunn, M.; Davis, R. (1974). The perceived effects of marijuana on spinal cord injured males. *Paraplegia,* 12:175.

Ehrenreich, H.; Rinn, T.; Kunert, H.J.; Moeller, M.R.; Poser, W.; Schilling, L.; Gigerenzer, G.; Hoehe, M.R. (1999). Specific attentional dysfunction in adults following early start of cannabis use. *Psychopharmacology (Berl),* 142:295-301.

Ellickson, P.; Bui, K.; Bell, R.; McGuigan, K.A. (1998). Does early drug use increase the risk of dropping out of high school? *J Drug Issues,* 28:357-380.

Ellingstad, V.S.; McFarling, L.H.; Struckman, D.L. (1973). *Alcohol, Marijuana, and Risk Taking.* Vermillion, SD: South Dakota University, Vermillion Human Factors Laboratory.

Fergusson, D.M.; Horwood, L.J. (1997). Early onset cannabis use and psychosocial adjustment in young adults. *Addiction,* 92(3):279-296.

Fergusson, D.M.; Horwood, L.J.; Beautrais, A.L. (2003). Cannabis and educational achievement. *Addiction,* 98:1681-1692.

Fergusson, D.M.; Horwood, L.J.; Swain-Campbell, N. (2002). Cannabis use and psychosocial adjustment in adolescence and young adulthood. *Addiction,* 97: 1123-1135.

Fergusson, D.M.; Lynskey, M.T.; Horwood, L.J. (1996). The short-term consequences of early cannabis use. *J Abnorm Child Psychol,* 24(4):499-512.

Fligiel, S.E.G.; Beals, T.F.; Tashkin, D.P.; Paule, M.G.; Scallet, A.L.; Ali, S.F.; Bailey, J.R.; Slikker, W. Jr. (1991). Marijuana exposure and pulmonary alterations in primates. *Pharmacol Biochem Behav,* 40:637-642.

Fligiel, S.E.G.; Roth, M.D.; Kleerup, E.C.; Barsky, S.H.; Simmons, M.S.; Tashkin, D.P. (1997). Tracheobronchial histopathology in habitual smokers of cocaine, marijuana, and/or tobacco. *Chest,* 112:319-326.

Foltin, R.W.; Brady, J.V.; Fischman, M.W. (1986). Behavioral analysis of marijuana effects on food intake in humans. *Pharmacol Biochem Behav,* 25:577-582.

Foltin, R.W.; Fischman, M.W. (1988). Effects of smoked marijuana on human social behavior in small groups. *Pharmacol Biochem Behav,* 30:539-541.

Foltin, R.W.; Fischman, M.W.; Brady, J.V.; Bernstein, D.J.; Capriotti, R.M.; Nellis, M.J.; Kelly, T.H. (1990). Motivational effects of smoked marijuana: Behavioral contingencies and low-probability activities. *J Exp Anal Behav,* 53(1):5-19.

Foltin, R.W.; Fischman, M.W.; Pippen, P.A.; Kelly, T.H. (1993). Behavioral effects of cocaine alone and in combination with ethanol or marijuana in humans. *Drug Alcohol Depend,* 32:93-106.

Fried, P.A. (1980). Marijuana use by pregnant women: Neurobehavioral effects in neonates. *Drug Alcohol Depend,* 6:415-424.

Fried, P.A.; Barnes, M.V.; Drake, E.R. (1985). Soft drug use after pregnancy compared to use before and during pregnancy. *Am J Obstet Gynecol,* 151:787-792.

Fried, P.A.; Watkinson, B. (1988). 12- and 24-month neurobehavioral follow-up of children prenatally exposed to marijuana, cigarettes, and alcohol. *Neurotoxicol Teratol,* 10:305-313.

Fried, P.A.; Watkinson, B. (1990). 36- and 48-month neurobehavioural follow-up of children prenatally exposed to marijuana, cigarettes, and alcohol. *J Dev Behav Pediatr,* 11:49-58.

Fried, P.A.; Watkinson, B. (2000). Visuoperceptual functioning differs in 9- to 12 year olds prenatally exposed to cigarettes and marihuana. *Neurotoxicol Teratol,* 22:11-20.

Fried, P.; Watkinson, B.; Gray, R. (2003). Differential effects on cognitive functioning in 13- to 16-year olds prenatally exposed to cigarettes and marihuana. *Neurotoxicol Teratol,* 25:427-436.

Fung, M.; Gallagher, C.; Machtay, M. (1999). Lung and aero-digestive cancers in young marijuana smokers. *Tumori,* 85:140-142.

Galanter, M.; Weingartner, H.; Vaughn,·T.B.; Roth, W.T.; Wyatt, R.J. (1973). Delta-9-transtetrahydrocannabinol and natural marijuana. *Arch Gen Psychiatry,* 28: 278-281.

Georgotas, A.; Zeidenberg, P. (1979). Observations on the effects of four weeks of heavy marijuana smoking on group interaction and individual behavior. *Compr Psychiatry,* 20:427-432.

Gibson, G.T.; Baghurst, P.A.; Colley, D.P. (1983). Maternal alcohol, tobacco and cannabis consumption and the outcome of pregnancy. *Aust NZ J Obstet Gynaecol,* 23:15-19.

Gil, E.; Chen, B.; Kleerup, E.; Webber, M.; Tashkin, D.P. (1995). Acute and chronic effects of marijuana smoking on pulmonary alveolar permeability. *Life Sci,* 56:2193-2199.

Goldschmidt, L.; Day, N.L.; Richardson, G.A. (2000). Effects of prenatal marijuana exposure on child behavior problems at age 10. *Neurotoxicol Teratol,* 22:325-336.

Gong, H.; Fligiel, S.; Tashkin, D.P.; Barbers, R.G. (1987). Tracheobronchial changes in habitual, heavy smokers of marijuana with and without tobacco. *Am Rev Respir Dis,* 136:142-149.

Gralla, R.J.; Tyson, L.B.; Bordin, L.A.; Clark, R.A.; Kelsen, D.P.; Kris, M.G.; Kalman, L.B.; Groshen, S. (1984). Antiemetic therapy: A review of recent studies and a report of a random assignment trial comparing metoclopramide with delta-9-tetrahydrocannabinol. *Cancer Treat Rep,* 68:163-172.

Grant, I.; Gonzalez, R.; Carey, C.L.; Natarajan, L.; Wolfson T. (2003). Non-acute (residual) neurocognitive effects of cannabis use: A meta-analytic study. *J Int Neuropsychol Soc,* 9(5):679-689.

Green, B.E.; Ritter, C. (2000). Marijuana use and depression. *J Health Soc Behav,* 41:40-49.

Greenberg, H.S.; Werness, S.A.; Pugh, J.E.; Andrus, R.O.; Anderson, D.J.; Domino, E.F. (1994). Short-term effects of smoking marijuana on balance in patients with multiple sclerosis and normal volunteers. *Clin Pharmacol Ther,* 55:324-328.

Greenburg, I.; Kuehnle, J.; Mendelson, J.H.; Bernstein, J.G. (1976). Effects of marijuana use on body weight and caloric intake in humans. *Psychopharmacology (Berl),* 49:79-84.

Greenwald, M.K.; Stitzer, M.L. (2000). Antinociceptive, subjective and behavioral effects of smoked marijuana in humans. *Drug Alcohol Depend,* 59:261-275.

Grinspoon, L.; Bakalar, J.B. (1997). *Marihuana, the Forbidden Medicine* (p. 296). New Haven, CT: Yale University Press.

Grunberg, S.M.; Hesketh, P.J. (1993). Control of chemotherapy-induced emesis. *N Engl J Med,* 329:1790-1796.

Haas, A.P.; Hendin, H. (1987). The meaning of chronic marijuana use among adults: A psychosocial perspective. *J Drug Issues,* 17:333-348.

Halikas, J.A.; Weller, R.A.; Morse, C.L.; Hoffman, R.G. (1983). Regular marijuana use and its effects on psychosocial variables: Longitudinal study. *Compr Psychiatry,* 24:229-235.

Halikas, J.A.; Weller, R.A.; Morse, C.; Shapiro, T. (1982). Incidence and characteristics of amotivational syndrome, including associated findings, among chronic marijuana users. *Marijuana and Youth: Clinical Observations on Motivation and Learning* (pp. 11-26). Rockville, MD: National Institute on Drug Abuse.

Hall, W. (1999). Assessing the health and psychological effects of cannabis use. In: Kalant, H.; Corrigall, W.A.; Hall, W.; Smart, R. G. (eds.), *The Health Effects of Cannabis* (pp. 1-18). Toronto: Centre for Addiction and Mental Health.

Hall, W.; Christie, M.; Currow, D. (2005). Cannabinoids and cancer: Causation, remediation, and palliation. *Lancet Oncology,* 6(1):35-42.

Hall, W.; Johnston, L.; Donnelly, N. (1999). Epidemiology of cannabis use and its consequences. In: Kalant, H.; Corrigall, W.A.; Hall, W.; Smart, R.G. (eds.), *The Health Effects of Cannabis* (pp. 69-126). Toronto: Centre for Addiction and Mental Health.

Hall, W.; Room, R.; Bondy, S. (1999). Comparing the health and psychological risks of alcohol, cannabis, nicotine, and opiate use. In: Kalant, H.; Corrigall, W.A.; Hall, W.; Smart, R.G. (eds.), *The Health Effects of Cannabis* (pp. 475-495). Toronto: Centre for Addiction and Mental Health.

Hall, W.; Solowij, N.; Lemon, J. (1994). *The Health and Psychological Consequences of Cannabis Use.* Canberra, Australia: Australian Government Publication Services.

Haney, M.; Comer, S.D.; Ward, A.S.; Foltin, R.W.; Fischman, M.W. (1999). Abstinence symptoms following oral THC administration to humans. *Psychopharmacology (Berl),* 14:385-394.

Haney, M.; Gunderson, E.W.; Rabkin, J.; Hart, L.L.; Vosburg, S.; Comer, S.; Foltin, R.W. (in press). Dronabinol and marijuana in HIV-positive marijuana smokers: Caloric intake, mood, and sleep. *J Acquired Immune Deficiency Syndrome.*

Haney, M.; Ward, A.S.; Comer, S.D.; Foltin, R.W.; Fischman, M.W. (1999). Abstinence symptoms following smoked marijuana in humans. *Psychopharmacology (Berl),* 14:395-404.

Hansteen, R.W.; Miller, R.D.; Lonero, L. (1976). Effects of cannabis and alcohol on automobile driving and psychomotor tracking. *Ann NY Acad Sci,* 282:240-256.

Hatch, E.E.; Bracken, M.B. (1986). Effect of marijuana use in pregnancy on fetal growth. *Am J Epidemiol,* 124:986-993.

Heishman, S.J.; Arasteh, K.; Stitzer, M.L. (1997). Comparative effects of alcohol and marijuana on mood, memory and performance. *Pharmacol Biochem Behav,* 58:93-101.

Heishman, S.J.; Stitzer, M.L.; Bigelow, G.E. (1988). Alcohol and marijuana: Comparative dose effect profiles in humans. *Pharmacol Biochem Behav,* 31:649-655.

Heishman, S.J.; Stitzer, M.L.; Yingling, J.E. (1989). Effects of tetrahydrocannabinol content on marijuana smoking behavior: Subjective reports and performance. *Pharmacol Biochem Behav,* 34:173-179.

Hendin, H.; Haas, A.P.; Singer, P.; Eller, M.; Ulman, R. (1987). *Living High: Daily Marijuana Use Among Adults.* New York: Human Sciences Press.

Higgins, S.T.; Stitzer, M.L. (1986). Acute marijuana effects on social conversation. *Psychopharmacology (Berl),* 89:234-238.

Hill, S.Y.; Schwin, R.; Goodwin, D.W.; Powell, B.J. (1974). Marijuana and pain. *J Pharmacol Exp Ther,* 188:415-418.

Hingson, R.; Alpert, J.; Day, N.; Dooling, E.; Kayne, H.; Morelock, S.; Oppenheimer, E.; Zuckerman, B. (1982). Effects of maternal drinking and marijuana use on fetal growth and development. *Pediatrics,* 70:539-546.

Hoffman, D.; Brunnemann, K.D.; Gori, G.B.; Wynder, E.L. (1975). On the carcinogenicity of marijuana smoke. In: Runeckles, V.C. (ed.), *Recent Advances in Phytochemistry* (pp. 63-81). New York: Plenum Press.

Hollister, L.E. (1971). Hunger and appetite after single doses of marijuana, alcohol, and dextroamphetamine. *Clin Pharmacol Ther,* 12:44-49.

Hollister, L.E. (2000). An approach to the medical marijuana controversy. *Drug Alcohol Depend,* 58:3-7.

Hooker, W.D.; Jones, R.T. (1987). Increased susceptibility to memory intrusions and the Stroop interference effect during acute marijuana intoxication. *Psychophamacologia,* 91:20-24.

Huber, G.L.; First, M.W.; Grubner, O. (1991). Marijuana and tobacco smoke gas-phase cytotoxins. *Pharmacol Biochem Behav,* 40:629-636.

Hutchings, D.E.; Fried, P.A. (1999). Cannabis during pregnancy: Neurobehavioral effects in animals and humans. In: Kalant, H.; Corrigall, W.A.; Hall, W.; Smart, R.G. (eds.), *The Health Effects of Cannabis* (pp. 401-434). Toronto: Centre for Addiction and Mental Health.

Institute of Medicine (1982). *Marijuana and Health.* Washington, DC: National Academy Press, Institute of Medicine.

Jablensky, A.; Sartorius, N.; Ernberg, G.; Anker, M.; Korten, A.; Cooper, J.E.; Day, R.; Bertelsen, A. (1991). *Schizophrenia: Manifestations, Incidence, and Course in Different Cultures. A World Health Organization Ten-Country Study.* Geneva: World Health Organization.

Jain, A.K.; Ryan, J.R.; McMahon, F.G.; Smith, G. (1981). Evaluation of intramuscular levonantradol and placebo in acute postoperative pain. *J Clin Pharmacol,* 21:320S-326S.

Jones, R.T. (1980). Human effects: An overview. In: Peterson, R.C. (ed.), *Marijuana Research Findings: 1980.* NIDA Research Monograph 31 (pp. 54-80). Washington, DC: U.S. Government Printing Office.

Jones, R.T. (1984). Marijuana: Health and treatment issues. *Psychiatr Clin North Am,* 7:703-712.

Jones, R.T.; Benowitz, N. (1976). The 30-day trip—Clinical studies of cannabis tolerance and dependence. In: Braude, M.C.; Szara, S. (eds.), *Pharmacology of Marihuana* (pp. 627-642). New York: Raven Press.

Jones, R.T.; Stone, G.C. (1970). Psychological studies of marijuana and alcohol in man. *Psychopharmacologia,* 18:108-117.

Joy, J.E.; Watson, S.J.; Benson, J.A. (1999). *Marijuana As Medicine: Assessing the Scientific Base.* Washington, DC: National Academy Press.

Kalant, H. (1999). *The Health Effects of Cannabis.* Toronto: Centre for Addiction and Mental Health.

Kalant, H. (2004). Adverse effects of cannabis on health: An update of the literature since 1996. *Progress in Neuro-Psychopharmacology and Biological Psychiatry,* 28:849-863.

Kamien, J.B.; Bickel, W.K.; Higgins, S.T.; Hughes, J.R. (1994). The effects of delta-9-tetrahydrocannabinol on repeated acquisition and performance of response sequences and on self-reports in humans. *Behav Pharmacol,* 5:71-78.

Kandel, D.B. (1984). Marijuana users in young adulthood. *Arch Gen Psychiatry,* 41:200-209.

Kandel, D.B.; Davies, M. (1992). Progression to regular marijuana involvement: Phenomenology and risk factors of near daily use. In: Glantz, M.; Pickens, R. (eds.), *Vulnerability to Drug Abuse* (pp. 221-253). Washington, DC: American Psychological Association.

Kandel, D.B.; Davies, M.; Karus, D.; Yamaguchi, K. (1986). The consequences in young adulthood of adolescent drug involvement. *Arch Gen Psychiatry,* 43:746-754.

Kaymakcalan, S. (1973). Tolerance to and dependence on cannabis. *Bull Narc,* 25:39-47.

Kelly, T.H.; Foltin, R.W.; Emurian, C.S.; Fischman, M.W. (1990). Multidimensional behavioral effects of marijuana. *Prog Neuropsychopharmacol Biol Psychiatry,* 14:885-902.

Kelly, T.H.; Foltin, R.W.; Fischman, M.W. (1993). Effects of smoked marijuana on heart rate, drug ratings, and task performance by humans. *Behav Pharmacol,* 4:167-178.

Kelly, T.H.; Foltin, R.W.; Mayr, M.T.; Fischman, M.W. (1994). Effects of delta 9-tetrahydrocannabinol and social context on marijuana self-administration by humans. *Pharmacol Biochem Behav,* 49:763-768.

Klein, T.W. (1999). Cannabis and immunity. In: Kalant, H.; Corrigall, W.A.; Hall, W.; Smart, R.G. (eds.), *The Health Effects of Cannabis* (pp. 347-374). Toronto: Centre for Addiction and Mental Health.

Klein, T.W.; Friedman, H.; Specter, S. (1998). Marijuana, immunity, and infection. *J Neuroimmunol,* 83:102-115.

Klonoff, H. (1974). Marijuana and driving in real-life situations. *Science,* 186: 317-324.

Koob, G.F.; Caine, S.B.; Parsons, L.; Markou, A.; Weiss, F. (1997). Opponent process model and psychostimulant addiction. *Pharmacol Biochem Behav,* 57:51-521.

Kouri, E.M.; Pope, H.G. (2000). Abstinence symptoms during withdrawal from chronic marijuana use. *Exp Clin Psychopharmacol,* 8:483-492.

Krohn, M.D.; Lizotte, A.J.; Perez, C.M. (1997). The interrelationship between substance use and precocious transitions to adult statuses. *J Health Soc Behav,* 38(1):87-103.

Kusher, D.I.; Dawson, L.O.; Taylor, A.C.; Djeu, J.Y. (1994). Effect of the psychoactive metabolite of marijuana, delta 9-tetrahydrocannabinol (THC), on the synthesis of tumor necrosis factor by human large granular lymphocytes. *Cell Immunol,* 154:99-108.

Leavitt, J.; Webb, P.; Norris, G.; Struve, F.; Straumanis, J.; Fitz-Gerald, M.; Nixon, F.; Patrick, G.; Manno, J. (1993). Performance of chronic daily marijuana users on neuropsychological tests. In: Harris, L. (ed.), *Problems of Drug Dependence 1992* (p. 179). Washington, DC: U.S. Government Printing Office.

Leon, S.C.; Lyons, J.S.; Christopher, N.J.; Miller, S.I. (1998). Psychiatric hospital outcomes of dual diagnosis patients under managed care. *Am J Addict,* 7:81-86.

Levitt, M.; Faiman, C.; Hawks, R.; Wilson, A. (1984). Randomized double blind comparison of delta-9-tetrahydrocannabinol (THC) and marijuana as chemotherapy antiemetics. *Proceedings of the Meeting of the American Society of Clinical Oncology,* 3:91.

Lezak, M.D. (1995). *Neurophysical Assessment,* Third Edition. New York: Oxford University Press.

Libman, E.; Stern, M.H. (1985). The effects of delta-9-tetrahydrocannabinol on cutaneous sensitivity and its relation to personality. *Pers Indiv Differ,* 6:169-174.

Lichtman, A.H.; Wiley, J.L.; LaVecchia, K.L.; Niviaser, S.T.; Arthur, D.B.; Wilson, D.M.; Martin, B.R. (1998). Effects of SR 141716A after acute or chronic cannabinoid administration in dogs. *J Pharmacol Exp Ther,* 278:1290-1295.

Liguori, A.; Gatto, C.P.; Jarrett, D.B. (2001). *Effects of Marijuana-Alcohol Combinations on Mood, Equilibrium and Simulated Driving.* Scottsdale, AZ: College on Problems of Drug Dependence.

Liguori, A.; Gatto, C.P.; Robinson, J.H. (1998). Effects of marijuana on equilibrium, psychomotor performance, and simulated driving. *Behav Pharmacol,* 9:599-609.

Linszen, D.H.; Dingemans, P.M.; Lenior, M.E. (1994). Cannabis abuse and the course of recent-onset schizophrenic disorders. *Arch Gen Psychiatry,* 51:273-279.

Linszen, D.H.; Dingemans, P.M.; Nugter, M.A.; Does, A.; Scholte, W.F.; Lenior, M.A. (1997). Patient attributes and expressed emotion as risk factors for psychotic relapse. *Schizophr Bull,* 23:119-130.

Lynskey, M.; Hall, W. (2000). The effects of adolescent cannabis use on educational attainment: A review. *Addiction,* 95:1621-1630.

MacPhee, D. (1999). Effects of marijuana on cell nuclei: A review of the literature relating to the genotoxicity of cannabis. In: Kalant, H.; Corrigall, W.A.; Hall, W.; Smart, R.G. (eds.), *The Health Effects of Cannabis* (pp. 291-310). Toronto: Centre for Addiction and Mental Health.

Maddock, R.; Farrell, T.R.; Herning, R.; Jones, R.T. (1979). Marijuana and thermoregulation in a hot environment. In: Cox, B.; Lomax, P.; Milton, A.S.; Schonbaum, E. (eds.), *Thermoregulatory Mechanisms and Their Therapeutic Implications* (pp. 62-64). Basel, NY: Karger.

Malec, J.; Harvey, R.F.; Cayner, J. (1982). Cannabis effect on spasticity in spinal cord injury. *Arch Phys Med Rehabil,* 63:116-118.

Mao, L.; Oh, Y. (1998). Does marijuana or crack cocaine cause cancer? [Comment] *J Natl Cancer Inst,* 90:1182-1183.

Marijuana Treatment Project Research Group. (2004). Brief Treatments for cannabis dependence: Findings from a randomized multisite trial. *J Consul Clin Psychol,* 72:455-466.

Marks, D.F.; MacAvoy, M.F. (1989). Divided attention performance in cannabis users and non-users following alcohol and cannabis separately and in combination. *Psychopharmacology (Berl),* 99:397-401.

Marks, W.H.; Florence, L.; Lieberman, J.; Chapman, P.; Howard, D.; Roberts, P.; Perkinson, D. (1996). Successfully treated invasive pulmonary aspergillosis associated with smoking marijuana in a renal transplant recipient. *Transplantation,* 61:1771-1774.

Marques-Magallanes, J.A.; Tashkin, D.P.; Serafian, T.; Stegeman, J.; Roth, M.D. (1997). In vivo and in vitro activation of cytochrome P4501A1 by marijuana smoke. *1997 Symposium on the Cannabinoids of the International Cannabinoid Research Society,* Stone Mountain, GA.

Martinez-Arevalo, M.J.; Calcedo-Ordonez, A.; Varo-Prieto, J.R. (1994). Cannabis consumption as a prognostic factor in schizophrenia. *Br J Psychiatry,* 164:679-681.

Mathers, D.C.; Ghodse, A.H.; Caan, A.W.; Scott, S.A. (1991). Cannabis use in a large sample of acute psychiatric admissions. *Br J Addict,* 86:779-784.

Mayor's Committee on Marijuana (1944). *The Marijuana Problem in the City of New York.* Lancaster, PA: Jacques Cattell Press.

McGee, R.; Williams, S.; Poulton, R.; Moffitt, T. (2000). A longitudinal study of cannabis use and mental health from adolescence to early adulthood. *Addiction,* 95:491-503.

McGlothlin, W.H.; West, L.J. (1968). The marijuana problem: An overview. *Am J Psychiatry,* 125:370-378.

Meinck, H.M.; Schonle, P.W.; Conrad, B. (1989). Effect of cannabinoids on spasticity and ataxia in multiple sclerosis. *J Neurol,* 236:120-122.

Mendelson, J.H.; Mello, N.K.; Cristofaro, P.; Ellingboe, J.; Benedikt, R. (1985). Acute effects of marijuana on pituitary and gonadal hormones during the periovulatory phase of the menstrual cycle. In: Harris, L.S. (ed.), *Problems of Drug Dependence* (pp. 24-31). Washington, DC: U.S. Government Printing Office.

Mendelson, J.H.; Mello, N.K.; Ellingboe, J.; Skupny, A.T.; Lex, B.W.; Griffin, M. (1986). Marijuana smoking suppresses luteinizing hormone in women. *J Pharmacol Exp Ther,* 237:862-866.

Mendelson, J.H.; Mello, N.K.; Lex, B.W.; Bavli, S. (1984). Marijuana withdrawal syndrome in a woman. *Am J Psychiatry,* 141:1289-1290.

Mendelson, J.H.; Rossi, A.M.; Meyer, R.E. (1974). *The Use of Marijuana: A Psychological and Physiological Inquiry.* New York: Plenum Press.

Miles, C.G.; Congreve, G.R.S.; Gibbins, R.J.; Marshman, J.; Devenyi, P.; Hicks, R.C. (1974). An experimental study of the effects of daily cannabis smoking on behaviour patterns. *Acta Pharmacol Toxicol,* 34(1):1-43.

Miller-Johnson, S.; Lochman, J.E.; Cone, J.D.; Terry, R.; Hyman, C. (1998). Comorbidity of conduct and depressive problems at sixth grade: Substance use outcomes across adolescence. *J Abnorm Child Psychol,* 26:221-232.

Millsaps, C.L.; Azrin, R.L.; Mittenberg, W. (1994). Neuropsychological effects of chronic cannabis use on the memory and intelligence of adolescents. *J Child Adolesc Sub Abuse,* 3:47-55.

Moore, B.A.; Augustson, E.M.; Moser, R.P.; Budney, A.J. (2005). Respiratory effects of marijuana and tobacco use in a U.S. Sample. *J Gen Intern Med,* 20(1):33-37.

Moore, B.A.; Budney, A.J. (2001). Tobacco smoking in marijuana dependent outpatients. *J Subst Abuse,* 13:585-598.

Moore, B.A.; Budney, A.J. (2003). Relapse in outpatient treatment for marijuana dependence. *J Substance Abuse Treat,* 25(2):85-89.

Mouzak, A.; Agathos, P.; Kerezoudi, E.; Mantas, A.; Vourdeli-Yiannakoura, E. (2000). Transient ischemic attack in heavy cannabis smokers—How "safe" is it? *Eur Neurol,* 44:42-44.

Mueser, K.T.; Yarnold, P.R.; Levinson, D.F.; Singh, H.; Bellack, A.S.; Kec, K.; Morrison, R.L.; Yadalam, K. G. (1990). Prevalence of substance abuse in schizophrenia: Demographic and clinical correlates. *Schizophr Bull,* 16:31-56.

Murphy, L. (1999). Cannabis effects on endocrine and reproductive function. In: Kalant, H.; Corrigall, W.A.; Hall, W.; Smart, R.G. (eds.), *Health Effects of Cannabis* (pp. 375-400). Toronto: Centre for Addiction and Mental Health.

Negrete, J.C. (1989). Cannabis and schizophrenia. *Br J Addict,* 84:349-351.

Negrete, J.C.; Gill, K. (1999). Cannabis and schizophrenia: An overview of the evidence to date. In: Nahas, G.G. (ed.), *Marijuana and Medicine* (pp. 671-681). Totowa, NJ: Humana Press.

Newton, C.A.; Klein, T.W.; Friedman, H. (1994). Secondary immunity to *Legionella pneumophila* and Th1 activity are suppressed by delta-9-tetrahydrocannabinol injection. *Infect Immun,* 62:4015-4020.

Nowlan, R.; Cohen, S. (1977). Tolerance to marijuana: Heart rate and subjective "high." *Clin Pharmacol Ther,* 22:550-556.

Noyes, R. Jr.; Brunk, S.F.; Avery, D.H.; Canter, A. (1975). The analgesic properties of delta-9-tetrahydrocannabinol and codeine. *Clin Pharmacol Ther,* 18:84-89.

Noyes, R. Jr.; Brunk, S.F.; Baram, D.; Canter, A. (1975). Analgesic effect of delta 9-tetrahydrocannabinol. *J Clin Pharmacol,* 15:139-143.

O'Connell, C.M.; Fried, P.A. (1984). An investigation of prenatal cannabis exposure and minor physical anomalies in a low risk population. *Neurotoxicol Teratol,* 6:345-350.

O'Connell, C.M.; Fried, P.A. (1991). Prenatal exposure to cannabis: A preliminary report of postnatal consequences in school-age children. *Neurotoxicol Teratol,* 13:631-639.

Patton, G.C.; Coffey, C.; Carlin, J.B.; Degenhardt, L.; Lynskey, M.; Hall, W. (2002). Cannabis use and mental health in young people: Cohort study. *Br Med J* 325:1195-1198.

Peck, R.C.; Biasotti, A.; Boland, P.N.; Mallory, C.; Reeve, V. (1986). The effects of marijuana and alcohol on actual driving performance. *Alcohol, Drugs and Driving,* 2:135-154.

Perez-Reyes, M.; Hicks, R.E.; Bumberry, J.; Jeffcoat, A.R.; Cook, C.E. (1988). Interaction between marijuana and ethanol: Effects on psychomotor performance. *Alcohol Clin Exp Res,* 12:268-276.

Perez-Reyes, M.; Lipton, M.A.; Timmons, M.C.; Walls, M.E.; Brine, D.R.; Davis, K.H. (1973). Pharmacology of administered delta-9-tetrahydrocannabinol. *Clin Pharmacol Ther,* 14:48-55.

Perez-Reyes, M.; White, W.R.; McDonald, S.A.; Hicks, R.E.; Jeffcoat, A.R.; Cook, C.E. (1991). The pharmocologic effects of daily marijuana smoking in humans. *Pharmacol Biochem Behav,* 40:691-694.

Petro, D.J.; Ellenberger, C. Jr. (1981). Treatment of human spasticity with delta 9-tetrahydrocannabinol. *J Clin Pharmacol,* 21:413S-416S.

Pickworth, W.B.; Rohrer, M.S.; Fant, R.V. (1997). Effects of abused drugs on psychomotor performance. *Exp Clin Psychopharmachol,* 5:235-241.

Pihl, R.O.; Sigal, H. (1978). Motivational levels and the marijuana high. *J Abnorm Psychol,* 87(2):280-285.

Plasse, T.F.; Gorter, R.W.; Krasnow, S.H.; Lane, M.; Shepard, K.V.; Wadleigh, R.G. (1991). Recent clinical experience with dronabinol. *Pharmacol Biochem Behav,* 40:695-700.

Polen, M.R.; Sidney, S.; Tekawa, I.S.; Sadler, M.; Friedman, G.D. (1993). Health care use by frequent marijuana smokers who do not smoke tobacco. *West J Med,* 158:596-601.

Pope, H.G. Jr.; Gruber, A.J.; Hudson, J.I.; Huestis, M.A.; Yurgelun-Todd, D. (2001). Neuropsychological performance in long-term cannabis users. *Arch Gen Psychiatry,* 58:909-915.

Pope, H.G.; Yurgelun-Todd, D. (1996). The residual cognitive effects of heavy marijuana use in college students. *JAMA,* 275:521-527.

Rachlinski, J.J.; Foltin, R.W.; Fischman, M.W. (1989). The effects of smoked marijuana on interpersonal distances in small groups. *Drug Alcohol Depend,* 24:183-186.

Raft, D.; Gregg, J.; Ghia, J.; Harris, L. (1977). Effects of intravenous tetrahydro-cannabinol on experimental and surgical pain: Psychological correlates of the analgesic response. *Clin Pharmacol Ther,* 21:26-33.

Rainone, G.A.; Deren, S.; Kleinman, P.H.; Wish, E.D. (1987). Heavy marijuana users not in treatment: The continuing search for the "pure" marijuana user. *J Psychoactive Drugs,* 19:353-359.

Ramaekers, J.G.; Berghaus, G.; van Laar, M.; Drummer, O.H. (2004). Dose related risk of motor vehicle crashes after cannabis use. *Drug Alcohol Depend,* 73:109-119.

Ramaekers, J.G.; Robbe, H.W.J.; O'Hanlon, J.F. (2000). Marijuana, alcohol, and actual driving performance. *Human Psychopharmacol,* 15:551-558.

Renaud, A.M.; Cormier, Y. (1986). Acute effects of marijuana smoking on maximal exercise performance. *Med Sci Sports Exerc,* 18:685-689.

Richardson, G.A.; Ryan, C.; Willford, J.; Day, N.L.; Goldschmidt, L. (2002). Prenatal alcohol and marijuana exposure: Effects on neuropsychological outcomes at 10 years. *Neurotoxicol Teratol,* 24:309-320.

Richardson, M.S.; Craig, T.J.; Haugland, G. (1985). Treatment patterns of young chronic schizophrenic patients in the era of deinstitutionalization. *Psychiatr Q,* 57:104-110.

Robbe, H.J.; O'Hanlon, J.F. (1999). *Marijuana and Actual Driving Performance.* Washington, DC: National Highway Transportation Administration.

Roffman, R.K.; Barnhart, R. (1987). Assessing need for marijuana dependence treatment through an anonymous telephone interview. *Int J Addict,* 22:639-651.

Roth, M.D.; Arora, A.; Barsky, S.H.; Kleerup, E.C.; Simmons, M.; Tashkin, D.P. (1998). Airway inflammation in young marijuana and tobacco smokers. *Am J Respir Crit Care Med,* 157:928-937.

Roth, M.D.; Baldwin, G.C.; Tashkin, D.P. (2002). Effects of delta-9-tetrahydro-cannabinol on human immune function and host defense. *Chem Phys Lipids,* 121(1-2):229-239.

Roth, M.D.; Whittaker, K.; Salehi, K.; Tashkin, D.P.; Baldwin, G.C. (2004). Mechanisms for impaired effector function in alveolar macrophages from marijuana and cocaine smokers. *J Neuroimmunol,* 147(1-2):82-86.

Rubin, F.; Comitas, L. (1976). *Ganja in Jamaica.* Garden City, NY: Doubleday.

Sallan, S.E.; Zinberg, N.E.; Freii, E. (1975). Antiemetic effect of delta-9-tetra-hydrocannabinol in patients receiving cancer chemotherapy. *N Engl J Med,* 293:795-797.

Sallan, S.E.; Cronin, C.; Zelen, M.; Zinberg, N.E. (1980). Antiemetics in patients receiving chemotherapy for cancer: A randomized comparison of delta-9-tetra-hydrocannabinol and prochlorperazine. *N Engl J Med,* 302:135-138.

Sasco, A.J.; Merrill, R.M.; Dari, I.; Benhaim-Luzon, V.; Carriot, F.; Cann, C.I.; Bartal, M. (2002). A case-control study of lung cancer in Casablanca, Morocco. *Cancer Causes Control,* 13(7):609-616.

Schuckit, M.A. (1990). *Drug Abuse and Alcohol Abuse: A Clinical Guide to Diagnosis and Treatment.* New York: Plenum Medical Book Company.

Schwartz, R.H. (1987). Marijuana: An overview. *Pediatr Clin North Am,* 34(2): 305-317.

Schwartz, R.H.; Beveridge, R.A. (1994). Marijuana as an antiemetic drug: How useful is it today? Opinions from clinical oncologists. *J Addict Dis,* 13:53-65.

Schwartz, R.H.; Gruenewald, P.J.; Klitzner, M.; Fedio, P. (1989). Short-term memory impairment in cannabis-dependent adolescents. *Am J Dis Child,* 143:1214-1219.

Shapiro, B.J.; Reiss, S.; Sullivan, S.F.; Tashkin, D.P.; Simmons, M.S.; Smith, R.T. (1976). Cardiopulmonary effects of marijuana smoking during exercise. *Chest,* 70:1351-1356.

Shay, A.H.; Choi, R.; Whittaker, K.; Salehi, K.; Kitchen, C.M.R.; Tashkin, D.P.; Roth, M.D.; Baldwin, G.C. (2003). Impairment of antimicrobial activity and nitric oxide production in alveolar macrophages from smokers of marijuana and cocaine. *J Infect Dis,* 187(4):700-704.

Sherman, M.P.; Aeberhard, E.E.; Wong, V.Z.; Simmons, M.S.; Roth, M.D.; Tashkin, D.P. (1995). Effects of smoking marijuana, tobacco, or cocaine alone or in combination on DNA damage in human alveolar macrophages. *Life Sci,* 56: 2201-2207.

Sherman, M.P.; Campbell, L.A.; Gong, H.J.; Roth, M.D.; Tashkin, D.P. (1991). Antimicrobial and respiratory burst characteristics of pulmonary alveolar macrophages recovered from smokers of marijuana alone, smokers of tobacco alone, smokers of marijuana and tobacco, and nonsmokers. *Am Rev Respir Dis,* 144: 1351-1356.

Sidney, S.; Quesenberry, C.P.; Friedman, G.D.; Tekawa, I.S. (1997). Marijuana use and cancer incidence (California, United States). *Cancer Causes Control,* 8:722-728.

Smiley, A.M.; Moskowitz, H.; Zeidman, K. (1981). Driving simulator studies of marijuana alone and in combination with alcohol. *Proceedings of the 25th Conference of the American Association for Automotive Medicine* (pp. 107-116), Amsterdam.

Smiley, A.M.; Noy, Y.I.; Tostowaryk, W. (1986). The effects of marijuana, alone and in combination with alcohol, on driving an instrumented car. *Proceedings of the 10th International Conference on Alcohol, Drugs, and Traffic Safety* (pp. 203-206), Amsterdam.

Solowij, N. (1999). Long-term effects of cannabis on the central nervous system. In: Kalant, H.; Corrigall, W.A.; Hall, W.; Smart, R.G. (eds.), *The Health Effects of Cannabis* (pp. 195-266). Toronto: Centre for Addictions and Mental Health.

Solowij, N.; Grenyer, B.F.S.; Chesher, G.; Lewis, J. (1995). Biopsychosocial changes associated with cessation of cannabis use: A single case study of acute and chronic cognitive effects, withdrawal, and treatment. *Life Sci,* 56:2127-2134.

Solowij, N.; Grenyer, B.F.S.; Peters, R.; Chesher, G. (1997). Long term cannabis use impairs memory processes and frontal lobe function. *1997 Symposium on the Cannabinoids* (p. 84). Burlington, VT: International Cannabinoid Research Society.

Solowij, N.; Stephens, R.S.; Roffman, R.A.; Kadden, T.; Miller, R.; Christiansen, M.; McRee, K.; Vendetti, B. (2002). Cognitive functioning of long-term heavy cannabis users seeking treatment. *J Am Med Assoc,* 287:1123-1131.

Soni, S.D.; Brownlee, M. (1991). Alcohol abuse in chronic schizophrenics: Implications for management in the community. *Acta Psychiatr Scand,* 84: 272-276.

Sridhar, K.S.; Raub, W.A.; Weatherby, N.L.; Metsch, L.R. (1995). Possible role of marijuana smoking as a carcinogen in the development of lung cancer at a young age. *J Psychoactive Drugs,* 26:285-288.

Staquet, M.; Gantt, C.; Machin, D. (1978). Effect of nitrogen analog of tetra hydrocannabinol of cancer pain. *Clin Pharmacol Ther,* 23:397-401.

Stefanis, C.; Dornbush, R.; Fink, M. (1977). *Hashish: Studies of Long-Term Use.* New York: Raven Press.

Stein, A.C.; Allen, R.W.; Cook, M.L.; Karl, R.L. (1983). *A Simulator Study of the Combined Effects of Alcohol and Marijuana on Driving Behaviour.* Hawthorne, CA: National Highway Traffic Safety Administration.

Stephens, R.S. (1999). Cannabis and hallucinogens. In: McCrady, B.S.; Epstein, E.E. (eds.), *Addictions* (pp. 121-140). New York: Oxford University Press.

Stephens, R.S.; Roffman, R.A.; Curtin, L. (2000). Comparison of extended versus brief treatments for marijuana use. *J Consult Clin Psychol,* 68:898-908.

Stephens, R.S.; Roffman, R.A.; Simpson, E.E. (1993). Adult marijuana users seeking treatment. *J Consult Clin Psychol,* 61(6):1100-1104.

Stephens, R.S.; Roffman, R.A.; Simpson, E.E. (1994). Treating adult marijuana dependence: A test of the relapse prevention model. *J Consult Clin Psychol,* 62:92-99.

Substance Abuse and Mental Health Services Administration (SAMHSA) (2005a). *Summary of Findings from the 1998 National Household Survey on Drug Abuse.* Rockville, MD: U.S. Department of Health and Human Services.

Substance Abuse and Mental Health Services Administration (SAMHSA) (2005b). *National Admissions to Substance Abuse Treatment Services—The Treatment Episode Data Set (TEDS).* http://www.icpsr.umich.edu/cocoon/SAMHDA/SERIES/00056.xml.

Tahir, S.K.; Zimmerman, A.M. (1991). Influence of marijuana on cellular structures and biochemical activities. *Pharmacol Biochem Behav,* 40:617-623.

Tanner, J.; Davies, S.; O'Grady, B. (1999). Whatever happened to yesterday's rebels? Longitudinal effects of youth delinquency on education and employment. *Soc Probl,* 46:250-274.

Tashkin, D.P. (1999). Cannabis effects on the respiratory system. In: Kalant, H.; Corrigall, W.A.; Hall, W.; Smart, R.G. (eds.), *The Health Effects of Cannabis* (pp. 311-346). Toronto: Centre for Addiction and Mental Health.

Tashkin, D.P.; Coulson, A.H.; Clark, V.A.; Simmons, M.; Borque, L.B.; Duann, S.; Spivey, G.H.; Gong, H. (1987). Respiratory symptoms and lung function in habitual heavy smokers of marijuana alone, smokers of marijuana and tobacco, smokers of tobacco alone, and nonsmokers. *Am Rev Respir Dis,* 135:209-216.

Tashkin, D.P.; Gliederer, F.; Rose, J.; Change, P.; Hui, K.K.; Yu, J.L.; Wu, T.C. (1991). Effects of varying marijuana smoking profile on disposition of tar and absorption of CO and delta-9-THC. *Pharmacol Biochem Behav,* 40: 651-656.

Tashkin, D.P.; Shapiro, B.J.; Frank, I.M. (1973). Acute pulmonary physiologic effects of smoked marijuana and oral delta-9-tetrahydrocannabinol in healthy young men. *N Engl J Med,* 289(7):336-341.

Tashkin, D.P.; Shapiro, B.J.; Lee, Y.E.; Harper, C.E. (1975). Effects of smoked marijuana in experimentally induced asthma. *Am Rev Respir Dis,* 112:377-386.

Taylor, D.R.; Fergusson, D.M.; Milne, B.J.; Horwood, L.J.; Moffitt, T.E.; Sears, M.R.; Poulton, R. (2002). A longitudinal study of the effects of tobacco and cannabis exposure on lung function in young adults. *Addiction,* 97(8): 1055-1061.

Taylor, D.R.; Poulton, R.; Moffitt, T.E.; Ramankutty, P.; Sears, M.R. (2000). The respiratory effects of cannabis dependence in young adults. *Addiction,* 95:1669-1677.

Taylor, F.M. (1988). Marijuana as a potential respiratory tract carcinogen: A retrospective analysis of a community hospital population. *South Med J,* 81:1213-1216.

Tennes, K.; Avitable, N.; Blackard, C.; Boyles, C.; Hassoun, B.; Holmes, L.; Kreye, M. (1985). Marijuana: Prenatal and postnatal exposure in the human. In: Pinkert, T.M. (ed.), *Current Research on the Consequences of Maternal Drug Abuse* (pp. 48-60). Washington, DC: U.S. Government Printing Office.

Thacore, V.R.; Shukla, S.P. (1976). Cannabis psychosis and paranoid schizophrenia. *Arch Gen Psychiatry,* 33:383-386.

Thomas, H. (1996). A community survey of adverse effects of cannabis use. *Drug Alcohol Depend,* 42:201-207.

Thornicroft, G. (1990). Cannabis and psychosis: Is there epidemiological evidence for association? *Br J Psychiatry,* 157:25-33.

Tilles, D.S.; Goldenheim, P.D.; Johnson, D.C.; Mendelson, J.A.; Mellow, N.K.; Hales, C.A. (1986). Marijuana smoking as cause of reduction in single-breath carbon monoxide diffusing capacity. *Am J Med,* 80:601-606.

Timpone, J.G.; Wright, D.J.; Egorin, M.J.; Enama, M.E.; Mayers, J.; Galetto, G. (1997). The safety and pharmacokinetics of single-agent and combination therapy with megestrol acetate and dronabinol for the treatment of HIV wasting syndrome. *AIDS Res Hum Retroviruses,* 13:305-315.

Ungerleider, J.T.; Andrysiak, Y.; Fairbanks, L.; Ellison, G.W.; Myers, L.W. (1987). Delta-9-THC in the treatment for spasticity associated with multiple sclerosis. *Adv Alcohol Subst Abuse,* 7:39-50.

Vachon, L.; Fitzgerald, M.X.; Solliday, N.F.; Gould, I.A.; Gaensler, E.A. (1973). Single-dose effect of marijuana smoke: Bronchial dynamics and respiratory center sensitivity in normal subjects. *N Engl J Med,* 288:985-989.

Vandrey, R.G.; Budney, A.J.; Hughes, J.R.; Liguori, A. (in press). A within-subject comparison of withdrawal symptoms during abstinence from cannabis, tobacco, and both substances. *Drug and Alcohol Dependence.*

Vandrey, R.G.; Budney, A.J.; Kamon, J.; Stanger, C. (2005). Cannabis withdrawal in adolescent treatment seekers. *Drug Alcohol Depend,* 78:205-210.

Vandrey, R.; Budney, A.J.; Moore, B.A.; Hughes, J.R. (2005). Comparison of tobacco and marijuana withdrawal. *Am J Addict,* 14:54-63.

VanHoozen, B.E.; Cross, C.E. (1997). Marijuana: Respiratory tract effects. *Clin Rev Allergy Immunol,* 15:243-269.

van Os, J.; Bak, M.; Hanssen, M.; Bijl, R.; de Graaf, R.; Verdoux, H. (2002). Cannabis use and psychosis: A longitudinal population-based study. *Am J Epidemiol,* 156:319-327.

Verweij, P.E.; Kerremans, J.J.; Voss, A.; Meis, J.F. (2000). Fungal contamination of tobacco and marijuana. *JAMA,* 384:2875.

Wallace, J.M.; Oishi, J.S.; Barbers, R.G.; Simmons, M.S.; Tashkin, D.P. (1994). Lymphocytic subpopulation profiles in bronchoalveolar lavage fluid and peripheral blood from tobacco and marijuana smokers. *Chest,* 105:847-852.

Walton, R.P. (1938). *Marijuana—America's New Drug Problem.* Philadelphia: J.P. Lippincott.

Wells, J.E.; Bushnell, J.A.; Joyce, P.R.; Oakley-Browne, M.A.; Hornblow, A.R. (1992). Problems with alcohol, drugs and gambling in Christchurch, New Zealand. In: Abbot, M.; Evans, K. (eds.), *Alcohol and Drug Dependence and Disorders of Impulse Control* (pp. 3-13). Auckland, New Zealand: Alcohol Liquor Advisory Council.

Wert, R.C.; Raulin, M.L. (1986a). The chronic cerebral effects of cannabis use: I. Methodological issues and neurological findings. *Int J Addict,* 21:605-628.

Wert, R.C.; Raulin, M.L. (1986b). The chronic cerebral effects of cannabis use: II. Psychological findings and conclusions. *Int J Addict,* 21:629-642.

Wetzel, C.D.; Janowsky, D.S.; Clopton, P.L. (1982). Remote memory during marijuana intoxication. *Psychopharmacology (Berl),* 76:278-281.

Witter, F.R.; Niebyl, J.R. (1990). Marijuana use in pregnancy and pregnancy outcome. *Am J Perinatol,* 7:36-38.

World Health Organization (WHO) (1992). Classification of mental and behavioural disorders: Clinical description and diagnostic guidelines. In: *International Statistical Classification of Diseases and Related Health Programs,* Tenth Revision. Geneva: WHO.

Wu, T.C.; Tashkin, D.P.; Djahed, B.; Rose, J.E. (1988). Pulmonary hazards of smoking marijuana as compared with tobacco. *N Engl J Med,* 318:347-351.

Zacny, J.P.; Chait, L.D. (1989). Breathhold duration and response to marijuana smoke. *Pharmacol Biochem Behav,* 33:481-484.

Zammit, S.; Allebeck, P.; Andreasson, S.; Lundberg, I.; Lewis, G. (2002). Self reported cannabis use as a risk factor for schizophrenia in Swedish conscripts of 1969: Historical cohort study. *Br Med J,* 325:1199-1201.

Zhang, Z.F.; Morgenstern, H.; Spitz, M.R.; Tashkin, D.P.; Yu, G.P.; Marshall, J.R.; Hsu, T.C. (1999). Marijuana use and increased risk of squamous cell carcinoma of the head and neck. *Cancer Epidemiol Biomarkers Prev,* 8:1071-1078.

Zhu, L.X.; Sharma, S.; Stolina, M.; Gardner, B.; Roth, M.D.; Tashkin, D.P.; Dubinett, S.M. (2000). Delta-9-tetrahydrocannabinol inhibits antitumor immunity by a CB2 receptor-mediated, cytokine-dependent pathway. *J Immunol,* 165:373-380.

Zuckerman, B.; Frank, D.; Hingson, R.; Amaro, H.; Levenson, S.; Kayne, H.; Parker, S. et al. (1989). Effects of maternal marijuana and cocaine use on fetal growth. *N Engl J Med,* 320:762-768.

Chapter 9

The Medical Consequences
of Opiate Abuse and Addiction
and Methadone Pharmacotherapy

Pauline F. McHugh
Mary Jeanne Kreek

INTRODUCTION AND OVERVIEW

The incomparable ability of opium and its derivatives to kill pain, both physical and mental, has led to their use throughout recorded history as much for medicinal as for "recreational" purposes. For as long as opiates have been used, they have also been abused, and the dangers inherent in opiate abuse and addiction have long been recognized. The introduction in 1898 of the highly lipid-soluble, injectable opiate diacetylmorphine, or heroin, has led to problems of opiate abuse and addiction on a large scale. The rapid onset of heroin and its powerful reinforcing properties have made it the most commonly abused opiate in the United States (Kreek, 1996). In recent reports from the National Institute of Drug Abuse and the Substance Abuse and Mental Health Services Administration, about 2.7 million people in the United States were reported to have used heroin at some time in their lives, and an estimated 800,000 to 1 million were currently hard-core addicts, only a fraction of whom were in methadone treatment programs (Karch and Stephens, 2000; Kreek, 1996). Although 1998 is the last year for which such statistics are available, reports indicate that these numbers are rising

Authors' note: Preparation of this chapter was supported in part by NIH grants NIDA P50-DA-05130, K05 DA00049, NCRR M01RR00102, and OASAS-NYS. Thanks to Dr. James Schluger for reviewing the manuscript.

Handbook of the Medical Consequences of Alcohol and Drug Abuse
doi:10.1300/6039_09

(Perrone, Shaw, and De Roos, 1999). The costs to society have been enormous. In 1996 alone, 70,500 emergency room visits in the United States were directly attributable to heroin use, while in 1993, heroin was held to be directly responsible for approximately 4,000 deaths by overdose (Sporer, 1999). The number of deaths for which heroin has been indirectly responsible, due to the transmission of HIV-1 or the development of other medical complications, as well as from high-risk psychosocial behavior associated with drug abuse and addiction, is much harder to calculate. The estimated cost to society in the United States of the medical and legal consequences of drug addiction was $246 billion in 1992, of which a significant percentage was due to heroin (Kreek, 1996). The cost in terms of human suffering is incalculable.

Apart from the vast psychosocial risks associated with drug abuse and addiction, the medical consequences of addiction to any drug can be attributed to several factors: the pharmacological properties of the drug itself, the problems inherent in the routes of self-administration, and the various diluents and adulterants that are used to extend the resale value of the drug on the streets or sometimes used to enhance the quality of the drug's intended effects (Furst, 2000; Kreek, 1973b; Kreek et al., 1972). Drugs can exacerbate underlying medical problems, or, alternatively, can cause medical problems to be neglected. In already dire social situations such as homelessness, the additional presence of a drug addiction significantly increases an individual's likelihood of premature death (Gunne and Gronbladh, 1981; Hwang et al., 1998).

Opiates are set apart from other drugs of abuse by the diverse sites of opiate receptors throughout human tissues and organ systems, including vital centers in the brain. Thus medical problems due to direct pharmacological effects of opiates involve multiple organ systems and have a higher lethality in the case of overdose than other drugs of abuse. Findings about the effects of opiates on specific biochemical functions, such as neuroendocrine functioning or immune response, suggest other ways in which opiates differ from other drugs of abuse. There appears to be an even greater risk for complications and infections in addicted individuals because of the suppressive effect opiates have on immune response and endocrine functioning (Kreek, 1990a,b; Kreek et al., 1990).

The opiates most commonly abused tend to be those with rapid onset and short half-lives, as is the case with heroin. The half-life of heroin in humans is about three minutes. The major metabolite of heroin, morphine, has a half-life of four to six hours (Inturrisi et al., 1984). The rapidity of onset of a drug is related not only to its rewarding or reinforcing effects, but also to its intoxicating effects. As such, rapidity of onset may also be involved in the neurobiological changes that occur in addiction. The short half-lives of heroin, morphine, and related short-acting opiates also result in a need for multiple doses to be self-administered throughout any given day, in order to maintain the rewarding effect or, as addiction progresses, to avoid the sickness of withdrawal. Multiple daily self-administrations of a drug in unhygienic conditions increase the risk of infection and other complications to the drug user. In addition, this short-acting pharmacokinetic profile results in peaks and troughs of serum opiate levels that are cycling several times a day, and the corresponding waxing and waning of functionality in an opiate-addicted individual (see Figure 9.1).

This cycling of serum opiate level in cases of abuse and addiction appears to cause some of the deleterious pharmacological effects of opiates. The "on-off" cycles of opiates lead to a dysregulation of those physiological systems which are at least partly modulated by opiate receptors. This is most striking in the immune system and the neuroendocrine system, both of which appear to be suppressed in opiate abuse and addiction (Cushman and Kreek, 1974a; Kreek, 1973a,b,c; Kreek et al., 1972). These systems may slowly recover when drug use is stopped, but in the hard-core addict for whom stopping opiate use is unlikely or impossible, pharmacotherapy with a long-acting opioid such as methadone or l-α-acetylmethadone (LAAM) may ameliorate physiological changes by eliminating the "on-off" cycle (Kreek, 1990a, 1996; Novick et al., 1993.)* The half-lives of these medications are significantly longer than those of the commonly abused opiates. Racemic methadone has a half-life of 36 to 48 hours, while LAAM has a half-life of two days or longer (Kreek, 1973c, 2000). The slow onset of times and long half-lives of these medications allow for a physiological steady-state of opioid stimulation in the hard-core addict. Thus, multiple daily cycles of euphoria and withdrawal are elimited and normal functioning is restored (see Figure 9.2).

This chapter is intended to describe the medical consequences attributable to abuse of and addiction to short-acting opiates such as heroin. The medical consequences of the pharmacotherapy of opiate addiction with long-acting opiates such as methadone and LAAM will also be discussed. As death is the worst direct medical consequence of heroin abuse and addiction, it is covered first, followed by the direct pathophysiological effects of opiates on tissues and organ systems that result in significant morbidity for this patient population. Indirect causes of medical illness resulting from heroin

---

*Buprenorphine, a mixed opioid agonist/antagonist with long-acting activity at opiate receptors, is also currently being investigated as another medication for the treatment of opiate addiction.

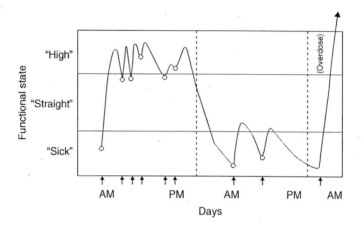

FIGURE 9.1. Diagrammatic summary of the functional state of a typical intravenous heroin user. Dashed lines indicate new days. Arrows show the repetitive injection of uncertain doses of heroin, usually 10 to 30 mg, but sometimes much more. The addict is hardly every in a state of normal function. *Source:* Adapted from Dole et al., 1966.

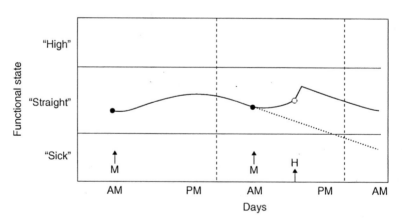

FIGURE 9.2. Methadone maintenance: functional state of a former heroin addict treated with a single daily oral dose of methadone pharmacotherapy (M). The effect of an intravenous injection of heroin (H) in the methadone-treated patient is shown in the second day. The dotted line indicates the course if methadone is omitted. *Source:* Adapted from Dole et al., 1966.

use, such as infection and contamination with adulterants used to cut the drug, are covered last. Psychosocial problems caused by drug abuse which affect the population, including prostitution and violence, are not specifically covered here, as these problems are common to all varieties of addictions and resolve with treatment of the addiction, including the methadone pharmacotherapy that is the current treatment of choice for people addicted to heroin. Finally, the medical consequences of methadone pharmacotherapy are included with each section, to provide a comparison with the medical problems so often seen in people addicted to short-acting opiates.

PHARMACOLOGICAL EFFECTS OF OPIATES: DEATH

The mortality rate for opiate abusers and addicts has been estimated at 6 to 20 times that of the non-drug-using population. Although much of the morbidity and mortality associated with opiate abuse and addiction is from secondary causes such as infection or other complications, a significant percentage is due to the direct effects of the drug itself. In people who regularly inject heroin, for example, the annual mortality rate is estimated to be 2 percent, half of which is attributable to overdose (Gunne and Gronbladh, 1981; Sporer, 1999). Although overdose is the most common acute cause of death in the opiate-abusing population, other physiological mechanisms have also been reported, although the rates of these causes of death are unclear. When opioid pharmacotherapy such as methadone is made available, the death rates from opiate abuse and addiction drop precipitously (Karch and Stephens, 2000).

Overdose Deaths

Overdose Deaths Due to Heroin and Other Short-Acting Opiates

Overdose of short-acting opiates results in central respiratory depression and coma due to the direct effects of opiate agonists on central nervous system opiate receptors. Overdose is most commonly reported in intravenous opiate abusers, although cases of fatal overdose by intranasal, subcutaneous, intramuscular, and oral self-administration have also been reported (Karch and Stephens, 2000; Sporer, 1999). The majority of opiate overdose deaths occur in experienced users and are due to unexpectedly high purity of the drug contained in the usual "dose" (or purchased packet), interactions between opiates and very large amounts of other drugs, especially alcohol and benzodiazepines (which can exacerbate the respiratory depression effects of the opiates) or, alternatively, the deliberate self-administration of an overdose in a suicide attempt (Karch and Stephens, 2000). Accidental overdoses have also been reported in naïve users and "body packers," people who transport quantities of drugs in packages by swallowing them or inserting them rectally. Body packers are susceptible to overdose if a package breaks en route (Utecht, Stone, and McCarron, 1993; Wetli, Rao, and Rao, 1997).

The mechanism of overdose death is respiratory depression. Most intravenous opiate deaths occur within one to three hours of intravenous administration, although some occur with the needle used to intravenously inject heroin still in the vein. Central respiratory depression is reversible with opiate antagonists such as naloxone or nalmefene, which are administered by bolus followed by continuous intravenous drip until the opiate agonist has been adequately cleared. Owing to the *different* half-lives of the various opiates, or the interactions of other drugs with the opiates, clearance rates may vary. In addition, the duration of antagonistic effects of opiate antagonists varies. The duration of effectiveness of naloxone is one to four hours, while the duration of effectiveness of nalmefene is four to ten hours. Clearance times of opiates as well as duration of action of opiate antagonists must be taken into account in the treatment of overdose, and overdose victims must be monitored for several hours before the opiate antagonist treatment can be discontinued (Finfer, 1996; Hartman and Kreek, 1983). Withdrawal symptoms following opiate antagonist administration can be severe and seizures (though rare) have been reported in connection with acute and severe opiate withdrawal (Delanty, Vaughan, and French, 1998; Kaplan et al., 1999).

Owing to the widespread use of opiates in both addictive diseases and the treatment of pain, opiate antagonists should be administered to anyone presenting with unconsciousness of unknown origin. Monitoring of the patient should continue following discontinuation of opiate antagonist therapy, as complications such as aspiration or recurrent respiratory depression with resultant hypoxia or anoxia can lead to further morbidity and mortality. About 3 to 7 percent of opiate overdose patients receiving emergency treatment will develop complications requiring hospitalization (Karch and Stephens, 2000; Kumar et al., 1999).

Overdose Deaths Due to Methadone

Deaths that have been reported as resulting from methadone or LAAM overdose have frequently been iatrogenic, secondary to a too-rapid increase in dose by methadone treatment providers in persons who have only a modest opioid tolerance. Other methadone-related overdose deaths are attributable to accidental causes, such as the combination of illicit methadone with very large amounts of alcohol or benzodiazepines or accidental ingestion, as well as deliberate causes such as overdose suicide attempts (Karch and Stephens, 2000; Perret et al., 2000). Death is again attributable to respiratory depression, with both pulmonary and cerebral edema found postmortem (Perret et al., 2000). Owing to the long half-life of these medications, opiate antagonist therapy must be instituted for up to twenty-four hours in the event of an overdose, and the patient must be monitored closely for at least one day, rather than a few hours (Finfer, 1996; Hartman and Kreek, 1983).

Positional Asphyxia and Muscular Necrosis

Positional Asphyxia Due to Heroin and Other Short-Acting Opiates

Owing to the rapid onset of short-acting opiates, the sedating effects of these drugs are profound and occur very quickly following self-administration of the drug. Numerous case reports describe unusual or awkward positions in which acutely intoxicated people have remained for long periods of time following self-administration. A mechanism for death in these individuals has been attributed to some form of respiratory compromise that can result from a compressed position, particularly in combination with the central respiratory depression characteristic of opiates. This cause of death has been presumed in many cases where serum levels of opiates measured postmortem were too low to be lethal by themselves and no other mechanism of death was apparent. However, in many other cases the sedated position in which the victim was found was more clearly involved in the mechanism of death. A syndrome consisting of hypoxia, vascular thromboses, and necrosis of skeletal muscle has been seen in case reports of deaths following acute intoxication while sitting in the lotus or other constricted positions (Howard and Reay, 1998; Klockgether et al., 1997; Rabl and Markwalder, 1996). A certain number of deaths of opiate addicts in police custody have been attributed to police procedures of restraining acutely intoxicated heroin addicts in "hogtie" positions, although this finding has been the subject of much debate (Howard and Reay, 1998; Karch and Stephens, 1999; Rabl and Markwalder, 1996).

Positional Asphyxia and Methadone

There are apparently no reports of positional asphyxia occurring in the presence of methadone pharmacotherapy alone. The sedating effects of methadone are less profound and of much slower onset than those of the short-acting opiates, and therefore the chances of an individual suddenly collapsing into an awkward position are very low.

"Anaphylactoid" Shock Due to Direct or Indirect Effects of Opiates

"Anaphylactoid" Shock Due to Heroin and Other Short-Acting Opiates

Some immediate deaths following opiate self-administration appear to have an acute hypersensitivity-like response as their cause. In one study of heroin addicts who died suddenly following injection of heroin, Edston and van Hage-Hamsten (1997) found increased levels of mast-cell tryptase in the serum and pulmonary tissue. This is sometimes described as an "anaphylactoid reaction" to the drug, due to the well-known effects of opioids in causing mast-cell degranulation and related histamine release. Alternatively, an adulterant in the drug may be present that causes an actual allergic response (Edston and van Hage-Hamsten, 1997).

It has been shown that in all individuals, morphine administered subcutaneously will cause a wheal-and-flare response secondary to mast-cell degranulation and histamine release (Novick et al., 1989). Likewise, acute opiate administration can also cause acute release of histamine in lung tissue, thus triggering an allergy-like response that can have rapid effects on pulmonary and systemic capillaries. This can lead to a drop in blood pressure and further respiratory compromise in a patient who already has central respiratory depression as a result of the direct effects of the opiate (Karch, 1998; Remskar et al., 1998). In these cases, death from respiratory failure appears to occur more rapidly than in uncomplicated overdose. Although it has been speculated that this mechanism may account for many opiate deaths that have been ascribed to overdose, the rate of "anaphylactoid" death for opiate abuses is unknown. Pulmonary edema due to this mechanism is implicated in many or most overdose deaths. True "allergic" response to heroin, morphine, and related drugs is probably rare.

"Anaphylactoid" Shock Due to Methadone

The oral route of administration of methadone and slow onset time markedly decrease the chance of an individual having a fulminant mast-cell degranulation and reaction to acute histamine release. Methadone induces histamine release to a modest extent, but again the slow onset time decreases the chances of acute bronchospasm, capillary insufficiency, and related sequelae.

DIRECT MEDICAL CONSEQUENCES OF OPIATES

It has been documented that opiates have no known direct toxic effect on tissues and organ systems in humans apart from the risk of overdose. Adulterants in the drugs and the unhygienic methods used in the course of their self-administration, as well as the relative hypoxia or anoxia resulting from central respiratory depression in overdose, are the principle causes of tissue damage in opiate addicts. However, the direct effects of short-acting opiates on opiate receptor systems when self-administered chronically can lead to physiological disruption of metabolic pathways and organ system functioning. Some of these opiate-induced tissue alterations in normal physiological function, while not potentially fatal or debilitating in and of themselves, may predispose an individual to be at greater risk for the indirect effects of drug addiction. One of the most clinically relevant functional alterations is the effect of opiates on immune response. Studies have suggested that this effect may functionally decrease an individual's resistance to infection when exposed to an infectious agent (Cherubin and Sapira, 1993; Thomas, House, and Bhargava, 1995). Other physiological changes resulting from opiate addiction may also have great clinical relevance, both in their effects on normal systemic and metabolic function, and perhaps also in the acquisition and perpetuation of the addiction itself (Kreek, 1996).

The Effects of Opiates on Immune Response

The Effects of Heroin and Other Short-Acting Opiates on Immune Response

Among the earliest indications that chronic opiate abuse had affected human immune response were the lymphadenopathy, lymphocytosis, hyper-immunoglobulinemia, and altered T-cell function noted in untreated heroin addicts in early studies prior to the advent of HIV-1 but after hepatitis B had been recognized (Kreek, 1973a,b, 1990a; Kreek et al., 1972). Although the actions of the opiates themselves were suspected, it was initially held that chronic bouts of bacteremia, repeated exposure to inert adulterants, and infection with hepatitis B virus, all results of intravenous drug use, could be the causes of immune system changes seen in heroin addicts. More recently, extensive studies performed in a variety of in vitro, animal, and a few human models suggest that opiates can directly modulate the immune response through opiate receptors located on immune cell surfaces. In laboratory models these effects appear to be dose dependent and are reversible by opiate antagonists such as naloxone (Singhal et al., 1995, 2000). A number of different mechanisms for these effects have been proposed, but the evidence from these models is often conflicting, and their relevance to human disease is unclear at this time.

In humans, short-acting opiates may additionally affect the immune system through modulation of the hypothalamic-pituitary-adrenal axis via changes in the levels of serum cortisol that are released through that endocrine cascade (Culpepper-Morgan and Kreek, 1997; Novick et al., 1989). Both of these actions result in changes in immune function that are generally suppressive in nature. However, specific immune cell activation induced by morphine and morphine withdrawal has also been reported (Singhal et al., 1999). Dose and chronicity of administration may play a role in the specific immune functions that are induced or suppressed. The immune alterations that have been found in humans to date include: attenuation of lymphocyte proliferation (Govitrapong et al., 1998); increased levels of serum immunoglobulins (Novick et al., 1989); suppression of bone marrow macrophage colony formation (Govitrapong et al., 1998); suppression of natural killer-cell activity (Yeager et al., 1995); suppression of phagocytosis of *Candida albicans* (Carr, Rogers, and Weber, 1996); the presence in the circulation of heroin addicts of elevated levels of immune complexes (Lazzarin et al., 1984); destruction of thymocytes (Glavina-Durdov and Definis-Gojanovic, 1999); and a change in the total number of B cells (Fletcher, Klimas, and Morgan, 1993; Novick et al., 1989). Such immune impairments have been seen in chronic, untreated heroin addicts, in the absence of any evidence of hepatitis B markers, HIV-1, HTLV-I, or HTLV-II infection (Fletcher, Klimas, and Morgan, 1993).

Natural killer-cell activity seems particularly vulnerable to the acute effects of opiates. Suppression occurs within hours of the initial dose, and will persist for some time following cessation of opiate administration in the opiate naïve subject. Natural killer-cell activity appears to be suppressed in opiate addicts in the absence of HIV-1 or other viral infections. This may, in fact, predispose opiate addicts to acquire a retroviral infection (Novick et al., 1989; Yeager et al., 1995).

The Effects of Methadone on the Immune Response

Some, although not all, of the functions altered in short-acting opiate addiction appear to return to normal when patients are treated with a long-acting opioid pharmacotherapy such as methadone. Natural killer-cell activity in particular appears to normalize with methadone treatment (Novick et al., 1989). Methadone does not appear to have the same immunosuppressive potential as heroin or other commonly abused short-acting opiates. This may be due to methadone's efficacy in preventing opiate withdrawal, a result of normalization of the hypothalamic-pituitary-adrenal HPA axis, or possibly due to pharmacokinetic *differences* at the level of immune cell surface opiate receptors (Kreek, 1996; Novick et al., 1989; Thomas, House, and Bhargava, 1995).

The Effects of Opiates on Neuroendocrine Functioning

The Effects of Heroin and Other Short-Acting Opiates on Neuroendocrine Functioning

The stress hormone cortisol is regulated by the hormone cascade produced by the HPA axis. The release of corticotrophin releasing factor (CRF) from the hypothalamus induces the synthesis and release of adrenocorticotrophin (ACTH) and beta-endorphin, major peptides derived from proopiomelanocortin (POMC) in the pituitary gland. ACTH then induces the release of cortisol from the adrenal glands. The major modulator of the HPA axis is cortisol, which acts at the levels of the pituitary and the hypothalamus in a negative feedback mode to reduce CRF release from the hypothalamus. Furthermore, endogenous opioids have been found to modulate this hormone axis by their inhibitory action on opiate receptors present in the pituitary gland and the hypothalamus (Kreek, 1987, 2000). Therefore, endogenous opioids are intimately involved with the regulation of the stress response.

Addiction to short-acting opiates results in a chronically fluctuating dysregulation of the HPA axis and abnormal release of cortisol throughout the course of the day. Irregular release of cortisol is a factor that may contribute to the immune response abnormalities seen in opiate addicts. The physiological dysregulation of stress hormones also leads to disruptions in the sleep-wake cycle as well as regulations of mood states, thus contributing to the decrease in daily functioning experienced by opiate addicts (Kreek, 1987, 2000; Novick and Kreek, 1992; Novick, Haverkos, and Teller, 1997).

The feedback mechanism for the hypothalamic-pituitary-gonadal (HPG) axis is similarly impaired. Acute administration of opiates can suppress pulsatile leuteinizing hormone (LH) release from the hypothalamus, resulting in irregularities of sex hormone levels (Mendelson and Mello, 1978). Therefore, ovarian function in women may be impaired, with resultant anovulation and amenorrhea, and in men decreased libido and erectile dysfunction are frequently reported (Melman and Gingell, 1999; Mendelson and Mello, 1978; Santen et al., 1975; Thomas, Shahid-Salles, and Donovan, 1977). Some evidence indicates that other hormone systems involving hypothalamic releasing factors, such as the thyroid and parathyroid hormone systems, are also subject to dysregulation in the presence of opiates. The mechanisms, though presumably similar to those for the HPA and HPG axes, have not been well established (Surks and Sievert, 1995; Tagliaro et al., 1984).

The Effects of Methadone on Neuroendocrine Functioning

Most of the dysregulations of the neuroendocrine axis occurring in heroin addiction appear to be normalized following the successful treatment of heroin addiction with methadone. The HPA axis in particular appears to normalize, in part due to the steady-state pharmacokinetics of the long-acting opioids, and in part due to the elimination of the stress-inducing lifestyle that accompanies heroin addiction (Kreek, 1973a, b, 1996; Novick and Kreek, 1992). Some reduction in pulsatile secretion of LH persists with methadone treatment, although absolute values are no different from those of normal controls. Nevertheless, some ovulatory or erectile dysfunction may persist with methadone treatment, although not to the degree that is seen in active heroin addiction (Cushman and Kreek, 1974a). Thyroid-stimulating hormone levels appear to be reduced with methadone treatment, as well as in active addiction. In neither case does this appear to have much clinical significance (Cushman and Kreek, 1974b; Surks and Sievert, 1995).

The Effects of Opiates on Organ Systems

The Effects of Heroin and Other Short-Acting Opiates on Organ Systems

The majority of toxic effects from opiate abuse and addiction come from adulterants and inert diluents used to cut the drug on the street or from the relative hypoxia or anoxia resulting from opiate overdose. However, some questions remain as to whether there are any toxic effects of the opiates themselves. In vitro and animal studies have suggested that there may be a specific toxicity of short-acting opiates such as pure morphine or pure heroin on various tissue types. However, direct toxic effects of opiates on organ systems are generally not seen in opiate-addicted humans. The organ system changes seen in opiate-addicted humans are instead due to an expected regulatory effect of endogenous opioids that is dysregulated in the presence of illicit opiates.

Neuropathies. The rate of peripheral neuropathies and plexopathies in HIV-negative intravenous heroin users is nearly 25 times higher than the general population (Berger et al., 1999). Mechanisms that have been proposed for opiate-related neuropathies have included chronic inflammation, neurotoxic adulterants, nutritional deficiencies, and comorbid alcoholism, all of which doubtlessly contribute to neurological damage in opiate addicts (Berger et al., 1999; Evans and Millington, 1993; Hillstrom, Cohn, and McCarroll, 1990). However, similar neuropathic symptoms may also be seen in nondrug-abusing cancer patients who are being treated for chronic pain with large doses of morphine. It has been hypothesized from a small series of patients that the morphine metabolite morphine-3-glucuronide (M-3-G), which constitutes a small percentage of the metabolites of morphine but is highly neuroexcitatory and possibly neurotoxic, is responsible for neuronal damage in patients who are regularly receiving large doses of morphine. In these patients, the neuropathies were reversible when the morphine doses were stopped (Inturrisi et al., 1984; Sjogren et al., 1998). Morphine is the primary metabolite of heroin. Diacetylmorphine breaks down to morphine in the liver, which is further broken down into M-3-G. Therefore, heroin users may also be subject to the direct neurotoxic effects from heroin's metabolites, compounded by or perhaps even predisposed to them by the nutritional deficiencies and other problems that commonly occur in addictions. However, this hypothesis has not been confirmed.

Pulmonary Effects. The acute, rapid administration of opiates directly triggers the release of histamines in lung tissue, causing acute bronchoconstriction, inflammation, and increased capillary permeability (Benson and Bentley, 1995; Cruz et al., 1998). By this mechanism, short-acting opiate use by asthmatic opiate users can result in sudden asphyxic asthma, although as with the "anaphylactoid" syndrome described earlier, asthma-like symptoms may similarly be triggered in opiate users who have no prior asthma history (Cygan, Trunsky, and Corbridge, 2000; Levenson et al., 1996).

Even in the absence of acute bronchoconstriction, the increased permeability of the pulmonary capillary bed caused by opiate-induced histamine release can result in noncardiogenic pulmonary edema. Pulmonary edema as a result of opiate abuse is most often described as a complication of overdose, independent of the route by which the overdose was administered. However, with the increasing popularity of inhaled heroin, cases of acute pulmonary edema following heroin inhalation or insufflation in the absence of overdose have been reported (Benson and Bentley, 1995; Cruz et al., 1998; Karne et al., 1999).

In some individuals, the inflammation accompanying pulmonary edema can present as acute pneumonia. The inflammation is often found by bronchial lavage to consist of eosinophils, thus attesting to the origin of the pneumonia as a hypersensitivity-like response rather than an infection (Pope-Harman et al., 1996). Circulating immune complexes have also been found deposited in alveolar capillary membranes in association with this edema (Smith et al., 1978). The infiltrates caused by eosinophilic pneumonia may persist as long as drug use persists. When chronic, this can eventually result in an interstitial pneumonitis that is responsive to steroids (Benson and Bentley, 1995; Brander and Tukiainen, 1993). The central respiratory depression characteristic of opiate abuse and addiction doubtless contributes to the development of such pulmonary problems (O'Donnell et al., 1995).

Skeletal-Muscle Toxicity. Rhabdomyolysis, a disease in which massive skeletal-muscle-cell breakdown causes the release of intracellular myoglobin into the bloodstream, is one cause of severe medical complications in drug addicts. Severe myoglobinemia resulting from acute rhabdomyolysis can cause renal damage, which can progress to end-stage renal failure (Deighan et al., 2000; Kumar et al., 1999). This has been reported in intravenous drug users, irrespective of the drug that is being injected. For this reason, rhabdomyolysis is often attributed to the use of contaminated needles, drug adulterants, or skeletomuscular injuries sustained while intoxicated.

In opiate-addicted individuals, rhabdomyolysis is again most commonly reported in intravenous heroin users. However, there have been reports of rhabdomyolysis also occurring in heroin addicts who inhale rather than inject heroin (Annane et al., 1990; Otero et al., 1992; Rabl and Markwalder, 1996). It is likely that the pharmacological properties of opiates contribute further risks for the development of rhabdomyolysis. The anoxia or hypoxia caused by opiate overdose and the muscular breakdown that can accompany long periods of immobility while intoxicated with opiates are predisposing factors for rhabdomyolysis (Novick, Haverkos, and Teller, 1997; Richards, 2000). Furthermore, recent animal model studies have suggested that short-acting opiates may have a direct toxic effect on skeletal-muscle cell membranes (Pena et al., 1990, 1993). Although the relevance of these findings is not clear in regard to human illness, they raise the possibility that short-acting opiates may play a more direct causal role in the development of rhabdomyolysis.

Renal Effects. Apart from the risk of renal failure secondary to rhabdomyolysis, renal illness is increased in heroin addicts, particularly among intravenous drug users. Heroin-associated nephropathy occurs as focal segmental glomerulosclerosis (predominantly in young African-American men who have been using heroin for several years, and as such may be related to a genetic predisposition), but may also present as a membranous glomerulopathy or a chronic interstitial nephritis irrespective of ethnicity or gender (Dettmeyer, Wessling, and Madea, 1998; Haskell, Glicklich, and Senitzer, 1988). Although the etiologies of heroin-associated nephropathies remain largely idiopathic, both in vitro and postmortem human studies have suggested that elevated amounts of circulating immune complexes formed in response to opiates may play a role in their genesis (Sanders and Marshall, 1989; Singhal et al., 1995). The mechanisms remain unclear, but may be due to mesangial deposition of circulating immune complexes or the formation of antiglomerulomembrane antibodies (Savige, Dowling, and Kincaid-Smith, 1989).

Teratogenicity and Fetal Development. Babies born to heroin-addicted mothers have been found to be significantly smaller in terms of head circumference and lower birth weight than babies born to nondrug-using mothers (Vance et al., 1997). However, it is not clear whether the low birth weight is an effect of heroin itself, or a consequence of nicotine dependence. The rate of cigarette smoking, which has been linked with low birth weight in numerous studies, is nearly 100 percent in the heroin-addicted population (Kenner and D'Apolito, 1997; Miller et al., 1991). Poor nutrition, also commonly seen in this population, may be another contributing factor to low birth weight.

Opiates, and heroin in particular, readily cross the placenta, and heroin will appear in fetal tissue within one hour of maternal use (Kenner and D'Apolito, 1997). For pregnant women who are addicted to short-acting opiates such as heroin, the fetus experiences multiple daily cycles of intoxication and withdrawal. The increased catecholamine release accompanying opiate withdrawal, which is generally well tolerated by the mother, can be fatal to the developing fetus. In addition, short-acting opiate abuse and dependence during pregnancy has been associated with a number of complications, including spontaneous abortion, placental insufficiency, preterm labor, premature rupture of membranes, breech presentation, chorioamnionitis, meconium passage, fetal distress during labor, pre-eclampsia, and eclampsia (Archie, 1998). The likelihood of a fetus surviving to term appears largely dependent on the pharmacokinetics of the opiate. Longer-acting opiates do not have the continuous cycle of intoxication and withdrawal of the short-acting opiates and are not associated with increased risk to fetal survival. For these reasons, a long-acting opiate pharmacotherapy such as methadone maintenance continues to be the treatment of choice for opiate-addicted mothers (American Academy of Pediatrics Committee on Drugs, 1998; Archie, 1998).

Neonates may undergo opiate withdrawal, usually beginning several hours after delivery. Infants have much greater difficulty than adults in tolerating withdrawal. The increased catecholamine release that accompanies opiate withdrawal causes central nervous system irritability, with seizures and respiratory difficulties that in rare instances can be fatal to the neonate. Subacute withdrawal symptoms may resemble colic: gastrointestinal distress, sleeplessness, continuous crying, fever, and weight loss may persist in infants for weeks or months after birth (American Academy of Pediatrics Committee on Drugs, 1998; Vance et al., 1997).

Development after birth proceeds at a normal pace, and generally by six months to a year, the infant's growth has "caught up" with its peers. Developmental abnormalities not attributable to social factors such as poverty, neglect, or comorbid alcohol or cocaine abuse have not been seen in children born to opiate-addicted mothers (Vance et al., 1997).

Gastrointestinal Effects. Opiate receptors found along the musculature of the gastrointestinal tract appear to play a regulatory role in gastrointestinal motility. Stimulation of these receptors leads to marked functional slowing of the gastrointestinal tract, resulting in decreased gastric emptying, prolonged transit time, and increased absorption of water by the large bowel. This frequently results in constipation that can be severe and debilitating. Tolerance to these effects does not appear to fully develop over time (Quigley, 1999; Yuan et al., 2000).

Drug-Drug Interactions. Many short-acting opiates are substrates of the 2D6 enzyme of the P450 enzyme system, an enzyme for which many common antidepressants and other medications are also substrates. Thus, opiates can act as competitive inhibitors of this enzyme system in the presence of other drugs. Conversely, other drugs may act as competitive inhibitors at this enzyme system with respect to the opiates. Other drugs may also interact with short-acting opiates by activating or inhibiting the P450 enzyme system's biotransformational properties (Goldberg, 1996). This can lead to drug-drug interactions in the medically or psychiatrically ill addict who is taking prescribed medications, and may increase the chances of accidental overdose. This effect is sometimes exploited by "street doctors," who use empirical knowledge of these drug-drug interactions to prolong the effects of heroin by cutting it with antidepressants or other competitive inhibitors, a practice which may also have lethal consequences (Furst, 2000). Presently, researchers have little knowledge of these interactions, and few drug-drug interactions with heroin and other short-acting opiates are well understood. Methadone-drug interactions are discussed later in this chapter and opiate drug interactions are discussed further in Chapter 16.

Street drugs and alcohol may also interact with short-acting opiates. Large amounts of alcohol used in combination with heroin may increase morbidity and mortality by inhibiting the P450 enzyme system (Goldberg, 1996). Cocaine's known attenuating effect on heroin intoxication and withdrawal is also exploited by "street doctors," and many heroin addicts will begin using cocaine as a means of "titrating" the effects of the opiate. The increasing appearance of heroin in nightclubs has encouraged the admixture of heroin and "club drugs" including amphetamines and hallucinogens, and at least one death associated with the concurrent use of heroin and the club drug γ-hydroxybutyrate (GHB) has been reported (Ferrara et al., 1995).

Antinociception, Tolerance, and Withdrawal. Some medical consequences of opiate abuse and addiction are inadvertent results of expected opiate effects. The most commonly expected, and indeed anticipated, effect of opiates is antinociception stemming from the activity of the abused opiate on central opioid receptors that mediate the perception of pain. Although lack of awareness of pain is one of the prime motivators in the induction of opiate abuse and addiction, it may also lead to neglect of injury and illness, particularly those sustained early in the course of an addiction. Tolerance developing over periods of chronic opiate use can diminish the antinociceptive effect of the opiates as well as interfere with induction of anesthesia, potential problems for an ill or injured opiate addict who may require surgery for an injury that has been neglected. The development of tolerance also predisposes opiate-addicted people to overdose, as greater amounts of the drug are needed to induce the same desired effect.

Physical dependence is the inevitable result of the chronic self-administration of opiates. Thus, withdrawal ensues when the opiates are stopped or when opiate antagonists are given. Withdrawal from opiates is not lethal in and of itself and rarely causes seizures or other significant morbidity. However, it is remarkably uncomfortable and frequently associated with feelings of desperation and a fear of dying, which is extraordinarily aversive to the patient experiencing it and is the other prime motivator for ongoing opiate use once addiction has been established. This may be due in part to the increased release of catecholamines that accompanies opiate withdrawal, although the dysregulation of the stress hormone axis and other physiological mechanisms may also play a role (Kreek, 1996).

The Effects of Methadone on Organ Systems

Some, although not all, of the physiological functions that are dysregulated by short-acting opiates appear to return to normal when patients are treated with a long-acting opiate pharmacotherapy such as methadone.

Neuropathies. Methadone is not broken down into any known neurotoxic metabolites, nor are there reports of neuropathies attributable to methadone seen in the literature. Neurological injury or impairment does not appear to be a result of methadone treatment.

Pulmonary Effects. Although methadone induces some modest histamine release from mast cells, its effects on histamine release in lung tissue are negligible, and rapid bronchospasm or clinically significant changes in capillary permeability are not seen in successful methadone treatment. Pulmonary morbidity does not appear in methadone pharmacotherapy (Novick, Haverkos, and Teller, 1997).

Skeletal-Muscle Toxicity. There are no reports of skeletal-muscle toxicity or rhabdomyolysis in successful methadone pharmacotherapy. Myoglobinuria and myoglobulinemia are not seen as a consequence of methadone treatment.

Renal Effects. As methadone and other long-acting opiates do not appear to precipitate the immune complexes seen in heroin addiction, there is no risk for immune- complex deposition in renal tissues once heroin use has stopped. Renal illness has not been identified as a consequence of chronic methadone pharmacotherapy (Novick, Haverkos, and Teller, 1997).

Teratogenicity and Fetal Development. Reports of low birth weight in some babies born to methadone-maintained mothers are confounded by the high prevalence of nicotine dependence and other drug comorbidities seen in methadone-treated populations. Although cigarette smoking is a known risk factor for decreased birth weight, methadone is not known to cause reduction of birth weight by itself. As mentioned previously, treatment of heroin-addicted pregnant women with methadone reduces the multiple daily cycles of intoxication and withdrawal experienced by the fetus, and thus increases the chances of the fetus surviving to term. The reduction of intravenous drug use by the mother occasioned by adequate treatment with methadone further decreases the risk to the fetus of viral and bacterial infections, as well as exposure to toxic adulterants that may cross the placental barrier or obstruct blood vessels.

Babies born to methadone-treated mothers may experience methadone withdrawal within the first few days of life. Methadone withdrawal is usually modest in severity, but more protracted in neonates because of the longer half-life of the drug. Methadone lacks the potential fatality that heroin withdrawal has, since catecholamine release is much less severe in methadone withdrawal. Owing to the increase in health benefits to the mother, as well as the increase in viability and health of the fetus and neonate, methadone remains the treatment of choice for heroin-addicted pregnant women (American Academy of Pediatrics Committee on Drugs, 1998; Vance et al., 1997).

Gastrointestinal Effects. As with other opiates, methadone does not appear to be hepatotoxic (Kreek et al., 1972; Novick et al., 1993). Gastrointestinal slowing persists in methadone pharmacotherapy, and chronic constipation is a significant problem for many patients treated with methadone. Tolerance to the gastrointestinal effects of methadone develops very slowly, however, with less than 20 percent of persons experiencing relief from gastrointestinal slowing and constipation after three years of moderate-to-high dose treatment (Kreek, 1973a, b). Methadone-induced constipation can be treated effectively by oral doses of naloxone or by methylated naltrexone, which are not readily absorbed into the bloodstream from the gut, and therefore reverse the gastrointestinal effects of methadone without placing an individual at risk for withdrawal (Culpepper-Morgan et al., 1992; Yuan et al., 2000).

Drug-Drug Interactions. Methadone is metabolized by different P450 enzymes than the shortacting opiates, and therefore, competitive-inhibition drug-drug-interaction profiles are somewhat *different* from those of the short-acting opiates (Goldberg, 1996; Kreek, 1990b). For example, while heroin may be more likely to interfere with the metabolism of tricyclic antidepressants, methadone has been found to interfere with the metabolism of selective serotonin reuptake inhibitors such as fluoxetine and fluvoxamine (Borg and Kreek, 1995). Significant drug-drug interactions between methadone and other medications include the antitubercular drug rifampin and the anticonvulsant phenytoin, both of which accelerate the biotransformation of methadone and result in lower plasma levels and mild-to-moderate withdrawal symptoms if the methadone dose is not adjusted (Kreek et al., 1976; Tong et al., 1981). Methadone may also interfere with the biotransformation of antiretroviral drugs such as retronavir or zidovudine (Borg and Kreek, 1995; McCance-Katz et al., 1998; Tooley et al., 1999), a significant issue for HIV-seropositive former heroin addicts whose addictions are being treated with methadone.

Street drugs and alcohol may also interact with methadone. Alcohol in particular may have a bimodal effect, that is, it may inhibit the metabolism of methadone when very high blood levels of alcohol are present. When people who were regular, heavy users of alcohol stop drinking, the metabolism of methadone may be accelerated due to the resultant enhancement of P450 enzymes (Kreek, 2000).

Antinociception, Tolerance, and Withdrawal. The antinociceptive effects of methadone are well documented. Through its long-acting properties, methadone can be used effectively for the management of chronic pain. Owing to its slow onset time and paucity of intoxicating effects, as well as the regular monitoring of former heroin addicts in methadone treatment programs, injuries and other pain-producing ailments are not neglected in methadone-maintained former addicts, and increased morbidity from untreated physical illness does not appear to be an issue in successfully treated addicted populations (Novick et al., 1993).

Tolerance does not appear to develop in former addicts being treated with methadone, in that larger doses of methadone are not continually required to produce the same opiate blockade effect, even in patients treated with methadone for 20 or 30 years. When adequate doses of methadone are administered to former heroin addicts, drug craving and symptoms of opiate withdrawal are eliminated. Barring changes in methadone serum level due to physical illness or drug-drug interactions, no further increase of methadone dose is necessary (Kreek, 2000).

Withdrawal from long-acting opiates may be protracted, because of their long half-lives, but also involves less acute catecholamine release, and may be somewhat less uncomfortable than withdrawal from short-acting opiates for that reason. However, withdrawal from methadone requires very slow dose reduction to avoid the signs and symptoms of opiate withdrawal (Kreek, 1996).

INDIRECT MEDICAL CONSEQUENCES OF OPIATE ABUSE AND ADDICTION

As described previously, the direct effects of opiate abuse and addiction on the immune system can predispose an individual to be at higher risk for indirect medical problems associated with drug addiction. Many of these problems stem from the means of self-administration of the drug. Intravenous drug use in particular has been associated with increases in morbidity and mortality in this population. The vast majority of medical problems associated with opiate addiction stem from exposure to microorganisms or foreign matter via the use of shared or contaminated needles in nonsterile environments. The suppressed immune response associated with short-acting opiate addiction may contribute to the development of disease following exposure. Exposure to infectious agents and contaminants is of equal likelihood in improperly used opioid pharmacotherapy, that is, if injectable methadone preparations (generally stolen from hospitals) are used illicitly or the oral methadone preparations used in clinics are solubilized and injected. It is unknown at this time whether persons injecting only long-acting opioids are at lesser risk for the development of disease than persons injecting short-acting opiates.

However, other routes of self-administration also have risks associated with them, as will be described; attempts to stave off medical consequences in the era of AIDS by avoiding needle use has unmasked other medical conditions that accompany intranasal use or inhalation of opiate smoke. In addition, methods of diluting and enhancing the effects of drugs with adulterants have become more complicated in the past decade, resulting in miniepidemics of medical syndromes in places where noxious adulterants are used. As these kinds of problems are seen so commonly with heroin use in particular, this section will focus specifically on the indirect medical consequences of heroin, in comparison with methadone pharmacotherapy.

It should be understood that "successful" methadone pharmacotherapy in these cases refers to the complete elimination of all illicit substance in the context of methadone treatment. In cases in which illicit drug use or other high-risk behavior persists despite methadone treatment (a possibility that is not rare: 20 to 30 percent of methadone-treated individuals in well-run programs using adequate doses of methadone report comorbid alcohol, cocaine, or other illicit drug use, which includes occasional heroin use), the risks of indirect medical consequences probably remain the same (Kreek et al., 1986). Patients successfully treated with methadone outlive their untreated counterparts. One study of long-term medical follow-ups of patients treated for eight or more years with methadone had difficulty finding an age-matched cohort of ongoing heroin addicts (Novick et al., 1993). The long-term methadone patients in this study showed medical problems consistent with a normal aging population with a sedentary lifestyle. Non-insulin-dependent diabetes mellitus, obesity, and hypertension were problems affecting these patients while debilitating infections, abscesses, renal failure, pulmonary compromise, and neurological complaints were not.

Viral Infections

Heroin and Viral Infections

Intravenous drug use in particular is associated with an increased risk of transmission of blood-borne viruses, particularly HIV, HTLV-I and HTLVII, hepatitis B virus (HBV), and hepatitis C virus (HCV). The considerable morbidity and mortality of illnesses caused by these viral infections have been well documented and are beyond the scope of this chapter. It has been demonstrated, however, that the complications of these viral infections tend to be more severe and more lethal in affected individuals whose abuse and addiction remain untreated (Borg et al., 1999; Des Jarlais et al., 1984; Friedman et al., 1996; Modahl et al., 1997; Muga et al., 2000; Novick, Khan, and Kreek, 1986). This may be a result of nutritional deficiencies and poor self-care seen in people with active addictions, although the additional immune function impairments seen in opiate addiction may also play a role.

The prevalence of these viral infections in intravenous (IV) drug users is high. At their peak periods, before the effect of AIDS awareness education and needle-exchange programs took hold in 1985-1986, 55 percent of IV drug users were HIV positive, 65 percent were hepatitis B and C (HBC) positive, and as many as 98 percent were positive for HCV when blood samples were tested retrospectively (Borg et al., 1999; Kreek, 1996; Novick et al., 1988). The high-risk sexual behaviors often associated with addictions may also predispose individuals to these infections in the presence of opiate-induced T-cell immunosuppression.

Methadone and Viral Infections

The number of blood-borne viral infections in opiate addiction currently appear to be decreasing, especially in the context of methadone pharmacotherapy (Novick et al., 1993; Piccolo et al., 2000). By eliminating the use of needles and decreasing the likelihood of high-risk sexual behaviors associated with active heroin addiction, methadone pharmacotherapy is associated with much lower risks for infection with HIV-1, HBC, and HCV in seronegative individuals (Des Jarlais et al., 1984; Piccolo et al., 2000). Whether the improved immune functioning seen in methadone-treated former heroin addicts is also a protective factor against viral infection is still unknown.

Bacterial and Fungal Infections

Heroin and Bacterial and Fungal Infections

Seeding of microorganisms into the bloodstream is produced by intravenous or subcutaneous drug use, or through injuries sustained in the course of an addiction. The sources of infective microorganisms may be skin or saliva, or they may be harbored in the drug itself. Repeated bouts of bacteremia or fungemia due to multiple daily intravenous self-administrations of the drug may lead to systemic infections and debilitating complications. The classic example of this is infective endocarditis caused most often by seeding of skin and oral flora directly into blood vessels by unsterilized needles, which can have a rate of serious cardiovascular complications as high as 70 percent (Mathew et al., 1995). Poor dentition, reduced brachio-tracheal clearance, and high-risk sexual behavior may also account for sources of infection (Scheidegger and Zimmerli, 1989).

More unusual varieties of infection, of the kind seen in immunocompromised patients and held to be opportunistic in nature, are also seen in HIV-seronegative opiate addicts. Systemic fungal infections, for example, can be seen in intravenous heroin abusers. Systemic candidiasis due to infection with *Candida albicans* in the absence of HIV seropositivity has been linked specifically with intravenous heroin abuse, as opposed to intravenous drug use in general (LaFont et al., 1994). More recently, outbreaks of systemic infections with a newly emerging fungal pathogen, *Scedosporium prolificans,* have been reported in heroin addicts in California, the United Kingdom, Australia, and Spain (Berenguer et al., 1997). Tuberculosis is endemic among opiate addicts in some areas, particularly among untreated homeless heroin addicts. Opiates may also interfere with the metabolism of antitubercular medications (Borg and Kreek, 1995; Friedman et al., 1996).

Relatively unusual presentations of bacterial infections may also be seen in opiate addicts. Group B streptococcal infections, generally quite rare in adult populations, are more common among intravenous opiate abusers (Garcia-Lechuz et al., 1999). Group B streptococcal infections and more common staphylococcal infections may present as osteomyelitis in the absence of any history of injury, or as septic arthritis, most notably in the knee and hip (Goldenberg, 1998; Lossos et al., 1998). Abscesses caused by any number of organisms have been reported in every organ in the bodies of intravenous heroin users, including the brain, liver, skin, and lungs (Cherubin and Sapira, 1993; Novick, Haverkos, and Teller, 1997).

Subcutaneous opiate use provides an anaerobic environment for other bacteria to propagate, notably *Clostridium tetani* and *Clostridium botulinum.* The prevalence of tetanus and botulism occurring in heroin addicts currently appears to be increasing (Shapiro, Hatheway, and Swerdlow, 1998; Talan and Moran, 1998). Street preparations of heroin can harbor *Clostridium* spores, which are not killed by the boiling process used to prepare the drug for injection. Injection of contaminated heroin into subcutaneous spaces provides an environment for spores to hatch and reproduce, resulting in systemic illness or death due to the toxins secreted. The fatality rate of tetanus in this population in one study was 25 percent (Sun et al., 1994). Preventative vaccination, at least to tetanus, may not be protective in this population. Cases of fatal tetanus in opiate-addicted patients with therapeutic antitetanus titer levels have been documented (Abrahamian et al., 2000).

Methadone and Bacterial and Fungal Infections

Again, the elimination of needle use in successful methadone pharmacotherapy markedly reduces the risk of exposure to bacterial and fungal pathogens. It is unknown whether the improved immune status of methadone-treated former heroin addicts provides additional protection against pathogens introduced by routes other than needle use. However, the unusual and opportunistic infections seen in heroin addiction are not reported in methadone-maintained populations (Kreek, 2000; Novick, Khan, and Kreek, 1986).

Handwritten annotation: Neurological Sequelae

Systemic Toxic/Metabolic Syndromes

Heroin and Systemic Toxic/Metabolic Syndromes

The presence of adulterants and contaminants in the needles used for intravenous administration or in the drug itself may lead to contaminant-specific toxic or metabolic syndromes. Many of these are poisonings due to deliberate adulteration of the street preparation with other drugs such as scopolamine. Street drugs are often cut with others to produce a specific drug-drug interaction and effect (Furst, 2000). Accidental poisonings due to contamination of needles with heavy metals such as lead or mercury have also been reported (Antonini et al., 1989; Haffner et al., 1991).

Talcosis is a systemic syndrome frequently reported in individuals who have injected opiates containing talc, particularly when oral preparations of opiates are ground and injected intravenously. The talc or other inert material used to bind opiate pills is disseminated widely by intravenous injection and lodges in capillary beds where granulomas form around talc deposits. Pulmonary capillary beds are particularly vulnerable to talc deposition and granuloma formation, and respiratory compromise or failure may result (Ben-Haim et al., 1988; Pare, Cote, and Fraser, 1989).

Repeated injection of inert materials as well as multiple bouts of bacteremia have been associated with the deposition of amyloid in tissues, leading to a systemic amyloidosis that is symptomatic depending on the size and locations of the amyloid deposits. Although the mechanism for this is unknown, a predisposing genetic factor appears to be required (Neugarten et al., 1986).

Methadone and Toxic/Metabolic Syndromes

The elimination of needle use and use of street drugs containing adulterants eliminates the risk for toxic and metabolic syndromes in persons successfully treated with methadone pharmacotherapy. Toxic/metabolic syndromes are not reported as a consequence of successful methadone treatment (Novick et al., 1993).

Neurological Sequelae

Neurological Sequelae of Heroin

Apart from the peripheral neuropathies and plexopathies seen in heroin addiction that may be due to a combination of alcohol or other drug comorbidities and/or nutritional deficiencies, indirect neurological complications of opiate addiction seem relatively rare. Seizures are rarely reported in the context of heroin use and, when present, have most often been attributed to other underlying causes. Cerebrovascular accidents are more commonly reported in heroin addicts and have been attributed to intracerebral vasculitis induced by opiate use or infarcts caused by infective emboli in patients with endocarditis stemming from intravenous drug use (Adams et al., 1995; Brust, 1998; Calabrese, Duna, and Lie, 1997; Niehaus and Meyer, 1998; Sloan et al., 1998).

Recently, reports of a progressive leukoencephalopathy have been seen in individuals who inhale the heated vapor of heroin, a practice known as "huffing" or "chasing the dragon," and which appears to be on the rise in an attempt by opiate abusers to avoid the risks of needle use. The leukoencephalopathy consists of a vacuolization of white matter, which can be generalized throughout the central nervous system, although some reports suggest lesions are more likely to be seen in regions of poor blood perfusion, particularly the basal ganglia and cerebellum. The mechanism of the leukoencephalopathy is not known. The fact that it is most often seen in miniepidemics suggests that a particular unidentified contaminant may be to blame, although reports that only a few individuals using a particular supply of heroin have been affected suggest that an underlying genetic predisposition may also be necessary to develop the syndrome. Speculation that a toxic metabolite of heroin produced by heat vaporization may be a causative factor seems to have been invalidated by a report of an identical progressive leukoencephalopathy in an addict who was using heroin intranasally. Initially seen as pockets of miniepidemics in Europe over the past decade, cases have recently been reported in the United States (Celius and Andersson, 1996; Hill, Cooper, and Perry, 2000; Kreigstein et al., 1998; Rizzuto et al., 1997).

Neurological Sequelae of Methadone

The elimination of intravenous or inhalation routes of administration of street drugs, as well as the elimination of exposure to toxic adulterants by successful treatment with orally administered methadone, appears to eliminate the risks of neurological complications. Neurological sequelae are not associated with successful methadone treatment (Brust, 1998; Novick et al., 1993).

Cardiovascular Sequelae

Cardiovascular Sequelae of Heroin

Postmortem studies of heroin addicts have revealed very little gross cardiac pathology (Kringsholm and Christoffersen, 1987). However, one study of asymptomatic intravenous heroin users showed changes in mitral and tricuspid heart valve function that were detectable by echocardiograph. It was speculated that contaminants found in heroin caused microscopic damage to heart valves that is cumulative over time, and may form toeholds for the bacteria that result in endocarditis (Pons-Llado et al., 1992). A combination of microscopic cardiovascular damage from adulterants, fungemia, and immune suppression may also contribute to the mycotic aneurysms that are sometimes seen in intravenous heroin addicts (Spirito et al., 1999; Tsao et al., 1999).

Cardiovascular Sequelae of Methadone

Cardiovascular tone may actually be improved with methadone pharmacotherapy, both because the catecholamine release accompanying multiple daily withdrawals is avoided, and because opiates when at steady-state appear to have a protective or preconditioning effect on cardiac function (Barron, 2000; Liang and Gross, 1999).

Renal Sequelae

Renal Sequelae of Heroin

Along with the direct opiate-induced interstitial injuries seen in renal tissue, and the potential for renal failure as a consequence of opiate-induced rhabdomyolysis, some of the adulterants contained in street opiates have been implicated in mechanisms of renal damage, particularly when injected intravenously. Much of this appears in the form of insoluble diluents that are deposited in the capillary beds of glomeruli, resulting in progressive glomerulonephropathy and consequent nephrotic syndrome. Tissue pathology is varied and tends to occur in miniepidemics seen in specific localizations, suggesting again that locally introduced adulterants are the culprits (Crowe et al., 2000; Lynn et al., 1998; Peces et al., 1998). Other immune related kidney damage including reports of mixed cryoglobulinemia and hemolytic uremic syndrome, necrotizing angiitis, and chronic interstitial nephritis have been speculated to be caused by adulterants found in injectable opiates although the action of opiates themselves on immune cells cannot be ruled out as a causative factor (Crowe et al., 2000; Peces et al., 1998; Ramos, Vinhas, and Carvalho, 1994).

Renal Sequelae of Methadone

The elimination of needle use and use of street drugs containing adulterants eliminates the risk for renal damage in persons successfully treated with methadone pharmacotherapy. Renal syndromes are not reported as a consequence of successful methadone treatment (Novick et al., 1993).

Dermatological Sequelae

Dermatological Sequelae of Heroin

The dermatological manifestations of heroin addiction are related to intravenous and subcutaneous heroin use. Bacterial infections and abscesses in the skin are a common finding in opiate addicts using needles in unhygienic conditions. Stigmata of chronic opiate use include multiple round scars resulting from abscesses caused by subcutaneous injection, as well as "track marks," scars resulting from repeated IV needle injury along the paths of veins. These marks are often darkened by a tattooing effect produced by the introduction of carbonized contaminants into the skin during injection (Novick, Haverkos, and Teller, 1997).

Dermatological Sequelae of Methadone

Methadone pharmacotherapy is administered orally, and thus no dermatological symptoms have been associated with methadone in the therapeutic setting.

SUMMARY AND CONCLUSIONS

As many of the medical problems seen as a result of opiate abuse and addiction are common with other drugs of abuse, and are clearly related to the mechanisms of administration of the drugs and psychosocial complications, it has been largely assumed that the opiates themselves were reasonably medically benign. More recent studies, however, have continued to support our findings that short-acting opiates such as heroin may directly alter normal physiological function (and also, as seen in animal models, molecular, neurobiological, and cellular functions) that not only lead to problems in and of themselves, but may also predispose an individual to some of the secondary effects of drug addiction. The most striking findings have been studies suggesting that short-acting opiates actively alter the immune response and neuroendocrine functioning, rendering opiate addicts more susceptible to infection, hypersensitivity-like responses, and organ damage from the deposition of immune complexes. In addition, microscopic damage to tissues caused by adulterants or inert substances in the drugs are less likely to be repaired with an altered immune response, especially when multiple daily self-administrations of the drug cause repeated injuries to the tissues.

Recent attempts by opiate addicts to avoid the medical problems associated with needle use, likely as a result of HIV-awareness education, have led to a recent increase in reports of medical complications associated with other routes of opiate self-administration, particularly smoking. Reports of heroin-associated pulmonary edema, interstitial pneumonitis, and progressive leukoencephalopathy appear to be on the rise as a result of the increasing popularity of smoking and intranasal use of heroin as substitutes for intravenous and subcutaneous needle use.

Whatever the route of administration, the harmful effects of short-acting opiates continue to be associated with their pharmacokinetics. The "on-off" pattern of multiple daily intoxications and withdrawals seem to place opiate addicts at greater risk for medical complications. The ameliorating effects of the steady-state pharmacokinetics of the long-term opiate pharmacotherapies such as methadone are associated with the prolongation of life and the diminution of morbidity. Methadone thus continues to be the treatment of choice for chronic opiate addiction.

REFERENCES

Abrahamian, F.M.; Pollack, C.V.; LoVecchio, F.; Nanda, R.; Carlson, R.W. (2000). Fatal tetanus in a drug abuser with "protective" antitetanus antibodies. *The Journal of Emergency Medicine,* 18(2):189-193.

Adams, H.P.; Kappelle, L.J.; Biller, J.; Gordon, D.L.; Love, B.B.; Gomez, F.; Heffner, M. (1995). Ischemic stroke in young adults. *Archives of Neurology,* 52:491-495.

American Academy of Pediatrics Committee on Drugs (1998). Neonatal drug withdrawal. *Pediatrics,* 101(6):1079-1088.

Annane, D.; Teboul, J.L.; Richard, C.; Auzepy, P. (1990). Severe rhabdomyolysis related to heroin sniffing [letter]. *Intensive Care Medicine,* 16(6):410.

Antonini, G.; Palmieri, G.; Spagnoli, L.G.; Millefiorini, M. (1989). Lead brachial neuropathy in heroin addiction. A case report. *Clinical Neurology and Neurosurgery,* 91(2):167-170.

Archie, C. (1998). Methadone in the management of narcotic addiction in pregnancy. *Current Opinion in Obstetrics and Gynecology,* 10:435-440.

Barron, B.A. (2000). Cardiac opioids. *Proceedings of the Society for Experimental Biology and Medicine,* 224:1-7.

Ben-Haim, S.A.; Ben-Ami, H.; Edoute, Y.; Goldstien, N.; Barzilai, D. (1988). Talcosis presenting as pulmonary infiltrates in an HIV-positive heroin addict. *Chest,* 94(3):656-658.

Benson, M.K.; Bentley, A.M. (1995). Lung disease induced by drug addiction. *Thorax,* 50:1125-1127.

Berenguer, J.; Rodriguez-Tudela, J.L.; Richard, C.; Alvarez, M.; Sanz, M.A.; Gaztelurrutia, L.; Ayats, J.; Martinez-Suarez, J.V. (1997). Deep infections caused by *Scedosporium prolificans.* A report on 16 cases in Spain and a review of the literature. *Scedosporium prolificans* Spanish Study Group. *Medicine,* 76:256-265.

Berger, A.R.; Schaumburg, H.H.; Gourevitch, M.N.; Freeman, K.; Herskovitz, S.; Arezzo, J.C. (1999). Prevalence of peripheral neuropathy in injection drug users. *Neurology,* 53:592-597.

Borg, L.; Khuri, E.; Wells, A.; Melia, D.; Bergasa, N.; Ho, A.; Kreek, M.J. (1999). Methadone-maintained former heroin addicts, including those who are antiHIV-1 seropositive, comply with and respond to hepatitis B vaccination. *Addiction,* 94(4):489-493.

Borg, L.; Kreek, M.J. (1995). Clinical problems associated with interactions between methadone pharmacotherapy and medications used in the treatment of HIV-1-positive and AIDS patients. *Current Opinion in Psychiatry,* 8:199-202.

Brander, P.E.; Tukiainen, P. (1993). Acute eosinophilic pneumonia in a heroin smoker. *European Respiratory Journal,* 6:750-752.

Brust, J.C.M. (1998). Acute neurologic complications of drug and alcohol abuse. *Neurologic Clinics of North America,* 16(2):503-519.

Calabrese, L.H.; Duna, G.F.; Lie, J.T. (1997). Vasculitis in the central nervous system. *Arthritis and Rheumatism,* 40(7):1189-1201.

Carr, D.J.J.; Rogers, T.J.; Weber, R.J. (1996). The relevance of opioids and opioid receptors on immunocompetence and immune homeostasis. *Proceedings of the Society for Experimental Biology and Medicine,* 213:248-257.

Celius, E.G.; Andersson, S. (1996). Leucoencephalopathy after inhalation of heroin: A case report. *Journal of Neurology, Neurosurgery, and Psychiatry,* 60(6):694-695.

Cherubin, C.E.; Sapira, J.D. (1993). The medical complications of drug addiction and the medical assessment of the intravenous drug user: 25 years later. *Annals Internal Medicine,* 119(10):1017-1028.

Crowe, A.V.; Howse, M.; Bell, G.M.; Henry, J.A. (2000). Substance abuse and the kidney. *Quarterly Journal of Medicine,* 93:147-152.

Cruz, R.; Davis, M.; O'Neil, H.; Tamarin, F.; Brandstetter, R.D.; Karetzky, M. (1998). Pulmonary manifestations of inhaled street drugs. *Heart and Lung,* 27(5):297-305.

Culpepper-Morgan, J.A.; Inturrisi, C.E.; Portenoy, R.K.; Foley, K.; Houde, R.W.; Marsh, F.; Kreek, M.J. (1992). Treatment of opioid-induced constipation with oral naloxone: A pilot study. *Clinical Pharmacology and Therapeutics,* 52(1): 90-95.

Culpepper-Morgan, J.A.; Kreek, M.J. (1997). Hypothalamic-pituitary-adrenal axis hypersensitivity to naloxone in opioid dependence: A case of naloxone-induced withdrawal. *Metabolism,* 46(2):130-134.

Cushman, P.; Kreek, M.J. (1974a). Methadone-maintained patients: Effect of methadone on plasma testosterone, FSH, LH, and prolactin. *New York State Journal of Medicine,* 74(11):1970-1973.

Cushman, P.; Kreek, M.J. (1974b). Some endocrinologic observations in narcotic addicts. In: Zimmerman, E.; George, R. (eds.), *Narcotics and the Hypothalamus* (pp. 161-173). New York: Raven Press.

Cygan, J.; Trunsky, M.; Corbridge, T. (2000). Inhaled heroin-induced status asthmaticus: Five cases and a review of the literature. *Chest,* 117(1):272-275.

Deighan, C.J.; Wong, K.M.; McLaughlin, K.J.; Harden, P. (2000). Rhabdomyolysis and acute renal failure resulting from alcohol and drug abuse. *Quarterly Journal of Medicine,* 93:29-33.

Delanty, N.; Vaughan, C.J.; French, J.A. (1998). Medical causes of seizures. *The Lancet,* 352:383-390.

Des Jarlais, D.C.; Marmor, M.; Cohen, H.; Yancovitz, S.; Garber, J; Friedman, S.; Kreek, M.J. et al. (1984). Antibodies to a retrovirus etiologically associated with acquired immunodeficiency syndrome (AIDS) in populations with increased incidences of the syndrome. *Morbidity and Mortality Weekly Report,* 33:377-379.

Dettmeyer, R.; Wessling, B.; Madea, B. (1998). Heroin associated nephropathy— A post-mortem study. *Forensic Science International,* 95(2):109-116.

Edston, E.; van Hage-Hamsten, M. (1997). Anaphylactoid shock—A common cause of death in heroin addicts? *Allergy,* 52(9):950-954.

Evans, P.A.; Millington, H.T. (1993). Atraumatic brachial plexopathy following intravenous heroin use. *Archives of Emergency Medicine,* 10(3):209-211.

Ferrara, S.D.; Tedeschi, L.; Frison, G.; Rossi, A. (1995). Fatality due to gammahydroxybutyric acid (GHB) and heroin intoxication. *Journal of Forensic Sciences,* 40(3):501-504.

Finfer, S. (1996). Fatal methadone overdose. Close observation in intensive care unit is required when naloxone infusion ends. *British Medical Journal,* 313(7070):1480.

Fletcher, M.A.; Klimas, N.G.; Morgan, R.O. (1993). Immune function and drug treatment in anti-retrovirus negative intravenous drug users. *Advances in Experimental Medicine and Biology,* 335:241-246.

Friedman, L.N.; Williams, M.T.; Singh, T.P.; Frieden, T.R. (1996). Tuberculosis, AIDS, and death among substance abusers on welfare in New York City. *The New England Journal of Medicine,* 334:828-833.

Furst, R.T. (2000). The re-engineering of heroin: An emerging heroin "cutting" trend in New York City. *Addiction Research,* 8(4):357-379.

Garcia-Lechuz, J.M.; Bachiller, P.; Vasallo, F.J.; Munoz, P.; Padilla, B.; Bouza, E. (1999). Group B streptococcal osteomyelitis in adults. *Medicine,* 78:191-199.

Glavina-Durdov, M.; Definis-Gojanovic, M. (1999). Thymus alterations related to intravenous drug abuse. *The American Journal of Forensic Medicine and Pathology,* 20(2):150-153.

Goldberg, R.J. (1996). The P-450 system. *Archives of Family Medicine,* 5:406-412.

Goldenberg, D.L. (1998). Septic arthritis. *The Lancet,* 351:197-202.

Govitrapong, R.; Suttitum, T.; Kotchabhakdi, N.; Uneklabh, T. (1998). Alterations of immune functions in heroin addicts and heroin withdrawal subjects. *The Journal of Pharmacology and Experimental Therapeutics,* 286(2):883-889.

Gunne, L.M.; Gronbladh, L. (1981). The Swedish methadone program: A controlled study. *Drug and Alcohol Dependence,* 7(3):249-256.

Haffner, H.T.; Erdelkamp, J.; Goller, E.; Schweinsberg, F.; Scmidt, V. (1991). Morphological and toxicological findings after intravenous injection of metallic mercury. *Deutsche Medizinische Wochenshrift,* 116(36):1342-1346.

Hartman, N.; Kreek, M.J. (1983). Narcotic poisoning. *Current Therapy,* 896-898.

Haskell, L.P.; Glicklich, D.; Senitzer, D. (1988). HLA associations in heroin associated nephropathy. *American Journal of Kidney Diseases,* 12(1):45-50.

Hill, M.D.; Cooper, P.W.; Perry, J.R. (2000). Chasing the dragon—Neurological toxicity associated with inhalation of heroin vapour: Case report. *Canadian Medical Association Journal,* 162(2):236-238.

Hillstrom, R.P.; Cohn, A.M.; McCarroll, K.A. (1990). Vocal cord paralysis resulting from neck injections in the intravenous drug use population. *Laryngoscope,* 100:503-506.

Howard, J.D.; Reay, D.T. (1998). Positional asphyxia [letter]. *Annals of Emergency Medicine,* 32(1):116-117.

Hwang, S.W.; Lebow, J.M.; Bierer, M.F.; O'Connell, J.J.; Orav, E.J.; Brennan, T.A. (1998). Risk factors for death in homeless adults in Boston. *Archives of Internal Medicine,* 158:1454-1460.

Inturrisi, C.E.; Max, M.B.; Foley, K.M.; Schultz, M.; Shin, S.U.; Houde, R.W. (1984). The pharmacokinetics of heroin in patients with chronic pain. *New England Journal of Medicine,* 310(19):1213-1217.

Kaplan, J.L.; Marx, J.A.; Calabro, J.J.; Gin-Shaw, S.L.; Spiller, J.D.; Spivey, W.L.; Gaddis, G.M.; Zhao, N.; Harchelroad, F.P. (1999). Double-blind, randomized study of nalmefene and naloxone in emergency department patients with suspected narcotic overdose. *Annals of Emergency Medicine,* 34(1):42-50.

Karch, S.B. (1998). Diphenhydramine toxicity: Comparisons of postmortem findings in diphenhydramine-, cocaine-, and heroin-related deaths. *The American Journal of Forensic Medicine and Pathology,* 19(2):143-147.

Karch, S.B.; Stephens, B.G. (1999). Drug abusers who die during arrest or in custody. *Journal of the Royal Society of Medicine,* 92:110-113.

Karch, S.B.; Stephens, B.G. (2000). Toxicology and pathology of deaths related to methadone: Retrospective review. *Western Journal of Medicine,* 172:11-14.

Karne, S.; D'Ambrosio, C.; Einarsson, O.; O'Connor, P.G. (1999). Hypersensitivity pneumonitis induced by intranasal heroin use. *The American Journal of Medicine,* 107:392-395.

Kenner, C.; D'Apolito, K. (1997). Outcomes for children exposed to drugs in utero. *Journal of Obstetric, Gynecologic, and Neonatal Nursing,* 26:595-603.

Klockgether, T.; Weller, M.; Haarmeier, T.; Kaskas, B.; Maier, G.; Dichgans, J. (1997). Gluteal compartment syndrome due to rhabdomyolysis after heroin abuse. *Neurology,* 48:275-276.

Kreek, M.J. (1973a). Medical safety and side effects of methadone in tolerant individuals. *The Journal of the American Medical Association,* 223(6):665-668.

Kreek, M.J. (1973b). Physiological implications of methadone treatment. Appendix D. In: *Methadone Treatment Manual* (pp. 85-91), U.S. Department of Justice Publication No.2700-00227. Washington, DC: U.S. Government Printing Office.

Kreek, M.J. (1973c). Plasma and urine levels of methadone: Comparison following four medication forms used in chronic maintenance treatment. *New York State Journal of Medicine,* 73(23):2773-2777.

Kreek, M.J. (1987). Multiple drug abuse patterns and medical consequences. In: Meltzer, H.Y. (ed.), *Psychopharmacology: The Third Generation of Progress* (pp. 1597-1604). New York: Raven Press.

Kreek, M.J. (1990a). Immune functions in heroin addicts and former heroin addicts in treatment: Pre- and post-AIDS epidemic. *NIDA Research Monograph,* 96:192-219.

Kreek, M.J. (1990b). Immunological function in active heroin addicts and methadone-maintained former addicts: Observations and possible mechanisms. *NIDA Research Monograph,* 105:75-80.

Kreek, M.J. (1996). Opiates, opioids, and addiction. *Molecular Psychiatry,* 1: 232-254.

Kreek, M.J. (2000). Methadone-related opioid agonist pharmacotherapy for heroin addiction: History, recent molecular and neurochemical research and future in mainstream medicine. *Annals of the New York Academy of Sciences,* 909:186-216.

Kreek, M.J.; Dodes, L.; Kane, S.; Knobler, J.; Martin, R. (1972). Long-term methadone maintenance therapy: Effects on liver function. *Annals of Internal Medicine,* 77(4):598-602.

Kreek, M.J.; Garfield, J.W.; Gutjahr, C.L.; Giusti, L.M. (1976). Rifampin-induced methadone withdrawal. *New England Journal of Medicine,* 294:1104-1106.

Kreek, M.J.; Khuri, E.; Fahey, L.; Miescher, A.; Arns, P.; Spagnoli, D.; Craig, J.; Millman, R.; Harte, E.H. (1986). Long-term followup studies of the medical status of adolescent former heroin addicts in chronic methadone maintenance treatment: Liver disease and immune status. *NIDA Research Monograph,* 67:307-309.

Kreek, M.J.; Khuri, E.; Flomenberg, N.; Albeck, H.; Ochshorn, M. (1990). Immune status of unselected methadone maintained former heroin addicts. *Progress in Clinical and Biological Research,* 328:445-448.

Kreigstein, A.R.; Armitage, B.A.; Millar, W.S.; Shungu, D.C.; Brust, J.C.M.; Goldman, J.E.; Lynch, T. (1998). Toxic heroin-induced spongiform leukoencephalopathy in two American patients [abstract]. *Neurology,* 50:A81-A82.

Kringsholm, B.; Christoffersen, P. (1987). Lung and heart pathology in fatal drug addiction: A consecutive autopsy study. *Forensic Science International,* 34:39-51.

Kumar, R.; West, D.M.; Jingree, M.; Laurence, A.S. (1999). Unusual consequences of heroin overdose: Rhabdomyolysis, acute renal failure, paraplegia, and hypercalcaemia. *British Journal of Anaesthesia,* 83:496-498.

Lafont, A.; Olive, A.; Gelman, M.; Roca-Burniols, J.; Cots, R.; Carbonell, J. (1994). *Candida albicans* spondylocystitis and vertebral osteomyelitis in patients with intravenous heroin drug addiction: Report of 3 new cases. *Journal of Rheumatology,* 21:953-956.

Lazzarin, A.; Mella, L.; Trombini, M.; Uberti-Foppa, C.; Franzetti, F.; Mazzoni, G.; Galli, M. (1984). Immunological status in heroin addicts: Effects of methadone maintenance treatment. *Drug and Alcohol Dependence,* 13(2):117-123.

Levenson, T.; Greenberger, P.A.; Donoghue, E.R.; Lifschultz, B.D. (1996). Asthma deaths confounded by substance abuse: An assessment of fatal asthma. *Chest,* 110:604-610.

Liang, B.T.; Gross, G.J. (1999). Direct preconditioning-of cardiac myocytes via opioid receptors and KATP channels. *Circulation Research,* 84:1396-1400.

Lossos, I.S.; Yossepowitch, O.; Kandel, L.; Yardeni, D.; Arber, N. (1998). Septic arthritis of the glenohumeral joint. *Medicine,* 77:177-187.

Lynn, K.L.; Pickering, W.; Gardner, J.; Bailey, R.R.; Robson, R.A. (1998). Intravenous drug use and glomerular deposition of lipid-like material. *Nephron,* 80:274-276.

Mathew, J.; Addai, T.; Anand, A.; Morrobel, A.; Maheshwari, P.; Freels, S. (1995). Clinical features, site of involvement, bacteriologic findings, and outcome of infective endocarditis in intravenous drug users. *Archives of Internal Medicine,* 155:1641-1648.

McCance-Katz, E.F.; Rainey, P.M.; Jatlow, P.; Friedland, G. (1998). Methadone effects on zidovudine disposition (AIDS Clinical Trials Group 262). *Journal of Acquired Immune Deficiency Syndromes and Human Retrovirology,* 18(5): 435-443.

Melman, A.; Gingell, J.C. (1999). The epidemiology and pathophysiology of erectile dysfunction. *The Journal of Urology,* 161:5-11.

Mendelson, J.H.; Mello, N.K. (1978). Plasma testosterone levels during chronic heroin use and protracted abstinence: A study of Hong Kong addicts. *NIDA Research Monograph,* (19):142-148.

Miller, A.; Taub, H.; Spinak, A.; Pilipski, M.; Brown, L.K. (1991). Lung function in former intravenous drug abusers: The effect of ubiquitous cigarette smoking. *The American Journal of Medicine,* 90:678-684.

Modahl, L.E.; Young, K.C.; Varney, K.F.; Khayam-Bashi, H.; Murphy, E.L. (1997). Are HTLV-II—Seropositive injection drug users at increased risk of bacterial pneumonia, abscesses, and lymphadenopathy? *Journal of Acquired Immune Deficiency Syndromes and Human Retrovirology,* 16:169-175.

Muga, R.; Roca, J.; Egea, J.M.; Tor, J.; Sirera, G.; Rey-Joly, C.; Munoz, A. (2000). Mortality of HIV-positive and HIV-negative heroin abusers as a function of duration of injecting drug use. *Journal of Acquired Immune Deficiency Syndromes,* 23:332-338.

Neugarten, J.; Gallo, G.R.; Buxbaum, J.; Katz, L.A.; Rubenstein, J.; Baldwin, D.S. (1986). Amyloidosis in subcutaneous heroin abusers ("skin poppers' amyloidosis"). *The American Journal of Medicine,* 81:635-640.

Niehaus, L.; Meyer, B.U. (1998). Bilateral borderzone brain infarctions in association with heroin abuse. *Journal of the Neurological Sciences,* 160:180-182.

Novick, D.M.; Farci, P.; Croxson, T.S.; Taylor, M.B.; Schneebaum, C.W.; Lai, M.E.; Bach, N.; Senie, R.T.; Gelb, A.M.; Kreek, M.J. (1988). Hepatitis D virus and human immunodeficiency virus antibodies in parenteral drug abusers who are hepatitis B surface antigen positive. *The Journal of Infectious Diseases,* 158(4): 795-803.

Novick, D.M.; Haverkos, H.W.; Teller, D.W. (1997). The medically ill substance abuser. In: Lowinson, J.H.; Ruiz, P.; Millman, R.B.; Langrod. J.G. (eds.), *Substance Abuse: A Comprehensive Textbook,* Third Edition (pp. 534-550). Baltimore: Williams and Wilkins.

Novick, D.M.; Khan, I.; Kreek, M.J. (1986). Acquired immunodeficiency syndrome and infection with hepatitis viruses in individuals abusing drugs by injection. *Bulletin on Narcotics,* 38(1/2):15-25.

Novick, D.M.; Kreek, M.J. (1992). Methadone and immune function [letter]. *The American Journal of Medicine,* 92:113-114.

Novick, D.M.; Ochshorn, M.; Ghali, V.; Croxson, T.S.; Mercer, W.D.; Chiorazzi, N.; Kreek, M.J. (1989). Natural killer cell activity and lymphocyte subsets in parenteral heroin abusers and long-term methadone maintenance patients. *The Journal of Pharmacology and Experimental Therapeutics,* 250(2):606-610.

Novick, D.M.; Richman, B.L.; Friedman, J.M.; Friedman, J.E.; Fried, C.; Wilson, J.P.; Townley, A.; Kreek, M.J. (1993). The medical status of methadone maintenance patients in treatment for 11-18 years. *Drug and Alcohol Dependence,* 33:235-245.

O'Donnell, A.E.; Selig, J.; Aravamuthan, M.; Richardson, M.S.A. (1995). Pulmonary complications associated with illicit drug use: An update. *Chest,* 108:460-463.

Otero, A.; Esteban, J.; Martinez, L.; Cejudo, C. (1992). Rhabdomyolysis and acute renal failure as a consequence of heroin inhalation. *Nephron,* 62:245.

Pare, J.P.; Cote, G.; Fraser, R.S. (1989). Long-term follow-up of drug abusers with intravenous talcosis. *American Review of Respiratory Diseases,* 139:233-241.

Peces, R.; Diaz-Corte, C.; Baltar, J.; Seco, M.; Alvarez-Grande, J. (1998). Haemolytic-uraemic syndrome in a heroin addict. *Nephrology Dialysis Transplantation,* 13:3197-3199.

Pena, J.; Aranda, C.; Luque, E.; Vaamonde, R. (1990). Heroin-induced myopathy in rat skeletal muscle. *Acta Neuropathologica,* 80(1):72-76.

Pena, J.; Luque, E.; Aranda, C.; Jimena, I.; Vaamonde, R. (1993). Experimental heroin-induced myopathy: Ultrastructural observations. *Journal of Submicroscopic Cytology and Pathology,* 25(2):279-284.

Perret, G.; Deglon, J.J.; Kreek, M.J.; Ho, A.; LaHarpe, R. (2000). Lethal methadone intoxications in Geneva, Switzerland from 1994-1998. *Addiction,* 95(11): 1647-1653.

Perrone, J.; Shaw, L.; De Roos, F. (1999). Laboratory confirmation of scopolamine co-intoxication in patients using tainted heroin. *Clinical Toxicology,* 37(4): 491-496.

Piccolo, P.; Borg, L.; Lin, A.; Khuri, E.T.; Wells, A.; Melia, D.; Kreek, M.J. (2000). Prevalence of hepatitis C and HIV-1 in former opioid addicts in methadone maintenance treatment [abstract]. *Problems of Drug Dependence, 2000: Proceedings of the 62nd Annual Scientific Meeting for the College on Problems on Drug Dependence.* National Institute of Drug Abuse Research Monograph Series. Washington, DC: US Government Printing Office.

Pons-Llado, G.; Carreras, F.; Borras, X.; Cadafalch, J.; Fuster, M.; Guardia, J.; Casas, M. (1992). Findings on Doppler echocardiography in asymptomatic intravenous heroin users. *The American Journal of Cardiology,* 69:238-241.

Pope-Harman, A.L.; Davis, W.B.; Allen, E.D.; Christofordis, A.J.; Allen, J.N. (1996). Acute eosinophilic pneumonia: A summary of 15 cases and review of the literature. *Medicine,* 75(6):334-342.

Quigley, E.M.M. (1999). Gastroduodenal motility. *Current Opinion in Gastroenterology,* 15:481-491.

Rabl, W.; Markwalder, C. (1996). Fatal posture- and heroin-related intestinal infarction and leg muscle necrosis after snorting heroin—A case report. *American Journal of Forensic Medicine and Pathology,* 17(2):163-166.

Ramos, A.; Vinhas, J.; Carvalho, M.F. (1994). Mixed cryoglobulinemia in a heroin addict. *American Journal of Kidney Diseases,* 23(5):731-734.

Remskar, M.; Noc, M.; Leskovsek, B.; Horvat, M. (1998). Profound circulatory shock following heroin overdose. *Resuscitation,* 38(1):51-53.

Richards, J.R. (2000). Rhabdomyolysis and drugs of abuse. *The Journal of Emergency Medicine,* 19(1):51-56.

Rizzuto, N.; Morbin, M.; Ferrari, S.; Cavallaro, T.; Sparaco, M.; Boso, G.; Gaetti, L. (1997). Delayed spongiform leukoencephalopathy after heroin abuse. *Acta Neuropathologica,* 94:87-90.

Sanders, M.M.; Marshall, A.P. (1989). Acute and chronic toxic nephropathies. *Annals of Clinical and Laboratory Science,* 19(3):216-220.

Santen, F.J.; Sofsky, J.; Bilic, N.; Lippert, R. (1975). Mechanisms of action of narcotics in the production of menstrual dysfunction in women. *Fertility and Sterility,* 26(6):538-548.

Savige, J.A.; Dowling, J.; Kincaid-Smith, P. (1989). Superimposed glomerular immune complexes in anti-glomerular basement membrane disease. *American Journal of Kidney Diseases,* 14(2):145-153.

Scheidegger, C.; Zimmerli, W. (1989). Infectious complications in drug addicts: Seven-year review of 269 hospitalized narcotics abusers in Switzerland. *Reviews of Infectious Diseases,* 11(3):486-493.

Shapiro, R.L.; Hatheway, C.; Swerdlow, D.L. (1998). Botulism in the United States: A clinical and epidemiological review. *Annals of Internal Medicine,* 129(3): 221-228.

Singhal, P.C.; Kapasi, A.A.; Franki, N.; Reddy, K. (2000). Morphine-induced macrophage apoptosis: The role of transforming growth factor-beta. *Immunology,* 100:57-62.

Singhal, P.C.; Kapasi, A.A.; Reddy, K.; Franki, N.; Gibbons, N.; Ding, G. (1999). Morphine promotes apoptosis in Jurkat cells. *Journal of Leukocyte Biology,* 66:650-658.

Singhal, P.C.; Pan, C.Q.; Sagar, S.; Gibbons, N.; Valderrama, E. (1995). Morphine enhances deposition of ferritin-antiferritin complexes in the glomerular mesangium. *Nephron,* 70:229-234.

Sjogren, P.; Thunedborg, L.P.; Christrup, L.; Hansen, S.H.; Franks, J. (1998). Is development of hyperalgesia, allodynia, and myoclonus related to morphine metabolism during long-term administration? *Acta Anaesthesiologica Scandinavica,* 42:1070-1075.

Sloan, M.A.; Kittner, S.J.; Feeser, B.R.; Gardner, J.; Epstein, A.; Wozniak, M.A.; Wityk, R.J. et al. (1998). Illicit drug-associated ischemic stroke in the Baltimore-Washington Young Stroke Study. *Neurology,* 50:1688-1693.

Smith, W.R.; Glauser, F.L.; Dearden, D.C.; Wells, I.D.; Novey, H.S.; McRae, D.M.; Reid, J.S.; Newcomb, K.A. (1978). Deposits of immunoglobulin and complement in the pulmonary tissue of patients with "heroin lung." *Chest,* 73(4):471-476.

Spirito, P.; Rapezzi, C.; Bellone, P.; Betocchi, S.; Autore, C.; Conte, M.R.; Bezante, G.P.; Bruzzi, P. (1999). Infective endocarditis in hypertrophic cardiomyopathy: Prevalence, incidence, and indications for antibiotic prophylaxis. *Circulation,* 99:2132-2137.

Sporer, K.A. (1999). Acute heroin overdose. *Annals of Internal Medicine,* 130: 584-590.

Sun, K.O.; Chan, Y.W.; Cheung, R.T.F.; So, P.C.; Yu, Y.L.; Li, P.C.K. (1994). Management of tetanus: A review of 18 cases. *Journal of the Royal Society of Medicine,* 87:135-137.

Surks, M.I.; Sievert, R. (1995). Drugs and thyroid function. *The New England Journal of Medicine,* 333(25):1688-1694.

Tagliaro, F.; Capra, F.; Dorizzi, R.; Luisetto, G.; Accordini, A.; Renda, E.; Parolin, A. (1984). High serum calcitonin levels in heroin addicts. *Journal of Endocrinological Investigation,* 7:331-333.

Talan, D.A.; Moran, G.J. (1998). Tetanus among injecting-drug users—California, 1997. *Annals of Emergency Medicine,* 32:385-386.

Thomas, J.A.; Shahid-Salles, K.S.; Donovan, M.P. (1977). Effects of narcotics on the reproductive system. *Advances in Sex Hormone Research,* 3:169-195.

Thomas, P.T.; House, R.V.; Bhargava, H.N. (1995). Direct cellular immunomodulation produced by diacetylmorphine (heroin) or methadone. *General Pharmacology,* 26(1):123-130.

Tong, T.G.; Pond, S.M.; Kreek, M.J.; Jaffery, N.F.; Benowitz, N.L. (1981). Phenytoin-induced methadone withdrawal. *Annals of Internal Medicine,* 94:349-351.

Tooley, A.; Rostami-Hodjegan, A.; Lennard, M.S.; Tucker, G.T. (1999). Acute inhibition of methadone metabolism by ritonavir: Projection of interindividual variability from in vitro data. *Journal of Clinical Pharmacology,* 48:883P-884P.

Tsao, J.W.; Garlin, A.B.; Marder, S.R.; Haber, R.J. (1999). Mycotic aneurysm presenting as Pancoast's syndrome in an injection drug user. *Annals of Emergency Medicine,* 34(4):546-549.

Utecht, M.J.; Stone, A.F.; McCarron, M.M. (1993). Heroin body packers. *The Journal of Emergency Medicine,* 11:33-40.

Vance, J.C.; Chant, D.C.; Tudehope, D.I.; Gray, P.H.; Hayes, A.J. (1997). Infants born to narcotic dependent mothers: Physical growth patterns in the first 12 months of life. *Journal of Paediatrics and Child Health,* 33:504-508.

Wetli, C.V.; Rao, A.; Rao, V.J. (1997). Fatal heroin body packing. *American Journal of Forensic Medicine and Pathology,* 18(3):312-318.

Yeager, M.P.; Colacchio, T.A.; Yu, C.T.; Hildebrandt, L.; Howell, A.L.; Weiss, J.; Guyre, P.M. (1995). Morphine inhibits spontaneous and cytokine-enhanced natural killer cell cytotoxicity in volunteers. *Anesthesiology,* 83:500-508.

Yuan, C.S.; Foss, J.F.; O'Connor, M.; Osinski, J.; Karrison, T.; Moss, J.; Roizen, M.F. (2000). Methylnaltrexone for reversal of constipation due to chronic methadone use. *Journal of the American Medical Association,* 283(3):367-372.

Chapter 10

Medical Consequences of the Use of Cocaine and Other Stimulants

Aaron B. Schneir

INTRODUCTION AND OVERVIEW

Once thought to be a benign, nonaddictive drug, cocaine now has well-recognized adverse effects. These adverse effects can manifest throughout the body, and in the following chapter will be summarized by an organ system classification. Although such a classification is helpful in organization, it is important to realize that multiple organs are often affected by similar mechanisms. In particular, the effects of cocaine on the cardiovascular system explain many of the effects on other organs throughout the body. In addition, certain adverse effects may be dependent on the route of administration, or dose of cocaine. The adverse effects of three other stimulant drugs, methamphetamine, phenylpropanolamine, and ephedra will be summarized at the end of the chapter.

HISTORY

The history of cocaine use has been well described by a number of authors (Karch, 1999; Warner, 1993). Peruvian Indians have a long history of chewing coca leaves to achieve euphoria, combat fatigue, and increase stamina. Sigmund Freud used cocaine and also prescribed it as treatment for alcohol or opioid addiction. At one time, cocaine was a common ingredient in many commercial products, including teas and patent medicines. Although no longer the case, when first introduced, Coca-Cola was formulated using extracts from coca leaves and actually contained a small amount of cocaine.

Handbook of the Medical Consequences of Alcohol and Drug Abuse
© 2008 by The Haworth Press, Taylor & Francis Group. All rights reserved.
doi:10.1300/6039_10 *341*

In the late nineteenth century, cocaine use was popular and reports of addiction and adverse effects became known. The Harrison Narcotic Tax Act of 1914 prohibited the importation of cocaine and coca leaves, except for pharmaceutical purposes. This legislation helped curtail much of the then burgeoning cocaine use. In 1970, passage of the Controlled Substances Act prohibited the manufacture, distribution, and possession of cocaine, except for limited medical purposes. However, with the advent of crack cocaine in the 1980s, a huge resurgence of cocaine use occurred. This epidemic helped reveal many of the adverse effects of cocaine use, yet its use remains popular.

FORMS OF COCAINE

Many review articles describe in depth the various forms and properties of cocaine (Boghdadi and Henning, 1997; Cregler and Mark, 1986; Warner, 1993). Cocaine is an alkaloid extracted from the leaves of the *Erythroxylon coca* plant, grown predominantly in Central and South America. The two *different* chemical forms in which cocaine is abused are cocaine hydrochloride and cocaine alkaloid. Cocaine hydrochloride is produced by adding hydrochloric acid to the cocaine base. The result is a water-soluble salt that is typically insufflated, but may also be administered intravenously. Freebase and crack cocaine are both cocaine alkaloids that are smoked, but are produced by *different* techniques. Freebase is a colorless, crystalline substance that is made by dissolving cocaine hydrochloride in water, alkalinizing the solution, and then adding ether as a solvent. The cocaine base dissolves in the ether layer and is extracted by evaporating the ether. Many adulterants are removed by this process, but the remaining flammable ether predisposes the user to burns. Crack cocaine is made by a simpler process that allows more adulterants to remain, but does not require the use of ether. Crack is made by dissolving cocaine hydrochloride in water, adding baking soda, and slowly heating it to allow the alkaloidal cocaine to precipitate. The name crack stems from the popping sound that is made when crack is smoked (see Brick and Erickson, 1999, for a review).

All forms of cocaine produce the desired effect of euphoria. However, the onset and duration of effect differs between the different cocaine forms and mode of administration. Both smoking and intravenous use of cocaine produce a rapid euphoria. Cocaine smoke is rapidly absorbed by the pulmonary vasculature, reaching the brain in six to eight seconds and producing a euphoric effect for about twenty minutes. When used intravenously cocaine reaches the brain in about double the time taken by smoked cocaine. The euphoria achieved with cocaine insufflation takes longer (three to five minutes), but lasts one to two hours. With insufflation, cocaine causes local vasoconstriction of the nasal mucosa which both delays and prolongs its absorption. Coadministration of cocaine with alcohol results in the production of an active metabolite, cocaethylene. This metabolite has a long half-life and may result in a more prolonged euphoria than that achieved from using cocaine alone (Hart et al., 2000). Prior to the late 1970s, cocaine hydrochloride was primarily used by nasal insufflation. At that time, the intravenous use of cocaine hydrochloride and the smoking of freebase cocaine became popular. Smoking of cocaine became even more popular with the introduction of crack cocaine in the 1980s.

PHYSIOLOGICAL MECHANISMS OF COCAINE'S EFFECT

The mechanism of action of cocaine helps to explain both the desired effects by users and also many of the adverse effects observed with its use. The effects of cocaine are mediated through both the central and peripheral nervous system and have been reviewed in depth (Boghdadi and Henning, 1997; Warner, 1993).

Centrally, cocaine blocks the reuptake of the neurotransmitters dopamine and serotonin into presynaptic neurons, which leads to their accumulation in synaptic clefts. Dopamine and serotonin receptors are stimulated and the desired effects of euphoria, enhanced alertness, increased energy, diminished appetite, and increased self-confidence are achieved. By suppressing the activity of two specific parts of the brain, the pontine nucleus and locus ceruleus, cocaine also suppresses feelings of fear and panic. When used repetitively, however, dopamine stores become depleted, leading to the compensatory increased production of dopamine receptors. It is believed that the ensuing cocaine craving experienced by the chronic user results from the "starvation" of these receptors for dopamine.

In the peripheral nervous system, cocaine blocks the reuptake of catecholamines, specifically norepinephrine, by sympathetic nerve terminals, leading to accumulation in the synaptic cleft. Norepinephrine acts on both the alpha- and beta-adrenergic receptors located in the heart and blood vessels. Stimulation of alpha-adrenergic receptors leads to constriction and in some cases spasm of blood vessels, whereas the stimulation of beta-adrenergic receptors leads to increased heart rate. These effects of norepinephrine on the heart and blood vessels combined with other systemic effects are referred to as the sympathomimetic effect. The term sympathomimetic derives from the "fight or flight" effect of the sympathetic nervous system. The resulting sympathomimetic presentation may include hypertension (elevated blood pressure), tachycardia (elevated heart rate), hyperthermia (elevated temperature), mydriasis (dilated pupils), and diaphoresis (sweating).

The local anesthetic effect of cocaine is also well known. In fact, cocaine was introduced as the first local anesthetic in Vienna, Austria, in 1884. Cocaine competitively inhibits fast sodium channels in neurons that normally allow sodium to enter cells to initiate the propagation of neural impulses. Blockage of these channels prevents nerve impulse formation and explains the anesthetic effect of cocaine. This effect is still used therapeutically with the use of topical cocaine used to provide local anesthesia to mucous membranes and to reduce bleeding through local vasoconstriction. Sodium channels are also located in the cells of the heart and blockage may result in conduction delays and dysrhythmias (abnormal heart rhythms).

ADVERSE EFFECTS OF COCAINE

Cocaine is one of the most frequently abused illicit drugs and the adverse effects of cocaine use have been well summarized (Boghdadi and Henning, 1997; Cregler, 1989; Cregler and Mark, 1986; Warner, 1993). According to the 1997 National Household Survey on Drug Abuse (NHSDA), an estimated 1.5 million Americans were using cocaine (National Institute on Drug Abuse, 1999). Of patients presenting to the emergency department following cocaine use, cardiopulmonary, neurologic, and psychiatric presentations have been shown to be the most common (Brody, Slovis, and Wrenn, 1990; Rich and Singer, 1991). Although the overall morbidity and mortality of patients presenting with cocaine-associated complaints appears to be low (Brody, Slovis, and Wrenn, 1990), devastating effects, including death, do occur. Of the New York City residents who died between 1990 and 1992 from intentional or unintentional injury, one-fourth of the cases showed evidence of recent cocaine use. Of these deaths, one-third were attributed to cocaine intoxication and two-thirds to traumatic injury (Marzuk et al., 1995). The psychiatric adverse effects of cocaine are likely contributory to trauma-related deaths. See Table 10.1 for a list of the adverse effects of cocaine.

Cardiovascular

The most significant adverse effects of cocaine use involve the cardiovascular system. In addition, many of the adverse effects in other organ systems are mediated cardiovascularly. Adverse effects include myocardial infarction, dysrhythmias, cardiomyopathies, aortic dissection, and endocarditis.

TABLE 10.1. Adverse effects of cocaine summary.

Central nervous system	"Agitated delirium," cerebrovascular accidents (ischemic, hemorrhagic), convulsions, movement disorders
Psychiatric	"Agitated delirium," poor judgment, psychosis, withdrawal symptoms
Head and neck	Chronic rhinitis, destructive facial processes, nasal septal perforations, thermal injuries
Ocular	Corneal abrasions ("crack eye"), opsoclonus, precipitation of acute angle closure glaucoma
Cardiovascular	Aortic dissection, atherosclerosis, cardiomyopathy, dysrhythmias, endocarditis, hypertension, myocardial infarction, tachycardia
Pulmonary	Barotraumas (pneumomediastinum, pneumoperi-cardium, pneumothorax), exacerbation of asthma, lung disease (eosinophilic, granulomatous), pulmonary edema
Genitourinary	Renal failure, sexual dysfunction, renal infarction
Gastrointestinal	Infarction, ischemia, ulcer perforation, liver failure
Musculoskeletal	Rhabomyolysis
Pregnancy	Intrauterine growth retardation, microcephaly, placental abruption, prematurity

Various pathophysiologic mechanisms help explain the adverse effect cocaine has on the heart. Cocaine use not only increases cardiac oxygen demand by causing hypertension and tachycardia, it also decreases cardiac oxygen supply by causing constriction of the coronary arteries and small intracardiac vessels (Lange et al., 1989; Vitullo et al., 1989). Vasospasm of such vessels explains why, in some cases, cocaine-associated myocardial infarctions occur in the absence of coronary artery disease (Howard, Heuter, and Davis, 1985; Minor et al., 1991; Zimmerman, Gustafson, and Kemp, 1987). Furthermore, when such atherosclerotic disease is present, the constriction is even more pronounced (Flores et al., 1990). In fact, cocaine is also associated with enhanced platelet aggregation (Heesch et al., 2000) and is a risk factor for the development of such atherosclerosis (Benzaquen, Cohen, and Eisenberg, 2001). These adverse combinations explain why myocardial infarctions are well described after cocaine use, and why even young individuals, in whom it would otherwise be unheard of to suffer a myocardial infarction, occasionally do so after cocaine use. Cocaine-induced myocardial ischemia may also precipitate dysrhythmias (Hollander and Hoffman, 1992). In addition, both cocaine and the metabolite it forms with ethanol cocaethylene have sodium channel blocking properties (Przywara and Dambach, 1989; Xu, Crumb, and Clarkson, 1994). This property is associated with cardiac conduction impairment, dysrhythmias, and in cases of massive overdose is likely to be a major factor in mediating death (Kabas et al., 1990). The combination of sodium channel blockage, cardiac ischemia, sympathetic excess, and structural heart disease is implicated in sudden cardiac death associated with cocaine use (Bauman et al., 1994). Chronic myocardial ischemia and systemic hypertension from cocaine may also explain the reported cases of cardiomyopathy (Wiener, Lockhart, and Schwartz, 1986). The acute hypertension seen with cocaine use has also been implicated in the development of aortic dissections (Chang and Rossi, 1995; Fisher and Holroyd, 1992; Hsue et al., 2002). The higher than expected incidence of endocarditis from intravenous cocaine administration suggests that, by an as yet unknown mechanism, cocaine increases the likelihood of this potentially devastating condition (Chambers et al., 1987).

Many of the most serious cardiovascular complications seem to be rare, considering the relatively common use of cocaine. However, when these adverse effects do occur with the use of cocaine, they can be life-threatening and must be taken seriously. For example, the presence of cocaine-associated chest pain in an otherwise healthy young patient should be taken seriously by the treating physician.

Neurologic

The adverse effects of cocaine on the neurologic system include all forms of stroke, convulsions, headache, and movement disorders. A retrospective study conducted by researchers at San Francisco General Hospital detailed that convulsions and focal neurological symptoms and signs were the two major presenting acute neurological complications of cocaine use (Lowenstein et al., 1987). Many of these complications can be severe and result in long-term morbidity and death.

A particularly devastating neurologic effect of cocaine use is stroke. Cocaine-related strokes have mostly been reported in patients younger than fifty years, an age group that otherwise has a very low incidence of these events. All types of strokes including subarachnoid hemorrhage, intracerebral hemorrhage, and ischemic infarcts have been reported from cocaine use. In addition, all major vascular territories of the brain have been involved and all routes of cocaine administration have been implicated (Rowbotham and Lowenstein, 1990).

Various etiologies have been postulated. The pharmacologic effect of cocaine to acutely increase blood pressure seems especially likely as an etiology resulting in hemorrhage. The rapid increase in blood pressure may rupture both normal and preexisting abnormal cerebrovasculature (Aggarwal et al., 1996; Lichtenfeld, Rubin, and Feldman, 1984; Nolte, Brass, and Fletterick, 1996; Wojak and Flamm, 1987). Vasospasm, platelet aggregation, and vasculitis may also be contributory to both ischemic and hemorrhagic strokes (Daras et al., 1994; Fredericks et al., 1991).

Generalized convulsions are another adverse effect associated with cocaine use (Myers and Earnest, 1984). Although the local anesthetic property of cocaine has traditionally been implicated, it is likely that various other mechanisms are responsible (Lason, 2001). Unlike many other adverse effects of cocaine, convulsions appear to be dose related (Rowbotham and Lowenstein, 1990).

Various movement disorders have been associated with cocaine use. The association of choreiform movements with crack cocaine use led to the term "crack dancing" (Daras, Koppel, and Atos-Radzion, 1994). Cocaine use may worsen preexisting movement disorders (Daniels, Baker, and Norman, 1996), increase the risk of acute dystonic reactions in patients taking dopamine-blocking agents, and occasionally induce an acute dystonic reaction without other contributing factors (Catalano, Catalano, and Rodriguez, 1997; Farrel and Diehl, 1991). The mechanism by which cocaine induces these effects remains unclear but is thought to be related to dopamine dysregulation (Catalano, Catalano, and Rodriguez, 1997).

Pulmonary

Pulmonary symptoms are a common presenting complaint of cocaine users and a wide variety of adverse pulmonary effects of cocaine use have been reported. In contrast to the adverse effects on many other organs, the route of cocaine administration seems particularly important in producing pulmonary problems. The vast majority of adverse effects reported result from smoking cocaine either as freebase or crack (Perper and Van Thiel, 1992) and have been reviewed elsewhere (Haim et al., 1995). Adverse effects range from acute respiratory irritation to asthma exacerbation, pulmonary edema, eosinophilic lung disease, granulomatous lung disease, and barotrauma.

Cough, hemoptysis, and shortness of breath are common acute respiratory symptoms after smoking cocaine. Often these symptoms are not the result of significant pulmonary damage and are likely from the local irritant effect of cocaine (Perper and Van Thiel, 1992). However, this irritant effect of cocaine has also been implicated in causing more serious pathology. Severe asthma exacerbations have been associated with cocaine smoking (Rebhun, 1988; Rome et al., 2000), and some evidence indicates that the increasing incidence of death from asthma may, in part, be related to cocaine use (Levenson et al., 1996). The fact that inhaled but not intravenous cocaine administration induces bronchoconstriction supports a local irritant effect (Tashkin et al., 1996). The irritant effect has also been implicated in the hypersensitivity-related eosinophilic lung disorder referred to as "crack lung," which involves diffuse alveolar infiltrates associated with fever and eosinophilia (Forrester et al., 1990; Kissner et al., 1987). The presence of cutting agents in cocaine may also cause irritation to the lungs and result in granulomatous lung disease. Both cellulose and talc granulomas in the lung have resulted from nasal insufflation of cocaine (Cooper, Bai, and Heyderman, 1983; Oubeid et al., 1990).

Pulmonary barotrauma including pneumomediastinum (Morris and Schuck, 1985), pneumothorax (Chan, Pham, and Reece, 1997; Shesser, Davis, and Edelstein, 1981) and pneumopericardium (Adrouny and Magnusson, 1985) have all been reported in association with cocaine inhalation. All three in fact have been reported in the same patient (Uva, 1997). Pneumomediastinum has also been reported with cocaine insufflation (Shesser, Davis, and Edelstein, 1981). Prolonged and repeated Valsalva maneuvers performed by individuals attempting to heighten the effect of the drug are thought to induce alveolar rupture. The escaped air then can induce a pneumothorax or move to the mediastinum or, rarely, the pericardium. The fact that similar barotrauma has been reported with the use of other drugs suggests that the etiology is not the result of an intrinsic property of cocaine (Miller, Spiekerman, and Hepper, 1972).

Much still remains to be learned about the effect of cocaine on the lungs. The etiology of noncardiogenic pulmonary edema seen in association with cocaine use is unknown. The majority of cases have occurred from smoking cocaine (Cucco et al., 1987; Hoffman and Goodman, 1989), but one report exists of fatal pulmonary edema from intravenous administration of "freebase" cocaine (Allred and Ewer, 1981). Cocaine has also been shown to decrease the effectiveness of alveolar macrophages, but the clinical significance of this is yet to be determined (Baldwin et al., 1997).

Psychiatric

Various psychiatric problems occur with cocaine use. Exactly what effect is observed depends on whether a patient is acutely intoxicated, in a state of withdrawal, or is suffering from the chronic effects of the drug. The exact mechanisms by which cocaine produces such effects are unclear.

Cocaine intoxication may be complicated by poor judgment, delirium, and, in severe cases, psychosis. Psychosis from cocaine use may occur both with acute intoxication and also more insidiously with chronic use. Psychosis with acute intoxication has been noted to be associated often with violent behavior (Manschreck et al., 1988). Cocaine use in individuals with a predisposition for, or preexisting, psychiatric illness may certainly make an accurate diagnosis difficult (Mendoza, Miller, and Mena, 1992).

Long thought not to occur, a triphasic abstinence syndrome observed in outpatients following chronic cocaine abuse has been described. Phase one of the withdrawal involves the "crash" of mood and energy following cocaine binge cessation. It is marked by dysphoria, anxiety, depression, and profound exhaustion, and may last for days. Cocaine craving is also typical. The crash is thought to reflect acute neurotransmitter depletion caused by cocaine. Following the crash, phase two, or cocaine withdrawal ensues. In contrast to the withdrawal associated with many other abused drugs, with cocaine there are no gross physiological alterations. However, significant dysphoria, anhedonia, and amotivation are noted. Memories of cocaine euphoria may prompt the individual to reuse cocaine. Finally, phase three (extinction) occurs, which may last years, in which anhedonia and further craving may prompt reuse (Gawin and Kleber, 1986). It must be noted that additional inpatient studies on cocaine withdrawal did not reveal distinct phases, but a gradually resolving dysphoria. It is currently thought that the characteristics of withdrawal *differ* from an outpatient to inpatient setting and may rest with the presence or absence of triggering cues that can prompt cravings (Weddington, 1993; Withers et al., 1995).

Genitourinary

Adverse effects of cocaine use on the genitourinary system are significant. Adverse effects include acute renal failure, renal infarction, and progression of chronic renal failure. In addition, various sexual dysfunctions have been described.

Cocaine-induced rhabdomyolysis (muscle breakdown) is well documented and may lead to acute renal failure (Herzlich et al., 1988; Merigram and Roberts, 1987; Roth et al., 1988; Welch, Todd, and Krause, 1991). In a retrospective review of emergency department patients with rhabdomyolysis, the most common etiology was found to be cocaine use (Fernandez et al., 2005). The mechanism by which cocaine induces rhabdomyolysis is unclear and may be multifactorial. Although often associated with convulsions and hyperthermia, rhabdomyolysis associated with cocaine use has been documented without either of these conditions being present (Roth et al., 1988; Welch, Todd, and Krause, 1991). A direct toxic effect of cocaine on skeletal muscle, increased muscular activity, and cocaine-induced vasospasm with resultant ischemia have all been suggested mechanisms (Richards, 2000). It is thought that renal damage occurs from the toxic effect of myoglobin on the renal tubules (Richards, 2000). Acute renal failure may also be the result of the severe hypertension precipitated by cocaine use (Thakur et al., 1996). Hypertension from cocaine use may also accelerate the progression of chronic renal failure (Dunea et al., 1995). It is not surprising that reports of renal infarction are associated with cocaine use (Goodman and Rennie, 1995; Wohlman, 1987), with the pathophysiology likely to be similar to that associated with myocardial infarction involving accelerated atherosclerosis, vasospasm, and enhanced platelet aggregation (Nzerue, Hewan-Lowe, and Riley, 2000). An aortic thrombosis associated with renal infarction has also been described (Mochizuki et al., 2003).

At low doses, cocaine can delay ejaculation and orgasm, which combined with its euphoric effects may be used to heighten the sexual experience (Smith, Wesson, and Apter-Marsh, 1984). However, chronic cocaine use has been associated with sexual dysfunction. Male users have difficulty maintaining erection and ejaculating (Cregler, 1989). Priapism has been associated with insufflation, intraurethral, intracavernous, and topical use of cocaine (Altman et al., 1999; Munarriz et al., 2003). The mechanisms responsible for sexual dysfunction and priapism remain unclear.

Gastrointestinal

Compared with the effect of cocaine use on other organ systems, there are relatively few reported adverse effects on the gastrointestinal tract (Hoang, Lee, and Anand, 1998). However, serious adverse effects of cocaine on the gastrointestinal tract have been observed, and include intestinal ischemia, intestinal infarction, and ulcer perforation. A particular problem with cocaine, related to the gastrointestinal tract, is the ingestion of cocaine in an effort to either hide evidence ("body stuffers") or transport large amounts of it ("body packers") (Hollander and Hoffman, 1998).

The occurrence of intestinal ischemia from cocaine use has been well documented and has occurred from all routes of exposure, including insufflation, intravenous injection, smoking, and ingestion (Herrine, Park, and Wechsler, 1998; Hon et al., 1990; Linder et al., 2000; Myers et al., 1996; Nalbandian et al., 1985). Ischemia in both the large and small intestines has been reported and has progressed to infarction and death in some cases (Hoang, Lee, and Anand, 1998). In many of the reported cases, the intestinal vasculature was normal on examination, suggesting vasospasm as the etiology of ischemia and infarction (Freudenberger, Cappell, and Hutt, 1990; Herrine, Park, and Wechsler, 1998; Mustard et al., 1992). In some cases, however, abnormalities have been documented in the arteries. Damage to small caliber arterioles has been observed, suggesting that the cocaine may have caused endothelial damage (Garfia et al., 1990). Thrombosis in the major mesenteric arteries has also been demonstrated angiographically (Myers et al., 1996). In some cases of gastrointestinal infarction, perforation of the gastrointestinal tract has occurred (Brown, Rosenholtz, and Marshall, 1994).

Perforations of gastric and duodenal ulcers are also known to occur in temporal relation to crack use (Feliciano et al., 1999; Lee et al., 1990; Muniz and Evans, 2001; Sharma et al., 1997). The mechanism for this remains unknown but may also be related to the vasoconstrictive effect and resulting ischemia on the stomach and duodenum (Feliciano et al., 1999; Sharma et al., 1997).

A potentially disastrous scenario occasionally encountered is the individual who has swallowed cocaine. This may have been done in an attempt to conceal evidence during imminent arrest ("body stuffing"), or as a means of concealment for drug smuggling ("body packing") (Caruana et al., 1984). When done in an attempt at rapid concealment the cocaine may be unwrapped, wrapped in a plastic bag, balloon, condom, paper, or in a crack vial (Hoffman et al., 1990; Sporer and Firestone, 1997). With smuggling, the cocaine is typically well packaged in balloons or condoms (Suarez, Arango, and Lester, 1977). Although many people pass the contained material uneventfully, release of the contents has resulted in convulsions and death (Fishbain and Wetli, 1981; June et al., 2000; Suarez, Arango, and Lester, 1977).

Liver

Liver damage is a relatively uncommon reported adverse effect associated with cocaine use (Mallat and Dhumeaux, 1991). Liver damage, and in some cases liver failure have been reported associated with cocaine use (Kanel et al., 1990; Perino, Warren, and Levine, 1987; Silva et al., 1991; Wanless et al., 1990). In addition, the lifestyle of cocaine users and the intravenous route of cocaine administration may predispose users to various viral causes of hepatitis (Van Thiel and Perper, 1992).

The mechanism for cocaine-induced liver damage is probably multifactorial (Mallat and Dhumeaux, 1991) and liver damage often occurs in the setting of cocaine-induced hyperthermia and shock, which are known causes of liver injury (Silva et al., 1991). Furthermore, the metabolism of cocaine may lead to toxic metabolites which may be directly injurious to liver cells. The majority of cocaine is metabolized in the blood by pseudo-cholinesterase and in the liver by hepatic esterase to nontoxic metabolites. Within the liver, the cytochrome P450 system metabolizes the remaining cocaine (Van Thiel and Perper, 1992) through a minor pathway that produces metabolites such as norcocaine nitroxide, a free radical that may initiate liver damage (Kloss, Rosen, and Rauckman, 1984; Ndikum-Moffor, Schoeb, and Roberts, 1998).

Pancreas

One study from Brazil associated chronic cocaine smoking with the development of pancreatic adenocarcinoma. Further study is required to confirm this association (Duarte et al., 1999).

Head and Neck, Nose and Throat

Head and neck complications from cocaine use are intimately related to the route of drug administration. Adverse effects include chronic rhinitis, nasal septal perforations, destructive facial processes, sinusitis, dental erosions, and thermal injuries.

Chronic nasal insufflation of cocaine may lead to various local effects on the nares. Rebound hyperemia after drug discontinuation may lead to a condition of chronic rhinitis similar to rhinitis medicamentosa (Schwartz et al., 1989). Nasal septal perforation is a well-known adverse effect of chronic cocaine insufflation that in some cases has progressed to nasal cartilage collapse and saddle-nose deformity (Deutsch and Millard, 1989; Vilensky, 1982). An even more devastating condition is an aggressive destructive facial process that may simulate Wegener's granulomatosis, neoplasms, or chronic infections (Carter and Grossman, 2000; Dagget, Haghighi, and Terkeltaub, 1990; Sittel and Eckel, 1998). A similar condition resulted when an individual was assaulted and had crack cocaine forcibly impacted in the nostrils (Tierney and Stadelmann, 1999). Nasal septal perforation and the more devastating conditions associated with chronic nasal insufflation all involve the progressive destruction of tissue. This is likely the result of a combination of chronic cocaine-induced vasoconstriction, irritation, and local trauma from nasal picking. Irritation from adulterants in the insufflated cocaine may also be contributory (Carter and Grossman, 2000; Dagget, Haghighi, and Terkeltaub, 1990). Insufflation has also been associated with bacterial sinusitis, including an unusual case in which the causative organism was *Clostridium botulinum* (Kudrow et al., 1988).

Dental erosions have been reported with insufflation and with an abuser who applied cocaine topically (Krutchkoff et al., 1990). Rapid gingival recession has also been reported in an individual who regularly applied cocaine to his gums (Kapila and Kashani, 1997).

Thermal injuries from smoking both freebase and crack have resulted in burns to the upper respiratory tract and esophagus (Meleca et al., 1997). Both the hot cocaine vapors and metal from the pipes used to smoke the cocaine have been implicated. One of the potentially life-threatening thermal injuries described is epiglottitis (Mayo-Smith and Spinale, 1997; Savitt and Colagiovanni, 1991). In one case, passive inhalation of crack smoke in a child was implicated in thermal epiglottitis (Karasch, Vinci, and Reece, 1990). Hot cocaine vapor has also caused loss of eyelash and eyebrow hair (Tames and Goldenring, 1986).

Ocular

Relatively few adverse effects of cocaine use on the eyes have been reported. The adverse effects include corneal epithelial defects, preseptal cellulitis, optic neuropathy, precipitation of acute angle-closure glaucoma, opsoclonus, and impaired color vision.

Corneal epithelial defects resulting from crack smoking have led to the term "crack eye" (McHenry et al., 1989). Multiple mechanisms postulated include a direct toxic effect of the cocaine alkaloid and a local anesthetic effect that disrupts normal blink mechanisms and causes an exposure keratopathy (Sachs, Zagelbaum, and Hersh, 1993). In some cases, the injuries led to a secondary bacterial infection (Zagelbaum, Tannenbaum, and Hersh, 1991). Another infection, preseptal cellulitis, has been reported in the setting of cocaine-induced bony orbit destruction (Underdahl and Chiou, 1998). The ability of chronic cocaine use to cause an osteolytic sinusitis leading to bilateral optic neuropathy has also been reported (Newman et al., 1988).

Nasal insufflation of cocaine has precipitated narrow angle-closure glaucoma. It is thought that cocaine may reach the eye by retrograde delivery via the nasolacrimal system or by inadvertent rubbing of the eye. The mydriatic (pupil-dilating) effect of cocaine appears to be a precipitating factor (Hari et al., 1999; Mitchell and Schwartz, 1996).

Opsoclonus, an abnormal movement disorder of the eye that involves rapid, irregular, nonrhythmic movements in horizontal and vertical directions, has been reported with cocaine use. The mechanism is unclear (Elkardoudi-Pijnenburg and Van Vliet, 1996). Studies have also shown impaired color vision in patients recovering from cocaine use. It is postulated that cocaine interferes with the retinal dopamine system, which affects retinal neurotransmission (Desai et al., 1997).

Pregnancy

Cocaine use during pregnancy is associated with various adverse effects both to the mother and fetus including an increased incidence of placental abruption, prematurity, intrauterine growth retardation, and microcephaly (small brain size). Various neurologic, cardiac, ophthalmic, and gastrointestinal defects have occurred in children who were exposed in utero to cocaine (Plessinger and Woods, 1998). A detailed review of the effects of cocaine on the fetus appears in Chapter 7.

OTHER STIMULANTS

Methamphetamine

Amphetamine was first synthesized in 1887 and introduced in the 1930s in the form of inhalers for treating rhinitis and asthma. Amphetamines and amphetamine derivatives are still prescribed for the treatment of attention deficit disorder and for the treatment of narcolepsy. Multiple drugs, both legal and illegal, have been synthesized by various modifications to the structure of amphetamine. Therapeutic medications include phenylpropanolamine, pseudoephedrine, and ephedrine. Illicit drugs include methamphetamine and the "designer" drug Ecstasy (3,4-methylenedioxymethamphetamine), also known as MDMA (Derlet and Heischober, 1990).

Both amphetamine and methamphetamine have become common drugs of abuse. Methamphetamine differs from amphetamine by the presence of a methyl group on the amine portion of the molecule, which affords improved central nervous system penetration. Amphetamines are abused through various routes of administration including intravenous, oral, insufflation, and inhalation (Albertson, Derlet, and Van Hoozen, 1999). Amphetamine and methamphetamine exert their clinical effects primarily by releasing the catecholamines dopamine, and norepinephrine from presynaptic nerve terminals. The resulting clinical effects are very similar to cocaine with a few notable exceptions. The duration of effect of amphetamines is up to 24 hours, which is much longer than that of cocaine. In addition, amphetamines lack the sodium channel blocking effect of cocaine and therefore may be less likely to precipitate cardiac dysrhythmias (Chiang, 1991). Last, amphetamines have not been associated with the platelet aggregation and atherosclerosis that cocaine has and therefore may be less likely to precipitate myocardial infarctions.

As predicted by the very similar mechanism of action and physiological response to cocaine, many of the reported associated adverse effects to amphetamines are also similar (Albertson, Derlet, and Van Hoozen, 1999). Associated cardiovascular adverse effects include hypertension, tachycardia, myocardial infarction (Bashour, 1994; Packe, Garton, and Jennings, 1990; Wijetunga et al., 2004), cardiomyopathy (Hong, Matsuyama, and Nur, 1991; Wijetunga et al., 1993), and aortic dissection (Davis and Stalwell, 1994). Central nervous system effects include intracerebral hemorrhages (Imanse and Vanneste, 1990), intracerebral ischemic strokes (Rothrock, Rubenstein, and Lyden, 1988), seizures, psychosis, and choreoathetoid movements (Lundh and Tunving, 1981). Ischemic colitis (Johnson and Berenson, 1991), rhabdomyolysis (Richards et al., 1999), hepatotoxicity (Jones et al., 1994), and various fetal anomalies (Plessinger, 1998) have also been reported. The medical literature detailing the associated adverse effects of cocaine use is much more extensive than that about amphetamine use. This is likely to change with continued abuse of amphetamines.

Phenylpropanolamine

Phenylpropanolamine is a synthetic stimulant that has a very similar structure to amphetamine. Until recently it was present in a multitude of both over-the-counter and prescription-only cold preparations, as well as weight loss formulations (Pentel, 1984). Adverse effects associated with its use, misuse, and intentional overdose have been known for many years, leading many to recommend removing it from the market. In 2000, the Food and Drug Administration (FDA) began taking steps to remove phenylpropanolamine from all drug products and requested that all drug companies discontinue marketing products containing the drug (FDA Talk Paper, 2000).

The major adverse effects associated with phenylpropanolamine are neurologic, particularly hemorrhagic strokes that have been lethal (Forman et al., 1989; Glick et al., 1987; Lake et al., 1990). Less commonly reported adverse effects include hypertension (Lake et al., 1988), myocardial infarction (Leo et al., 1996; Oosterbaan and Burns, 2000), dysrhythmias (Conway, Walsh, and Palomba, 1989), ischemic bowel (Johnson, Stafford, and Volpe, 1985), seizures, and psychosis (Marshall and Douglas, 1994). Most of the adverse effects are explained by the pharmacologic action of phenylpropanolamine. Phenylpropanolamine primarily works as a direct alpha-1 agonist causing constriction of arterioles. Through this mechanism the commonly desired therapeutic effect of nasal decongestion is achieved. With slightly higher than therapeutic doses, however, the alpha-1 agonist can cause potentially severe hypertension which may require treatment and lead to lethal complications such as hemorrhagic stroke (Pentel, 1984).

Ephedra

Ephedra refers to the stems and leaves derived from various plants of the genus *Ephedra*. Often referred to by its Chinese name, ma huang, ephedra has been used for thousands of years for various ailments (Scheindlin, 2003). Ephedrine, an amphetamine-like substance, is one of the major active constituents of ephedra, and has significant sympathomimetic properties. Prior to a recent, and what may be temporary, withdrawal from the market, ephedra had become a popular component in various supplements that were marketed for weight loss and athletic performance enhancement. However, various associated adverse effects, as could be predicted by its amphetamine-like structure and mechanism of action, became more frequently reported. In a review of adverse events reported to the FDA that were deemed definitely, probably, or possibly related to the use of ephedra alkaloid containing dietary supplements, hypertension was found to be the most frequent. Strokes, myocardial infarctions, and cardiac arrest or sudden death, were also found to be definitely or probably related to use (Haller and Benowitz, 2000). In a recent analysis of reported convulsions associated with dietary supplements, ephedra use was implicated in the majority of cases (Haller, Meier, and Olson, 2005). Ephedrine and ephedra have also been associated with an increased risk of both minor and more serious psychiatric symptoms, such as psychosis (Maglione et al., 2005; Shekelle et al., 2003). The death of a professional baseball player that was attributed partly to his use of an ephedra-containing dietary supplement helped prompt the FDA in 2004 to ban ephedra as a dietary supplement.

SUMMARY AND CONCLUSIONS

Cocaine use is fairly common in the United States and is associated with a variety of serious adverse effects. Many of these effects seem to occur by means of the physiological effects of cocaine on the cardiovascular system. Methamphetamine is becoming a more popular drug of abuse whose mechanism of action and adverse effects are very similar to those of cocaine. Phenylpropanolamine and ephedra are both amphetamine-like agents that until recently were found in numerous nonprescription formulations. Recognition that both are associated with severe side effects led to significant restrictions on their use.

REFERENCES

Adrouny, A.; Magnusson, P. (1985). Pneumopericardium from cocaine inhalation (letter). *New England Journal of Medicine* 313:48-49.

Aggarwal, S.K.; Williams, V.; Levine, S.R.; Cassin, B.J.; Garcia, J.H. (1996). Cocaine-associated intracranial hemorrhage: Absence of vasculitis in 14 cases. *Neurology* 46:1741-1743.

Albertson, T.E.; Derlet, R.W.; Van Hoozen, B.E. (1999). Methamphetamine and the expanding complications of amphetamines. *Western Journal of Medicine* 170: 214-219.

Allred, R.J.; Ewer, S. (1981). Fatal pulmonary edema following intravenous "free base" cocaine use. *Annals of Emergency Medicine* 10:441-442.

Altman, A.L.; Seftel, A.D.; Brown, S.L.; Hampel, N. (1999). Cocaine associated priapism. *Journal of Urology* 161:1817-1818.

Baldwin, G.C.; Tashkin, D.P.; Buckley, D.M.; Park, A.N.; Dubinett, S.M.; Roth, M.D. (1997). Marijuana and cocaine impair alveolar macrophage function and cytokine production. *American Journal of Respiratory and Critical Care Medicine* 156:1606-1613.

Bashour, T.T. (1994). Acute myocardial infarction resulting from amphetamine abuse: A spasm-thrombus interplay? *American Heart Journal* 128:1237-1239.

Bauman, J.L.; Grawe, J.J.; Winecoff, A.P.; Hariman, R.J. (1994). Cocaine-related sudden cardiac death: A hypothesis correlating basic science and clinical observations. *Journal of Clinical Pharmacology* 34:902-911.

Benzaquen, B.S.; Cohen, V.; Eisenberg, M.J. (2001). Effects of cocaine on the coronary arteries. *American Heart Journal* 142:402-410.

Boghdadi, M.S.; Henning, R.J. (1997). Cocaine: Pathophysiology and clinical toxicology. *Heart and Lung* 26:466-483.

Brick, J.; Erickson, C. (1999). *Drugs, the Brain, and Behavior: The Pharmacology of Abuse and Dependence.* Binghamton, NY: The Haworth Medical Press.

Brody, S.L.; Slovis, C.M.; Wrenn, K.D. (1990). Cocaine-related medical problems: Consecutive series of 233 patients. *American Journal of Medicine* 88:325-331.

Brown, D.N.; Rosenholtz, M.J.; Marshall, J.B. (1994). Ischemic colitis related to cocaine abuse. *The American Journal of Gastroenterology* 89:1558-1560.

Carter, E.L.; Grossman, M.E. (2000). Cocaine-induced centrofacial ulceration. *Cutis* 65:73-76.

Caruana, D.S.; Weinbach, B.; Goerg, D.; Gardner, L.B. (1984). Cocaine-packet ingestion. *Annals of Internal Medicine* 100:73-74.

Catalano, G.; Catalano, M.C.; Rodriguez, R. (1997). Dystonia associated with crack cocaine use. *Southern Medical Journal* 90:1050-1052.

Chambers, H.F.; Morris, D.L.; Tauber, M.G.; Modin, G. (1987). Cocaine use and the risk for endocarditis in intravenous drug users. *Annals of Internal Medicine* 106:833-836.

Chan, L.; Pham, H.; Reece, E.A. (1997). Pneumothorax in pregnancy associated with cocaine use. *American Journal of Perinatology* 14:385-388.

Chang, R.A.; Rossi, N.F. (1995). Intermittent cocaine use associated with recurrent dissection of the thoracic and abdominal aorta. *Chest* 108:1758-1762.

Chiang, W.K. (1991). Amphetamines. In: Goldfrank, L.R.; Flomenbaum, N.E.; Lewin, N.A.; Weisman, R.S.; Howland, M.A.; Hoffman, R.S. (eds.), *Goldfrank's Toxicological Emergencies* (pp. 1091-1103). Stamford, CT: Simon and Schuster.

Conway, E.E.; Walsh, C.A.; Palomba, A.L. (1989). Supraventricular tachycardia following the administration of phenylpropanolamine in an infant. *Pediatric Emergency Care* 5:173-174.

Cooper, C.B.; Bai, T.R.; Heyderman, E. (1983). Cellulose granulomas in the lungs of a cocaine sniffer. *British Medical Journal* 286:2021-2022.

Cregler, L.L. (1989). Adverse health consequences of cocaine abuse. *Journal of the National Medical Association* 81:27-38.

Cregler, L.L.; Mark, H. (1986). Medical complications of cocaine abuse. *New England Journal of Medicine* 315:1495-1500.

Cucco, R.A.; Yoo, O.H.; Cregler, L.; Chang, J.C. (1987). Nonfatal pulmonary edema after "freebase" cocaine smoking. *American Review of Respiratory Diseases* 136:179-181.

Dagget, R.B.; Haghighi, P.; Terkeltaub, R.A. (1990). Nasal cocaine abuse causing an aggressive midline intranasal and pharyngeal destructive process mimicking midline reticulosis and limited Wegener's granulomatosis. *Journal of Rheumatology* 17:838-840.

Daniels, J.; Baker, D.G.; Norman, A.B. (1996). Cocaine-induced tics in untreated Tourette's syndrome (letter). *American Journal of Psychiatry* 153(7):965.

Daras, M.; Koppel, B.S.; Atos-Radzion, E. (1994). Cocaine-induced choreoathetoid movements ("crack dancing"). *Neurology* 44:751-752.

Daras, M.; Tuchman, A.J.; Koppel, B.S.; Samkoff, L.M.; Weitzner, I.; Marc, J. (1994). Neurovascular complications of cocaine. *Acta Neurologica Scandinavica* 90:124-129.

Davis, G.G.; Swalwell, C.I. (1994). Acute aortic dissections and ruptured berry aneurysms associated with methamphetamine abuse. *Journal of Forensic Sciences* 39:1481-1485.

Derlet, R.W.; Heischober, B. (1990). Methamphetamine: Stimulant of the 1990s? *Western Journal of Medicine* 153:625-628.

Desai, P.; Roy, M.; Roy, A.; Brown, S.; Smelson, D. (1997). Impaired color vision in cocaine-withdrawn patients. *Archives of General Psychiatry* 54:696-699.

Deutsch, H.L.; Millard, R. (1989). A new cocaine abuse complex. *Archives of Otolaryngology Head and Neck Surgery* 115:235-237.

Duarte, J.G.C.; Pantoja, A.F.; Pantoja, J.G.; Chaves, C.P. (1999). Chronic inhaled cocaine abuse may predispose to the development of pancreatic adenocarcinoma. *American Journal of Surgery* 178:426-427.

Dunea, G.; Arruda, J.; Bakir, A.A.; Share, D.S.; Smith, E.C. (1995). Role of cocaine in end-stage renal disease in some hypertensive African Americans. *American Journal of Nephrology* 15:5-9.

Elkardoudi-Pijnenburg, Y.; Van Vliet, A. (1996). Opsoclonus: A rare complication of cocaine misuse (letter). *Journal of Neurology, Neurosurgery, and Psychiatry* 60:592.

Farrel, P.E.; Diehl, A.K. (1991). Acute dystonic reaction to crack cocaine. *Annals of Emergency Medicine* 20:322.

FDA Talk Paper (2000). FDA issues public health warning on phenylpropanolamine. November 6.

Feliciano, D.V.; Ojukwu, J.C.; Rozycki, G.S.; Ballard, R.B.; Ingram, W.L.; Salomone, J.; Narnias, N.; Newman, P.G. (1999). The epidemic of cocaine-related juxtapyloric perforations. *Annals of Surgery* 229(6):801-806.

Fernandez, W.G.; Hung, O.; Bruno, G.R.; Galea, S.; Chiang, W.K. (2005). Factors predictive of acute renal failure and need for hemodialysis among ED patients with rhabdomyolysis. *American Journal of Emergency Medicine* 23:1-7.

Fishbain, D.A.; Wetli, C.V. (1981). Cocaine intoxication, delirium, and death in a body packer. *Annals of Emergency Medicine* 10:531-532.

Fisher, A.; Holroyd, B.R. (1992). Cocaine-associated dissection of the thoracic aorta. *Journal of Emergency Medicine* 10:723-727.

Flores, E.D.; Lange, R.A.; Cigarroa, R.G.; Hillis, L.D. (1990). Effect of cocaine on coronary artery dimensions in atherosclerotic coronary artery disease: Enhanced vasoconstriction at sites of significant stenoses. *Journal of the American College of Cardiology* 16:74-79.

Forman, H.P.; Levin, S.; Stewart, B.; Patel, M.; Feinstein, S. (1989). Cerebral vasculitis and hemorrhage in an adolescent taking diet pills containing phenylpropanolamine: Case report and review of literature. *Pediatrics* 83:737-741.

Forrester, J.M.; Steele, A.W.; Waldron, J.A.; Parsons, P.E. (1990). Crack lung: An acute pulmonary syndrome with a spectrum of clinical and histopathologic findings. *American Review of Respiratory Diseases* 142:462-467.

Fredericks, R.K.; Lefkowitz, D.S.; Challa, V.R.; Troost, T. (1991). Cerebral vasculitis associated with cocaine abuse. *Stroke* 22:1437-1439.

Freudenberger, R.S.; Cappell, M.S.; Hutt, D.A. (1990). Intestinal infarction after intravenous cocaine administration. *Annals of Internal Medicine* 113:715-716.

Garfia, A.; Valverde, J.L.; Borondo, J.C.; Candenas, I.; Lucena, J. (1990). Vascular lesions in intestinal ischemia induced by cocaine-alcohol abuse: Report of a fatal case due to overdose. *Journal of Forensic Sciences* 35:740-745.

Gawin, F.H.; Kleber, H.D. (1986). Abstinence symptomatology and psychiatric diagnosis in cocaine abusers. *Archives of General Psychiatry* 43:107-113.

Glick, R.; Hoying, J.; Cerullo, L.; Perlman, S. (1987). Phenylpropanolamine: An over-the-counter drug causing central nervous system vasculitis and intracerebral hemorrhage. Case report and review. *Neurosurgery* 20:969-974.

Goodman, P.E.; Rennie, P.M. (1995). Renal infarction secondary to nasal insufflation of cocaine. *American Journal of Emergency Medicine* 13:421-423.

Haim, D.Y.; Lippmann, M.L.; Goldberg, S.K.; Walkenstein, M.D. (1995). The pulmonary complications of crack cocaine: A comprehensive review. *Chest* 107:233-240.

Haller, C.A.; Benowitz, N.L. (2000). Adverse cardiovascular and central nervous system events associated with dietary supplements containing ephedra alkaloids. *New England Journal of Medicine* 343:1833-1838.

Haller, C.A.; Meier, K.H.; Olson, K.R. (2005). Seizures reported in association with use of dietary supplements. *Clinical Toxicology* 43:23-30.

Hari, C.K.; Roblin, D.G.; Clayton, M.I.; Nair, R.G. (1999). Acute angle closure glaucoma precipitated by intranasal application of cocaine. *Journal of Laryngology and Otology* 113:250-251.

Hart, C.L.; Jatlow, P.; Sevarino, K.A.; McCance-Katz, E.F. (2000). Comparison of intravenous cocaethylene and cocaine in humans. *Psychopharmacology* 149: 153-162.

Heesch, C.M.; Wilhelm, C.R.; Ristich, J.; Bontempo, F.A.; Wagner, W.R. (2000). Cocaine activates platelets and increases the formation of circulating platelet containing microaggregates in humans. *Heart* 83:688-695.

Herrine, S.K.; Park, P.K.; Wechsler, R.J. (1998). Acute mesenteric ishchemia following intranasal cocaine use. *Digestive Diseases and Sciences* 43:586-589.

Herzlich, B.C.; Arsura, E.L.; Pagala, M.; Grob, D. (1988). Rhabdomyolysis related to cocaine abuse. *Annals of Internal Medicine* 109:335-336.

Hoang, M.P.; Lee, E.L.; Anand, A. (1998). Histologic spectrum of arterial and arteriolar lesions in acute and chronic cocaine-induced mesenteric ischemia. *The American Journal of Surgical Pathology* 22:1404-1410.

Hoffman, C.K.; Goodman, P.C. (1989). Pulmonary edema in cocaine smokers. *Radiology* 172:463-465.

Hoffman, R.S.; Chiang, W.K.; Weisman, R.S.; Goldfrank, L.R. (1990). Prospective evaluation of "crack-vial" ingestions. *Veterinary and Human Toxicology* 32:164-167.

Hollander, J.E.; Hoffman, R.S. (1992). Cocaine-induced myocardial infarction: An analysis and review of the literature. *Journal of Emergency Medicine* 10:169-177.

Hollander, J.E.; Hoffman, R.S. (1998). Cocaine. In: Goldfrank, L.R.; Flomenbaum, N.E.; Lewin, N.A.; Weisman, R.S.; Howland, M.A.; Hoffman, R.S. (eds.), *Goldfrank's Toxicologic Emergencies* (pp. 1072-1089). Stamford, CT: Simon and Schuster.

Hon, D.C.; Salloum, L.J.; Hardy, H.W.; Barone, J.E. (1990). Crack-induced enteric ischemia. *New Jersey Medicine* 87:1001-1002.

Hong, R.; Matsuyama, E.; Nur, K. (1991). Cardiomyopathy associated with the smoking of crystal methamphetamine. *Journal of the American Medical Association* 265:1152-1154.

Howard, R.E.; Heuter, D.C.; Davis, G.J. (1985). Acute myocardial infarction following cocaine abuse in a young woman with normal coronary arteries. *Journal of the American Medical Association* 254:95-96.

Hsue, P.Y.; Salinas, C.L.; Bolger, A.F.; Benowitz, N.L.; Waters, D.D. (2002). Acute aortic dissection related to crack cocaine. *Circulation* 105:1592-1595.

Imanse, J.; Vanneste, J. (1990). Intraventricular hemorrhage following amphetamine abuse. *Neurology* 40:1318-1319.

Johnson, D.A.; Stafford, P.W.; Volpe, R.J. (1985). Ischemic bowel infarction and phenylpropanolamine use. *Western Journal of Medicine* 142:399-400.

Johnson, T.D.; Berenson, M.M. (1991). Methamphetamine-induced ischemic colitis. *Journal of Clinical Gastroenterology* 13:687-689.

Jones, A.L.; Jarvie, D.R.; McDermid, G.; Proudfoot, A.T. (1994). Hepatocellular damage following amphetamine intoxication. *Clinical Toxicology* 32:435-444.

June, R.; Aks, S.E.; Keys, N.; Wahl, M. (2000). Medical outcome of cocaine bodystuffers. *Journal of Emergency Medicine* 18:221-224.

Kabas, J.S.; Blanchard, S.M.; Matsuyama, Y.; Long, J.D.; Hoffman G.W. Jr.; Ellinwood, E.H.; Smith, P.K.; Strauss, H.C. (1990) Cocaine-mediated impairment of cardiac conduction in the dog: A potential mechanism for sudden death after cocaine. *Journal of Pharmacology and Experimental Therapeutics* 252: 185-191.

Kanel, G.C.; Cassidy, W.; Shuster, L.; Reynolds, T.B. (1990). Cocaine-induced liver cell injury: Comparison of morphological features in man and in experimental models *Hepatology* 11:646-651.

Kapila, Y.L.; Kashani, H. (1997). Cocaine-associated rapid gingival recession and dental erosion. A case report. *Journal of Periodontology* 68:485-488.

Karasch, S.; Vinci, R.; Reece, R. (1990). Esophagitis, epiglottitis, and cocaine alkaloid ("crack"): "Accidental" poisoning or child abuse? *Pediatrics* 86:117-119.

Karch, S.B. (1999). Cocaine: History, use, abuse. *Journal of the Royal Society of Medicine* 92:393-397.

Kissner, D.G.; Lawrence, W.D.; Selis, J.E.; Flint, A. (1987). Crack lung: Pulmonary disease caused by cocaine abuse. *American Review of Respiratory Diseases* 136:1250-1252.

Kloss, M.W.; Rosen, G.M.; Rauckman, E.J. (1984). Cocaine-mediated hepatotoxicity: A critical review. *Biochemical Pharmacology* 33:169-173.

Krutchkoff, D.J.; Eisenberg, E.; O'Brien, J.E.; Ponzillo, J.J. (1990). Cocaine induced dental erosions (letter). *New England Journal of Medicine* 320:408.

Kudrow, D.B.; Henry, D.A.; Haake, D.A.; Marshall, G.; Mathisen, G. (1988). Botulism associated with *Clostridium botulinum* sinusitis after intranasal cocaine abuse. *Annals of Internal Medicine* 109:984-985.

Lake, C.R.; Gallant, S.; Masson, E.; Miller, P. (1990). Adverse drug effects attributed to phenylpropanolamine: A review of 142 case reports. *American Journal of Medicine* 89:195-208.

Lake, C.R.; Zaloga, G.; Clymer, R.; Quirk, R.; Chernow, B. (1988). A double dose of phenylpropanolamine causes transient hypertension. *American Journal of Medicine* 85:339-343.

Lange, R.A.; Cigarroa, R.G.; Yancy, C.W.; Willard, J.E.; Popma, J.J.; Sills, M.N.; McBride, W.; Kim, A.S.; Hillis, L.D. (1989). Cocaine-induced coronary-artery vasoconstriction. *New England Journal of Medicine* 321:1557-1562.

Lason, W. (2001). Neurochemical and pharmacological aspects of cocaine-induced seizures. *Polish Journal of Pharmacology* 53:57-60.

Lee, H.S.; LaMaute, H.R.; Pizzi, W.F.; Picard, D.L.; Luks, F.I. (1990). Acute gastroduodenal perforations associated with use of crack. *Annals of Surgery* 211:15-17.

Leo, P.J.; Hollander, J.E.; Shih, R.D.; Marcus, S.M. (1996). Phenylpropanolamine and associated myocardial injury. *Annals of Emergency Medicine* 28:359-362.

Levenson, T.; Greenberger, P.A.; Donoghue, E.R.; Lifschultz, B.D. (1996). Asthma deaths confounded by substance abuse. *Chest* 110:604-610.

Lichtenfeld, P.J.; Rubin, D.B.; Feldman, R.S. (1984). Subarachnoid hemorrhage precipitated by cocaine snorting. *Archives of Neurology* 41:223-224.

Linder, J.D.; Monkemuller, K.E.; Raijman, I.; Johnson, L.; Lazenby, A.J.; Wilcox, C.M. (2000). Cocaine-associated ischemic colitis. *Southern Medical Journal* 93:909-913.

Lowenstein, D.H.; Massa, S.M.; Rowbotham, M.C.; Collins, S.D.; McKinney, H.E.; Simon, R.P. (1987). Acute neurologic and psychiatric complications associated with cocaine abuse. *American Journal of Medicine* 83:841-846.

Lundh, H.; Tunving, K. (1981). An extrapyramidal choreiform syndrome caused by amphetamine addiction. *Journal of Neurology, Neurosurgery, and Psychiatry* 44:728-730.

Maglione, M.; Miotto, K.; Iguchi, M.; Jungvig, L.; Morton, S.C.; Shekelle, P.G. (2005). Psychiatric effects of ephedra use: An analysis of food and drug administration reports of adverse events. *American Journal of Psychiatry* 162:189-191.

Mallat, A.; Dhumeaux, D. (1991). Cocaine and the liver. *Journal of Hepatology* 12:275-278.

Manschreck, T.C.; Laughery, J.A.; Weisstein, C.C.; Allen, D.; Humblestone, B.; Neville, M.; Podlewski, H.; Mitra, N. (1988). Characteristics of freebase cocaine psychosis. *Yale Journal of Biology and Medicine* 61:115-122.

Marshall, R.D.; Douglas, C.J. (1994). Phenylpropanolamine-induced psychosis: Potential predisposing factors. *General Hospital Psychiatry* 16:358-360.

Marzuk, P.M.; Tardiff, K.; Leon, A.C.; Hirsch, C.S.; Stajic, M.; Portera, L.; Hartwell, N.; Iqbal, I. (1995). Fatal injuries after cocaine use as a leading cause of death among young adults in New York City. *New England Journal of Medicine* 332:1753-1757.

Mayo-Smith, M.F.; Spinale, J. (1997). Thermal epiglottitis in adults: A new complication of illicit drug abuse. *Journal of Emergency Medicine* 15:483-485.

McHenry, J.G.; Zeiter, J.H.; Mandion, M.P.; Cowden, J.W. (1989). Corneal epithelial defects after smoking crack cocaine. *American Journal of Ophthalmology* 108:732.

Meleca, R.J.; Burgio, D.L.; Carr, R.M.; Lolachi, C.M. (1997). Mucosal injuries of the upper aerodigestive tract after smoking crack or freebase cocaine. *Laryngoscope* 107:620-625.

Mendoza, R.; Miller, B.L.; Mena, I. (1992). Emergency room evaluation of cocaine-associated neuropsychiatric disorders. *Recent Developments in Alcoholism* 10: 73-87.

Merigram, K.S.; Roberts, J.R. (1987). Cocaine intoxication: Hyperpyrexia, rhabdomyolysis and acute renal failure. *Clinical Toxicology* 25:135-148.

Miller, W.E.; Spiekerman, R.E.; Hepper, N.G. (1972). Pneumomediastinum resulting from performing Valsalva maneuvers during marijuana smoking. *Chest* 62:233-234.

Minor, R.L.; Scott, B.D.; Brown, D.D.; Winniford, M.D. (1991). Cocaine-induced myocardial infarction in patients with normal coronary arteries. *Annals of Internal Medicine* 115:797-806.

Mitchell, J.D.; Schwartz, A.L. (1996). Acute angle-closure glaucoma associated with intranasal cocaine abuse. *American Journal of Ophthalmology* 122:425-426.

Mochizuki, Y.; Zhang, M.; Golestaneh, L.; Thananart, S.; Coco, M. (2003) Acute aortic thrombosis and renal infarction in acute cocaine intoxication: A case report and review of literature. *Clinical Nephrology* 60:130-133.

Morris, J.B.; Shuck, J.M. (1985). Pneumomediastinum in a young male cocaine user (letter). *Annals of Emergency Medicine* 14:164-166.

Munarriz, R.; Hwang, J.; Goldstein, I.; Traish, A.M.; Kim, N.N. (2003). Cocaine and ephedrine-induced priapism: Case reports and investigation of potential adrenergic mechanisms. *Urology* 62:187-192.

Muniz, A.E; Evans, T. (2001). Acute gastrointestinal manifestations associated with use of crack. *American Journal of Emergency Medicine* 19:61-63.

Mustard, R.; Gray, R.; Maziak, D.; Deck, J. (1992). Visceral infarction caused by cocaine abuse: A case report. *Surgery* 112:951-955.

Myers, J.A.; Earnest, M.P. (1984). Generalized seizures and cocaine abuse. *Neurology* 34:675-676.

Myers, S.I.; Clagett, P.; Valentine, J.; Hansen, M.; Anand, A.; Chervu, A. (1996). Chronic intestinal ischemia caused by intravenous cocaine use: Report of two cases and review of the literature. *Journal of Vascular Surgery* 23:724-729.

Nalbandian, H.; Sheth, N.; Dietrich, R.; Georgiou, J. (1985). Intestinal ischemia caused by cocaine ingestion: Report of two cases. *Surgery* 97:374-376.

National Institute on Drug Abuse (1999). NIDA *Research Report Series: Cocaine Abuse and Addiction.* NIH Publication No. 99-4342. Rockville, MD: National Institutes of Health.

Ndikum-Moffor, F.M.; Schoeb, T.R.; Roberts, S.M. (1998). Liver toxicity from norcocaine nitroxide: An N-oxidative metabolite of cocaine. *The Journal of Pharmacology and Experimental Therapeutics* 284:413-419.

Newman, N.M.; DiLoreto, D.A.; Ho, J.T.; Klein, J.C.; Birnbaum, N.S. (1998). Bilateral optic neuropathy and osteolytic sinusitis complications of cocaine abuse. *Journal of the American Medical Association* 259:72-74.

Nolte, K.B.; Brass, L.M.; Fletterick, C.F. (1996). Intracranial hemorrhage associated with cocaine abuse: A prospective autopsy study. *Neurology* 46:1291-1296.

Nzerue, C.M.; Hewan-Lowe, K.; Riley, L.J. (2000). Cocaine and the kidney: A synthesis of pathophysiologic and clinical perspectives. *American Journal of Kidney Diseases* 35:783-795.

Oosterbaan, R.; Burns, M.J. (2000). Myocardial infarction associated with phenyl propanolamine. *Journal of Emergency Medicine* 18:55-59.

Oubeid, M.; Bickel, J.T.; Ingram, E.A.; Scott, G.C. (1990). Pulmonary talc granulomatosis in a cocaine sniffer. *Chest* 98:237-239.

Packe, G.E.; Garton, M.J.; Jennings, K. (1990). Acute myocardial infarction caused by intravenous amphetamine abuse. *British Heart Journal* 64:23-24.

Pentel, P. (1984). Toxicity of over-the-counter stimulants. *Journal of the American Medical Association* 252:1898-1903.

Perino, L.E.; Warren, G.H.; Levine, J.S. (1987). Cocaine-induced hepatotoxicity in humans. *Gastroenterology* 93:176-180.

Perper, J.A.; Van Thiel, D.H. (1992). Respiratory complications of cocaine abuse. *Recent Developments in Alcoholism* 10:363-377.

Plessinger, M.A. (1998). Prenatal exposure to amphetamines: Risks and adverse outcomes in pregnancy. *Obstetrics and Gynecology Clinics of North America* 25:119-138.

Plessinger, M.A.; Woods, J.R. (1998). Cocaine in pregnancy: Recent data on maternal and fetal risks. *Obstetrics and Gynecology Clinics of North America* 25:99-118.

Przywara, D.A.; Dambach, G.E. (1989). Direct actions of cocaine on cardiac cellular electrical activity. *Circulation Research* 65:185-192.

Rebhun, J. (1988). Association of asthma and freebase smoking. *Annals of Allergy* 60:339-342.

Rich, J.A.; Singer, D.E. (1991). Cocaine-related symptoms in patients presenting to an urban emergency department. *Annals of Emergency Medicine* 20:616-621.

Richards, J.R. (2000). Rhabdomyolysis and drugs of abuse. *Journal of Emergency Medicine* 19:51-56.

Richards, J.R.; Johnson, E.B.; Stark, R.W.; Derlet, R.W. (1999). Methamphetamine abuse and rhabdomyolysis in the ED: A 5-year study. *American Journal of Emergency Medicine* 17:681-685.

Rome, L.A.; Lippmann, M.L.; Dalsey, W.C.; Taggart, P.; Pomerantz, S. (2000). Prevalence of cocaine use and its impact on asthma exacerbation in an urban population. *Chest* 117:1324-1329.

Roth, D.; Alarcon, F.J.; Fernandez, J.A.; Preston, R.A.; Bourgoignie, J.J. (1988). Acute rhabdomyolysis associated with cocaine intoxication. *New England Journal of Medicine* 319:673-677.

Rothrock, J.F.; Rubenstein, R.; Lyden, P.D. (1988). Ischemic stroke associated with methamphetamine inhalation. *Neurology* 38:589-592.

Rowbotham, M.C.; Lowenstein, D.H. (1990). Neurologic consequences of cocaine use. *Annual Review of Medicine* 41:417-422.

Sachs, R.; Zagelbaum, B.M.; Hersh, P.S. (1993). Corneal complications associated with the use of crack cocaine. *Opthalmology* 100:187-191.

Savitt, D.L.; Colagiovanni, S. (1991). Crack cocaine-related epiglottitis (letter). *Annals of Emergency Medicine* 20:322-323.

Scheindlin, S. (2003). Ephedra: Once a boon, now a bane. *Molecular Interventions* 3:358-360.

Schwartz, R.H.; Estroff, T.; Fairbanks, D.; Hoffmann, N.G. (1989). Nasal symptoms associated with cocaine abuse during adolescence. *Archives of Otolaryngology—Head and Neck Surgery* 115:63-64.

Sharma, R.; Organ, C.H.; Hirvela, E.R.; Henderson, V.J. (1997). Clinical observation of the temporal association between crack cocaine and duodenal ulcer perforation. *American Journal of Surgery* 174:629-633.

Shekelle, P.G.; Hardy, M.L.; Morton, S.C.; Maglione, M.; Mojica, W.A.; Suttorp, M.J.; Rhodes, S.L.; Jungvig, L.; Gagne, J. (2003). Efficacy and safety of ephedra and ephedrine for weight loss and athletic performance: a meta-anaylsis. *Journal of the American Medical Association* 289:1537-1545.

Shesser, R.; Davis, C.; Edelstein, S. (1981). Pneumomediastinum and pneumothorax after inhaling alkaloidal cocaine. *Annals of Emergency Medicine* 10:213-215.

Silva, M.O.; Roth, D.; Reddy, K.R.; Fernandez, J.A.; Albores-Saavedra, J.; Schiff, E.R. (1991). Hepatic dysfunction accompanying acute cocaine intoxication. *Journal of Hepatology* 12:312-315.

Sittel, C.; Eckel, H.E. (1998). Nasal cocaine abuse presenting as a central facial destructive granuloma. *European Archives of Otorhinolaryngology* 255:446-447.

Smith, D.E.; Wesson, D.R.; Apter-Marsh, M. (1984). Cocaine- and alcohol-induced sexual dysfunction in patients with addictive diseases. *Journal of Psychoactive Drugs* 16:359-361.

Sporer, K.; Firestone, J. (1997). Clinical course of crack cocaine body stuffers. *Annals of Emergency Medicine.* 29:596-601.

Suarez, C.A.; Arango, A.; Lester, L. (1977). Cocaine-condom ingestion. *Journal of the American Medical Association* 238:1391-1392.

Tames, S.M.; Goldenring, J.M. (1986). Madarosis from cocaine use (letter). *New England Journal of Medicine* 314(20):1324.

Tashkin, D.P.; Kleerup, E.C.; Koyal, S.N.; Marques, J.A.; Goldman, M.D. (1996). Acute effects of inhaled and i.v. cocaine on airway dynamics. *Chest* 110:904-910.

Thakur, V.K.; Godley, C.; Weed, S.; Cook, M.E.; Hoffman, E. (1996). Case reports: Cocaine-associated accelerated hypertension and renal failure. *American Journal of Medical Science* 312(6):295-298.

Tierney, B.P.; Stadelmann, W.K. (1999). Necrotizing infection of the face secondary to intranasal impaction of "crack" cocaine. *Annals of Plastic Surgery* 43(6): 640-643.

Underdahl, J.P.; Chiou, A. (1998). Preseptal cellulites and orbital wall destruction secondary to nasal cocaine abuse. *American Journal of Ophthalmology* 125: 266-267.

Uva, J.L. (1997). Spontaneous pneumothoraces, pneumomediastinum, and pneumoperitoneum: Consequences of smoking crack cocaine. *Pediatric Emergency Care* 13:24-26.

Van Thiel, D.H.; Perper, J.A. (1992). Hepatotoxicity associated with cocaine abuse. *Recent Developments in Alcoholism* 10:335-341.

Vilensky, W. (1982). Illicit and licit drugs causing perforation of the nasal septum. *Journal of Forensic Sciences* 27:958-962.

Vitullo, J.C.; Karam, R.; Mekhail, N.; Wicker, P.; Engelmann, G.L.; Khairallah, P.A. (1989). Cocaine-induced small vessel spasm in isolated rat hearts. *American Journal of Pathology* 135:85-91.

Wanless, I.R.; Dore, S.; Gopinath, N.; Tan, J.; Cameron, R.; Heathcote, E.J.; Blendis, L.M.; Levy, G. (1990). Histopathology of cocaine hepatotoxicity report of four patients. *Gastroenterology* 98:497-501.

Warner, E.A. (1993). Cocaine abuse. *Annals of Internal Medicine* 119:226-235.

Weddington, W.W. (1993). Cocaine diagnosis and treatment. *Psychiatric Clinics of North America* 16:87-95.

Welch, R.D.; Todd, K.; Krause, G.S. (1991). Incidence of cocaine-associated rhabdomyolysis. *Annals of Emergency Medicine* 20:154-157.

Wiener, R.S.; Lockhart, J.T.; Schwartz, R.G. (1986). Dilated cardiomyopathy and cocaine abuse. Report of two cases. *American Journal of Medicine* 81:699-701.

Wijetunga, M.; Bhan, R.; Lindsay, J.; Karch, S. (2004). Acute coronary syndrome and crystal methamphetamine use: A case series. *Hawaii Medical Journal* 63:8-13, 25.

Wijetunga, M.; Seto, T.; Lindsay, J.; Schatz, I. (2003). Crystal methamphetamine-associated cardiomyopathy: Tip of the iceberg? *Journal of Toxicology and Clinical Toxicology* 41:981-986.

Withers, N.W.; Pulvirenti, L.; Koob, G.F.; Gillin, J.C. (1995). Cocaine abuse and dependence. *Journal of Clinical Psychopharmacology* 15:63-78.

Wohlman, R.A. (1987). Renal artery thrombosis and embolization associated with intravenous cocaine injection. *Southern Medical Journal* 80:928-930.

Wojak, J.C.; Flamm, E.S. (1987). Intracranial hemorrhage and cocaine use. *Stroke* 18:712-715.

Xu, Y.Q.; Crumb, W.J. Jr.; Clarkson, C.W. (1994). Cocaethylene, a metabolite of cocaine and ethanol, is a potent blocker of cardiac sodium channels. *Journal of Pharmacology and Experimental Therapeutics* 271:319-325.

Zagelbaum, B.M.; Tannenbaum, M.H.; Hersh, P.S. (1991). *Candida albicans* corneal ulcer associated with crack cocaine. *American Journal of Ophthalmology* 111:248-249.

Zimmerman, F.H.; Gustafson, G.M.; Kemp, H.G. Jr. (1987). Recurrent myocardial infarction associated with cocaine abuse in a young man with normal coronary arteries: Evidence for coronary artery spasm culminating in thrombosis. *Journal of the American College of Cardiology* 9:964-968.

Chapter 11

Inhalant Abuse

Paul Kolecki
Richard Shih

INTRODUCTION AND OVERVIEW

The intentional inhalation of fumes derived from solvents (e.g., spray paint, glue, gasoline, nitrous oxide) is extremely common in youth culture (Banken, 2004; Spiller and Krenzelok, 1997; Watson et al., 2004). Ease of availability, administration, titration, and low cost have all contributed to this widespread and growing epidemic. A case series from two poison control centers noted the typical inhalant user to be between the ages of 10 and 24 and typically male. The two most abused inhalants were spray paint and gasoline (Spiller and Krenzelok, 1997). In 2003, the American Association of Poison Control Centers reported more than 55,000 cases of hydrocarbon exposure (Watson et al., 2004). Approximately 12 cases of mortality associated with intentional inhalant abuse were reported (Watson et al., 2004). The exact incidence and mortality rate from inhalant abuse, however, is unknown.

Two distinct groups of adolescents who sniff glue have been identified: those who do it for experience and experimentation as part of a peer group, and a smaller group who become dependent, chronic users (Masterton, 1979). Prior physical and/or sexual child abuse is suspected to be one important correlate for extensive involvement of inhalant use (Fendrich et al., 1997). Several studies have reported significant past inhalant abuse among youths in juvenile detention or correctional facilities (McGarvey, Clavet, and Mason, 1999; Young, Longstaffe, and Tenebein, 1999). A majority of these youths preferred using the inhalants in the presence of friends and

Handbook of the Medical Consequences of Alcohol and Drug Abuse
© 2008 by The Haworth Press, Taylor & Francis Group. All rights reserved.
doi:10.1300/6039_11

abusing inhalants at the home of a friend (McGarvey, Clavet, and Mason, 1999). Studies also report significant inhalant abuse (e.g., volatile nitrites) among males in their workplace, including homosexual males, Native Americans, and Hispanic youths (Cohen, 1984; Craib et al., 2000). To prevent illegal use, many stores that sell inhalants keep these products behind locked screens (see Figure 11.1).

It is a commonly held belief that most inhalant abusers usually engage in this activity for short periods of time. Some reports, however, cite patients who chronically abuse inhalants, such as prisoners who work with industrial solvents (Davies, Thorley, and O'Connor, 1985; Lewis, Moritz, and Mellis, 1981). These workers inhale the fumes of accessible solvents periodically during their daily shifts in an attempt to maintain euphoria throughout the workweek (Cohen, 1984). Inhalant abusers have also been reported to proceed to chronic alcohol and illicit drug abuse. Recent evidence suggests that early-onset inhalant use by females signals an excess risk of suicide attempt (Wilcox and Anthony, 2004).

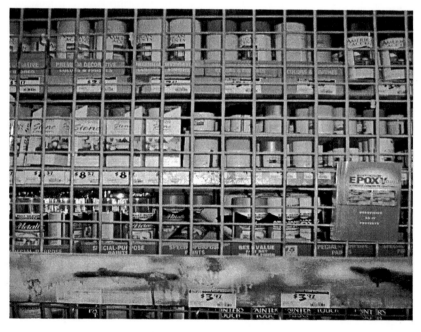

FIGURE 11.1. To prevent on-site abuse, commercially available inhalants are frequently stored behind locked screens.

HISTORY

The inhalation of intoxicants is not new. The early Greeks used inhalants to mark the rites of passage of the young. The intentional inhalation of volatile substances (e.g., gasoline) was first observed in the United States before World War II (Morton, 1987; Nicholi, 1983). In the United States, a number of communities in widely separated areas began reporting a relatively high incidence of "glue sniffing" around 1960 (Kupperstein and Susman, 1968). Concern about the abuse of inhalants have since been expressed from many countries around the world (Morton, 1987; Nicholi, 1983).

Inhalation abuse is classically described as "the deliberate inhalation of solvent vapors to induce sensations of euphoria and exhilaration" (Glaser and Massengale, 1962, p. 179). Inhalation is usually continued until the desired sensation is achieved or until all of the toxic fumes have evaporated (Kupperstein and Susman, 1968). "Huffing" and "sniffing" are two of the more common methods of inhaling toxic fumes. Huffing involves nasally inhaling the fumes from a solvent-saturated rag (Barker and Adams, 1963). Sniffing involves the act of directly sniffing the fumes from the container or squeezing the toxic substance onto a rag and nasally sniffing the fumes from the rag. Another method, "bagging," involves the act of transferring the toxic substance into a paper bag, placing the bag over the nose and mouth, and inhaling deeply. Some abusers transfer the toxic substance into a pan or other vessel which is then heated. This results in a more rapid and concentrated vapor (Kupperstein and Susman, 1968). Finally, some toxic substances (e.g., nitrous oxide) are inhaled after being transferred into a balloon. This form of inhalant abuse, called "ballooning," is very common at tailgate parties before and after sporting events and rock concerts.

SUBSTANCES

The inhaled substances of abuse are aromatic and short-chained volatile hydrocarbons that, upon inhalation, have a rapid onset of intoxicating effects Common inhalants are shown in Table 11.1. The volatilized inhalant used is absorbed well from the lungs and rapidly distributed to the central nervous system. One or two large inhalations of the inebriating substance intoxicates the user very quickly, and the effects can last for hours. Some chronic inhalant abusers maintain a prolonged state of inebriation by periodically inhaling a substance. It is very difficult to clinically differentiate an inhalant-induced inebriation from ethanol-induced inebriation, although

TABLE 11.1. Inhalants of abuse and their main chemical constituents.

Inhalants of abuse	Chemical constituents
Acrylic paint	Toluene
Aerosol propellant	Fluorocarbons
Anesthetics	Chloroform, nitrous oxide
Fire-extinguishing agent	Bromochlorodifluoromethane
Fuel, lighter fluid, torches	Propane, butane
Gasoline	Hydrocarbons, tetraethyl lead
Glues, plastic cement, rubber cement	Benzene, carbon tetrachloride, methylethyl ketone, n-hexane, toluene, trichloroethylene, trichloroethane, xylene
Inks	Toluene, xylene
Paint stripper	Methylene chloride
Paints, varnishes, lacquer	Trichloroethylene, toluene
Refrigerants	Fluorocarbons
Shoe polish	Chlorinated hydrocarbons, toluene
Spot remover	Trichloroethane, trichloroethylene, carbon tetrachloride
Typewriter correction fluid (e.g., Wite-Out)	Tetrachloroethylene, trichloroethane, trichloroethylene

Source: Adapted from LoVecchio and Gerkin, 1997.

toxic inhalation inebriation is usually of shorter duration as compared with alcohol. Two distinguishing signs of inhalant abuse include the smell of solvents on the patient's hands or breath and skin discoloration secondary to paint sniffing (LoVecchio and Gerkin, 1997; Shih, 1998).

TOXIC EFFECTS BY ORGAN SYSTEM

Patients who abuse inhalants typically experience the anticipated euphoria and suffer no long-term physiologic consequences. However, the intentional abuse of inhalants is potentially dangerous, as patients can acutely die and/or suffer severe permanent organ damage. The following paragraphs detail both the acute and chronic effects of commonly abused inhalants based on organ system.

Acute Toxic Effects of Inhalant Abuse

Central Nervous System

Patients abuse inhalants for the expected euphoria. This intoxication has been reported as a feeling of lightheadedness, stupor, lethargy, excitation, and occasional hallucinations (e.g., auditory and visual) (Spiller and Krenzelok, 1997). Profound relaxation and deep sleep usually follow this initial euphoric phase (LoVecchio and Gerkin, 1997). Unpleasant symptoms reported after the use of inhalants include agitation, seizures, ataxia, headache, and dizziness (Shih, 1998; Spiller and Krenzelok, 1997).

Pulmonary

Pulmonary effects following inhalant abuse are rare but deadly. High concentrations of an inhalant have resulted in oxygen displacement, hypoxia, asphyxiation, and suffocation (Linden, 1990). Symptoms of hypoxia develop when the inspired oxygen concentration suddenly falls below 17 percent, while loss of consciousness often occurs when inspired oxygen concentrations fall below 10 percent (Linden, 1990). Most victims were found with a paper bag over their head (Press and Done, 1967).

Cardiac

During the 1960s and late 1950s, an epidemic of sudden deaths occurred among teenagers who recently inhaled volatile hydrocarbons. This scenario, termed "sudden sniffing death" (SSD), was initially believed to result from plastic-bag suffocation (Press and Done, 1967). However, a comprehensive review in 1970 questioned this theory (Bass, 1970). In this study, 110 cases of SSD were reviewed. Common scenarios among these patients were the inhalation of a volatile hydrocarbon, then a scream or a vocalized impending sense of doom, followed by the victim running away from the agent of abuse. In many cases, the dead patient was found more than 100 feet from the abused substance or object used to transfer the inhalant (e.g., a paper bag). In this report, fluorocarbon propellants (pressurized aerosol containers) and trichloroethane (spot remover) were the two most common agents associated with SSD (Bass, 1970). Anoxia was thought not to be the cause of death, as many of these patients were well oxygenated after dashing several hundred feet before collapsing. Rather, it was postulated that SSD resulted from the volatile hydrocarbons sensitizing the myocardium to catecholamines, which subsequently produced lethal cardiac arrhythmias (Bass, 1970).

In 1972, a revealing animal study demonstrated that dogs exposed to fluorinated hydrocarbons suffered a chain of arrhythmias (e.g., sinus bradycardia, junctional or ventricular escape, ventricular fibrillation, asystole) and death (Flowers and Horan, 1972). These arrhythmias occurred in the setting of normal oxygenation. In addition, these arrhythmias continued despite halting exposure to the hydrocarbon at the first sign of rhythm change. This data concluded that SSD occurs secondary to cardiac arrhythmias and not anoxia. It has also been suggested that SSD can occur after the inhalant "senses doom" and discontinues the action of abuse (Flowers and Horan, 1972). For example, a typical scenario of SSD postulated by some toxicologists occurs when teenagers are caught abusing inhalants by parents or police. After being caught, a rush of catecholamines occurs in these teenagers as they sense a fear of parental punishment or they run to escape legal complications. It has been suggested that the catecholamine rush then "excessively stimulates" the inhalant-sensitized myocardium, leading to lethal arrhythmias and death in some teenagers.

There are numerous other reports of human SSD associated with the recent abuse of inhalants. Some inhalants reported to cause lethal arrhythmias and SSD include freon, bromochlorodifluoromethane, butane, propane, 1,1,1-trichloroethane, gasoline, and trichloroethylene (Bass, 1978; Brady et al., 1994; Heath, 1986; King, Smialek, and Troutman, 1985; Morita et al., 1977; Siegel and Wason, 1990; Smeeton and Clark, 1985).

Hematologic

Methemoglobinemia and carboxyhemoglobinemia, two abnormal hemoglobin states, are associated with the abuse of certain inhalants. Methemoglobinemia occurs when oxidant stress is placed on the hemoglobin molecule and thus causes the iron moiety of the hemoglobin molecule to exist in the ferric state. When the iron moiety exists in the ferric state, methemoglobinemia occurs and the resulting abnormal hemoglobin molecule known as methemoglobin is unable to bind oxygen. Abuse of alkyl nitrites (amyl, butyl, and isobutyl) have been reported to cause methemoglobinemia and male patients abuse these nitrites mainly for their supposed aphrodisiac properties (Cohen, 1979; Linden, 1990). The aphrodisiac properties reportedly occur because of the vasodilatory effects on the cerebral blood vessels, which subsequently causes an increase in intracranial pressure and a euphoric effect (Haverkos and Dougherty, 1988). In addition, abuse of these alkyl nitrites "slows the sense of time." Abusers inhale these nitrites before sexual climax in an attempt to prolong and enhance the sensation of orgasm (Cohen, 1979). Other reported aphrodisiac properties include penile erection and dilation of the anal sphincter (Forsyth and Moulden, 1991). Amyl nitrite is a yellowish, volatile, flammable liquid with a fruity odor. Amyl nitrite was initially introduced in medical practice as a coronary vasodilator. It is not used for this purpose today, however, and has since been replaced by organic nitrates. Amyl nitrite continues to be marketed as fragile glass pearls covered with a woven absorbent material. These pearls are available in cyanide antidote kits.

When used to treat a cyanide overdose, the pearls are crushed in the hand and the vapors from the liquid are inhaled. Common street names for amyl nitrite pearls are "poppers" and "snappers," derived from the sound made by the pearls when they are broken. Butyl and isobutyl nitrites are volatile hydrocarbons marketed as room odorizers and advertised as aphrodisiacs. They are often sold in "adult bookstores" in bottles containing 10 to 30 ml of liquid. Common names for butyl and isobutyl nitrites are "Bullet," "Rush," and "Satan's Scent" (Linden, 1990).

Carboxyhemoglobinemia occurs when carbon monoxide (CO) binds to hemoglobin and thus impairs further oxygen binding to hemoglobin and oxygen delivery to tissues. Poisoning by CO has frequently been reported after exposure to methylene chloride, a volatile hydrocarbon commonly found in paint strippers. Methylene chloride is metabolized slowly (over a three-to-eight hour time period) to CO. Methylene chloride poisoning has been frequently reported while the patient was stripping paint in a semienclosed area (Rioux and Myers, 1989; Stewart and Hake, 1976). There are also reports of intentional abuse of methylene chloride products (Horowitz, 1986; Sturmann, Mofenson, and Caraccio, 1985). Interestingly, methylene chloride exposure has not been associated with lethal arrhythmias in the human or animal literature (LoVecchio and Gerkin, 1997).

Hepatic

Liver injury secondary to hepatocellular necrosis has been reported after exposure to certain chlorinated hydrocarbons, mainly trichloroethylene, carbon tetrachloride, and 1,1,1-trichloroethane. Tricloroethylene (TCE) was originally used as an obstetric general anesthetic but has been banned in the United States because of an association with trigeminal neuropathies (Cavanagh and Buxton, 1989; Mitchell and Parsons-Smith, 1969). TCE is used in typewriter correction fluid, paint removers, spot removers, furniture strippers, and degreasers. Carbon tetrachloride was widely used as a dry-cleaning agent and a constituent of fire extinguishers in the 1930s. Fatalities from thermal decomposition of carbon tetrachloride to phosgene gas led to the banning of its use in fire extinguishers in the 1960s. The FDA banned the use of carbon tetrachloride as a dry-cleaning agent in the 1970s. Presently, carbon tetrachloride is used in the production of solvents, aerosol propellants, and fluorocarbon refrigerants. Although carbon tetrachloride poisoning is commonly associated with chronic abuse, acute poisoning does not frequently occur. 1,1,1-trichloroethane is one of the most commonly abused solvents and is presently used as a metal cleaner, degreaser, aerosol propellant, and pesticide.

Inhalant abusers of these chlorinated hydrocarbons have been labeled as "solvent sniffers." However, reports of hepatic toxicity involve cases not only of inhalational abuse but also of occupational exposure and suicide attempts (Thiele, Eigenbrodt, and Ware, 1982). The histopathologic liver damage associated with certain chlorinated hydrocarbon poisonings is centrolobular hepatic necrosis. This histopathologic pattern is also the pattern seen with severe acetaminophen (Tylenol) and poisonous mushroom *(Amanita phalloides)* toxicity. In all three poisonings (e.g., chlorinated hydrocarbons, acetaminophen, and *Amanita phalloides*), the liver damage occurs secondary to toxic metabolites produced during metabolism of the parent compounds by the cytochrome p450 system. Tetrachloroethylene, the chlorinated hydrocarbon used presently in most dry-cleaning industries, has rarely been reported to cause liver damage (Wax, 1997). Mothball abuse has also been reported to cause abnormal mild elevations of the hepatic transaminases (Kong and Schmiesing, 2004).

Chronic Toxic Effects of Inhalant Abuse

Metabolic/Renal

Metabolic abnormalities have been classically described in patients who abuse toluene. Toluene is a hydrocarbon found in a variety of household products, including adhesives, spray paints, paint thinners, and varnishes.

Chronic toluene abuse may cause metabolic acidosis with and without an anion gap (Taher et al., 1974). The elevated anion gap results from an accumulation of acidic metabolites, mainly hippuric and benzoic acid (Fischman and Oster, 1979). The electrolyte abnormalities include hypokalemia, hypochloremia, and hypophosphatemia. These electrolyte abnormalities occur due to the induction of a distal renal tubular acidosis by toluene (Fischman and Oster, 1979; Kamijo et al., 1998). The hypokalemia may be so great that patients suffer muscle weakness severe enough to cause rhabdomyolysis, paralysis, and respiratory failure (Kao et al., 2000). These metabolic abnormalities typically occur after chronic abuse of toluene. Complete recovery has been reported in patients during periods of avoidance (Taher et al., 1974). Severe hypokalemia and death associated with chronic toluene abuse have been reported (Kirk, Anderson, and Martin, 1984). Patients suffering the medical consequences of toluene abuse are often found in a severely weakened state with paint still on their faces and fingers.

Acute ingestion of toluene has been reported to cause central nervous system depression and diarrhea severe enough to cause a non-anion-gap metabolic acidosis (Caravati and Bjerk, 1997).

Neurologic

Permanent cerebral and cerebellar neurologic disability is a major toxic effect following chronic inhalant abuse (Lazar et al., 1983; Streicher et al., 1981). Long-term abusers or those who have been occupationally exposed have been reported to develop a neurobehavioral syndrome consisting of memory loss, cognitive impairment, sleep disturbance, depression, anxiety, and personality changes (Hormes, Filley, and Rosenberg, 1986). In addition, painters chronically exposed to solvents have developed encephalopathy, cerebral atrophy, and abnormal electroenchephalograms (EEGs) (Larsen and Leira, 1988). Permanent cognitive disorders are also well described in patients who chronically sniff gasoline (Poklis and Burkitt, 1977).

Chronic abuse of n-hexane, a commonly abused solvent found in glue, and nitrous oxide is known to cause peripheral neurologic deficits. Long-term abuse or occupational exposure of n-hexane can produce a profound sensorimotor polyneuropathy (Herskowitz, Ishii, and Schaumburg, 1971; Prockop, 1979). This neuropathy typically begins with sensory involvement in the distal extremities and progresses proximally to the motor system, eventually causing weakness. Many of these effects are reversible over weeks to months with discontinuation of abuse or exposure. Chronic n-hexane abuse is also associated with memory loss. Methyl n-butyl ketone, a similar industrial solvent, has also been reported to cause peripheral neuropathy following chronic exposure (Allen et al., 1975).

Nitrous oxide is an anesthetic agent used by medical practitioners, especially dentists, for pain control during procedures. Transient euphoria and central nervous system (CNS) depression occur when nitrous oxide is inhaled. Excluding intoxication, the acute side effects are minimal. Chronic inhalation of nitrous oxide can cause significant side effects. With chronic abuse, nitrous oxide can produce a demyelinating polyneuropathy and extremity weakness (Layzer, 1987; Pema, Horak, and Wyatt, 1998). The neurologic sequelae associated with chronic abuse occurs secondary to vitamin B_{12} inactivation (Pema, Horak, and Wyatt, 1998). Nitrous oxide abuse is very common today among younger drug abusers because of its ease of availability. Nitrous oxide abuse is very common at sporting event and rock concert tailgaters parties, where the gas is transferred from large containers into balloons and then inhaled. On a smaller scale, compressed nitrous oxide is present in cartridges for whipped cream dispensers and easily obtained in many supermarkets. Abusers discharge the cartridge into an empty cream dispenser and inhale the nitrous oxide (Lai et al., 1997). The slang term for abuse of nitrous oxide in this fashion is "whippets." Nitrous oxide–induced peripheral neuropathy is reversible following avoidance.

Hematologic

Chronic use and/or abuse of nitrous oxide can also cause hematologic abnormalities, specifically megaloblastic anemia (Amess et al., 1978; Amos et al., 1982; Lassen et al., 1956). This disorder occurs because chronic nitrous oxide abuse inactivates B_{12}, an important vitamin needed in bone marrow for the proper production of red blood cells. This anemia has been reported to reverse with B_{12} replacement therapy and discontinuation of nitrous oxide abuse (Layzer, 1987).

The major organic solvent of paints, paint thinners, and glues used to be benzene. The use of benzene as a solvent has been abandoned because of severe bone marrow toxicity (e.g., leukemia, aplastic anemia, multiple myeloma) (Decouffle, Blattner, and Blair, 1983; Rinsky et al., 1987; Vigliani and Saita, 1964). Toluene and n-hexane have replaced benzene as a constituent of these compounds (Lazar et al., 1983).

Miscellaneous

Gasoline, a mixture of hydrocarbons with various additives, is frequently inhaled in an attempt to get intoxicated. Patients who chronically abuse leaded gasoline are at risk for the neurologic complications associated with organic lead poisoning. These complications include mental confusion, poor short-term memory, psychosis, and encephalopathy (Law and Nelson, 1968). Elements of inorganic lead poisoning (headache, abdominal pain, hepatic injury, and renal damage) have also been reported in patients who chronically inhale gasoline (Hansen and Sharp, 1978; Robinson, 1978).

TREATMENT OF THE TOXIC EFFECTS
OF INHALANT ABUSE

Abuse of inhalants may produce significant morbidity, including respiratory depression and life-threatening arrhythmias. Securing an airway and ensuring adequate ventilation are first priority. The patient should also be placed on a cardiac monitor with the establishment of intravenous access. Gastrointestinal decontamination (gastric lavage and/or activated charcoal) should be considered, if it is suspected that the patient also ingested drugs or toxins. Excluding methylene chloride, patients who are asymptomatic for four to six hours after abusing an inhalant are generally considered safe for medical discharge. Specific management issues of caring for the acute and chronic toxic effects of inhalant abuse, including methylene chloride, are discussed in the following paragraphs.

Treatment of the Acute Toxic Effects of Inhalant Abuse

Central Nervous System and Pulmonary

The main treatment of central nervous system depression is adequate ventilation until the effects of the inhalant terminate. Patients who become aggressive or agitated after abusing an inhalant may need to be physically restrained and pharmacologically sedated. Hypoxic patients need adequate oxygenation and ventilation. If necessary, a definitive airway (e.g., endotracheal or nasotracheal airway) should be established.

Cardiac

Sudden sniffing death occurs because the inhalants sensitize the myocardium of the patient to catecholamines, which subsequently leads to lethal ventricular arrhythmias and death. In human reports of SSD, standard cardiac pharmacologic treatment and electrotherapy were unsuccessful (King, Smialek, and Troutman, 1985; Smeeton and Clark, 1985). Beta-adrenergic blocking agents have been proposed as a treatment option for life-threatening arrhythmias induced by inhalants (LoVecchio and Gerkin, 1997; Moritz et al., 2000). Should conventional cardiac resuscitation fail in treating inhalant abusers suffering lethal cardiac arrhythmias, the use of beta-adrenergic blocking agents (i.e., esmolol, propanolol) should be considered. Most patients who suffer cardiac consequences of inhalant abuse usually die at the scene or convert back to a normal sinus-cardiac rhythm prior to medical intervention.

Hematologic

Patients who sustain significant methemoglobinemia after alkyl nitrites abuse often suffer from cyanosis. Other signs and symptoms of methemoglobinemia include headache, dyspnea on exertion, tachycardia, tachypnea, confusion, coma, seizures, lethal cardiac arrhythmias, and death. The anti-dote for methemoglobinemia induced by alkyl nitrite, or by any drug or chemi-cal, is methylene blue.

Methylene chloride, when metabolized, produces carbon monoxide. The production of carbon monoxide occurs over three to eight hours. Signs and symptoms of carbon monoxide poisoning include headache, dizziness, ataxia, seizures, lethal cardiac arrhythmias, coma, and death. A treatment recommended by many physicians for significant carbon monoxide poison-ing is hyperbaric oxygen therapy, as there are many reports of successful treatment of methylene chloride-induced carbon monoxide poisoning with hyperbaric oxygen therapy (Horowitz, 1986; Rioux and Myers, 1989; Rudge, 1990). Testing for carbon monoxide poisoning over an eight-hour time is very important in caring for patients exposed to methylene chloride.

Hepatic

Due to the limited number of human cases, there is no standard treatment for chlorinated hydrocarbon-induced hepatotoxicity. *N*-acetylcysteine, an ac-cepted antidote for acetaminophen poisoning, has been recommended as a treatment option for carbon tetrachloride-induced hepatotoxicity (Agency for Toxic Substances and Disease Registry, 1992). Limited data exists show-ing *N*-acetylcysteine's efficacy in reversing chlorinated hydrocarbon-indu-ced hepatoxicity. Immediate oxygen therapy, including hyperbaric oxygen, has also been recommended for carbon tetrachloride poisoning (Bernacchi et al., 1984; Tomaszewski and Thom, 1994). Again, limited data exists showing oxygen therapy as efficacious in reversing chlorinated hydrocarbon-induced hepatoxicity.

Treatment of the Chronic Toxic Effects of Inhalant Abuse

Metabolic/Renal

The treatment for chronic toluene-induced electrolyte abnormalities is discontinuation of exposure, airway management if necessary, and fluid and electrolyte replacement. Specific attention to hypokalemia is necessary and significant deficits should be corrected, as metabolic acidosis, rhabdo-myolysis, lethal arrhythmias, and death have all been reported secondary to prolonged toluene abuse. Hemodialysis along with aggressive potassium replacement has been reported as a successful treatment option for severe chronic toluene poisoning (Gerkin and LoVecchio, 1998).

Neurologic and Hematologic

The most important treatment option for patients suffering central and peripheral neurologic deficits from chronic inhalant abuse is discontinuation of exposure. Vitamin B_{12} replacement therapy may be helpful for both chronic nitrous oxide-induced peripheral neuropathy and megaloblastic anemia.

Miscellaneous

Standard lead chelation techniques should be considered for chronic gasoline abusers who are suffering from the signs and symptoms of inorganic lead poisoning.

SUMMARY AND CONCLUSIONS

Inhalant abuse is a significant problem, especially among the youth population. This form of substance abuse occurs mainly because the common inhalants of abuse are easily attainable, easily administered, and very cheap to buy. Acute abusers of inhalants are at risk for serious pulmonary, cardiac, hematologic, and hepatic toxicity. Chronic abusers of inhalants are potentially at risk of suffering not only severe metabolic abnormalities, but also permanent neurologic and hematologic damage. Knowledge of the pharmacology and toxicology of these inhalants is necessary not only for the successful diagnosis and treatment of poisoned patients, but also for future study of medicinal and addiction therapeutic protocols.

REFERENCES

Agency for Toxic Substances and Disease Registry (1992). Carbon tetrachloride toxicity. *American Family Physician* 46(4):1199-1207.

Allen, N.; Mendell, J.R.; Billmaier, D.J.; Fontaine, R.E.; O'Neill, J. (1975). Toxic polyneuropathy due to methyl n-butyl ketone. *Archives of Neurology* 32:209-218.

Amess, J.A.L.; Burman, J.F.; Rees, G.M.; Nancekievill, D.G.; Mollin, D.L. (1978). Megaloblastic haemopoiesis in patients receiving nitrous oxide. *Lancet* 2(8085): 339-342.

Amos, R.J.; Amess, J.A.L.; Hinds, C.J.; Mollin, D.L. (1982). Incidence and pathogenesis of acute megaloblastic bone-marrow change in patients receiving intensive care. *Lancet* 2(8303):835-838.

Banken, J.A. (2004). Drug abuse trends among youth in the United States. *Annals of the New York Academy of Sciences* 1025:465-471.

Barker, G.H.; Adams, W.T. (1963). Glue sniffers. *Sociology and Social Research* 47(3):45.

Bass, M. (1970). Sudden sniffing death. *Journal of the American Medical Association* 212(12):2075-2079.

Bass, M. (1978). Death from sniffing gasoline [letter]. *New England Journal of Medicine* 299:203.

Bernacchi, A.; Myers, R.; Trump, B.F.; Marzella, L. (1984). Protection of hepatocytes with hyperoxia against carbon tetrachloride-induced injury. *Toxicologic Pathology* 12(4):315-323.

Brady, W.J.; Stremski, E.; Eljaiek, L.; Aufderheide, T.P. (1994). Freon inhalational abuse presenting with ventricular fibrillation. *American Journal of Emergency Medicine* 12:533-536.

Caravati, E.M.; Bjerk, P.J. (1997). Acute toluene ingestion toxicity. *Annals of Emergency Medicine* 30(6):838-839.

Cavanagh, B.; Buxton, P.H. (1989). Trichloroethylene cranial neuropathy: Is it really a toxic neuropathy or does it activate latent herpes virus? *Journal of Neurology, Neurosurgery, and Psychiatry* 52:297-303.

Cohen, S. (1979). The volatile nitrite. *Journal of the American Medical Association* 241:2077-2078.

Cohen, S. (1984). The hallucinogens and the inhalants. *Psychiatric Clinics of North America* 7(4):681-688.

Craib, K.J.P.; Weber, A.C.; Cornelisse, P.G.A.; Martindale, S.L.; Miller, M.L.; Schechter, M.T.; Strathdee, S.A.; Schilder, A.; Hogg, R.S. (2000). Comparison of sexual behaviors, unprotected sex, and substance use between two independent cohorts of gay and bisexual men. *Official Journal of the International AIDS Soceity* 14(3):303-311.

Davies, B.; Thorley, A.; O'Connor, D. (1985). Progression of addiction careers in young adult solvent misusers. *British Medical Journal* 290:109-110.

Decouffle, P.; Blattner, W.A.; Blair, A. (1983). Mortality among chemical workers exposed to benzene and other agents. *Environmental Research* 30:16-25.

Fendrich, M.; Mackesy-Amiti, M.E.; Wislar, J.S.; Goldstein, P.J. (1997). Childhood abuse and the use of inhalants: Differences by degree of use. *American Journal of Public Health* 87(5):765-769.

Fischman, C.M.; Oster, J.R. (1979). Toxic effects of toluene: A new cause of high anion gap metabolic acidosis. *Journal of the American Medical Association* 241(16):1713-1715.

Flowers, N.C.; Horan, L.G. (1972). Nonanoxic aerosol arrhythmias. *Journal of the American Medical Association* 219(1):33-37.

Forsyth, R.J.; Moulden, A. (1991). Methaemoglobinaemia after ingestion of amyl nitrite. *Archives of Disease in Childhood* 66:152.

Gerkin, R.D.; LoVecchio, F. (1998). Rapid reversal of life-threatening toluene-induced hypokalemia with hemodialysis. *Journal of Emergency Medicine* 16(4): 723-725.

Glaser, H.H.; Massengale, O.N. (1962). Glue sniffing in children—Deliberate inhalation of vaporized plastic cements. *Journal of the American Medical Association* 181:300-303.

Hansen, K.S.; Sharp, F.R. (1978). Gasoline sniffing, lead poisoning, and myoclonus. *Journal of the American Medical Association* 240(13):1375-1376.

Haverkos, J.W.; Dougherty, J. (1988). Health hazards of nitrite inhalants. *American Journal of Medicine* 84:479-482.

Heath, M.J. (1986). Solvent abuse using bromochlorodifluoromethane from a fire extinguisher. *Medical Science Law* 26(1):33-34.

Herskowitz, A.; Ishii, N.; Schaumburg, H. (1971). *N*-hexane neuropathy: A syndrome occurring as a result of industrial exposure. *New England Journal of Medicine* 285(2):82-85.

Hormes, J.T.; Filley, C.M.; Rosenberg, N.L. (1986). Neurologic sequelae of chronic solvent abuse. *Neurology* 36:698-702.

Horowitz, B.Z. (1986). Carboxyhemoglobinemia caused by inhalation of methylene chloride. *American Journal of Emergency Medicine* 4(1):48-51.

Kamijo, Y.; Soma, K.; Hasegawa, I.; Ohwada, T. (1998). Fatal bilateral adrenal hemorrhage following acute toluene poisoning: A case report. *Journal of Toxicology—Clinical Toxicology* 36(4):365-368.

Kao, K.-C.; Tsai, Y.-H.; Lin, M.-C.; Huang, C.-C.; Tsao, T.C.-Y.; Chen, Y.-C. (2000). Hypokalemia muscular paralysis causing acute respiratory failure due to rhabdomyolysis with renal tubular acidosis in a chronic glue sniffer. *Journal of Toxicology—Clinical Toxicology* 38(6):679-681.

King, G.S.; Smialek, J.E.; Troutman, W.G. (1985). Sudden death in adolescents resulting from the inhalation of typewriter correction fluid. *Journal of the American Medical Association* 253(11):1604-1606.

Kirk, L.M.; Anderson, R.; Martin, K. (1984). Sudden death from toluene abuse. *Annals of Emergency Medicine* 13(1):68-69.

Kong, J.T.; Schmiesing, C. (2004). Concealed mothball abuse prior to anesthesia: Mothballs, inhalants, and their management. *Acta Aneaesthesiologica Scandinavica* 49:113-116.

Kupperstein, L.; Susman, R.M. (1968). A bibliography on the inhalation of glue fumes and other toxic vapors—A substance abuse practice among adolescents. *International Journal of the Addictions* 3(1):177-197.

Lai, N.Y.; Silbert, P.L.; Erber, W.N.; Rijks, C.J. (1997). "Nanging": Another cause of nitrous oxide neurotoxicity. *Medical Journal of Australia* 166(3):166.

Larsen, F.; Leira, H.L. (1988). Organic brain syndrome and long-term exposure to toluene: A clinical psychiatric study of vocationally active printing workers. *Journal of Occupational Medicine* 30:875-878.

Lassen, H.C.A.; Henriksen, E.; Neukirch, F.; Kristensen, H.S. (1956). Treatment of tetanus. Severe bone-marrow depression after prolonged nitrous-oxide anesthesia. *Lancet* 270(6922):527-530.

Law, W.R.; Nelson, E.R. (1968). Gasoline-sniffing by an adult. *Journal of the American Medical Association* 204(11):144-146.

Layzer, R.B. (1987). Myeloneuropathy after prolonged exposure to nitrous oxide. *Lancet* 2:1227-1230.

Lazar, R.B.; Ho, S.U.; Melen, O.; Daghestani, A.N. (1983). Multifocal central nervous system damage caused by toluene abuse. *Neurology* 33:1337-1340.

Lewis, J.D.; Moritz, D.; Mellis, L.P. (1981). Long-term toluene abuse. *American Journal of Psychiatry* 138(3):368-370.

Linden, C.H. (1990). Volatile substances of abuse. *Emergency Medicine Clinics of North America* 8(3):559-578.

LoVecchio, F.; Gerkin, R. (1997). Inhalants of abuse. *Topics in Emergency Medicine* 19(4):44-52.

Masterton, G. (1979). Management of solvent abuse. *Journal of Adolescence* 2:65-75.

McGarvey, E.L.; Clavet, G.J.; Mason, W. (1999). Adolescent inhalant abuse: Environments of use. *American Journal of Drug and Alcohol Abuse* 25(4):731-741.

Mitchell, A.B.S.; Parsons-Smith, B.G. (1969). Trichloroethylene neuropathy. *British Medical Journal* 1:422-423.

Morita, M.; Miki, A.; Kazama, H.; Sakata, M. (1977). Case report of deaths caused by freon gas. *Forensic Science* 10:253-260.

Moritz, F.; de La Chapelle, A.; Bauer, F.; Leroy, J.-P.; Goullé, J.P.; Bonmarchand, G. (2000). Esmolol in the treatment of severe arrhythmia after acute trichloroethylene poisoning. *Intensive Care Medicine* 26(2):256.

Morton, H.G. (1987). Occurrence and treatment of solvent abuse in children and adolescents. *Pharmacology and Therapeutics* 33:449-469.

Nicholi, A.M. (1983). The inhalants: An overview. *Psychosomatics* 24(10):914-921.

Pema, P.J.; Horak, H.A.; Wyatt, R.H. (1998). Myelopathy caused by nitrous oxide toxicity. *American Journal of Neuroradiology* 19:894-896.

Poklis, A.; Burkitt, C.D. (1977). Gasoline sniffing: A review. *Clinical Toxicology* 11:35-41.

Press, E.; Done, A.K. (1967). Solvent sniffing: Physiologic effects and community control measure for intoxication from intentional inhalation of organic solvents. *Pediatrics* 39:451-461.

Prockop, L. (1979). Neurotoxic volatile substances. *Neurology* 29:862-865.

Rinsky, R.A.; Smith, A.B.; Hornung, R.; Filloon, T.G.; Young, R.J.; Okun, A.H.; Landrigan, P.J. (1987). Benzene and leukemia: An epidemiologic risk assessment. *New England Journal of Medicine* 316(17):1044-1050.

Rioux, J.P.; Myers, R.A.M. (1989). Hyperbaric oxygen for methylene chloride poisoning: Report on two cases. *Annals of Emergency Medicine* 18:691-695.

Robinson, R.O. (1978). Tetraethyl lead poisoning from gasoline sniffing. *Journal of the American Medical Association* 240(13):1373-1374.

Rudge, F.W. (1990). Treatment of methylene chloride induced carbon monoxide poisoning with hyperbaric oxygenation. *Military Medicine* 155(11):570-572.

Shih, R. (1998). Hydrocarbons. In: Goldfrank, L.R.; Flomenbaum, N.E.; Lewin, N.A. (eds.), *Goldfrank's Toxicologic Emergencies,* Sixth Edition (pp. 1383-1398). Stamford, CT: Appleton & Lange.

Siegel, E.; Wason, S. (1990). Sudden death caused by inhalation of butane and propane. *New England Journal of Medicine* 323(23):1638.

Smeeton, W.M.I.; Clark, M.S. (1985). Sudden death resulting from inhalation of fire extinguishers containing bromochlorodifluoromethane. *Medical Science Law* 25(4):258-262.

Spiller, H.A.; Krenzelok, E.P. (1997). Epidemiology of inhalant abuse reported to two regional poison centers. *Journal of Toxicology—Clinical Toxicology* 35(2): 167-173.

Stewart, R.D.; Hake, C.L. (1976). Paint-remover hazard. *Journal of the American Medical Association* 235(4):398-401.

Streicher, H.Z.; Gabow, P.A.; Moss, A.H.; Kono, D.; Kaehny, W.D. (1981). Syndromes of toluene sniffing in adults. *Annals of Internal Medicine* 94:758-762.

Sturmann, K.; Mofenson, H.; Caraccio, T. (1985). Methylene chloride inhalation: An unusual form of drug abuse. *Annals of Emergency Medicine* 14:903-905.

Taher, S.M.; Anderson, R.J.; McCartney, R.; Popovtzer, M.M.; Schrier, R.W. (1974). Renal tubular acidosis associated with toluene "sniffing." *New England Journal of Medicine* 290(14):765-768.

Thiele, D.L.; Eigenbrodt, E.H.; Ware, A.J. (1982). Cirrhosis after repeated trichloroethylene and 1,1,1-trichloroethane exposure. *Gastroenterology* 83:925-929.

Tomaszewski, C.A.; Thom, S.R. (1994). Use of hyperbaric oxygen in toxicology. *Emergency Medicine Clinics of North America* 12(2):437-459.

Vigliani, E.C.; Saita, G. (1964). Benzene and leukemia. *New England Journal of Medicine* 217(17):872-876.

Watson, W.A.; Litovitz, T.L.; Klein-Schwartz, W.; Rodgers, G.C. (2004). 2003 Annual report of the American Association of Poison Control Centers Toxic Exposure Surveillance System. *American Journal of Emergency Medicine* 22(5): 335-404.

Wax, P.M. (1997). Dry cleaners. In: Greenberg, M.I.; Hamilton, R.J.; Phillips, S.D. (eds.), *Occupational, Industrial, and Environmental Toxicology* (pp. 73-82). St. Louis, MO: Mosby.

Wilcox, H.C.; Anthony, J.C. (2004). The development of suicide ideation and attempts: An epidemiologic study of first graders followed into young adulthood. *Drug and Alcohol Dependence* 76 Suppl:S53-S67.

Young, S.J.; Longstaffe, S.; Tenebein, M. (1999). Inhalant abuse and the abuse of other drugs. *American Journal of Drug and Alcohol Abuse* 25(2):371-375.

Chapter 12

Medical Consequences
of Anabolic Steroids

James Langenbucher
Thomas Hildebrandt
Sasha J. Carr

INTRODUCTION AND OVERVIEW

Substance use that promotes strength gain, muscle synthesis, fat loss, and increased metabolic capacity in order to improve athletic performance, perceived cosmetic appearance, and social opportunity and self-esteem—so-called anabolic-androgenic steroids or AAS—is prevalent among both competitive and, increasingly, recreational athletes (Goldfield, Harper, and Blouin, 1998; Gridley and Hanrahan, 1994; Monaghan, 2002). These drugs are, for the most part, used within a broad context of operant drug-taking that includes the use of ergogenics, thermogenics, anorexigents, and ancillary drugs. Their use also generally involves larger lifestyle elements (Evans, 2004) that constellate around participation in arduous physical exercise (generally, weight-training and/or endurance or team sports) and, often, dietary restraint.

Steroidal and nonsteroidal anabolics are valued by users for several reasons. Most centrally, anabolic compounds promote better utilization of dietary protein and shift the body's "nitrogen balance" by increasing retention of nitrogen, an element essential to protein synthesis and, thus, to muscle growth. Anabolic compounds also stimulate the RNA-polymerase complex within muscle cells themselves, increasing protein synthesis, and potentiating cell multiplication. In addition, anabolic steroid molecules have a potent anticatabolic effect by competing for glucocorticoid receptors, which oth-

Handbook of the Medical Consequences of Alcohol and Drug Abuse
© 2008 by The Haworth Press, Taylor & Francis Group. All rights reserved.
doi:10.1300/6039_12

erwise act to inhibit protein synthesis after intense exercise by aiding in the secretion of the "stress hormone" cortisol. And finally, anabolic compounds, perhaps through placebo effect or perhaps through effects on central neural pathways, stimulate mood states characterized by euthymia and a feeling of personal power, enabling athletes who use them to train for longer periods of time, with more intensity, with less pause for recovery between training sessions, and with a greater feeling of well-being, overall.

The following is a review of the medical consequences of only a part of the lifestyle wherein people seek these benefits: the medically unsupervised use of anabolic steroids. The actions, unwanted side effects, and long-term consequences of their use, to the extent that these are known, will be described in the following text. However, it should be understood at the outset that when unauthorized use of anabolics was criminalized in the United States in 1990, little was known about these agents. Scientists had never monitored their positive and negative outcomes, the preferred combinations and doses in which they are used, and so on. Virtually no clinician had ever treated a patient whose chief complaint was use of anabolics. It is now a decade and a half later, little is still known, and where the literature once promised the emergence of solid findings, it now appears more and more replete with inconsistencies. These concern the proper attribution of cardiovascular side effects (Evans, 2004), the role of anabolic use, if any, in depression (Pope, Kouri, and Hudson, 2000), and even whether or not anabolics do, in fact, promote hypertrophy (Bhasin et al., 1996). This level of scientific ambiguity is unacceptable as an environment in which rational policy on this important issue can flourish. A great deal of new research is required to accurately map both the dimensions and consequences of anabolic steroid use.

However, first, because very few readers, even drug abuse specialists, are familiar with anabolic steroids, the history of their development and pharmacology will be briefly surveyed, in order to develop the context for the discussion of medical consequences to follow.

HISTORY AND PHARMACOLOGY

The Discovery of Androgens

Testosterone is synthesized primarily in testicular Leydig cells by the action of 17- and 3-hydroxysteroid dehydrogenase on the precursor molecules, androstenedione and androstenediol. Thecal cells in women, and the adrenal cortex in both sexes, are minor production sites. The role of the testes in the development, not only of secondary sex characteristics, but also of strength, muscle mass, and aggressivity, has been suspected since Greek warriors seeking greater strength and sexual appetite added animal testicles to their diet. Testicular action was linked to circulating blood fractions—now understood to be a family of anabolic/androgenic hormones—in the early work on castration and testicular transplantation in fowl by Arnold Berthold (1803-1861), who found that the "results [masculinization in the cockerel] . . . are determined by the productive function of the testes . . . by their action on the blood stream, and then by corresponding reaction of the blood upon the entire organism" (Berthold, 1849, n.p.). Research on the action of testosterone received a brief boost in 1889, when the former Harvard professor, Charles-Edouard Brown-Séquard (1817-1894), 72 years old and then residing in Paris, self-injected subcutaneously a "rejuvenating elixir" consisting of an extract of dog and guinea pig testicle. He reported in *The Lancet* (Brown-Séquard, 1889) that his vigor and feeling of well-being were markedly restored but, predictably, the effects were transient (and likely based on placebo), and Brown-Séquard's hopes for the compound were dashed. Suffering the ridicule of his colleagues, work on the mechanisms and effects of androgenic hormones in human beings was abandoned by Brown-Séquard and succeeding generations of biochemists for nearly 40 years.

The "Golden Age of Steroid Chemistry"

The trail remained cold until the University of Chicago's Professor of Physiologic Chemistry, Fred C. Koch, established easy access to a large source of bovine testicles—the Chicago stockyards—and to students willing to endure the ceaseless toil of extracting their isolates. In 1927, Koch and his student, Lemuel McGee, derived 20mg of a substance from a supply of 40 pounds of bull testicles that, when administered to castrated roosters, pigs and rats, remasculinized them (Gallagher and Koch, 1929; McGee, 1927). The group of Emil Laquer at the University of Amsterdam, later the scientific core of the famed Dutch steroid house Organon, purified this substance—testosterone—from bovine testicles in a similar manner in 1934, but isolation of the hormone from animal tissues in amounts permitting serious study in humans was clearly not feasible.

The game changed entirely when three European pharmaceutical giants—companies that are still heavily involved in the manufacture of anabolic steroids, namely Schering (then of Berlin, Germany; producer of injectible testosterone esters), Organon (Oss, Netherlands; producer of nandrolone esters), and Ciba (Basel, Switzerland; developer of the most popular oral steroid, Dianabol)—began full-scale steroid research and development programs in the 1930s. These pharmaceutical houses eventually combined with Roussel (Paris, France) and Bohringer (Mannheim, Germany) to form the European Hormone Cartel, sharing in common reciprocal rights to exploit each other's inventions and proprietary processes that lasted well into the 1950s; similar collaborative arrangements distinguish the history of domestic American steroid hormone development, with corteges involving Upjohn, Merck, and many other companies. In the 1930s, however, at about the same time that Koch was collecting his research assistants at the University of Chicago, it was Schering that harnessed the most scientific horsepower, under the leadership of Adolf Butenandt (1903-1995). Schering scientists worked out the chemical structure of testosterone, leading to its independent partial-synthesis from a cholesterol base in 1935 by both Butenandt at Schering/Berlin and Leopold Ruzicka (1887-1976) at the Federal Institute of Technology in Zurich; the two shared the 1939 Nobel Prize in Chemistry for this work, an almost unbelievably prompt acknowledgment of their work's importance. Testosterone (see Figure 12.1) was identified as 17beta-hydroxandrost-4-en-3-one ($C_{19}H_{28}O_2$), a solid polycyclic alcohol with a hydroxyl group at the seventeenth carbon atom (C-17). The presence of the hydroxyl group proved important, for two reasons.

First, the hydroxyl side chain made it obvious that testosterone could be *esterified,* or altered by the substitution of an acid group for the hydroxyl

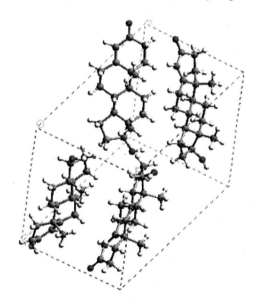

FIGURE 12.1. Stereoscopic view of testosterone molecule.

group at the C-17 position. Esterification lowers the water solubility of the molecule and increases its lipid solubility, permitting a sterile oil-based injectible to form a "depot" in the muscle, from which it is gradually released. Esterification temporarily deactivates the steroid molecule, because the presence of the large acid chain in place of the tiny hydroxyl group blocks the ability of the steroid to bind to androgen receptor (AR) molecules within muscle cells that promote protein synthesis. However, as the esterified steroid is gradually leached from the oily depot into the blood, naturally circulating esterases (acid-cleaving molecules) liberate the steroid, replacing the acid chain with a hydroxyl group as in the virgin molecule, permitting the steroid to bind to AR. The overall effect of esterification is to lengthen the steroid's half-life, ease its administration, and alter its anabolic/androgenic ratio (AAR), or the degree to which it affects striated muscle versus sexual organ tissues such as the testes or prostate.

The partial synthesis in the 1930s of abundant, potent, stable, oil-based testosterone esters permitted the characterization of the hormone's effects, so that Kochakian (1937) was able to show that testosterone raised nitrogen retention (a mechanism central to anabolism) in the dog, after which Charles Kenyon's group (Kenyon et al., 1938) was able to demonstrate both the anabolic and androgenic effects of testosterone propionate in eunuchoidal men, boys, and women. The period of the early 1930s to the 1950s has been called the "Golden Age of Steroid Chemistry" (Schwarz, Onken, and Schubert, 1999), and work during this period progressed quickly. The class of oil-based testosterone esters developed then that are still familiar include testosterone propionate, phenylpropionate, caproate, isocaproate, cypionate, enanthate, undecanoate, and many others. They differ principally in rapidity of action; esterases require more time to cleave away long acid chains (e.g., cypionate) than shorter ones (e.g., propionate).

The second important implication of the hydroxyl side chain at the C-17 position was that it permitted, not just esterification, but also *alkylation* of the steroid molecule (substitution of an ethyl or methyl group for the hydroxyl group). Alkylation was to permit the development of oral steroids, the so-called 17-α-alkylated steroids, a family of androgens such as methyltestosterone, which could be taken up by the digestive track, and so be easily administered in pill form.

Research in the Golden Age of Steroid Chemistry proved that this newly synthesized compound—testosterone—or rather family of compounds (for many derivatives were developed in the 1940s, 1950s and 1960s), was a potent multiplier of muscle, strength, and well-being. Much more than that, in fact: in *The Male Hormone* (1945), the Rockefeller University biochemist and science writer Paul de Kruif (himself, an early and unapologetic experimenter with synthetic testosterone) described how testosterone

> did more than give [clinical test subjects] more energy and a gain in weight . . . It changed them, and fundamentally . . . after many months on testosterone, their chest and shoulder muscles grew much heavier and stronger . . . in some mysterious manner, testosterone caused the human body to synthesize protein, it caused the human body to be able to build the very stuff of its own life. (cited in Todd, 1987, pp. 125-130; 152-156).

However, as is so often the case with remarkable, Nobel-winning discoveries, it was first employed, not in health as de Kruif (1945) would have it, but in conflict.

Androgens and the "Chemical Cold War"

Some of the first applications of the newly discovered class of anabolic compounds were made by the Nazi war machine. As indicated previously, German scientists at Schering had done much of the early work on anabolics, stoking the Wehrmacht's interest in testosterone's potential to provoke aggressivity, as well as its ability to stimulate tissue synthesis to repair battle wounds, and to restore body bulk in soldiers who had survived prolonged captivity or seige. Research on anabolics in Hitler's Germany moved in the Schering laboratories and elsewhere from animal to human applications before the war, using both military volunteers and prisoners. Hitler himself received testosterone injections, though reports that Nazi SS troops were injected with testosterone to increase their fierceness in battle appear to be apocryphal. However, following the war, recognizing the manifest advantages that abnormally large and powerful athletes enjoy when matched against chemically unassisted competitors, hungry for international recognition, and possessing much of the original Nazi-era research and scientific expertise, East Germany (DDR) intensified its interest in anabolics to garner the political capital that flows from success at prestigious sports venues. The DDR identified women's track and swimming events as being especially medal-rich, and so its special focus was on "androgenizing" young girls in a very aggressive steroid-based sports program.

Most of the anabolics were developed and manufactured by JEV Jenapharm (Jena, Germany), adapting technical expertise from the Schott-Zeiss Institute for Microbiology at the University of Jena. Much of the program was concentrated around the daily administration of 0.125 mg per kilo of bodyweight of an oral steroid, Turinabol, a close relative of methandrostenolone was first produced by Jenapharm in 1961. The drug was administered in five annual blocks or "cycles" of four to six weeks duration. Injectible anabolics, too, were administered, but for some reason have not been as widely discussed. The DDR program was astonishingly successful. An East German steroid-fueled national sports federation captured 181 Olympic medals 1968-1976, including 90 in the Montreal games alone, transforming a small country into an athletics powerhouse that consistently rivaled both the United States and the Soviet Union for medal supremacy. Some of the abuses of the DDR anabolic-sports federation have been revealed in formerly secret documents (Franke and Berendonk, 1997), and numerous DDR officials have faced both civil and criminal penalties for providing "vitamin cocktails" to naïve female adolescents whose deep voices, broad shoulders, and masculine-level power intimidated and amazed their international competition.

Even prior to this, the Soviet Union and other Eastern Bloc countries such as Bulgaria had a flourishing steroid program for male athletes in the Olympic "explosive strength" events of weightlifting, wrestling, hammer throw, and shot put. Much of the Soviet program remains wrapped in mystery, but its effects are not: steroid-assisted Soviet weightlifters completely dominated and demoralized the competition at their Olympic debut at Helsinki in 1952, fielding enormously muscular and powerful athletes in even the smaller weight classes. The rookie Soviet team practically swept the field at Helsinki, capturing three gold, three silver, and one bronze medal in the weightlifting events, prompting the suspicions of many officials, who were well aware of the earlier German research initiatives. Two years later, their suspicions were fully confirmed at the World Weightlifting Championship in Vienna, when American team physician Dr. John Ziegler was informed by his Soviet counterpart that regular injections with testosterone esters were an essential part of the Russian training program. Ziegler was aware of both the anabolic (tissue-creating) and androgenic (masculinizing) properties of the testosterone-based compounds with which the Soviets had achieved success. Soon after his return from Vienna, Ziegler himself obtained small quantities of testosterone propionate and administered it to himself, to American weightlifting coach Bob Hoffman, and to a number of his team members at York Barbell in Pennsylvania, an influential weightlifting club that had hosted the first World Weightlifting Championship in 1947. Dissatisfied with some of the androgenic side-effects of testosterone he saw in the men, including prostatic enlargement, Ziegler assisted the Swiss pharmaceutical house CIBA (with laboratories in Summit, New Jersey) in the development of derivatives of synthetic testosterone such as methandrostenolone (Dianbol, which the East Germans would soon clone in their favored compound, Turinabol) that would maximize anabolism, minimize androgenesis, and be available for oral administration, unlike testosterone, which is degraded by stomach and hepatic processes. The success of all parties—Russians, East Germans, Americans, and other Western athletes—sparked a "chemical Cold War" between East and West for athletic supremacy. American track and field athletes, French cyclists, Dutch speed skaters, Soviet wrestlers, Bulgarian powerlifters, and East German swimmers were the shock troops, and a steadily burgeoning array of anabolic steroids provided the ammunition.

The "Breakfast of Champions"

Methandrostenolone, debuted by CIBA in 1956, was the first fruit of Ziegler's "Chemical Cold War" program. Originally marketed to assist the recovery of burn and postoperative patients, the "little pink pills" produced excellent results on the elite powerlifters at York Barbell. As its clone Turinabol moved to the heart of the East German steroid program, "d-bol" was to become so popular with Western strength athletes that by 1969 it earned for itself, by the reckoning of *Track and Field News,* the sobriquet "Breakfast of Champions," based in part on athletes' practice of taking d-bol with heavy doses of caffeine and amphetamines on an empty stomach prior to their morning workouts, to increase "pump" and feelings of vigor. Meanwhile, another powerful injectable androgen, nandrolone decanoate (Deca-Durabolin), was synthesized in 1953 by Organon (Oss, Netherlands), and another Schering product, methenolone acetate (Primobolan Depot), a derivative of dihydrotestosterone, was approved for use in 1961. By 1964, most of the current array of anabolic steroids was available to athletes and, by the early 1970s, though most maintained a studious *omerta,* some athletes openly discussed their steroid use. Contemplating his upcoming challenge of the Soviet superheavyweight lifter Vasily Alexeev at the 1972 Munich Games, American champion weightlifter Ken Patera could barely contain his glee: "Last year, the only difference between me and him was that I couldn't afford his pharmacy bill. Now I can. When I hit Munich next year . . . we'll see which are better—his steroids or mine."

MEDICAL CONSEQUENCES

Unbiased scholarly review of the medical consequences of the use of these agents is inhibited from the start by one little-understood fact: that, unaccounted for in the design and conduct of what little research has so far accumulated, is the sense that the use of anabolics is very different from other illicit drug use patterns, as we hope the foregoing review makes clear. "Steroid abuse" is not just another variety of *drug abuse,* but is atypical in nearly every way. As shown, use patterns for steroidal and nonsteroidal anabolics have evolved gradually over the course of about 50 years in an intelligent, well planned, problem-focused, and thoroughly goal-oriented way, sometimes with government assistance and always with the cooperation of major pharmaceutical houses. Use patterns have developed not within a shady, outlaw culture of hedonistic drug users, but rather within an international subculture of strength, endurance, and fitness athletes and bodybuilders with an Apollonian rather than Dionysian pleasure ethic (e.g., pleasure through structure, discipline, and achievement rather than through chaos, release, and sensation), principally adult males but with an increasing number of youth and females (National Institute on Drug Abuse [NIDA], 2000). This is in sharp contrast to both the other patterns of illicit drug use, which tend to be opportunistic and chaotic, and it is in contrast to the anabolic use patterns that have been the object of controlled study, which are generally suspected as being of much lower doses, and simpler drug combinations, than are found "on the street," among athletes in situ.

Thus, to a dismaying extent, our knowledge about steroidal and nonsteroidal anabolics and related drugs as they are used on the street and in the gym is severely limited and almost certainly unrealistic. This is because, unlike most gregarious drug use, steroid use, particularly since criminalization in the United States, is an intensely solitary practice. Many users hide evidence of drug involvement even from one another, to promote the impression that "gains" were achieved "naturally." Furthermore, because use is proscribed by both law (in the United States) and by many sports federations, and because users recurrently experience periods of demonization by both government and media, use is insulated by many layers of privacy. Finally, like nicotine and caffeine in most cases, anabolics are relatively *transparent* in their effects, producing no obvious intoxication syndrome. Simply put, appearance- and performance-enhancing drugs lend themselves to undetected use, and are exceedingly difficult to study as used "on the street."

The result of this is that, as a scientist, a practitioner, or merely as a citizen or athlete yourself, there is a good chance that you know someone who uses appearance- and performance-enhancing drugs, including anabolic steroids. You probably just do not know that you do. The true proportion, chronicity, and health trajectories—both positive and negative—of these substance users is unknown.

Effects on the Endocrine System

The introduction to a stable metabolism of large exogenous doses of steroidal anabolics has no physical effect more important than perturbation of the endocrine system. It is for this reason that we choose to begin the review of the medical consequences of anabolic steroid use with a survey of effects on the endocrine system.

As already shown, all steroidal anabolics have, in addition to anabolic (tissue-building) properties, androgenic (masculinizing) properties as well. This is a balance of properties often referred to as the anabolic/androgenic ratio or AAR, a drug parameter established by the repeated administration of the steroid to rats, and then the measurement (by increase in weight) of the effects of the steroid on different tissue structures. The anabolic effect of a particular steroid molecule is measured by the increase in weight of the *levator ani* muscle in rats; the androgenic effect of the molecule is measured by increase in weight of rodent prostate tissue and, in some studies, seminal vesicles (Chaudry et al., 1976). Therefore, both the anabolic and androgenic properties of a drug are scaled by proxy measures, not by effects an athlete would easily recognize. Despite the limitations of the method, this is the assay used in steroid chemistry. Testosterone propionate as first developed by Schering in the 1930s, assigned an AAR of 1:1, is the basis of comparison for other anabolics.

As masculinizing effects are often associated with androgens, as well as feminizing effects when androgens are broken down or "aromatized," much effort in steroid chemistry has been devoted to maximizing the AAR of new drugs in order to obviate the untoward effects first noted by John Ziegler in the 1950s. Some drugs have been developed with much higher AARs than testosterone—10:1 in the case of nandrolone decanoate, and up to 30:1 for stanozolol. Still, the goal of developing an anabolic steroid with null androgenic effects remains elusive.

Therefore, use of AAS always involves the introduction of exogenous androgens to the system, resulting in a cascade of endocrinological events downstream (Carvalho et al., 2000): serum testosterone levels increase short-term; due to limited levels of androgen-binding globulin, the proportion of free androgen increases; spikes in the levels of free androgens, mostly testosterone and androstenedione, stimulate the secretion of *aromatases* which break down the androgen molecules and clear them from the system, a process known as *aromatization;* the availability of aromatases causes circulating androgens to be converted to estradiol and other estrogens, leading to an increase of estrogens circulating in the system (Calzada, 2000); finally, the presence of estrogens in male subjects triggers its own cascade of endocrinological events.

In males, this cascade caused by an excess of estrogens has a profoundly paradoxical and untoward effect, given the results most steroid users are seeking. This effect is physical *feminization,* including the development of breast tissue (gynecomastia), female-pattern fat deposition, and water retention. Gynecomastia is a frequently reported side effect of AAS use and is often a cause of psychological distress among those who experience it (Pope and Katz, 1994). It is in most cases transient, but when fatty gynecomastic deposits fail to resolve naturally, the sufferer may opt for costly surgical intervention, as removal of the fatty breast tissue is often the only way to eliminate cosmetic flaws of a type that can be profoundly embarrassing to men (Reyes et al., 1995).

Aromatization—or the transmutation of masculinizing androgens into feminizing estrogens by the action of circulating enzymes known as aromatases—can have profound effects in males. In their study of male AAS-using powerlifters, Alen et al. (1987) found levels of serum estradiol (the estrogen into which testosterone aromatizes) similar to those found in ovulating females. Cessation of AAS use usually results in a return of blood estradiol to normal levels, and most AAS users experience a concomitant reversal of gynecomastia. However in others, the condition persists well after cessation of AAS use (Friedl and Yesalis, 1989; Pope and Katz, 1994) and can result, as already discussed, in serious and permanent cosmetic flaws that can only be reversed surgically.

This persistence appears to occur not as a result of increased estrogen, but rather because of a short-term disruption of the estrogen/androgen balance due to a downregulation of endogenous testosterone production. Although the mechanisms underlying this process are not altogether clear, it appears that AAS use results temporarily in a decrease of endogenous testosterone release as a consequence of inhibitory feedback to the hypothalamic-pituitary-testicular axis (HPTA). The introduction of exogenous androgens in the form of AAS leads to a downregulation of the HPTA neuroendocrine pathway and a decreased release of endogenous testosterone (Alen and Rahkila, 1988; van Breda et al., 2003). This lack of endogenous testosterone results in such symptoms as short-term testicular shrinkage (Evans, 1997; Pope and Katz, 1994), a persistence of feminizing effects like gynecomastia due to an estrogen/testosterone imbalance (Gonzalez, McLachlan, and Keaney, 2001), and, in the absence of exogenous testosterone, loss of libido. In extreme cases, medical intervention including hormone supplementation may be required to return the HPTA to normal functioning (van Breda et al., 2003), which usually results in a return to normal testicular volume and restoration of libido.

These are well-documented endocrine effects of the administration of steroidal anabolics to males, particularly ones with low AARs—testicular shrinkage, loss of libido, and feminizing effects. They are widely reported in both professional literatures and in lay documents intended to discourage steroid use. However, it should be emphasized that, with the exception of some cases of gynecomastia, these effects are transient, and remit shortly upon cessation of AAS use. In addition, something that is not generally well understood outside of the user community is that users are often well educated about side effects and have adapted from various areas of medicine a sophisticated array of agents to combat them (Hildebrandt et al., 2006). Thus tamoxifen, used to treat estrogen-dependent tumors by competitively binding to estrogen receptors, is used by male steroid users at the first symptoms of gynecomastia to suppress emerging aromatization effects; aromatase inhibitors like anastrozole or letrozole, also used in the treatment of breast cancer, address aromatization effects prophylactically by reducing aromatase availability; clomiphene citrate, a follicle stimulant used in reproductive medicine, is used at the end of a cycle of anabolic steroids to stimulate release of follicle stimulating hormone and luteinizing hormone, thus speeding recovery of endogenous testosterone production. Human chorionic gonadotropin (HCG), another fertility aid, is used for the same purpose. Diuretics to suppress water retention, antihypertensives to normalize blood pressure, all and more have found their way into the anabolic pharmacopeia. As a result, very few steroid users appear to experience side effects that are more than mild and transitory, and most report high levels of satisfaction with their steroid use (Hildebrandt et al., 2006); Langenbucher et al., 2005).

If most endocrine effects for males are temporary and readily reversible, they are not so for women. The relatively small number of women who use anabolic steroids for athletic and cosmetic purposes favor those, like Stanozolol, with extremely high AARs, and so with more favorable (less androgenic) side effect profiles. However, highly androgenic compounds, including testosterone and even trenbolone, the most powerful androgen ever developed, are also sometimes observed in the tool kits of very hard-core female competitors, particularly female bodybuilders who are most concerned with visible muscularity and muscle density.

It should be noted that there has been a great deal of recent interest in the therapeutic effect of even low-AAR steroids, including testosterone, in older women, with generally positive findings for their effects on cognitive status, mood, body composition, bone mineralization, and other health indices (e.g., Davis et al., 1995; Shifren, Braunstein, and Simon, 2000). Androgens are secreted in the female body by the adrenal glands and ovaries, and play an important precursor role in the secretion of estrogens. They are thus, indirectly, of crucial importance in the expression of female sexuality, as well as in the maintenance of bone mineralization, immune function, and other vital physiologic processes.

However, studies of the effects on women of moderate to high doses of the generally more potent drugs with low AARs, like testosterone, have never been attempted, though an important source of longitudinal data on the effects of long-term administration of AAS to young, healthy females exists in reports on the formerly "secret doping program" of the DDR discussed in previous text, revealed in classic papers by Werner Franke and one of the affected athletes herself, Brigitte Berendonk (Franke and Berendonk, 1997). These and other authors (e.g., Gruber and Pope, 2000) clearly document a variety of serious, disfiguring, and typically permanent masculinizing side effects in females of large, sustained doses of AAS, including hirsutism (especially growth of facial hair), changes in or cessation of the menstrual cycle, clitoral enlargement, deepening of the voice, male-pattern baldness, reduction in breast size, and genitourinary effects including intractable infertility. This is particularly problematic as young girls, principally those with aspirations for excellence in speed and strength sports, are the demographic group with the highest recent increase in incidence of steroid use (NIDA, 2000).

Effects on the Hepatic and Gastrointestinal System

AAS and Liver

Animal studies have demonstrated the harmful effects of AAS on the liver, including impaired excretion function, cholestasis, peliosis hepatis, and liver cancer. These results from animal research have raised concerns that patients treated with AAS and individuals who self-administer these drugs at high doses are subject to liver damage (Bronson and Matherne, 1992; Ishak, 1981). In addition, a number of case studies have reported the occurrence of liver disorders (principally transient and fairly mild elevation in transamenase levels) in young, healthy athletes who used AAS (Cabasso, 1994; Creagh, Rubin, and Evans, 1988). However, it should be realized that most other orally administered medications have similar effects on the liver and that, in the case of anabolic steroids, these effects are associated only with the use of 17-α-alkylated steroids, a particular subset of orally administered AAS that are less aromatizable and thus sought after by some users wishing to avoid the androgenic effects related to excess estrogen. AAS in this group include methyltestosterone, oxymetholone, fluoxymesterone, norethandrolone, and metandienone.

Elevated transaminase levels have never been associated with the use of injectible steroids, which are the most commonly used anabolics and comprise the bulk of most user's cycles (Langenbucher et al., 2005). It should also be recognized that the activity engaged in by individuals in these case reports—weightlifting—itself causes elevation of transamenase levels, because weightlifting breaks down tissue, freeing transamenase molecules previously resident in muscle cells. Despite a great deal of furor over the liver effects of anabolic steroids, and the high profile given to these effects in many exhortatory documents, caution requires us to conclude that systematic research has shown mild and reversible elevations in transamenase levels due to oral 17-α-alkylated steroid use, but has not shown a relationship between serious liver pathology and AAS use in healthy adult humans.

AAS use has also been linked in animal models to the growth of tumors (particularly in the liver) and carcinoma in case reports (Creagh, Rubin, and Evans, 1988; Kosaka et al., 1996; Velazquez and Alter, 2004), but Friedl (2000) has argued that an exogenous administration AAS is not carcinogenic per se, but is rather more likely to interact with other carcinogenic effects to accelerate the growth of tumors. Some have argued that long-term AAS use increases the risk of developing carcinomas and tumors and may ultimately contribute to early mortality among some AAS users (Pärssinen and Seppälä, 2002). However, the long-term effects of AAS use have not been examined prospectively, so the link between tumor growth, carcinomas, and AAS remains unclear.

hGH and Intestinal Growth

Individuals wishing to increase muscle mass often take human growth hormone (hGH) or, much more rarely, insulin-like growth factor-I (IGF-I). Although these are not anabolic steroids in the strict sense because they are not steroid molecules (gonadohormones) but rather pituitary hormones, and as they are not androgenic at all, they are worth reviewing here because their unsupervised use tends to reside in the same group as the use of anabolic steroids. Taking hGH is attractive to many athletes because no test is currently available to determine its abuse. It can therefore be, and often is, used with legal and regulatory impunity by competitive athletes.

First isolated from pituitary tissue by C. H. Li in 1956, hGH is now produced by rDNA technology. hGH is a potent anabolic and strengthener of connective tissues, as well as a drug that has been shown to help users shed abdominal fat (Rudman et al., 1991). Produced in very large quantities by recombinant DNA technology in People's Republic of China, and in part responsible for the recent dominance of Chinese athletes in many sports requiring leanness and explosive power, hGH is a favorite with gymnasts, swimmers, and track and field athletes, so much so that the 1996 games in Atlanta were nicknamed, by the athletes themselves, as the "the hGH Games" (Blair, 1998).

Regular administration of hGH has been shown to emulate some of the effects of AAS, particularly increased cellular nitrogen retention (Yarasheski, 1994), a precursor for anabolic growth. However, their self-administration appears to result in marked growth of the small intestine, leading to a distension of the abdomen ("'roid gut," in popular parlance; De Palo et al., 2001). Additional effects of hGH on the musculoskeletal system are reviewed in following text.

Effects on the Circulatory System

AAS and Hypertension

Although the American College of Sports Medicine (1987) declared in a position paper that there was a clear relationship between AAS use and hypertension, this conclusion was based on the results of a single study that has not been replicated, while others have failed to find any effect at all (Friedl et al., 1990; Mauss et al., 1975; Pope and Katz, 1994). It is possible that anabolic steroids with marked effects on water retention (such as most oral anabolics, particularly methandrostenolone and oxymetholone) boost blood pressure, but this has yet to be demonstrated in humans, partly because these agents cannot be administered legally to human beings, at least in the United States. It is also possible that anabolic steroids with marked erythropoietic effects, such as boldenone undecylante (Equipoise, a veterinary steroid), raise blood pressure, because they increase blood volume in order to support the greater number of red cells. Certainly, lore among steroid users supports the idea that both oral anabolics and boldenone increase blood volume and cause events associated with hypertension, such as nosebleed, but this has yet to be demonstrated empirically.

AAS and Cholesterol

A relationship between the use of some forms of AAS and lowered serum high-density lipoprotein (HDL), an identified risk factor for heart disease, has been well established (Alen, Rahkila, and Marniemi, 1985; Hurley et al., 1984; Pope and Katz, 1994), while low-density lipoprotein

levels often increase in the presence of AAS. This effect on serum cholesterol levels is one of the most widely cited negative health effects of the use
of AAS. However, there is no evidence that the effect is more than mild and
transient, as all research indicates that serum cholesterol levels return to
normal after cessation of AAS use (Lenders et al., 1988; Pope and Katz,
1994). In addition, lowered HDL has been linked only to orally administered 17-α-alkylated steroids. Conversely, research on the use of AAS with
strong androgenic effects such as injectible nandralone and testosterone esters shows little or no change in HDL levels (Friedl et al., 1990, 1991), and a
large, controlled study comparing AAS-using to nonusing athletes who reported using a wide variety of AAS found no difference in HDL between
the two groups (Pope and Katz, 1994).

The possible difference between types of AAS in their effect on HDL
may be due to the tendency not of testerone, per se, but rather its metabolite
after aromatization—estrogen—to affect HDL levels (Furman et al., 1958).
In addition, Friedl et al. (1991) found a decrease of HDL among users who
added an antiestrogenic compound to their dose of injectible testosterone,
whereas those who took the testosterone alone maintained steady HDL levels, further indicating a relationship between androgen/estrogen balance
and HDL response. Thus, users who take low-aromatization AAS or add
antiestrogenics to their regimen in order to avoid negative androgenic effects may be at greater risk for lowered HDL.

AAS and Cardiomyopathy

Some cases of pathological remodeling of the heart muscle have been reported among AAS-using athletes (Melchert and Welder, 1995; Schollert
and Bendixen, 1993). One of the more notable of these cases is that of professional football player Steve Courson, who has publicly attributed his diagnosis of hypertrophic cardiomyopathy (HCM) to his use of AAS during
his professional career (Courson and Schrieber, 1991). HCM is characterized by a thickening and rigidity of the wall of the heart's left ventricle, the
chamber in the heart that pushes blood out of the heart and into the arterial
system. HCM is also called "enlarged heart" or "athlete's heart," a condition with grave implications because the thickening of the ventricular wall
is on the interior surface, thus reducing the size of the left ventricle and reducing the heart's pumping capacity.

Although it is possible that AAS, as a stimulant to muscle growth, may
also stimulate the growth of heart muscle taxed during exercise—the left ventricular wall—it is equally likely that HCM of this description may be related
to the intensity and specific types of training and exercise involved in strength

sports (Haykowsky et al., 2002; Pluim et al., 2000), rather than to the use of AAS per se. When a strength athlete performs the *Valsalva maneuver* (attempting to breathe out against a closed glottis, or "holding one's breath" while under load), thoracic blood pressure skyrockets momentarily; repeated elevations of thoracic blood pressure, against which the left-ventricle must push as it tries to perform its work of pumping blood out of the heart and into the thorax, may cause the muscle performing that work—the left ventricular wall—to compensate by becoming thicker and more powerful.

Currently, the contribution, perhaps an additive one, of AAS to HCM is unclear. Two studies comparing AAS-using to nonusing bodybuilders found no difference in left-ventricular size between the two groups (Salke, Rowland, and Burke, 1985; Zuliani et al., 1989), while a different study comparing AAS-using bodybuilders to nonusing strength athletes found significantly greater left-ventricular size among the bodybuilders (Urhausen, Albers, and Kindermann, 2004). In addition, work by Pärssinen et al. (2000) showed a marked secular trend (a period effect) in mortality risk for Finnish powerlifters, with risk increasing for lifters who competed in the postanabolic period (roughly 1955 to the present) compared with lifters who competed in the preanabolic period. As much of the excess mortality was due to cardiac problems, and because the pre-/postanabolic athletes had roughly similar lifestyles, diets, and training practices, a suspicion that the excess mortality may have been due to steroid-induced remodeling of the left ventricle is not unreasonable.

Although some types of AAS may be linked to an increase in risk factors for cardiovascular disease, others may actually reduce independent risk factors for heart disease such as Lp(a) and fibrinogen (Albers et al., 1984; Crook et al., 1992, Cohen, Hartford, and Rogers, 1996). It is possible that the cardiac risks posed by some of these drugs are offset by the benefits conferred by others. It is also possible that the potential risks incurred by AAS-using athletes such as lowered HDL levels may be offset by protective factors frequently present among athletes, such as frequent exercise, an avoidance of most kinds of recreational drugs, excellent diet, and a low incidence of smoking. However, only well-designed epidemiological research, which has yet to be undertaken, can determine with certainty what link, if any, exists between heart disease and AAS in general, or specific types of AAS in particular.

AAS and Stroke

A number of case studies involving AAS users indicate a possible relationship between taking high doses of AAS and thrombotic stroke among athletes (Laroche, 1990; Lommi and Harkonen, 1991). Shiozawa et al. (1982) observed in a group study a high frequency of thrombotic stroke among male patients receiving AAS as treatment for aplastic anemia. Ferenchick et al. (1995) identified a possible mechanism for thrombotic stroke among AAS users when they observed that clotting abnormalities were more frequent among AAS-using versus nonusing weightlifters. As with other effects discussed here previously, such clotting abnormalities may be related not to androgens, per se, but rather to a disturbance of the androgen/estrogen balance resulting from the aromatization of excess androgen into estrogens, as research has related elevated estrogen/androgen ratios to higher risk for stroke among both women and men receiving estrogen therapy.

In summary, potential cardiac risk is often discussed as the greatest health threat posed by AAS use, but the links between AAS use and various cardiac conditions have yet to be fully determined.

Effects on the Central Nervous System

The activity of AAS and other appearance- and performance-enhancing drugs on the central nervous system (CNS) is widespread and involves direct effects through androgen receptor binding. However, AAS also exerts indirect effects through increases in estrogen (Shahidi, 2001). Specific neurochemical effects for AAS and its metabolites have been observed throughout the brain and include effects on GABA, monoamines, serotonin, and sigma receptors in particular (Clark and Henderson, 2003; Kashkin and Kleber, 1989; Stoffel-Wagner, 2001, 2003).

The wealth of information about AAS from animal studies has yet to provide conclusive evidence of a primary reinforcement model of AAS abuse or dependence, although research on the interaction of AAS with other drugs of abuse such as stimulants (Clark, Lindenfeld, and Gibbons, 1996) and ethanol (Lukas, 1996; Pahlen, 2005) suggests that AAS use may increase the reinforcing effects of other drugs of abuse (Clark and Henderson, 2003). Stimulants often used by AAS users such as clenbuterol and ephedrine are thought to have similar effects on the CNS as amphetamines; thus, they have direct effects on the sympathetic nervous system and norepinephrine metabolism in the brain (Koch, 2002). The resulting medical impact of performance enhancing drugs on the CNS includes a range of behavioral and psychiatric disturbances as well as milder symptoms related to autonomic arousal.

Autonomic Effects

Although anabolic steroids themselves have no clear effect on the autonomic system, other drugs used by many steroid users, such as ergogenics and thyroid hormones, do, and are discussed briefly here.

The autonomic effects of performance-enhancing drugs are related to activation of the sympathetic nervous system. Regular use of milder stimulants such as caffeine may result in acute intoxication, anxiety, sleep disorders, or a withdrawal syndrome when discontinued (Silverman et al., 1992; Spriet, 2002). However, other stimulants such as ephedrine, which act on adrenergic receptors and affect vasoconstriction, cardiac function, and which stimulate energy metabolism, may have more severe consequences such as psychosis (Maglione et al., 2005; Philibert and Mack, 2004; Walton and Manos, 2003). The mechanism for this effect is thought to be related to stimulant effects on the sigma receptors (Karch, 2002), although the exact mechanism for the effects of ephedrine and other herbal stimulants remain undetermined (Rawson and Clarkson, 2002). As Karch (2002) has pointed out, stimulants acting as thermogenics also have a dehydrating effect, although there appears to be a mediating effect of the environment with hot humid conditions also increasing the metabolism of substances such as ephedrine and consequently exacerbating the risk of adverse effects (Vanakoski, Stromberg, and Seppala, 1993).

Use of thyroid hormones such as T3, common among users of AAS (Langenbucher et al., 2005), also has direct and indirect effects on the central nervous system with long-term continuous use mimicking the effects of hyperthyroidism. Among the symptoms of hyperthyroidism are increased body temperature, trouble sleeping despite being fatigued, and tremors, although the main effects of increased T3 are on cardiac functioning (Cooper, 2005). Unfortunately, there is no controlled research on prolonged use of exogenous thyroid hormones, so it is unclear whether T3 use can result in permanent alterations in thyroid functioning.

Some researchers have noted increased levels of thyroid hormones in persons exhibiting aggressive and violent behavior (Stalenheim, von Knorring, and Wide, 1998), although this relationship has been found mainly in cross-sectional study designs, leaving the question of causality unanswered. The interaction of thyroid hormones with AAS and other performance-enhancing drugs is unknown, although there is evidence that high doses of AAS raise endogenous thyroid hormone levels and may be the mechanism by which AAS relates to aggression (Daly et al., 2003). In this connection, one case-control study indicated that men with severe hyperthyroidism exhibit elevated levels of sex hormones including testosterone and estradiol (Zahringer et al., 2000). However, the overall psychiatric effects of thyroid hormone use remain unclear, particularly when used with other substances such as AAS, where the potential exists for increases in aggressive responding.

Psychiatric Effects

Along with effects on the endocrine system, liver, and circulatory system, the negative effects of AAS on the psychological bearing of users have been widely touted as one of the main reasons to avoid this group of agents. However, careful review shows that the extent to which AAS and other appearance- and performance-enhancing drugs cause or even exacerbate psychiatric conditions is unknown.

Several proposed relationships have been examined or described in the literature including the link between testosterone and hypomania/mania (Pope, Kouri, and Hudson, 2000; Pope and Katz, 1988, 1994; Freinhar and Alvarez, 1985), increased aggression (Clark and Hendersen, 2003; Daly, 2001; Daly et al., 2003; Pahlen, 2005; Perry et al., 2003), substance use disorders (Brower, 2002; Kanayama et al., 2003), and, especially, depression (Dickerman and McConathy, 1997; Francis, 1981; Gray, Singh, Woodhouse, et al., 2005; Perry et al., 2002; Rubin et al., 1999; Sachar et al., 1973; Schweiger et al., 1999; Seidman and Walsh, 1999; Weber et al., 2000; Yates et al., 1999). All of these relationships are highly confounded and unclear. Evidence for a relationship between psychiatric states such as these and other appearance- and performance-enhancing drugs is even more limited. Perhaps the strongest association is between ephedra or other stimulants and psychotic symptoms (Boerth and Caley, 2003; Jacobs and Hirsch, 2000; Maglione et al., 2005; Philibert and Mac, 2004; Traboulsi, Viswanathan, and Coplan, 2002; Walton and Manos, 2003), a topic covered elsewhere in this volume.

Hypomania, mania, increased violence, and suicide attempts preceded by acute or extended use of AAS have been observed in several case reports (Conacher and Workman, 1989; Freinhar and Alverez., 1985; Schulte, Hall, and Boyer, 1993; Thiblin and Parlklo, 2002; Thiblin, Runeson, and Rajs, 1999; Weiss, Bowers, and Mazure, 1999), but there is mixed support from cross-sectional, experimental, and especially longitudinal research for a causal relationship between these psychiatric states, problematic behaviors, and AAS use. Only four blinded randomized controlled trials have indicated an increase in psychiatric symptoms, aggression, or adverse overt behavior (Hannan et al., 1991; Kouri et al., 1995; Pope, Kouri, and Hudson, 2000; Su et al., 1993), most of these trials used a very low or ambiguous standard of abnormal behavior (it must be noted that many "manic" symptoms are merely indicators of elevated mood, even well-being, and these may be regarded as benefits, rather than as untoward consequences, of AAS use), and still other studies have found no effect at all. In a recent study, Pope, Kouri, and Hudson (2000) found greater increases in "manic symptoms" in participants using 600 mg/wk of testosterone cypionate, but concluded that very few, only 4.0 percent, became markedly hypomanic. Su et al. (1993) investigated the effects of two doses (40 and 240 mg/day) of methyl-testosterone and found a 10.0 percent incidence of mania or hypomania in normal, non-weight-training male volunteers. The greater incidence in manic or hypomanic states in the Su et al. study using methyltestosterone is of some clinical significance; an often overlooked factor is the chemical structure of the specific AAS used, as some have argued based on the animal literature that specific AAS chemistry is likely to be an important determinant of the specific psychiatric and psychological effects that remain has not been studied sufficiently in humans (Clark, Harrold, and Fast, 1997; Martinez-Sanchis, 1996).

The relationship between aggression and AAS has been explored in a number of cross-sectional and case-control studies comparing steroid users and nonusing controls (Galligani, Renck, and Hansen, 1996; Lefavi, Reeve, and Newland, 1990; Moss, Panazak, and Tarter, 1992; Parrot, Choi, and Davies, 1994; Perry, Andersen, and Yates 1990; Perry et al., 2003; Pope et al., 1994). However, many of these studies are limited by selection biases and do not adequately control for dietary practices, training identities, or personality differences between comparison groups. In one well-controlled experimental study, Kouri et al. (1995) found higher rates of aggressive responding (button pressing) in a double-blind, randomized, crossover design study with normal male volunteers prescribed AAS. Animal studies supporting aggressive responses indicate that dominant animals are much more likely to exhibit aggression and have higher basal testosterone levels than subordinate animals, suggesting that the social context interacts with testosterone levels in meaningful ways that have not been explored in human research (Rejeski et al., 1988). Thus, there are several case-controlled studies reporting elevated aggression on self-report questionnaires and one experimental study supporting the causal effects of steroid use and a laboratory analogue of aggressivity in men, but animal studies suggest that these effects are likely context dependent.

Despite some support for a link between aggression and AAS use, a number of studies have failed to find differences in aggressivity between AAS users and nonusers (Bahrke et al., 1992; Bond, Choi, and Pope, 1995; Perry, Andersen, and Yates, 1990). In fact, a well controlled experiment using high doses of testosterone for four weeks on normal volunteers found that partner ratings as well as self-report ratings of aggression did not differ as a function of testosterone, independent of involvement in exercise routines (Bhasin et al., 1996). Similar results were obtained from a short-term increasing dose testosterone administration trial in normal men (Fingerhood et al., 1997), and several other placebo controlled experiments (Ellingrod et al., 1997; Yates et al., 1999) suggesting that the causal role of AAS in mood disturbance, either hypomania, mania, or aggression, is not direct and is probably more likely the result of an interaction effect with other variables including environmental context, history of mood disorder, or personality. One alternative hypothesis is that AAS use is associated with large expectancy effects of aggression and hostility. Accordingly, some have argued that culturally generated beliefs about steroid use, beliefs to some extent modeled on public service drug prevention messages, contribute to an observed increase in negative mood symptoms among AAS users (Bjorkqvist et al., 1994).

Depressive symptoms and AAS use have also been described in the literature, mainly with the onset of steroid withdrawal. There have been several case reports of both suicide and increased suicidal ideation and depressive symptoms such as loss of libido, lethargy, sleep disturbance, and irritability during AAS discontinuation (Allnutt and Chaimowitz, 1994; Cowan, 1994; Malone and Dimeff, 1992). Pope and Katz (1988) also diagnosed depressive symptoms in many AAS users who were "off-cycle," and thus were experiencing temporarily suppressed testosterone levels. Evidence from treatment trials involving testosterone replacement in hypogonadal men support the relationship between low testosterone levels and decreased mood, as would be found in steroid users who have gone off-cycle, an effect that recedes with the return of normal levels of testosterone (Seidman et al., 2001; Wang et al., 2000). However, there is some evidence that increased depression following discontinuation of testosterone administration occurs only in a small number of men (approximately 10 percent of normal men), and may be more likely in men with greater natural libido and energy levels (Schmidt et al., 2004).

The exact mechanisms that support mood and aggressive effects of AAS are poorly understood. Current research suggests that increased testosterone indirectly affects pituitary-adrenal hormones such as thyroxine, which are better predictors of aggressive responses than testosterone levels per se (Daly et al., 2003). Some have argued that the link between aggression and testosterone is explained by levels of testosterone metabolites such as 5alpha-dihydrotestosterone (DHT) and estradiol (Pahlen, 2005; Pinna, Costa, and Guidotti, 2005), although these are preliminary models in need of further evaluation. Increased estrogen from aromatized testosterone is a key suspect in the relationship between testosterone and depressive symptoms, as estrogen is argued to play a key role in sensitivity to stress and susceptibility to anxiety and depression (Seeman, 1997). Thus, secondary hormone effects rather than direct effects per se are likely indicated in the expression of negative mood symptoms in men and women who use supraphysiological doses of AAS.

Effects on the Musculoskeletal System

The consequences of AAS and other performance enhancing drug use on the musculoskeletal system have not been well documented in athletic or weight lifting populations. Many of the consequences have been derived from medical observations of conditions such as acromegaly (oversecretion of hGH by the pituitary gland) and thus the prevalence of many of these effects in athletes is unknown. As with other systems, many of the consequences are also subject to interaction effects which to date are poorly understood given the wide range of performance enhancing substances used by many athletes.

Negative effects on bone typically associated with acromegaly (and thought to be associated with exogenous hGH use) include excess bone growth, particularly mandibular, frontal sinus, verterbral, and phalangeal overgrowth, and other consequences such as joint widening and accelerated osteoarthritis (Kraemer, Nindl, and Rubin, 2002). Evidence from treatment trials of individuals receiving hGH for deficiency states suggest that side effects are relatively rare (Carvalho et al., 2003; Grumbach, Bin-Abbas, and Kaplan, 1998), although some evidence suggests that hGH administration may be associated with increased risk for leukemia in individuals with preexisting risk factors (Wantabe et al., 1989).

Thyroid hormones are thought to have important effects on bone mineral density, and hyperthyroidism has been linked to osteoporosis and increased fractures (Parle et al., 1991). A recent review suggests that the mechanisms for such effects are still unclear but may involve both increased T3 and suppressed thyroid stimulating hormone (Murphy and Williams, 2004). Thus, the chronic use of thyroid hormones such as T3 may lead to early bone loss, although it is unclear what effect the simultaneous use of AAS or hGH may have.

AAS use in adolescents is argued to increase the risk of premature closing of epiphysial plates, which is likely due to the presence of androgen and estrogen receptors in growth plates (Nilsson et al., 2003). Some have also argued based on the animal literature that AAS use is associated with increased rate of tendon ruptures, although this effect may be associated with muscle hypertrophy even in non-AAS users (Friedl, 2000). The mechanisms for increased tendon rupturing is thought to be related to decreasing tendon elasticity, which has been observed in several animal studies (e.g., Miles et al., 1992) as well as case reports of AAS users (Liow and Tavares, 1995; Stannard and Bucknell, 1993), as well as to the simple fact that muscles grow more quickly than tendons and ligaments, so that the muscular strength obtained by AAS-using athletes may outstrip the ability of tendons and ligaments to support that level of muscularity, leaving the athlete vulnerable to numerous athletic injuries (Bryant, 2005).

Hazards from Routes of Supply and Mode of Administration

Though apparently rare, a number of dangers are associated with both routes of supply and routes of administration of AAS (Dickinson et al., 1999; Scott and Scott, 1989; Slarek et al., 1984). These include chemical impurities in the drugs themselves, biological contamination of the drugs during the manufacturing process, risks associated with needle sharing and multiuse vials, and abscess from nonsterile injection technique.

Historically, steroidal and nonsteroidal anabolics were manufactured by large pharmaceutical companies, such as Organon (Netherlands; developer of Deca-Durabolin), Schering (Berlin; developer of testosterone esters), and others with licenses to produce human-grade products. However, tightening controls on the distribution of these pharmaceuticals following the criminalization of anabolic steroids in 1990, and the wide use of anabolics in veterinary and agricultural settings—along with the legality of nearly all anabolic steroids in the large agricultural country immediately south of the United States, Mexico—has caused many users to turn to veterinary and agricultural sources, or to manufacture their own injectibles in their homes, using powdered hormone easily purchased over the internet. Most oral anabolics are human-grade pharmaceutical products, but their use is a small part of total exposure. Injectibles are used mostly (Langenbucher et al., 2005), where a very large proportion of testosterone stock, as well as all of the stock of the next two most popular injectibles, boldenone and trenbolone (compounds not in the human pharmacopeia), are veterinary. Some manufacturers use loose production controls, home-manufactured or "underground laboratory" steroids are nearly always poorly produced, and occasional cases of deep-muscle abscess from bacterial infiltrate are found in the weightlifting community. Such cases are rarely mentioned in medical journals (e.g., Evans, 1997; Rich et al., 1998), suggesting that they are rare. However, occasional cases of bacterial infection from poor injection technique are also noted among AAS users (Maropis and Yesalis, 1994; Plaus and Hermann, 1991), as is the sharing of multiuse vials, and very occasional incidents of needle-sharing (Midgley et al., 2000). All of these—the use of veterinary-grade or home-manufactured injectibles, the sharing of needles and multiuse vials, and the use of nonsterile injection practices—remains the cause of some concern, particularly given the reluctance of users to present for necessary treatment out of a fear of discovery.

SUMMARY AND CONCLUSIONS

As the foregoing review indicates, the use of appearance- and performance-enhancing drugs is ubiquitous, involving not only competitive athletes but recreational and occupational users of both sexes (Monaghan, 2002). The imagery of the anabolic user adorns a mounting proportion of advertisements using the partially clad human form (Pope et al., 1997). Anabolics loom large in the chemically augmented bodies of film stars in theaters across the country, bulge from the photo sidebars of fitness "how-to" articles in thousands of periodicals, surge powerfully down football grid-irons, baseball diamonds and sprint tracks on satellite television, swell the size of roll call ranks in police stations and firehouses around the country, and have come to exert a strong pull on the aesthetics and lifestyle perspectives of an increasing number of Americans (Pope, Kouri, and Hudson, 2000), especially the young. The presumption that many of these athletes, models, performers and protectors are devotees of "natural" training and dietary practices is naive to informed observers, who recognize many, perhaps most, of these figures as what they are: users of anabolic steroids and of other appearance- and performance-enhancing drugs.

Yet, despite the vigor of respected branches of medicine (endocrinology) and the behavioral sciences (sports psychology) that bear it within their province, probably not much is known about the actual "street use" of anabolic steroids and related drugs, their consequences—both positive and negative—than is known about any other drug use phenomenon on which policy is even debated, much less settled. Were caregivers to encounter anabolic users in their practices, or were the scientific community to recognize the scope and intricacy of appearance- and performance-enhancing drug use, more would be known. However, society is only fitfully concerned with anabolic use, growing vocal only when the occasional "scandal" erupts in a highly visible sports venue. This episodic concern unfortunately serves to equate anabolic steroid use with unethical behavior ("cheating" in sports) and, more important, builds the impression that anabolic use is limited to sports superstars seeking to boost 70 homeruns out of the ballpark, or to gullible youth seeking to emulate them. None of these impressions are accurate but, consequent to them, misunderstanding, not rational policy, and much less sensitive patient care, has flourished.

In this chapter, the medical consequences of the use of anabolic steroids and, very briefly, nonsteroidal anabolics and thermogenics associated with anabolic use, were reviewed according to the effects of these drugs on the endocrine, gastrointestinal, circulatory, musculoskeletal, and central nervous systems, with note of hazards having to do with the mode of supply and routes of administration of these compounds. Although numerous exhortatory pieces highlight grave, even mortal, risks for the use of these drugs even in healthy young males, a critical review finds risks, for most users, to be modest, immediately reversible and, very often, through the concurrent use of the appropriate ancillaries, preventable or controllable. Thus, anabolic steroids do, in fact, cause testicular atrophy, but this is in most cases a modest decline in testicular mass that reverses immediately upon cessation of steroid use and that can be prevented by proper use of clomiphene citrate and HCG; thus, anabolic steroids do, in fact, cause increases in transamenase levels that many take to be evidence of liver "pathology," but these increases are immediately reversible, of about the same level as those observed with many other medications, and to be expected anyway in athletes with rapid muscle cell turnover, as is found in people who use anabolic steroids within an ambitious program of weightlifting. For healthy males, most of the other "serious side effects" of anabolic use—effects of aromatization, downregulation of the HPTA neuroendocrine pathway, loss of libido, hypertension, effects on serum cholesterol, risk for thrombotic stroke, addictive potential, autonomic effects, negative effects of AAS on the psychological bearing of users including hypomania, aggression, and depression—are ambiguously related to the use of anabolic steroids or, where the relationship is clear, the effects are mild, reversible, and either preventable or manageable by the correct use of ancillary agents, many of which are widely discussed and available among users.

However, if these are unworrisome findings, others breed concern. Most oral anabolics are human-grade pharmaceutical products, but their use is a small part of total exposure. Most use is of injectibles, where a very large proportion of testosterone stock, as well as all of the stock of the next two most popular injectibles, boldenone and trenbolone, are veterinary, and where an increasing amount of steroids is coming from "underground labs" rather than established pharmaceutical houses with established manunfacturing protocols. The risks of infection and deep muscle abscess from "dirty gear" (steroids with bacterial infiltrate) or, for that matter, from unsterile injection technique are a cause for concern.

In addition, other serious health concerns may arise during the course of anabolic use. These include nonremitting gynecomastia requiring surgery (in a tiny number of users), intestinal growth in cases of long-term high-dose use of hGH, pathological remodeling of the heart leading to hypertrophic cardiomyopathy, depressive symptomatology arising in steroid withdrawal, a tendency to increased tendon rupturing when increased muscular strength outstrips the mechanical strength of connective tissue, and, of course, many of the masculinizing effects on women.

Much additional research is required to clarify these and other, related, issues. In fact, phenomena now prevalent in both athletic and fitness circles that warrant scientific study because of possible medical risks, as well as benefits, are extraordinarily complex, involving

1. the use of anabolic steroids;
2. the use of nonsteroidal anabolics such as insulin, human growth hormone, and insulin-like growth factor;
3. the use of hormone precursor molecules (e.g., androstenediol/dione, norandrostenediol/dione), sold until recently as "dietary supplements" but easily convertible into injectible steroids;
4. the use of ergogenic, thermogenic, and anorexigent compounds, many available over-the-counter, used to boost metabolism, raise body temperature, reduce appetite, and "burn fat";
5. the use of antianemics such as erythropoietin, used to increase vital capacity by packing blood with red corpuscles;
6. the use of ancillary drugs used to correct the side effects of anabolics, such as antiestrogenics used to combat aromatization of androgens into estrogen;
7. comorbid recreational and operant drug use;
8. anorexia-like eating aimed at achieving super-low body fat levels;
9. polypharmacy through a high comfort level with self-medicating a variety of conditions, mostly side effects and complications of AAS use, but often unrelated conditions as well;
10. esthetic/prosthetic implants; and
11. dangerous and catabolic exercise regimes, hazardous skin darkening, and others.

All of these phenomena are likely to grow in scope in the next decades, and to infiltrate other, non-gym-oriented strata of society, where they are not yet in evidence. Society would be wise to anticipate their emergence and move proactively to govern them, rather than take the reactive and hasty course that has so far characterized its approach to anabolic steroids.

REFERENCES

Albers, J.; Taggart, H.; Applebaum-Bowden, D.; Haffner, S.; Chesnut, C.; and Hazzard, W. (1984). Reduction of lecithincholesterol acyltransferase, apolipoprotein D and the Lp(a) with the anabolic steroid stanozolol. *Biochimica et Biophysica Acta* 79, 293-296.

Alen, M. and Rahkila, P. (1988). Anabolic-androgenic steroid effects on endocrinology and lipid metabolism in athletes. *Sports Medicine* 6, 327-332.

Alen, M.; Rahkila, P.; and Marniemi, J. (1985). Serum lipids in power athletes self-administering testosterone and anabolic steroids. *International Journal of Sports Medicine* 6, 139-144.

Alen, M.; Rahkila, P.; Reinila, M.; and Vihko, R. (1987). Androgenic-anabolic steroid effects on serum thyroid, pituitary and steroid hormones in athletes. *American Journal of Sports Medicine* 15, 357-361.

Allnutt, S. and Chaimowitz, G. (1994). Anabolic steroid withdrawal depression: A case report. *Canadian Journal of Psychiatry* 39, 317-318.

American College of Sports Medicine (1987). Position stand on the use of anabolic-androgenic steroids in sport. *Medical Science in Sports and Exercise* 19, 534-539.

Bahrke, M.S.; Wright, J.E.; Strauss, R.H.; and Catlin, D.H. (1992). Psychological moods and subjectively perceived behavioral and somatic changes accompanying anabolic-androgenic steroid usage. *American Journal of Sports Medicine* 20, 717-724.

Berthold, A.A. (1849). Transplantation der Hoden [The transplantation of the testes]. *Archives der Anatomie Physiologie Wissenschaft Medicina* 42-46.

Bhasin, S.; Storer, T.W.; Berman, N.; Callgari, C.; Clevenger, B.; and Phillips, J. (1996). The effects of supraphysiological doses of testosterone on muscle size and strength in normal men. *New England Journal of Medicine* 335, 1-7.

Bjorkqvist, K.; Nygren, T.; Bjorklund, A.-C.; and Bjorkqvist, S.-E. (1994). Testosterone intake and aggressiveness: Real effect or anticipation. *Aggressive Behavior* 20, 17-26.

Blair, T. (1998). Just say go. *Time.com* July 27, No. 30.

Boerth, J.M. and Caley, C.F. (2003). Possible case of mania associated with ma-huang. *Pharmacotherapy* 23, 380-383.

Bond, A.J.; Choi, P.Y.L.; and Pope, H.G. (1995). Assessment of attentional bias and mood in users and non-users of anabolic-androgenic steroids. *Drug and Alcohol Dependence* 37, 241-245.

Bronson, F.H. and Matherne, C.M. (1997). Exposure to anabolic-androgenic steroids shortens life span of male mice. *Medicine and Science in Sports and Exercise* 29, 615-619.

Brower, K.J. (2002). Anabolic steroid abuse and dependence. *Current Psychiatry Report* 4, 377-387.

Brown-Séquard, C.E. (1889). The effects produced on man by subcutaneous injections of a liquid obtained from the testicles of animals. *Lancet* 2, 105-107.

Bryant, H. (2005). *Juicing the Game.* New York: Viking.

Cabasso, A. (1994). Peliosis hepatis in a young adult bodybuilder. *Medical Science in Sports and Exercise* 26, 2-4.

Calzada, L.T. (2000). Measurement of androgen and estrogen receptors in breast tissue from subjects with anabolic steroid-dependent gynecomastia. *Life Sciences* 69, 1465-1479.

Carvalho, L.R.; de Faria, M.E.J.; Osorio, M.G.F.; Estefan, V.; Jorge, A.A.L.; Arnhold, I.G.P.; and Mendonca, B.B. (2003). Acromegalic features in growth hormone (GH)-deficient patients after long-term GH therapy. *Clinical Endocrinology* 59, 788-792.

Chaudry, M.A.; James, K.C.; Ng, C.T.; and Nicholls, P.J. (1976). Anabolic and androgenic activities, in rat, of some nandrolone and androstanolone esters. *Journal of Pharmacy and Pharmacology* 28, 882-885.

Clark, A.S.; Harrold, E.V.; and Fast, A.S. (1997). Anabolic-androgenic steroid effects on the sexual behavior of intact male rats. *Hormones and Behavior* 31, 35-46.

Clark, A.S. and Henderson, L.P. (2003). Behavioral and physiological responses to anabolic-androgenic steroids. *Neuroscience and Biobehavior Review* 27, 413-436.

Clark, A.S.; Lindenfeld, R.C.; and Gibbons, C.H. (1996). Anabolic-androgenic steroids and brain reward. *Pharmacology, Biochemistry and Behavior* 53, 741-745.

Cohen, L.; Hartford, C.; and Rogers, G. (1996). Lipoprotein (a) and cholesterol in bodybuilders using anabolic androgenic steroids. *Medicine and Science in Sports and Exercise* 8, 176-179.

Conacher, G.N. and Workman, D.G. (1989). Violent crime possibly associated with anabolic steroid use. *American Journal of Psychiatry* 146, 679.

Cooper, D.S. (2005). Antithyroid drugs. *New England Journal of Medicine* 352, 905-917.

Courson, S. and Schrieber, L. (1991). *False Glory: Steelers and Steroids: The Steve Courson Story.* Stamford, CT: Longmeadow Press.

Cowan, C.B. (1994). Depression in anabolic steroid withdrawal. *Irish Journal of Psychological Medicine* 11, 27-28.

Creagh, T.; Rubin, A.; and Evans, D. (1988). Hepatic tumours induced by anabolic steroids in an athlete. *Journal of Clinical Pathology* 41, 441-443.

Crook, D.; Sidhu, M.; Seed, M.; O'Donnell, M.; and Stevenson, J. (1992). Lipoprotein Lp (a) levels are reduced by danazol, an anabolic steroid. *Atherosclerosis* 92, 41-47.

Daly, R.C. (2001). Anabolic steroids, brain and behaviour. *Irish Medical Journal* 94, 102.

Daly, R.C.; Su, T.P.; Schmidt, P.J.; Pagliaro, M.; Pickar, D.; and Rubinow, D.R. (2003). Neuroendocrine and behavioral effects of high-dose anabolic steroid administration in male normal volunteers. *Psychoneuroendocrinology* 28, 317-331.

Davis, S.R.; McCloud, P.; Strauss, B.J.; and Burger, H. (1995). Testosterone enhances estradiol's effects on postmenopausal bone density and sexuality. *Maturitas* 21, 227-236.

de Kruif, P. (1945). *The Male Hormone.* New York: Harcourt, Brace & Co.

De Palo, E.; Gatti, R.; Lancerin, F.; Cappellin, E.; and Spinella, P. (2001). Correlations of growth hormone (GH) and insulin-like growth factor I (IGF-I): Effects of exercise and abuse by athletes. *Clinica Chimica Acta* 305, 1-17.

Dickerman, R.D. and McConathy, W.J. (1997). Testosterone, vasopressin and depression. *Progress in Neuro-Psychopharmacology and Biological Psychiatry* 21, 247-248.

Dickinson, B.P.; Mylonakis, E.; Strong, L.L.; and Rich, J.D. (1999). Potential infections related to anabolic steroid injection in young adolescents. *Pediatrics* 103, 694.

Ellingrod, V.; Perry, P.J.; Yates, W.R.; MacIndoe, J.; Watson, G.; and Arndt (1997). The effects of anabolic steroids on driving performance as assessed by the Iowa Driver Simulator. *American Journal of Drug and Alcohol Abuse* 23, 623-636.

Evans, N.A. (1997). Local complications of self administered anabolic steroid injections. *British Journal of Sports Medicine* 31, 349-350.

Evans, N.A. (2004). Current concepts in anabolic-androgenic steroids. *American Journal of Sports Medicine* 32, 534-542.

Ferenchick, G.S.; Hirokawa, S.; Mammen, E.F.; and Schwartz, K.A. (1995). Anabolic-androgenic steroid abuse in weight lifters: Evidence for activation of the hemostatic system. *American Journal of Hematology* 49, 282-288.

Fingerhood, M.I.; Sullivan, J.T.; Testa, M.; and Janinski, D.R. (1997). Abuse liability of testosterone. *Journal of Psychopharmacology* 11, 59-63.

Francis, K.T. (1981). The relationship between high and low trait psychological stress, serum testosterone, and serum cortisol. *Experientia* 37, 1296-1297.

Franke, W. and Berendonk, B. (1997). Hormonal doping and androgenization of athletes: A secret program of the German Democratic Republic government. *Clinical Chemistry* 43, 1262-1279.

Freinhar, J.P. and Alvarez, W. (1985). Androgen-induced hypomania. *Journal of Clinical Psychiatry* 46, 354-355.

Friedl, K.E. (2000). Effects of anabolic steroids on physical health. In: C.E. Yesalis (Ed.), *Anabolic Steroids in Sport and Exercise* (pp. 175-224). Champaign, IL: Human Kinetics.

Friedl, K.; Dettori, J.; Hannan, C.; Patience, T.; and Plymate, S. (1991). Comparison of the effects of high dose testosterone and 19-nortestosterone to a replacement dose of testosterone on strength and body composition in normal men. *Journal of Steroid Biochemistry and Molecular Biology* 40, 607-612.

Friedl, K.; Hannan, C.; Jones, R.; and Plymate, S. (1990). High-density lipoprotein cholesterol is not decreased if an aromatizable androgen is administered. *Metabolism: Clinical and Experimental* 39, 69-74.

Friedl, K. and Yesalis, C. (1989). Self-treatment of gynecomastia in bodybuilders who use anabolic steroids. *The Physician and Sportsmedicine* 17, 67-79.

Furman, R.; Howard, R.; Norcia, L.; and Keaty, E. (1958). The influence of androgens, estrogens and related steroids on serum lipids and lipoproteins. *American Journal of Medicine* 24, 80-97.

Gallagher, T.F.; and Koch, F.C. (1929). The testicular hormone. *Journal of Biological Chemistry* 84, 495-500.

Galligani, N.; Renck, A.; and Hansen, S. (1996). Personality profile of men using anabolic androgenic steroids. *Hormones and Behavior* 30, 170-175.

Goldfield, G.S.; Harper, D.W.; and Blouin, A.G. (1998). Are bodybuilders at risk for an eating disorder? *Eating Disorders* 6, 133-158.

Gonzalez, A.; McLachlan, S.; and Keaney, F. (2001). Anabolic steroid misuse: How much should we know? *International Journal of Psychiatry in Clinical Practice* 5, 159-167.

Gray, P. B.; Singh, A. B.; Woodhouse, L. J.; Storer, T. W.; Casaburi, R.; Dzekov, J. et al. (2005). Dose-dependent effects of testosterone on sexual function, mood, and visuospatial cognition in older men. *Journal of Clinical Endocrinology and Metabolism, 90,* 3838-3846.

Gridley, D.W. and Hanrahan, S.J. (1994). Anabolic-androgenic steroid use among male gymnasium participants: Dependence, knowledge and motives. *Sport Health* 12, 11-14.

Gruber, A.J. and Pope, H.G., Jr. (2000). Psychiatric and medical effects of anabolic-androgenic steroid use in women. *Psychotherapy and Psychosomatics* 69, 19-26.

Grumbach, M.M.; Bin-Abbas, B.S.; and Kaplan, S.L. (1998). The growth hormone cascade: Progress and long-term results of growth hormone treatment in growth hormone deficiency. *Hormone Research* 49, 41-57.

Hannan, C.J., Jr.; Friedl, K.E.; Zold, A.; Kettler, T.M.; and Plymate, S.R. (1991). Psychological and serum homovanillic acid changes in men administered androgenic steroids. *Psychoneuroendocrinology* 16, 335-343.

Haykowsky, M.; Dressendorfer, R.; Taylor, D.; Madic, S.; and Humen, D. (2002). Resistance training and cardiac hypertrophy: Unravelling the training effect. *Sports Medicine* 32, 837-849.

Hildebrandt, T.; Langenbucher, J.W.; Carr, S.; Sanjuan, P.; and Tung, K. (2006). Predicting intentions for long-term anabolic-androgenic steroid use among males: A covariance structure model. *Psychology of Addictive Behaviors* 20, 234-240.

Hurley, B.; Seals, D.; Hagberg, J.; Goldberg, A.; Ostrove, S.; Holloszy, J.; Wiest, W.; and Goldberg, A. (1984). High-density-lipoprotien cholesterol in bodybuilders vs. powerlifters: Negative effects of androgen use. *Journal of the American Medical Association* 425, 507-513.

Ishak, K. (1981). Hepatic lesions caused by anabolic and contraceptive steroids. *Seminars in Liver Disease* 1, 116-128.

Jacobs, K.M. and Hirsch, K.A. (2000). Psychiatric complications of Ma-huang. *Psychosomatics* 41, 58-62.

Kanayama, G.; Cohane, G.H.; Weiss, R.D.; and Pope, H.G. (2003). Past anabolic-androgenic steroid use among men admitted for substance abuse treatment: An underrecognized problem? *Journal of Clinical Psychiatry* 64, 156-160.

Karch, S.B. (2002). Stimulants. In: M.S. Bahrke and C.E. Yesalis (Eds.), *Performance-Enhancing Substances in Sport and Exercise* (pp. 257-265). Champiagn, IL: Human Kinetics.

Kashkin, K.B. and Kleber, H.D. (1989). Hooked on hormones? An anabolic steroid addiction hypothesis. *Journal of the American Medical Association* 262, 3166-3170.

Kenyon, A.T.; Sandiford, I.; Bryan, A.H.; and Koch, F. (1938). The effect of testosterone propionate on nitrogen, electrolyte, water and energy metabolism in eunuchoidism. *Endocrinology* 23, 135-153.

Koch, J.J. (2002). Performance-enhancing: Substances and their use among adolescent athletes. *Pediatrics Review* 23, 310-317.

Kochakian, C.D. (1937). Testosterone and testosterone acetate and the protein and energy metabolism of castrate dogs. *Endocrinology* 21, 750-755.

Kosaka, A.; Takahashi, H.; Yajima, Y.; Tanaka, M.; and Okamura, K. (1996). Hepatocellular carcinoma associated with anabolic steroid therapy: Report of a case and review of the Japanese literature. *Journal of Gastroenterology* 31, 450-454.

Kouri, E.M.; Lukas, S.E.; Pope, H.G., Jr.; and Oliva, P.S. (1995). Increased aggressive responding in male volunteers following the administration of gradually increasing doses of testosterone cypionate. *Drug and Alcohol Dependence* 40, 73-79.

Kraemer, W.J.; Nindl, B.C.; and Rubin, M.R. (2002). Growth hormone: Physiological effects of exogenous administration. In: M.S. Bahrke and C.E. Yesalis (Eds.), *Peformance-Enhancing Substances in Sport and Exercise* (pp. 151-179). Champaign, IL: Human Kinetics.

Laroche, G. (1990). Steroid anabolic drugs and arterial complications in an athlete—A case history. *Angiology* 41, 964-969.

Lefavi, R.G.; Reeve, T.G.; and Newland, M.C. (1990). Relationship between anabolic steroid use and selected psychological parameters in male bodybuilders. *Journal of Sports Behavior* 13, 157-166.

Lenders, J.; Denmacker, P.; Vos, J.; Jansen, P.; and Hoitsma, A. (1988). Deleterious effects of anabolic steroids on serum lioproteins, blood pressure, and liver function in amateur body builders. *International Journal of Sports Medicine* 9, 19-23.

Liow, R.Y. and Tavares, S. (1995). Bilateral rupture of the quadriceps tendon associated with anabolic steroids. *British Journal of Sports Medicine* 29, 77-79.

Lommi, J. and Harkonen, M. (1991). Temporary paralysis in a 17-year-old bodybuilder. *Duodecim; lääketieteellinen aikakauskirja* 107, 1723-1725.

Lukas, S.E. (1996). CNS effects and abuse liability of anabolic-androgenic steroids. *Annual Review of Pharmacology and Toxicology* 36, 333-357.

Maglione, M.; Miotto, K.; Iguchi, M.; Jungvig, L.; Morton, S.C.; and Shekelle, P.G. (2005). Psychiatric effects of ephedra use: An analysis of Food and Drug Administration reports of adverse events. *American Journal of Psychiatry* 162, 189-191.

Malone, D.A. and Dimeff, R.J. (1992). The use of fluoxetine in depression associated with anabolic steroid withdrawal: A case series. *Journal of Clinical Psychiatry* 53, 130-132.

Maropis, C. and Yesalis, C.E. (1994). Intramuscular abscess: Another anabolic steroid danger. *The Physician and Sportsmedicine* 22, 105-110.

Martinez-Sanchis, S.; Brain, P.F.; Salvador, A.; and Simon, V.M. (1996). Long-term chronic treatment with stanozolol lacks significant effects on aggression and activity in young and adult male laboratory mice. *General Pharmacology* 27, 293-298.

Mauss, J.; Borsch, G.; Bormacher, K.; Picheter, E.; Leyendecker, G.; and Nocke, W. (1975). Effect of long-term testosterone oenanthate administration on male reproductive function: Clinical evaluation, serum FSH, LH, testosterone, and seminal fluid analyses in normal men. *Acta Endocrinologica* 78, 373-384.

McGee, L.C. (1927). The effect of an injection of a lipoid fraction of bull testicle in capons. *Proceedings of the Institute of Medicine of Chicago* 6, 242-254.

Melchert, R. and Welder, A. (1995). Cardiovascular effects of androgenic-anabolic steroids. *Medicine and Science in Sports and Exercise* 27, 1252-1262.

Midgley, S.J.; Heather, N.; Best, D.; Henderson, D.; McCarthy, S.; and Davies, J.B. (2000). Risk behaviours for HIV and hepatitis infection among anabolic-androgenic steroid users. *AIDS Care* 12, 163-170.

Miles, J.W.; Grana, W.A.; Egle, D.; Min, K.W.; and Chitwood, J. (1992). The effect of anabolic steroids on the biomechanical and histological properties of rat tendon. *Journal of Bone and Joint Surgery* 74, 411-422.

Monaghan, L.F. (2002). Vocabularies of motive for illicit steroid use among bodybuilders. *Social Science and Medicine* 55, 695-708.

Moss, H.B.; Panazak, G.L.; and Tarter, R.E. (1992). Personality, mood, and psychiatric symptoms among anabolic steroid users. *American Journal of the Addictions* 1, 315-324.

Murphy, E. and Williams, G.R. (2004). The thyroid and the skeleton. *Clinical Endocrinology* 61, 285-298.

National Institute on Drug Abuse (2000). *NIDA Research Report Series: Anabolic Steroid Abuse*. NIH Publication No. 00-3721. Rockville, MD: National Institutes of Health.

Nilsson, O.; Chrysis, D.; Pajulo, O.; Boman, A.; Holst, M.; Rubinstein, J.; Ritzen, E.M.; and Savendahl, L. (2003). Localization of estrogen receptors-alpha and beta and androgen receptor in the human growth plate at different pubertal stages. *Journal of Endocrinology* 177, 319-326.

Pahlen, B. (2005). The role of alcohol and steroid hormones in human aggression. *Vitamins and Hormones* 70, 415-437.

Parle, J.V.; Franklyn, J.A.; Cross, K.W.; Jones, S.C.; and Sheppard, M.C. (1991). Prevalence and follow-up of abnormal TSH concentrations in the elderly in the United Kingdom. *Clinical Endocrinology* 34, 77-85.

Parrot, A.C.; Choi, P.Y.L.; and Davies, M. (1994). Anabolic steroid use by amateur athletes: Effects upon psychological mood states. *Journal of Sports Medicine and Physical Fitness* 34, 292-298.

Pärssinen, M.; Kujala, U.; Vartiainen, E.; Sarna, S.; and Seppälä, T. (2000). Increased premature mortality of competitive powerlifters suspected to have used anabolic agents. *International Journal of Sports Medicine* 21, 225-227.

Pärssinen, M. and Seppälä, T. (2002). Steroid use and long-term health risks in former athletes. *Sports Medicine* 32, 83-94

Perry, P.J.; Andersen, K.H.; and Yates, W.R. (1990). Illicit anabolic steroid use in athletes: A case series analysis. *American Journal of Sports Medicine* 18, 422-428.

Perry, P.J.; Kutscher, E.C.; Lund, B.C.; Yates, W.R.; Holman, T.L.; and Demers, L. (2003). Measures of aggression and mood changes in male weightlifters with and without androgenic anabolic steroid use. *Journal of Forensic Science* 48, 646-651.

Perry, P.J.; Yates, W.R.; and Andersen, K.H. (1990). Psychiatric symptoms associated with anaoblic steroids: A controlled, retrospective study. *Annals of Clinical Psychiatry* 2, 11-17.

Perry, P.J.; Yates, W.R.; Williams, R.D.; Andersen, A.E.; MacIndoe, J.H.; and Lund, B.C. (2002). Testosterone therapy in late-life major depression in males. *Journal of Clinical Psychiatry* 63, 1096-1101.

Philibert, R. and Mac, J. (2004). An association of Ephedra use with psychosis and autonomic hyperactivity. *Annals of Clinical Psychiatry* 16, 167-169.

Pinna, G.; Costa, E.; and Guidotti, A. (2005). Changes in brain testosterone and allopregnanolone biosynthesis elicit aggressive behavior. *Proceedings of the National Academy of Sciences* 102, 2135-2140.

Plaus, W.J.; and Hermann, G. (1991). The surgical management of superficial infections caused by atypical mycobacteria. *Surgery* 110, 99-105.

Pluim, B.; Zwinderman, A.; van der Laarse, A.; and van der Wall, E. (2000). The athlete's heart: A meta-analysis of cardiac structure and function. *Circulation* 101, 336-344.

Pope, H.G., Jr.; Gruber, A.J.; Choi, P.; Olivardia, R.; and Phillips, K.A. (1997). Muscle dymorphia. An underrecognized form of body dysmorphic disorder. *Psychosomatics* 38, 548-557.

Pope, H.G., Jr. and Katz, D.L. (1988). Affective and psychotic symptoms associated with anabolic steroid use. *Americal Journal of Psychiatry* 145, 487-490.

Pope, H.G., Jr. and Katz, D.L. (1994). Psychiatric and medical effects of anabolic-androgenic steroid use. A controlled study of 160 athletes. *Archives of General Psychiatry* 51, 375-382.

Pope, H.G., Jr.; Kouri, E.M.; and Hudson, J.I. (2000). Effects of supraphysiologic doses of testosterone on mood and aggression in normal men: A randomized controlled trial. *Archives of General Psychiatry* 57, 133-140.

Rawson, E.S. and Clarkson, P.M. (2002). Ephedrine as an ergogenic aid. In: M.S. Bahrke and C.E. Yesalis (Eds.), *Peformance-Enhancing Substances in Sport and Exercise* (pp. 289-298). Champaign, IL: Human Kinetics.

Rejeski, W.J.; Burbaker, P.H.; Herb, R.A.; Kaplan, J.R.; and Kortinik, D.J. (1988). Anabolic steroids and aggressive behaviour in cynomolgus monkeys. *Behavioral Medicine* 11, 95-105.

Reyes, R.J.; Zicchi, S.; Hamed, H.; Chaudary, M.A.; and Fentiman, I.S. (1995). Surgical correction of gynaecomastia in bodybuilders. *British Journal of Clinical Practice* 49, 177-179.

Rich, J.D.; Dickinson, B.P.; Merriman, N.A.; and Flanigan, T.P. (1998). Hepatitis C virus infection related to anabolic-androgenic steroid injection in a recreational weight lifter. *American Journal of Gastroenterology* 93, 1598.

Rubin, R.T.; O'Toole, S.M.; Rhodes, M.E.; Sekula, L.K.; and Czambel, R.K. (1999). Hypothalamo-pituitary-adrenal cortical responses to low-dose physostigmine and arginine vasopressin administration: Sex differences between major depressives and matched control subjects. *Psychiatry Research* 89, 1-20.

Rudman, D.; Feller, A.G.; Cohn, L.; Shetty, K.R.; Rudman, I.W.; and Draper, M.W. (1991). Effects of human growth hormone on body composition in elderly men. *Hormone Research* 36 (Supplement 1), 73-81.

Sachar, E.J.; Halpern, F.; Rosenfeld, R.S.; Galligher, T.F.; and Hellman, L. (1973). Plasma and urinary testosterone levels in depressed men. *Archives of General Psychiatry* 28, 15-18.

Salke, R.; Rowland, T.; and Burke, E. (1985). Left ventricular size and function in body builders using anabolic steroids. *Medicine and Science in Sports and Exercise* 17, 701-704.

Schmidt, P.J.; Berlin, K.L.; Danaceau, M.A.; Neeren, A.; Haq, N.A.; Roca, C.A.; and Rubinow, D.R. (2004). The effects of pharmacologically induced hypogonadism on mood in healthy men. *Archives of General Psychiatry* 61, 997-1004.

Schollert, P. and Bendixen, P. (1993). Dilated cardiomyopathy in a user of anabolic steroids [Danish]. *Ugeskrift for Laeger* 155, 1217-1218.

Schulte, H.M.; Hall, M.J.; and Boyer, M. (1993). Domestic violence associated with anabolic steroid abuse. *American Journal of Psychiatry* 150, 348.

Schwarz, S.; Onken, D.; and Schubert, A. (1999). The steroid story of Jenapharm: From the late 1940s to the early 1970s. *Steroids* 64, 439-445.

Schweiger, U.; Deuschle, M.; Weber, B.; Korner, A.; Lammers, C.H.; Schmider, J.; Gotthardt, U.; and Heuser, I. (1999). Testosterone, gonadotropin, and cortisol secretion in male patients with major depression. *Psychosomatic Medicine* 61, 292-296.

Scott, M.J. and Scott, M.J., Jr. (1989). HIV infection associated with injections of anabolic steroids. *Journal of the American Medical Association* 262, 207-208.

Seeman, M.V. (1997). Psychopathology in women and men: Focus on female hormones. *American Journal of Psychiatry* 154, 1641-1647.

Seidman, S.N.; Spatz, E.; Rizzo, C.; and Roose, S.P. (2001). Testosterone replacement therapy for hypogonadal men with major depressive disorder: A randomized, placebo-controlled clinical trial. *Journal of Clinical Psychiatry* 62, 406-412.

Seidman, S.N. and Walsh, B.T. (1999). Testosterone and depression in aging men. *American Journal of Geriatric Psychiatry* 7, 18-33.

Shahidi, N.T. (2001). A review of the chemistry, biological action, and clinical applications of anabolic-androgenic steroids. *Clinical Therapeutics* 23, 1355-1390.

Shifren, J.L.; Braunstein, G.D.; and Simon, J.A. (2000). Transdermal testosterone treatment in women with impaired sexual function after oophorectomy. *New England Journal of Medicine* 343, 682-688.

Shiozawa, Z.; Yamada, H.; Mabuchi, C.; Hotta, T.; Saito, M.; Sobue, I.; and Huang, Y.P. (1982). Superior sagittal sinus thrombosis associated with androgen therapy for hypoplastic anemia. *Annals of Neurology* 12, 578-580.

Silverman, K.; Evans, S.M.; Strain, E.C.; and Griffiths, R.R. (1992). Withdrawal syndrome after the double-blind cessation of caffeine consumption. *New England Journal of Medicine* 327, 1109-1114.

Slarek, H.M.; Mantovani, R.P.; Erens, E.; Heisler, D.; Niederman, M.S.; and Fein, A.M. (1984). AIDS in a bodybuilder using anabolic steroids. *New England Journal of Medicine* 311, 1701.

Spriet, L.L. (2002). Caffeine. In: M.S. Bahrke and C.E. Yesalis (Eds.), *Performance-Enhancing Substances in Sport and Exercise* (pp. 267-278). Champaign, IL: Human Kinetics.

Stalenheim, E.G.; von Knorring, L.; and Wide, L. (1998). Serum levels of thyroid hormones as biological markers in a Swedish forensic psychiatric population. *Biological Psychiatry* 43, 755-761.

Stannard, J.P. and Bucknell, A.L. (1993). Rupture of the triceps tendon associated with steroid injections. *American Journal of Sports Medicine* 21, 482-485.

Stoffel-Wagner, B. (2001). Neurosteroid metabolism in the human brain. *European Journal of Endocrinology* 145, 669-679.

Stoffel-Wagner, B. (2003). Neurosteroid biosynthesis in the human brain and its clinical implications. *Annals of the New York Academy of Sciences* 1007, 64-78.

Su, T.P.; Pagliaro, M.; Schmidt, P.J.; Pickar, D.; Wolkowitz, O.; and Rubinow, D.R. (1993). Neuropsychiatric effects of anabolic steroids in male normal volunteers. *Journal of the American Medical Association* 269, 2760-2764.

Thiblin, I. and Parlklo, T. (2002). Anabolic androgenic steroids and violence. *Acta Psychiatrican Scandinavica,* 19 (Suppl.), 125-128.

Thiblin, I.; Runeson, B.; and Rajs, J. (1999). Anabolic androgenic steroids and suicide. *Annals of Clinical Psychiatry* 11, 223-231.

Todd, T. (1987). Anabolic steroids: The gremlins of sport. *Journal of Sport History* 14, 87-107.

Traboulsi, A.S.; Viswanathan, R.; and Coplan, J. (2002). Suicide attempt after use of herbal diet pill. *American Journal of Psychiatry* 159, 318-319.

Urhausen, A.; Albers, T.; and Kindermann, W. (2004). Are the cardiac effects of anabolic steroid abuse in strength athletes reversible? *Heart* 90, 496-501.

Vanakoski, J.; Stromberg, C.; and Seppala, T. (1993). Effects of a sauna on the pharmacokinetics of pharmacodynamics of midazolam and ephedrine in healthy young women. *European Journal of Clinical Pharmacology* 45, 377-381.

van Breda, E.; Keizer, H.; Kuipers, H.; and Wolffenbuttel, B. (2003). Androgenic anabolic steroid use and severe hypothalamic-pituitary dysfunction: A case study. *International Journal of Sports Medicine* 24, 195-196.

Velazquez, I. and Alter, B.P. (2004). Androgens and liver tumors: Fanconi's anemia and non-Fanconi's conditions. *American Journal of Hematology* 77, 257-266.

Walton, R. and Manos, G.H. (2003). Psychosis related to ephedra-containing herbal supplement use. *Southern Medical Journal* 96, 718-720.

Wang, C.; Swerdloff, R.S.; Iranmanesh, A.; Dobs, A.; Snyder, P.J.; Cunningham, G.; Matsumoto, A.M.; Weber, T.; and Berman, N. (2000). Transdermal testosterone gel improves sexual function, mood, muscle strength, and body composition parameters in hypogonadal men. Testosterone Gel Study Group. *Journal of Clinical Endocrinology and Metabolism* 85, 2839-2853.

Wantabe, S.; Yamaguchi, N.; Tsunematsu, Y.; and Komiyama, A. (1989). Risk factors for leukemia occurence among growth hormone users. *Japanese Journal of Cancer* 80, 822-825.

Weber, B.; Lewicka, S.; Deuschle, M.; Colla, M.; and Heuser, I. (2000). Testosterone, androstenedione and dihydrotestosterone concentrations are elevated in female patients with major depression. *Psychoneuroendocrinology* 25, 765-771.

Weiss, E.L.; Bowers, M.B., Jr.; and Mazure, C.M. (1999). Testosterone-patch-induced psychotic mania. *American Journal of Psychiatry* 156, 969.

Yarasheski, K. (1994). Growth hormone effects on metabolism, body composition, muscle mass, and strength. *Exercise and Sport Sciences Reviews* 22, 285-312.

Yates, W.R.; Perry, P.J.; MacIndoe, J.; Holman, T.; and Ellingrod, V. (1999). Psychosexual effects of three doses of testosterone cycling in normal men. *Biological Psychiatry* 45, 254-260.

Zahringer, S.; Tomova, A.; von Werder, K.; Brabant, G.; Kumanov, P.; and Schopohl, J. (2000). The influence of hyperthyroidism on the hypothalamic-pituitary-gonadal axis. *Experimental Clinical Endocrinology and Diabetes* 108, 282-289.

Zuliani, U.; Bernardini, B.; Catapano, A.; Campana, M.; Cerioli, G.; and Spattini, M. (1989). Effects of anabolic steroids, testosterone, and HGH on blood lipids and echocardigraphic parameters in bodybuilders. *International Journal of Sports Medicine* 10, 62-66.

Chapter 13

Health Effects
of Tobacco, Nicotine, and Exposure
to Tobacco Smoke Pollution

Jonathan Foulds
Cristine Delnevo
Douglas M. Ziedonis
Michael B. Steinberg

INTRODUCTION AND OVERVIEW

This chapter reviews the medical consequences of tobacco and nicotine use. This chapter focuses on the effects of chronic cigarette smoking (the most prevalent type of nicotine use) on specific diseases and overall mortality. It also discusses the effects of different types of tobacco, evidence for dose-response effects, the effects of reduction and cessation of cigarette use, the effects of passive exposure to tobacco smoke, and the psychiatric effects of tobacco use.

THE NATURE AND HISTORY OF TOBACCO USE

Tobacco use has been known since around the first century BC when Native Americans used it for ceremonial purposes, and was widespread in the

Authors' note: The authors are supported by a grant from the New Jersey Department of Health and Senior Services, as part of New Jersey's Comprehensive Tobacco Control Program. The authors are also supported by the Cancer Institute of New Jersey (JF, MS), the Robert Wood Johnson Foundation (JF, MS, CD), the National Institute on Drug Abuse (DZ, JF), National Cancer Institute (CD), National Institute of Mental Health (CD), and the Substance Abuse and Mental Health Services Administration (DZ).

American continent when Europeans first arrived there in the fifteenth century. However, it was the invention of the cigarette making machine and subsequently the mass manufacture and distribution of machine-made cigarettes that led to the massive rise in cigarette smoking as the predominant form of nicotine consumption at the end of the nineteenth century and throughout the twentieth century. During the 1990s approximately one billion people (47 percent of all adult men and 12 percent of all adult women in the world) were daily smokers (Collishaw and Lopez, 1996).

Part of the reason for the slowness of many countries to react to the "tobacco epidemic" is that for many tobacco-caused diseases there is a 30-year lag between the increase in smoking prevalence and the increase in deaths from smoking-caused diseases (e.g., lung cancer). This delayed effect means that for some decades after an increase in national smoking prevalence it is possible to have high smoking prevalence but low (if increasing) smoking-caused death rates. Figure 13.1 describes the recognized stages in the epidemic of smoking-caused deaths that follow the increase in smoking rates in a country, and also indicates examples of countries at each stage at the end of the twentieth century.

The pattern of tobacco consumption in the United States throughout the twentieth century is shown in Figure 13.2. This pattern is fairly typical of

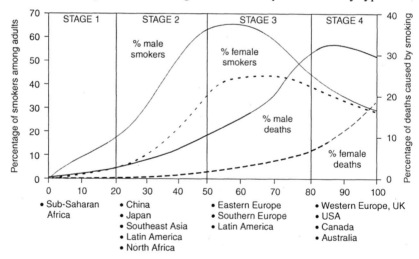

FIGURE 13.1. Four stages of the tobacco epidemic. A descriptive model of the cigarette epidemic in developed countries. *Tobacco Control,* 3, pp. 242-247. *Source:* From Lopez, A.D., Collishaw, N.E., and Piha, T. (1994). Reproduced with permission from the BMJ Publishing Group.

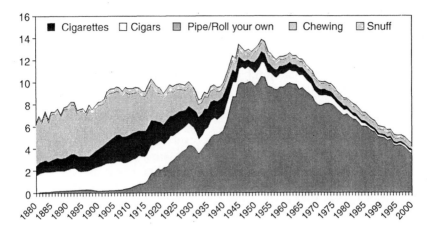

FIGURE 13.2. Per capita consumption of various tobacco products (in pounds)—United States, 1880-2000. *Source:* Tobacco Situation and Outlook Report, U.S. Department of Agriculture, U.S. Census. Adapted from Gerlach et al. (1998). Courtesy of Gary Giovino. *Note:* Among persons >18 years old. Beginning in 1982, fine-cut chewing tobacco was reclassified as snuff.

"mature" tobacco markets such as northern Europe, North America, and Australia, showing a mixed pattern of tobacco use, including significant amounts of smokeless tobacco until the beginning of the twentieth century, followed by the growing dominance of cigarettes by the 1930s and then a steady reduction in tobacco consumption overall since the 1960s, coinciding with increasing awareness of its harmful effects on health (Giovino, 2002).

Prior to the seminal publications on the effects of smoking on lung cancer risks in the 1950s (Doll and Hill, 1950; Wynder and Graham, 1950), relatively few people were aware that tobacco smoking caused serious illnesses. Medical consensus on the serious health effects of smoking was achieved and publicized during the early 1960s (Royal College of Physicians of London, 1962; U.S. Department of Health, Education and Welfare, 1964). However, the tobacco industry continued to deny or sow doubts about these health effects throughout the rest of the twentieth century (Cummings, Morley, and Hyland, 2002; Tobacco Industry Research Committee, 1954). For example, in 1971, Chairman of Philip Morris Joseph Cullman appeared on a TV news show (*Face the Nation*) and declared,

> "we do not believe that cigarettes are hazardous; we don't accept that." Joseph Cullman, chairman, Philip Morris, 1971 (Herman et al., 1971).

In a 1972 interview with the *Wall Street Journal,* Philip Morris Vice President James Bowling repeated the company's promise to consumers two decades earlier that,

> "if our product is harmful, we'll stop making it." James Bowling, vice president, Philip Morris, 1972. (Kwitny, 1972)

He repeated the company's position in a 1976 interview when he noted:

> "from our standpoint, if anyone ever identified any ingredient in tobacco smoke as being hazardous to human health or being something that shouldn't be there, we could eliminate it. But no one ever has." James Bowling, vice president Philip Morris, 1976. (Bowling and Taylor, 1976)

As recently as 1998, Philip Morris Chairman Geoffrey Bible responded to the question "Has anyone died from smoking cigarettes?" in the following manner:

> "I don't know if anyone dies from smoking tobacco. I just don't know." Geoffrey Bible, chairman, Philip Morris, 1998. (Geyelin, 1998)

The tobacco industry also reacted to the evidence on the harmfulness of tobacco by providing consumers with a series of adapted products that were perceived by the public as being less harmful ways of continuing to smoke (primarily via addition of filters and reductions in the machine-measured tar and nicotine yields of cigarettes).

In 1963, Addison Yeaman, executive vice president of Brown and Williamson Tobacco Company, and president of the Committee for Tobacco Research, wrote thus:

> Moreover nicotine is addictive. We are then in the business of selling nicotine, an addictive drug . . . But cigarettes . . . despite the beneficient effect of nicotine, have certain unattractive side effects:
>
> 1. They cause, or predispose to, lung cancer.
> 2. They contribute to certain cardiovascular diseases.
> 3. They may well be truly causative in emphysema etc.

However, these insights were not shared with the committee preparing the 1964 U.S. Surgeon General's Report on Tobacco and Health, and it was not until the late 1980s that scientific consensus was reached that tobacco use is addictive in the same way as heroin and cocaine, and that those who become addicted to tobacco are primarily addicted to nicotine (Royal College of Physicians, 2000; U.S. Department of Health and Human Services [USDHHS], 1988). Although people primarily use tobacco for the psychological and dependence-forming effects of nicotine, it is the other components in tobacco—the "tar," volatile oxidant gases and carbon-monoxide—that cause most (at least 90 percent) of the harm to health. The rest of this chapter reviews these health effects of tobacco use, before returning to discuss the addictiveness of tobacco.

DISEASES CAUSED BY TOBACCO

The recent review of the health effects of tobacco smoking published by the U.S. Surgeon General in 2004 (USDHHS, 2004) expanded the list of diseases known to be caused by smoking to include virtually every organ in the body. The conclusions about these causal relationships were made on the basis of the consistency, specificity, temporality, and strength of the observed associations, together with evidence on the biological plausibility, observed dose-response relationship, and results from experimental data (whether laboratory-based or "naturally occurring" experiments). Table 13.1 lists some of the deadly diseases known to be caused by tobacco smoking and the relative risks of death from each of these causes in continuing and former smokers compared with never smokers. It should be noted that in all of the diseases listed in the table, the evidence (which is thoroughly reviewed in the 2004 Surgeon General's report and associated documents) has been judged to be sufficient to infer a causal relationship between tobacco smoking and

TABLE 13.1. Age-adjusted relative risk of death from smoking-related diseases from CPS-II, comparing continuing and former smokers to never smokers.

| | CPS-II (1982-1988) | | | |
| | Males | | Females | |
Disease category	Continuing smokers	Former smokers	Continuing smokers	Former smokers
Neoplasms				
Lip, oral cavity, pharynx	10.9	3.4	5.1	2.3
Esophagus	6.8	4.5	7.8	2.8
Stomach	2	1.5	1.4	1.3
Pancreas	2.3	1.2	2.3	1.6
Larynx	14.6	6.3	13	5.2

TABLE 13.1 *(continued)*

Disease category	CPS-II (1982-1988)			
	Males		Females	
	Continuing smokers	Former smokers	Continuing smokers	Former smokers
Trachea, bronchus, lung	23.3	8.7	12.7	4.5
Cervix uteri			1.6	1.1
Urinary bladder	3.3	2.1	2.2	1.9
Kidney, other urinary diseases	2.7	1.7	1.3	1.1
Acute myeloid leukemia	1.9	1.3	1.1	1.4
Cardiovascular diseases				
Ischemic heart disease				
Aged 35-64 years	2.8	1.6	3.1	1.3
Aged $\geq$ 65 years	1.5	1.2	1.6	1.2
Other heart disease	1.8	1.2	1.5	1.1
Cerebrovascular diseases				
Aged 35-64 years	3.3	1	4	1.3
Aged $\geq$ 65 years	1.6	1	1.5	1
Atherosclerosis	2.4	1.3	1.8	1
Aortic aneurysm	6.2	3.1	7.1	2.1
Other arterial disease	2.1	1	2.2	1.1
Respiratory diseases				
Pneumonia, influenza	1.8	1.4	2.2	1.1
Bronchitis, emphysema	17.1	15.6	12	11.8
Chronic airway obstruction	10.6	6.8	13.1	6.8
Perinatal conditions				
Short gestation/low birth weight			1.8	
Respiratory distress syndrome			1.3	
Other respiratory conditions			1.4	
Sudden infant death syndrome			2.3	

Source: Adapted from Table 7-1.1, 2004 U.S. Surgeon General's Report (USDHHS, 2004).

Note: A relative risk of one implies no increased risk in smokers, and a relative risk of two implies a doubling of the risk of death due to that disease in smokers compared with never smokers.

that disease (rather than a noncausal statistical association or "risk factor"). Interestingly, the 2004 Surgeon General's report did not list nicotine dependence as a smoking-caused illness, although that conclusion had been reached in a prior report (USDHHS, 1988).

Smoking is also the established cause of a number of other nonfatal diseases and conditions including cataracts, periodontitis, acute respiratory infections in people with COPD, acute respiratory symptoms in adults and children (e.g., coughing and wheezing), adverse surgical outcomes related to wound healing and respiratory complications, hip fractures, and peptic ulcer disease in persons who are *Helicobacter pylori* positive (USDHHS, 2004).

In addition, there is considerable evidence suggesting (but not yet conclusively) that numerous other conditions may be caused or exacerbated by tobacco smoking. These diseases include colorectal cancer, impaired lung function, ectopic pregnancy, spontaneous abortion, and oral clefts in children whose mothers smoked during pregnancy, childhood asthma, bronchial hyper-responsiveness, low bone density, root-surface caries, erectile dysfuntion, age-related macular degeneration, Graves' disease, and peptic ulcer disease (USDHHS, 2004).

It has been estimated that tobacco smoking causes around 400,000 premature deaths per year in the United States (Thun, Apicella, and Henley, 2000), and 4.9 million deaths per year worldwide (8.8 percent of all global deaths) (World Health Organization [WHO], 1997). In developed countries, the largest number of these deaths are due to cardiovascular diseases, followed by cancer (predominantly of the lung), and then chronic obstructive pulmonary disease (COPD). Tobacco smoking causes more premature deaths each year in the United States than alcohol, illegal drugs, AIDS, road traffic accidents, microbial infections, homicide and suicide all added together (McGinnus and Foege, 1993). However, for every smoking-caused death each year in the United States, there are approximately twenty cases of nonfatal serious smoking-caused illness (CDC, 2003). The vast majority (59 percent) of these are chronic respiratory diseases, which consequently comprise a large part of the estimated $157 billion smoking-attributable economic costs per year in the United States. $82 billion of these costs are due to lost productivity and $75 billion are direct medical care to adults (USDHHS, 2004). The net effect of these smoking-caused diseases is that the continuing smoker is likely to die an average of ten years earlier than a never smoker, as reported by Doll et al. (2004) and shown in Figure 13.3. The approximate doubling of mortality risks for smokers is evident at age 50 (6 percent of smokers already died, versus 3 percent of never smokers) and continues past age 70 (by which 42 percent of smokers have died, versus 19 percent of never smokers).

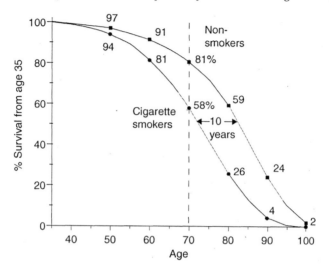

FIGURE 13.3. U.K. male doctors born 1900-1930: continuing cigarette versus never smokers. Fifty-year follow-up of mortality, 1951-2001. *Source:* Doll, Peto, et al. (2004). Mortality in relation to smoking: 50 years' observations on male British doctors. *British Medical Journal,* 328(7455):1519. Reproduced with permission from the BMJ Publishing Group.

DOSE-RESPONSE RELATIONSHIP BETWEEN CIGARETTE SMOKING AND DISEASE

For most of the smoking-caused diseases mentioned in previous text, there is also evidence of a significant dose-response relationship between the total amount of smoking and the risk of contracting the disease. The most striking dose-response relationship is typically found in lung cancer, as shown in Figure 13.4.

Thun et al. (1997) examined mortality from COPD in the second Cancer Prevention Study (CPS-II) and found that the relative risks increased from 5.9 in women smoking 1-9 cigarettes per day, to 25.2 for women smoking 40 or more cigarettes per day (relative to never-smoking women). Similarly, the Nurses Health Study (Stampfer et al., 2000) found adjusted relative risks of Coronary Heart Disease of 3.1 for women smoking up to 14 cigarettes per day and 5.5 for those smoking 15 or more per day.

However, it should be noted that reductions in some disease and mortality risks tend to be disappointingly small or nonexistent when smokers cut down their cigarette consumption per day (Godtfredsen et al., 2002). This is

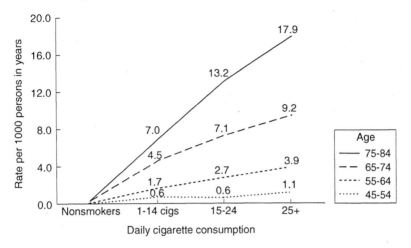

FIGURE 13.4. Lung cancer risk by age and cigarette consumption in CPS-II. *Source:* Thun et al., 1997.

likely because smokers who cut down cigarettes per day "compensate" by inhaling more from each cigarette in order to obtain their preferred dose of nicotine (Benowitz, 2001). It has also been established that the duration of smoking (i.e., number of years of smoking) is a much larger determinant of some disease risks (e.g., lung cancer) than the number of cigarettes smoked per day (Knoke et al., 2004). Thus, many epidemiological studies use the term "pack years" (packs of cigarettes per day multiplied by the number of years of smoking) as a crude measure of smoking "dose" and this measure is often significantly related to disease risk.

Although age itself is frequently a potent predictor of risk of many of the smoking-caused diseases, nonetheless it is clear that the earlier the smoker quits, the lower their risk of disease, independently of age. This relationship is shown in Figure 13.5, which indicates the cumulative risk of death from lung cancer by age for never smokers, continuing smokers, and smokers who quit at various ages.

REDUCTIONS IN DISEASE FOLLOWING SMOKING CESSATION

The 1990 U.S. Surgeon General's report reviewed the health benefits of ceasing tobacco use and concluded that smoking cessation has major health benefits, for men and women of all ages. For example, smokers who quit

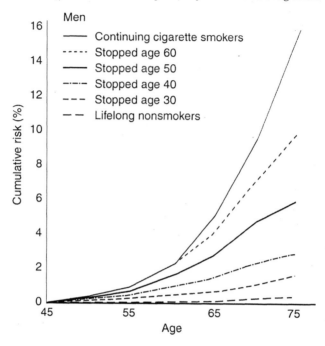

FIGURE 13.5. Effects of smoking cessation at various ages on the cumulative risk (%) of death from lung cancer up to age 75, at death rates for United Kindgom, 1990. *Source:* Peto et al. (2000). Smoking, smoking cessation, and lung cancer in the UK since 1950: Combination of national statistics with two case control studies. *British Medical Journal,* 321(7257):323-329. Reproduced with permission from the BMJ Publishing Group.

smoking by age 50 have one-half the risk of dying in the next 15 years, compared with continuing smokers (USDHHS, 1990).

The timescale for reduction in risks of disease after smoking cessation varies with each disease and even with the stage of the disease. Thus the excess risk of death from coronary heart disease will be cut in half within a year of stopping smoking, but the same level of risk reduction may take 10 to 15 years for lung cancer (USDHHS, 1990).

Lung function declines with age after reaching adulthood in nonsmokers, but it declines at a significantly faster rate for smokers. However, when a smoker stops smoking, the rate of decline of lung function normalizes to a rate similar to that for never-smokers. The effects of smoking cessation in the U.S. Lung Health Study were slightly better than described in previous text, and produced an absolute improvement in lung function within the first year of stopping smoking, as shown in Figure 13.6.

TOXINS IN CIGARETTE SMOKE
AND RELATIONSHIP TO DISEASE

The cigarette itself typically contains a large number of ingredients, including the tobacco leaf, tobacco paper, and filter (fibers of which may be inhaled—Pauly et al., 2002), and over 500 potential additives (e.g., acetaldehyde, ammonia, cocoa, levulinic acid, and menthol). When the cigarette is lit, and the tip burns, it reaches extremely high temperatures (over 400 degrees centigrade), rising to over 600 degrees centigrade as air is sucked into the cone (White et al., 2001). The resulting smoke is composed of a complex mixture of over 4,000 chemicals resulting from pyrolysis. Many of these chemicals exist in very small quantities just above the detection limits of sensitive toxicology assays, but many highly toxic chemicals are present in large measurable concentrations in tobacco smoke and are known to be involved in causing a variety of diseases. Exhibit 13.1 provides a list of some of the main toxic smoke constituents (see also Hoffman and Hoffman, 1998).

Many of the mechanisms whereby this complex mixture of toxins contained in tobacco smoke leads to specific diseases have been identified. For example, a large number of these chemicals have been shown to cause can-

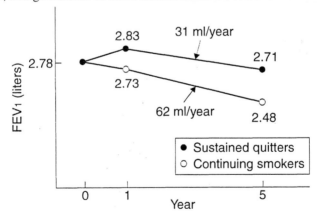

FIGURE 13.6. Change in lung function (FEV1—forced expiratory volume in one second) in smokers who quit versus those continuing to smoke in the U.S. Lung Health Study. *Source:* Scanlon et al. (2000). Reprinted with permission from American Thoracic Society.

EXHIBIT 13.1. Examples of Toxic Constituents in Tobacco Smoke (from over 4,000 identified chemicals)

Volatile organic substances
  1,3-butadiene
  Benzene
  Toluene
Gaseous substances
  Ammonia
  Hydrogen cyanide
  Carbon monoxide
  Nitrogen oxides
Metals
  Lead
  Cadmium
  Arsenic
Aromatic amines
  4-aminobiphenyl
  1-aminoaphthalene

Polycyclic aromatic hydrocarbons
  Benzo(a)pyrene
  Pyrene
  Benz(a)anthracene
Nitrosamines
  NNN
  NAB
  NNK
  N-Nitrosodimethylamine
Carbonyls
  Formaldehyde
  Acetaldehyde
  Acrolein
Aza-arenes
  Quinoline
  Dibenz(a,j)acridine

cer in animals and/or humans (e.g., benzo(a)pyrene, NNK, and NNN). These chemicals in the smoke cause DNA damage, inflammation, and oxidative stress, which promote the initiation and growth of tumors (Hecht, 1999).

The deposition of particles of tar in the lungs and upper airways leads to the blocking of airways and COPD. The toxic chemicals stimulate oxidative stress, inflammation, and a reduction in elastin, inhibiting the elasticity of the lungs and hence the ability to inhale and exhale normally. Irritants such as nitric oxide cause hypersecretion of mucus and substances such as acrolein, acetone, and acetaldehyde damage the cilia (inhibiting the ability of the cilia to clear mucus) which also contributes to chronic decrements in respiratory function. Years of smoking and daily coating of the lungs and airways in tar leads to irreversible lung damage and ultimately death from COPD (Barnes, 1999).

The carbon monoxide in smoke replaces oxygen in the hemoglobin, adversely affecting oxygen transport and energy supply, and requiring the heart to do more work to supply the same amount of oxygen to the body. A large number of smoke constituents, and particularly the volatile components of the gaseous phase of tobacco smoke, cause oxidative stress, immunologic responses, and inflammation in the endothelial cells (Powell, 1998). The resultant platelet aggregation, plaque formation, and inhibition of vasorelaxation contribute to endothelial malfunction and thrombosis. These processes increase the likelihood of a myocardial infarction, stroke, or other problems with the cardiovascular system. Acute nicotine administration increases heart rate, blood pressure, and causes peripheral vasoconstriction (i.e., impairs peripheral circulation and thus exacerbates Raynaud's disease and erectile dysfunction). However, studies of smokeless tobacco users (who have high nicotine exposure like smokers, but without the smoke) compared with smokers, suggest that most of the cardiovascular problems are not caused by nicotine. For example, smoking but not snuff use is associated with femoral artery intima-media thickness (Wallenfeldt et al., 2001), and snuff users have consistently been found to have lower risks of myocardial infarction than smokers (Critchley and Unal, 2003). It therefore appears that it is the thrombogenic effects of tobacco smoke exposure (primarily oxidant gases), combined with reduced oxygen supply (carbon monoxide), and increased myocardial oxygen demand (nicotine) that cause cardiovascular harm from smoking (USDHHS, 2004).

TAR AND NICOTINE DELIVERY FROM "LIGHT" CIGARETTES

In 1967, the U.S. Federal Trade Commission (FTC) began the systematic measurement of the yields of tar, nicotine, and carbon monoxide from cigarettes marketed in the United States using a standardized smoking-machine test, now referred to as the "FTC method" in the United States and the "ISO method" (International Organization for Standardization) in most other countries (National Cancer Institute, 1996). In the United States, this procedure measures the amount of toxins that are absorbed when the machine takes a two-second, 35 ml puff per minute until the cigarette has reached a specified distance from the butt (23 mm or overwrap plus 3 mm), with the number of puffs being variable. Tar is the term used for all of the particulate matter collected on the filter of a smoking machine, minus the moisture and alkaloids (e.g., nicotine). Since the 1950s, it has become widely known that a number of chemicals contained in the tar from cigarettes are carcinogenic and so there has been an effort to reduce exposure to cigarette tar. However, the FTC machine-smoked yields of tar and nicotine are typically very highly correlated (e.g., the correlation between FTC tar and FTC nicotine yield in a range of U.S. cigarette brands reported by Kozlowski et al., 1998, was 0.98), meaning that as one increases, the other typically increases in a direct linear relationship.

Although tar category cut-points are somewhat arbitrary and can vary over time and across countries, in the United States cigarette brands yielding 15 mg tar or greater using the FTC method are often referred to as "regular" or "full flavor," whereas brands yielding 6.5 mg to 14.5 mg tar have frequently been referred to by manufacturers as "lights," and those yielding less than 6.5 mg tar are often called "ultra-lights."

In order to exemplify some of the differences and similarities between a full flavor and a same-brand light cigarette, this discussion will focus on the Marlboro brand. Marlboro Reds is the name often given to the leading regular length full-flavor brand within the Marlboro portfolio, reflecting the distinctive red Marlboro logo on the pack (*note:* there can be over 20 different varieties of "Marlboros" available in the United States at any one time). In 1971, Philip Morris launched "Marlboro Lights." The pack and advertising were markedly different from Marlboro Reds, using a gold colored logo instead of red, and stating *"LOWERED TAR & NICOTINE"* on the pack. The advertising at that time stated,

> For the smokers of America who prefer low tar and nicotine cigarettes . . . Marlboro Lights: 14 mg "tar," 1.1 mg Nicotine av. Per cigarette by FTC method.

By 1995, Marlboro Reds (full flavor, soft pack) had FTC method yields of 16 mg tar and 1.1 mg nicotine, whereas Marlboro Lights (soft pack) had FTC method yields of 10 mg tar and 0.8 mg nicotine (Kozlowski et al., 1998).

Interestingly, however, the nicotine content of light and regular cigarettes bear little relation to their FTC yields and some lights actually contain more nicotine than their full-flavor same-brand counterparts. In the case of Marlboro, Kozlowski et al. reported in 1998 that Marlboro Lights contained only 2.8 percent less nicotine than regular Marlboros (10.6 mg versus 10.9 mg).

Unfortunately, however, the FTC yields also bare very little relation to the amount of nicotine or tar absorbed by a smoker. The reason for this is that unlike machines, humans can adjust their smoking behavior in a variety of ways that alter the amount of smoke, nicotine, and tar they absorb from each cigarette. Although a number of factors can potentially influence the FTC yields for different cigarettes (e.g., the amount and type of tobacco in the cigarette column, or the type, porosity, and burn characteristics of the cigarette paper), it has become clear that the main factor used by cigarette manufacturers to reduce the FTC measured nicotine and tar yields has been by adding ventilation holes to the filter design. These vents are typically small holes that are added to the filter (using laser or electrostatic technology) to enable air to be drawn into and through the filter with the main effect being to dilute the smoke drawn out of the filter. Percentage air dilution/filter ventilation is defined as the percentage of a standard puff (35 ml in two seconds) that is air taken into the puff through filter vents. Thus the "light" cigarettes are able to "trick" the FTC method by enabling the machine (and the smoker) to easily draw air out of the filter that was not drawn through the cigarette column. Kozlowski et al. (1998) reported that full flavor Marlboros had 10.2 percent filter ventilation whereas lights had 22.5 percent filter ventilation. Therefore the reason Marlboro Lights get lower FTC machine-smoked tar and nicotine yields is primarily that they have more vents added to the filter to dilute the smoke sucked out by the machine.

There are a number of reasons why the FTC machine-smoked yields bare little resemblance to the amounts inhaled by a smoker. One reason is that it is possible and indeed likely that some of the vent holes will be blocked by the smoker in the act of smoking (e.g., by covering with the fingers or lips (Martin and Dunn, 1967)). In addition, unlike a smoking machine, human smokers do not smoke in a standardized way, taking one 35 ml puff per minute. Rather, human smoking behavior is highly variable and is primarily determined by the smokers' need for nicotine (which tends to be rather consistent). Smokers primarily smoke cigarettes for the psychopharmacological and addictive effects of nicotine. Smokers therefore smoke in order to get a sufficient dose of nicotine to provide the desired psychological effects. When a smoker switches from regular to light cigarettes, they typically adjust their smoking behavior (often without being aware of it) to inhale more smoke in order to absorb their usual (preferred) dose of nicotine—a phenomenon often referred to as "compensation" (Benowitz, 2001).

Filter ventilation makes it easy to "compensate" by facilitating the inhalation of larger puffs (Goodman, 1975; Kozlowski and O'Connor, 2002). This is often referred to in the tobacco industry literature as a decreased "resistance to draw (RTD)." The ventilated cigarette requires a lower amount of pressure to be exerted against the filter to initiate inhalation, meaning that the smoker can easily take a larger puff without extra effort and so receives more smoke from the cigarette. Other methods of "compensatory" smoking behavior include taking more puffs per cigarette, blocking the vents in the filters, smoking more cigarettes, or simply removing the filter.

As a result of the fact that smokers regulate their intake of nicotine and that Lights (via filter vents) facilitate "elastic" nicotine (and therefore tar) dosing by smokers (if not by machines), there is often no reduction in nicotine or tar absorption when a smoker switches from regular to light cigarettes (Benowitz, 2001).

HEALTH EFFECTS OF "LIGHT"
VERSUS REGULAR CIGARETTES

A large number of epidemiological studies have now been conducted to assess the health effects of smoking "lights" as opposed to regular cigarettes. Such studies require careful analysis and interpretation because there is good evidence that smokers who choose or switch to "lights" differ in a number of ways from those smoking "regular" cigarettes (e.g., Light smokers tend to more likely to be women, older, better educated, have a higher income, and have a higher interest in smoking cessation and other health behaviors than smokers of regular cigarettes.). Another issue for such studies is whether or not to statistically "control for" the number of cigarettes smoked in the two comparison groups (i.e., those smoking regular cigarettes and those smoking "low-tar" cigarettes). Given the evidence that "light" smokers may increase the number of cigarettes smoked in order obtain their usual nicotine dose, such adjustments may unintentionally reduce the disease risk that should properly be attributed to switching to "lights."

Burns et al. (2001) reviewed the evidence to date on health risks from cigarettes with differing tar yields. Although there are some published studies finding reduced lung cancer risks for smokers of lower tar yielding cigarettes (using FTC method), these have typically not been able to measure and control for all potential confounding variables, or properly assess whether those using lower yielding cigarettes had increased their daily cigarette consumption. Other studies found no reduction in cancer risk among smokers of lower yielding cigarettes and some found increased lung cancer risks. Burns et al. (2001) analyzed a subsample of participants in the American Cancer Society Cancer Prevention Study I (CPS-I), who kept their cigarettes per day and FTC tar category constant throughout the follow-up period of the study. In this group, there was no significant reduction in lung cancer among those smoking cigarettes with lower tar yields.

The mortality risks from coronary heart disease and chronic respiratory disease was also reviewed by Burns et al., again finding no convincing evidence that switching to lower FTC-method tar or nicotine yielding cigarettes reduces disease risks. Burns et al. concluded:

> Existing disease risk data do not support making a recommendation that smokers switch cigarette brands . . .

> Widespread adoption of lower yield cigarettes by smokers in the United States has not prevented the sustained increase in lung cancer among older smokers . . .

Epidemiological studies have not consistently found lesser risk of diseases, other than lung cancer, among smokers of reduced yield cigarettes. Some studies have found lesser risks of lung cancer among smokers of reduced yield cigarettes. Some or all of this reduction in lung cancer risk may reflect differing characteristics of smokers of reduced-yield compared with higher-yield cigarettes.

A review of the epidemiological evidence on lower machine-yielding cigarettes published by the Royal College of Physicians in 2000, concluded:

Smokers of low yield cigarettes actually achieve little, if any, reduction in intake of nicotine and tar, and the health benefit accrued from switching to such cigarettes is, if anything, small. (RCP, 2000, "Key Points")

Harris et al. (2004) recently reported on the six-year follow-up of CPS-II participants and found that the lung cancer risk among smokers of very low tar cigarettes (machine-measured tar <7 mg/cig) was no different from the risks of smokers of low tar (8-14 mg/cig) and medium tar (15-21 mg/cig.) cigarettes. The main results from this study are shown in the Figure 13.7, demonstrating that those smoking cigarettes in the "light" category were no less likely to suffer lung cancer, than those smoking regular cigarettes.

As mentioned previously, smokers smoke light and regular cigarettes differently, and generally take larger puff volumes from cigarettes with lower machine-measured tar and nicotine yields. However, the changed inhalation pattern also alters the burn characteristics of the cigarette and hence also the precise mixture of toxic chemicals in the smoke. Harris (2004) has used data from the 1999 Massachusetts Benchmark Study to demonstrate that even if nicotine compensation is not 100 percent (even if smokers does not increase their puff volume sufficiently to absorb precisely the same amount of nicotine from the Light as the regular cigarette), the smoker may actually obtain a higher dosage of certain smoke toxins from the light cigarette. Overall, it is clear that light or "low-tar" cigarettes are not less harmful to health.

NONCIGARETTE TOBACCO PRODUCTS

Cigars

U.S. federal regulations define a cigar as "any roll of tobacco wrapped in leaf tobacco or in any substance containing tobacco" (26 USC Sec. 5702a).

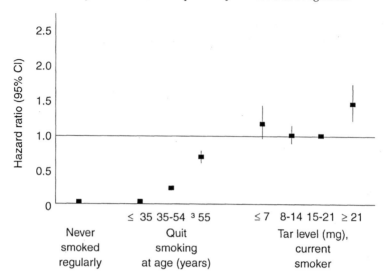

FIGURE 13.7. Hazard ratios for lung cancer in men, 1982-1988, by smoking status and tar yield of brand smoked relative to current smokers of 15-21 mg tar cigarettes. *Source:* Harris, J.E.; Thun, M.J.; Mondul, A.M.; Calle, E.E. (2004). Cigarette tar yields in relation to mortality from lung cancer in the Cancer Prevention Study II prospective cohort, 1982-8. *British Medical Journal,* 328(7431):72. Reproduced with permission from the BMJ Publishing Group.

In contrast, a cigarette is defined as "any roll of tobacco wrapped in paper or in any substance *not* containing tobacco" (26 USC Sec. 5702b). There are many different types of cigars, including large premium cigars, cigarillos, and small or little cigars. Despite the wide variety of cigar products, there is no universally accepted classification system (Baker et al., 2000). Alternatively, Hoffman and Hoffman (1998) classify cigars into four groups (see Table 13.2). This classification system is useful because it illustrates the fact that little and small cigars have characteristics other than weight that set them apart from large cigars. Most notably these cigars have features common to cigarettes, such as shape, size (length 70 to 100 mm), and frequent use of filter tips. In addition, a little or small cigar is sometimes wrapped in paper that contains tobacco or tobacco extract.

Cigar use is often dismissed as a health issue. Indeed, former cigarette smokers incorrectly perceive cigars as safe alternatives to cigarettes (Nyman, Taylor, and Biener, 2002). However, even moderate cigar use carries significant health risks, including increased risk for heart and lung disease, and cancer, including but not limited to oral, esophageal, larynx, and lung,

TABLE 13.2. Cigar types by weight, length, and description.

Classification	Weight in grams	Length in millimeters	Description
Little	0.9-1.3	70-100	Shaped like a cigarette, some with filter tip
Small	1.3-2.5	70-120	Also known as cigarillo, some with wood/plastic mouthpiece
Regular	5-17	110-150	Rolled to a tip, banded, machine, or handmade
Premium	≤ 22	127-214	Most handrolled

Source: Adapted from Hoffman and Hoffman (1998).

compared with nonsmokers. Although the risks for lung and laryngeal cancers are lower for cigar smokers compared with cigarette smokers, oral and esophageal cancer risks are similar in both cigar smokers and cigarette smokers. Like other carcinogenic products, risk increases with consumption (i.e., number of cigars smoked) and depth of inhalation (Baker et al., 2000). Smokers who quit cigarettes but substitute cigars will continue to face risks for tobacco-caused diseases. Of particular concern is that former cigarette smokers typically inhale when smoking cigars (Ockene et al., 1987) and thus are at higher risk for tobacco-caused diseases than cigar smokers who have never smoked cigarettes (National Cancer Institute, 1998). Indeed, cigar smokers who inhale have increased risk for chronic obstructive pulmonary disease and coronary heart disease compared with nonsmokers (Baker et al., 2000). Last, cigars have higher total nicotine content than cigarettes and can deliver nicotine both through smoke and/or direct oral contact with the tobacco wrapper. The potential for cigars to create nicotine addiction is unquestionable (Henningfield et al., 1999).

Pipe Smoking

Pipe smoking carries significant health risks, similar to that of cigar smoking. Compared with no tobacco use, pipe smoking is associated with increased risk for cancer (oral, esophageal, larynx, and lung), coronary heart disease, stroke, and chronic obstructive pulmonary disease (Henley et al., 2004; Shaper, Wannamethee, and Walker, 2003). Like other smoked tobacco products, risk increases with depth of inhalation and consumption (i.e., number of pipes smoked and years of smoking). Pipe smoke is more alkaline than cigarettes, dissolving more easily in saliva, thus reducing inhalation. Thus, pipes deliver nicotine without the need to inhale and are capable of providing levels of nicotine high enough to produce addiction and dependence. Pipe smokers, who formerly smoked cigarettes and continue their cigarette inhalation behaviors, are at greater risk for tobacco-caused disease than pipe cigar smokers who have never smoked cigarettes (Ockene et al., 1987).

Bidis

Bidis are small, brown, hand-rolled unfiltered cigarettes, consisting of tobacco flakes rolled in a tendu leaf and tied with a small string. Manufactured primarily in India and other Southeast Asian countries, bidis have been imported into the United States for the past 20 years. Bidis are frequently enhanced with appealing flavors like cherry, root beer, and vanilla.

Much of the available toxicological and epidemiological data on bidis are derived from research in India, where bidis are referred to as the "poor man's cigarette." Bidis must be puffed more often than regular cigarettes to keep the product lit. Consequently, the smoke from a bidi produces greater amounts of nicotine and tar than a regular cigarette (Pakhale and Maru, 1998). Owing to the higher concentration of nicotine, bidi smokers are at risk for nicotine dependence (Malson, Sims, and Murty, 2001). Bidi smokers also have increased risks for cancers of the throat, oral cavity, pharynx, larynx, lungs, esophagus, stomach, and liver, compared with nonsmokers (Gupta, Hamner, and Murti, 1992).

Kreteks

Kreteks are clove cigarettes, produced primarily in Indonesia, that blend tobacco and ground clove buds. It is believed that the name kretek comes from the crackling sound the cloves make when they are burned. Eugenol, an analgesic, naturally occurs in cloves and thus is present in kretek cigarettes. It is believed that eugenol (like menthol) may minimize the harshness of cigarette smoke (Malson et al., 2003). Kreteks seem to carry tobacco-related health risks similar to conventional cigarettes (Anonymous, 1988). Although the health effects above and beyond normal cigarette smoking are unclear, it is plausible that the eugenol in the kreteks may introduce additional risks (e.g., facilitate initiation or inhibit quitting).

Smokeless Tobacco

The use of smokeless tobacco of various varieties is common throughout the world, with chewing tobacco and snuff being commonly used in North America, snus (a form of moist snuff that is low in nitrosamines and other toxins) is common in Sweden, and paan and Gutka are common in Southeast Asia. All of the commonly used varieties deliver pharmacologically active doses of nicotine, primarily via the lining of the mouth (with nasal snuff occasionally used in Europe). These different varieties vary as much as 130-fold in their content and delivery of tobacco toxins (McNeill et al., 2006). Some (primarily the Asian varieties) have very high concentrations of nitrosamines and are therefore a significant cause of oral cancer (Stepanov et al., 2005), whereas others, including the snus used in Sweden have relatively low concentrations of nitrosamines and appear not to cause cancer. Given the harmful effects of nicotine on the fetus, all of these products are potentially harmful in pregnancy. It has been proposed that the low-nitrosamine variety in Sweden is around 90 percent less harmful to health than smoking (Levy et al., 2005) and has had a net beneficial effect on the health of men in Sweden by helping to reduce the number of daily smokers (Foulds et al., 2003).

EFFECTS OF SMOKING ON THE FETUS AND EARLY CHILD DEVELOPMENT

One of the most dramatic and emotional impacts that tobacco smoke can have is the effect on fetal and child development. Unfortunately, with the stigma associated with smoking in pregnancy, current estimates of maternal tobacco use and their effects on health may not be accurate (and more likely to underestimate the health effects) unless combined with biochemical measures of smoke intake (Webb et al., 2003). Although the majority of women who continue to smoke in pregnancy report decreasing their cigarette consumption, it is likely that compensatory inhalation patterns may serve to maintain the exposure of the mother and fetus to nicotine and the multitude of toxins in tobacco smoke.

The general effects that smoke has on pregnancy are through several mechanisms. Vascular effects, such as constriction of blood vessels, lead to decreased blood supply and thus oxygen to the fetus via the placenta. Decreased delivery of oxygen to the fetus also occurs because carbon monoxide replaces oxygen in the maternal circulation. Through its effects as an appetite suppressant, maternal smoking can lead to decreased nutritional intake and relative maternal malnutrition, which can impact on fetal development. Finally, direct cellular damage can result from exposure to such chemicals as arsenic, cadmium, cyanide, and lead.

Based on the 2004 U.S. Surgeon General's report, there is evidence sufficient to conclude that there is a causal relationship between maternal smoking in pregnancy and low birth weight, preterm labor, premature rupture of membranes, placental abnormalities (e.g., abruption) as well as a reduced risk of preeclampsia. The protective effect of smoking on preeclampsia appears to be mediated via components of tobacco smoke other than nicotine because it does not occur in women using smokeless tobacco during pregnancy, who have an increased risk of preeclampsia (England et al., 2003). In addition, there is evidence that is suggestive of an increased risk of miscarriage/spontaneous abortion, ectopic pregnancy, and birth defects such as cleft lip (USDHHS, 2004).

These and many other risks continue after birth and are borne by the new infant and child. Many other linked conditions have been suggested, including SIDS, childhood respiratory infections, childhood ear infections, asthma, learning difficulties and behavior problems, childhood cancers, and higher blood pressure (through age six) (Castles et al., 1999; Higgins, 2002; USDHHS, 2004). Other effects influence the mother's body and subsequently the child such as toxins in breast milk and reduction of breast milk production.

Based on the wide range of the effects of smoking during and after pregnancy, it is critical to encourage women to quit at all stages of pregnancy. Whether they quit smoking in early pregnancy during organogenesis, midpregnancy during fetal growth and development, late in pregnancy prior to delivery, or even following delivery, the benefit of cessation to the mother and fetus/child is a large one. The earlier the woman can stop smoking, the greater the magnitude of harm reduction.

The health effects listed are related to the 4,000 toxins found in tobacco smoke. A difficult issue related to maternal smoking is consideration of the use of pharmacological treatments for tobacco dependence in pregnancy. Nicotine itself has been shown to have detrimental effects to the developing fetus, and therefore its use as a cessation aid has been limited in pregancy. However, in deciding how to most appropriately treat pregnant smokers, most clinical practice guidelines and professional organizations recognize the potential benefit of pharmacotherapy, and recommend consideration of medications if other treatments have not been successful (American College of Obstetricians and Gynecologists, 2000; Benowitz et al., 2000; Fiore et al., 2000).

EXPOSURE TO TOBACCO SMOKE POLLUTION (ENVIRONMENTAL TOBACCO SMOKE/SECONDHAND SMOKE)

Despite continued claims from the tobacco industry, environmental tobacco smoke (ETS) has emerged as a major preventable health hazard in our society. As with other major pollutants, ETS exposure is often involuntary and frequently unavoidable. Smoke that is produced by combustion of tobacco and is inhaled directly by the smoker is referred to as mainstream smoke. Mainstream smoke is 92 percent gaseous compounds and 8 percent tar (Pryor and Stone, 1993). ETS is mostly sidestream smoke but also contains some exhaled mainstream smoke. The sidestream smoke contains higher concentrations of certain toxins as they are produced by tobacco burning at lower temperatures. This composition may influence the types and rates of health effects caused by ETS.

Much of the evidence relating ETS to health effects comes from large epidemiological studies and determining a causal link between the two frequently requires the combination of data sets in meta-analyses. A point of contention in recent analyses of certain studies is the accuracy of exposure assessment. Some studies include residential exposures, such as living with a spouse who smokes or having parents that had smoked, while others include occupational exposures. The "misclassification" of exposure can potentially have a significant impact on the interpretation of ETS exposure data (Johnson and Letzel, 1984), and should be considered in reviewing the evidence.

As tobacco smoke is one of the most potent toxic compounds, ETS pollution can impact on many health problems, even at low levels of exposure. It is estimated that at least 50,000 deaths are attributable to secondhand smoke each year in the United States (California Air Resources Board [CAR], 2005). Exhibit 13.2 lists some of the most common health effects of those that have been causally linked to ETS.

Exposure to ETS can increase the relative risks of the diseases listed in Exhibit 13.2 in the range of 1.2 to 1.7 for heart disease to as high as a relative risk of 1.7 to 3 for nasal sinus cancer, and 3.5 for sudden infant death syndrome (CAR, 2005). The range of diseases influenced by ETS is related to the vast array of toxic compounds found in this pollutant. The causal relationship between ETS and breast cancer may appear surprising, given that some prior reports had not found active smoking to be causally related to breast cancer. The California Air Resources Board came to their conclusion primarily by focusing on the studies with the most careful measurement of lifetime ETS exposure, so as to avoid diluting the effect by including exposed

EXHIBIT 13.2. Effects Causally Associated with Exposure to Environmental Tobacco Smoke

Developmental Effects
Low birthweight
Sudden infant death syndrome (SIDS)
Preterm delivery

Respiratory Effects
Acute lower respiratory tract infections in children (e.g., bronchitis and pneumonia)
Asthma induction and exacerbation in children and adults
Chronic respiratory symptoms in children
Middle ear infections in children

Carcinogenic Effects
Lung cancer
Nasal sinus cancer
Breast cancer in younger, primarily premenopausal women

Cardiovascular Effects
Coronary artery disease

Source: California Air Resources Board (2005).

individuals in the "unexposed" control group. They also restricted their finding to premenopausal breast cancer.

With cardiovascular diseases representing such a high proportion of deaths, factors that increase risk of cardiovascular mortality have a substantial societal impact. ETS results in smoke exposure of about 1 percent to mainstream smoking, but increases cardiovascular risk by 30 percent (Glantz and Parmley, 1991; Law, Morris, and Wald, 1997; Law et al., 1997). Exposure to ETS has numerous effects on the cardiovascular system, including activating platelets and causing endothelial dysfunction via exposure to oxidant gases (Knight-Lozano et al., 2002; Law and Wald, 2003; Valkonen and Kussi, 1998). Some of these effects occur at relatively low levels of exposure, with a nonlinear dose-response curve (Barnoya and Glantz, 2005).

Recent evidence suggests that policy regarding ETS can have substantial effects on cardiovascular events. A study conducted in Helena, Montana, found that implementation of a comprehensive local ordinance on clean air was related to a 40 percent reduction in admissions for acute myocardial infarction, which subsequently rebounded after the ordinance was suspended (Sargent, Shephard, and Glantz, 2004). This study demonstrates the potential health benefit of establishing smoke-free environments.

Exposure to ETS has also been linked to increased risk of cancer, listed as a carcinogen by the U.S. Environmental Protection Agency and the U.S. Department of Health and Human Services. It is understandable that as there appears to be no safe threshold level above which carcinogens need to reach to induce genetic damage and subsequent abnormal cell cycle growth, relatively high increases in risk can be seen with low levels of exposure. However, it is often difficult to demonstrate causal effects for cancer-related exposures as there is often a long latency period (i.e., 20-30 years) between the exposure and the diagnosis of a malignancy. It has been demonstrated that nonsmokers have statistically greater risk of lung cancer if their spouses are smokers. Meta-analyses show the increased risk of lung cancer was about 25 percent greater than expected in women and 35 percent greater in men if their spouses smoked (National Cancer Institute, 1999). Although acute exposure may be variable in these settings, it is clear that the cumulative exposure over years of living in a smoke-exposed environment can lead to malignant transformation.

The evidence currently available demonstrates that ETS exposure poses a serious public health problem and policies designed to protect the public from secondhand smoke need to be continued to limit its deadly impact.

PSYCHIATRIC AND PSYCHOLOGICAL EFFECTS OF TOBACCO/NICOTINE USE

Nicotine dependence is one of the first tobacco-caused disorders experienced by most people who start regular tobacco use. Unsuccessful attempts to stop smoking, difficulty controlling use, and previous experience of withdrawal symptoms during a period of abstinence are criteria for nicotine dependence in both the American Psychiatric Association's *Diagnostic and Statistical Manual of Mental Disorders* (Fourth Edition) (DSM-IV) and the World Health Organization's *International Classification of Diseases and Related Health Problems* (Tenth Revision) (ICD-10) (American Psychiatric Association, 2000; World Health Organization, 1992). The Fagerstrom Test for Nicotine Dependence (FTND) is a six-item scale that has been shown to predict withdrawal symptom and craving severity, and is the most widely used questionnaire measure of tobacco dependence (Heatherton et al., 1991). The items and scoring for the FTND are shown in Exhibit 13.3.

Epidemiological studies using research diagnostic criteria suggest that between 50 percent and 90 percent of current tobacco users meet diagnostic criteria for nicotine dependence, and 21 to 46 percent meet criteria for nicotine withdrawal when abstaining for at least 24 hours (Grant et al., 2004; Hughes, Gust, and Pechacek, 1987). Clinicians frequently view nicotine dependence in dimensional rather than categorical terms and there has been a general consensus that smokers of at least 10 cigarettes per day (or those smoking within 60 minutes of waking) are moderately nicotine dependent

EXHIBIT 13.3. The Fagerstrom Test for Nicotine Dependence

Question	Answer	Score
How soon after you wake up do you smoke your first cigarette?	Within 5 minutes	3
	6-30 minutes	2
	31-60 minutes	1
	>60 minutes	0
Do you find it difficult to refrain from smoking in places where it is forbidden?	Yes	1
	No	0
Which cigarette would you hate to give up most?	The first one in the morning	1
	Others	0
How many cigarettes per day do you smoke?	<10	0
	11-20	1
	21-30	2
	>31	3
Do you smoke more frequently during the first hours after waking than during the rest of the day?	Yes	1
	No	0
Do you smoke if you are so ill that you are in bed most of the day?	Yes	1
	No	0

Scores are totaled to yield a single value, with scores of 6 or more indicating high nicotine dependence.

Source: Heatherton et al. (1991).

and those smoking over 20 cigarettes per day (or within 30 minutes of waking) are highly nicotine dependent. More recent studies of the development of dependence in young people have suggested that loss of autonomy over one's smoking (as a central criteria for dependence) develops at much lower levels of smoking, including less than one cigarette per day. DiFranza et al. have developed a scale called the "Hooked on Nicotine Checklist" (HONC) that is particularly useful in predicting the development of dependence in young people and may potentially be a useful index of dependence in adults as well (see Exhibit 13.4; DiFranza et al., 2002; O'Loughlin et al., 2002; Wellman et al., 2005).

Nicotine withdrawal symptoms are believed to be a key factor making it hard for smokers to abstain and are an important medical consequence of tobacco use. The DSM-IV criteria for nicotine withdrawal are shown in Exhibit 13.5 (American Psychiatric Association, 2000).

EXHIBIT 13.4. The Hooked on Nicotine Checklist (HONC)

1. Have you ever tried to quit but couldn't?
2. Do you smoke *now* because it is really hard to quit?
3. Have you ever felt like you were addicted to tobacco?
4. Do you ever have strong cravings to smoke?
5. Have you ever felt like you really needed a cigarette?
6. Is it hard to keep from smoking in places where you are not supposed to?

When you tried to stop smoking or when you haven't used tobacco for a while . . .

7. Did you find it hard to concentrate because you couldn't smoke?
8. Did you feel more irritable because you couldn't smoke?
9. Did you feel a strong need or urge to smoke?
10. Did you feel nervous, restless, or anxious because you couldn't smoke?

The number of items checked "yes" give a total score with zero indicating no dependence, 1 = low dependence, and 10 = high dependence.

Source: DiFranza et al. (2002).

EXHIBIT 13.5. DSM-IV Criteria for Nicotine Withdrawal

A. Daily use of nicotine for at least several weeks.

B. Abrupt cessation of nicotine use, or reduction in the amount of nicotine used, followed within 24 hours by four (or more) of the following:

    (1) dysphoric or depressed mood

    (2) insomnia

    (3) irritability, frustration, or anger

    (4) anxiety

    (5) difficulty concentrating

    (6) restlessness

    (7) decreased heart rate

    (8) increased appetite or weight gain.

C. The symptoms in criterion B cause clinically significant distress or impairment in social, occupational, or other important areas of functioning.

D. The symptoms are not due to a general medical condition and are not better accounted for by another mental disorder.

    Associated features:

      Craving for nicotine

      Desire for sweets

      Impaired performance on tasks requiring vigilance

      EEG slowing

      Decrease in catecholamine and cortisol levels

      Decreased metabolism of medications and other substances

Source: American Psychiatric Association (2000).

Smoking is banned from many workplaces and other indoor areas in order protect against passive exposure to secondhand smoke, and so many smokers may be forced into a state of nicotine withdrawal on an almost daily basis. Mental health professionals in particular, should assess and treat nicotine dependence and withdrawal in their patients, to ensure that these symptoms are not exacerbating or being mistaken for other mental health problems.

There remains considerable debate over the extent to which tobacco use may be a form of self-medication for people with a range of psychiatric disorders. It is clear that once an individual becomes dependent on nicotine, then continued tobacco use is partly motivated by the need to medicate nicotine withdrawal symptoms (many of which overlap with symptoms of psychiatric disorders). However, it is less clear that nicotine and/or tobacco use does not provide any direct and primary beneficial effects (other then mild stimulant and appetite suppressant effects) or worsening effects (e.g., other than via nicotine withdrawal or as secondary to other tobacco caused illness) in any psychiatric condition.

To take just one disorder, there is evidence that people with a history of depression are more likely to smoke. Smokers are also more likely to have an episode of major depression after stopping smoking, as compared with similar individuals who keep smoking (Glassman et al., 2001). There is also evidence that chemicals in tobacco other than nicotine may reduce depressive symptoms through their effect on reducing the monoamine oxidase enzyme (MAO B) in a manner similar to MAO inhibitor antidepressant medications. Reducing MAO B enzyme levels, which is a goal of some antidepressants, slows the breakdown of catecholamines. Studies have shown that the brains of living smokers had 40 percent less MAO B compared with nonsmokers or former smokers (Fowler et al., 1996). These kinds of studies appear to lay a foundation for concluding that smoking may have beneficial effects on depression. However, a number of studies have also demonstrated that smoking frequently predates the onset of psychiatric illnesses such as depression. For example, the National Longitudinal Study of Adolescent Health revealed that current cigarette smoking was the strongest predictor of developing depressive symptoms at follow-up (Goodman and Capitman, 2000). Nondepressed teens who smoked at least one pack per week during the study were four times more likely to develop depression than their nonsmoking peers. The relationship between tobacco use and mental health clearly warrants further study. What is very clear, however, is that tobacco use is particularly common among people with psychiatric comorbidity or chemical dependence, with around 44 percent of all the cigarettes smoked in the United States being consumed by people who have suffered from a psychiatric problem within the past 30 days (Lasser et al., 2000).

Health Consequences of Tobacco Use in Psychiatric Patients

In some categories of behavioral health provision (e.g., inpatient substance abuse services) patients are more likely to ultimately be killed by their tobacco use than by the problem being presented for treatment (Hurt et al., 1996).

The rates of cancer, cardiovascular, and respiratory diseases among individuals with severe mental illness (SMI) are double those of age-matched controls, due to the two to three times increased rate of tobacco addiction (Brown, Inskip, and Barraclough, 2000; Stroup, Gilmore, and Jarskog, 2000). In addition to increased medical comorbidity, smokers with SMI experience increased psychiatric symptoms, hospitalizations, and need for higher medication doses compared with non-smokers with SMI. Heavy smokers with SMI have increased positive symptoms (hallucinations and delusions) and reduced negative symptoms (anhedonia, alogia, flat affect, low motivation, and poor social skills) compared with nonsmokers and light smokers (Goff, Henderson, and Amico, 1992).

Effects of Tobacco Smoking on Metabolism of Psychiatric Medications

Some researchers speculate that the high rates of tobacco dependence in those suffering from another mental illness may be secondary to some patients managing medication side effects by changing their intake of cigarettes. The tars of tobacco are metabolized in the liver and are very potent inducers of the CYP 1A2 cytochrome isoenzyme in the P450 liver enzymes. The induction of the 1A2 isoenzyme has a clinically significant impact on increasing the metabolism of many antipsychotics and some antidepressants and antianxiety medications (e.g., oxazepam, desipramine, haloperidol, clozapine, and olanzapine). The medications are metabolized quicker in smokers and and so smokers typically need twice the dosage of medications as non-smokers. When smokers initially abstain from tobacco, medication blood levels increase, and there is a risk for increased side-effects if the medication dosage is not adjusted (Desai, Seabolt, and Jann, 2001). Of note, nicotine is not metabolized through the 1A2 isoenzyme, but has a small clinically insignificant effect on the 2D6 isoenzyme.

SUMMARY AND CONCLUSIONS

Tobacco remains the only legal consumer product that is lethal when used as intended. It causes serious damage to practically every organ in the body, but is particularly harmful to the lungs and the cardiovascular system. Approximately half of long-term smokers are killed prematurely by their smoking (Peto et al., 1994), and on average, the continuing smoker will lose ten years of life (Doll et al., 2004). However, there is a one in four chance of losing a much larger part of ones life (e.g., 30 years). It has been estimated that, on average, each cigarette will reduce life expectancy by around 11 minutes (Shaw, Mitchell, and Dorling, 2000). Thus, time spent smoking translates almost one minute for one minute into premature death. It is important for smokers to know that those years of life lost are healthy years, as smokers have fewer years in health (free from disability) and more years in sickness/disability (Nusselder et al., 2000). In addition to these dramatic health effects, tobacco is highly addictive, and has a complex relationship with mental health. For all of these reasons, it is important that society, the health care system and behavioral health professionals in particular, start to address tobacco use with the seriousness its lethal nature deserves.

REFERENCES

American College of Obstetricians and Gynecologists (2000). *Smoking Cessation During Pregnancy.* ACOG Educational Bulletin 260. Washington, DC: ACOG.

American Psychiatric Association (2000). *Diagnostic and Statistical Manual of Mental Disorders,* 4th ed., Text Revision. Washington, DC.

Anonymous (1988). Evaluation of the health hazard of clove cigarettes. Council on Scientific Affairs. *JAMA* 260(24):3641-3644.

Baker, F.; Ainsworth, S.R.; Dye, J.T.; Crammer, C.; Thun, M.J.; Hoffmann, D.; Repace, J.L. et al. (2000). Health risks associated with cigar smoking. *JAMA* 284(6):735-740.

Barnes, P.J. (1999). Molecular genetics of chronic obstructive pulmonary disease. *Thorax* 54(3):245-252.

Barnoya, J.; Glantz, S.A. (2005). Cardiovascular effects of secondhand smoke: Nearly as large as smoking. *Circulation* 111:2684-2698.

Benowitz, N.L. (2001). Compensatory smoking of low-yield cigarettes. In: National Cancer Institute, Smoking and Tobacco Control Monograph No. 13, *Risks Associated with Smoking Cigarettes with Low Machine-Measured Yields of Tar and Nicotine.* Bethesda, MD: NCI.

Benowitz, N.L.; Dempsey, D.A.; Goldenberg, R.L.; Hughes, J.R.; Dolan-Mullen, P.; Ogburn, P.L.; Oncken, C.; Orleans, C.T.; Slotkin, T.A.; Whiteside, H.P., Jr; Yaffe, S. (2000). The use of pharmacotherapies for smoking cessation during pregnancy. *Tob Control* 9(Suppl 3):III91-4.

Bowling, J.; Taylor, P. (1976). *This Week: Philip Morris.* Mr. James Bowling, vice president, Philip Morris Inc. being interviewed by Mr. Peter Taylor, Thames Broadcasting Co., London, August 16. Bates Number: 1002410318-1002410351.

Brown, S.; Inskip, H.; Barraclough, B. (2000). Causes of the excess mortality of schizophrenia. *Br J Psychiatry* 177:212-217.

Burns, D.M.; Major, J.M.; Shanks, T.G.; Thun, M.J. (2001). Smoking lower yield cigarettes and disease risk. In: National Cancer Institute, Smoking and Tobacco Control Monograph No. 13, *Risks Associated with Smoking Cigarettes with Low Machine-Measured Yields of Tar and Nicotine.* Bethesda, MD: NCI.

California Air Resources Board. (2005). *Proposed Identification of Environmental Tobacco Smoke as a Toxic Air Contaminant.* SRP Approved Version. http://www.arb.ca.gov/toxics/ets/finalreport/finalreport.htm.

Castles, A.; Adams, K.; Melvin, C.L.; Kelsch, C.; Boulton, M.L. (1999). Effects of smoking during pregnancy: Five meta-analyses. *Am J Prev Med* 16(3):208-215.

CDC (2003). Cigarette smoking-attributable morbidity—United States, 2000. *MMWR Morb Mortal Wkly Rep* 52(35):842-844.

Collishaw, N.E.; Lopez, A.D. (1996). *The Tobacco Epidemic: A Global Public Health Emergency.* Geneva: World Health Organization.

Critchley, J.A.; Unal, B. (2003). Health effects associated with smokeless tobacco: A systematic review. *Thorax* 58(5):435-443.

Cummings, K:M.; Morley, C.P.; Hyland, A. (2002). Failed promises of the cigarette industry and its effect on consumer misperceptions about the health risks of smoking. *Tob Control* (Suppl 1):I110-I117.

Desai, H.D.; Seabolt, J.; Jann, M.W. (2001). Smoking in patients receiving psychotropic medications: A pharmacokinetic perspective. *CNS Drugs* 15(6):469-494.

DiFranza, J.R.; Savageau, J.A.; Fletcher, K.; Fletcher, K.; Ockene, J.K.; Rigotti, N.A.; McNeill, A.D.; Coleman, M.; Wood, C. (2002). Measuring the loss of autonomy over nicotine use in adolescents: The DANDY (Development and Assessment of Nicotine Dependence in Youths) study. *Arch Pediatr Adolesc Med* 156(4):397-403.

Doll, R.; Hill, A.B. (1950). Smoking and carcinoma of the lung. Preliminary report. *BMJ* 2:739-748.

Doll, R.; Peto, R.; Boreham, J.; Sutherland, I. (2004). Mortality in relation to smoking: 50 years' observations on male British doctors. *BMJ* 328(7455):1519.

England, L.J.; Levine, R.J.; Mills, J.L.; Klebanoff, M.A.; Yu, K.F.; Cnattingus, S. (2003). Adverse pregnancy outcomes in snuff users. *Am J Obstet Gynecol* 189(4):939-943.

Fiore, M.C.; Bailey, W.C.; Cohen, S.J.; Dorfman, S.F.; Goldstein, M.G.; Gritz, E.R.; Heyman, R.B. et al. (2000). *Treating Tobacco Use and Dependence: Clinical Practice Guideline.* Rockville, MD: U.S. Department of Health and Human Services, Public Health Service.

Foulds, J.; Ramstrom, L.; Burke, M.; Fagerstrom, K. (2003). The effect of smokeless tobacco (snus) on public health in Sweden. *Tob Control* 12:349-359.

Fowler, J.S.; Volkow, N.D.; Wang, G.J.; Pappas, N.; Logan, J.; MacGregor, R.; Alexoff, D. et al. (1996). Inhibition of MAO B in the brains of smokers. *Nature* 379:733-738.

Gerlach, K.K.; Cummings, K.M.; Hyland, A.; Gilpin, E.; Johnson, M.D.; Pierce, J.P. (1998). Trends in cigar consumption and smoking prevalence. In: National Cancer Institute, Smoking and Tobacco Control Monograph No. 9, NIH publication 98-4302, *Cigars: Health Effects and Trends.* Bethesda, MD: U.S. Department of Health and Human Services, Public Health Service.

Geyelin, M. (1998). Tobacco executive doubts product risks. *Wall Street Journal.* March 3rd, 1998.

Giovino, G.A. (2002). Epidemiology of tobacco use in the United States. *Oncogene* 21(48):7326-7340.

Glantz, S.A.; Parmley, W.W. (1991). Passive smoking and heart disease: Epidemiology, physiology, and biochemistry. *Circulation* 83:1-12.

Glassman, A.H.; Covey, L.S.; Stetner, F.; Rivelli, S. (2001). Smoking cessation and the course of major depression: A follow-up study. *Lancet* 357(9272):1929-1932.

Godtfredsen, N.S.; Holst, C.; Prescott, E.; Vestbo, J.; Osler, M. (2002). Smoking reduction, smoking cessation, and mortality: A 16-year follow-up of 19,732 men and women from The Copenhagen Centre for Prospective Population Studies. *Am J Epidemiol* 156(11):994-1001.

Goff, D.C.; Henderson, D.C.; Amico, B.S. (1992). Cigarette smoking in schizophrenia: Relationship to psychopathology and medication side effects. *Am J Psychiatry* 149:1189-1194.

Goodman, B. (1975). *Marlboro-Marlboro Lights Study Delivery Data*. Philip Morris; Bates No. 1001900842.

Goodman, E.; Capitman, J. (2000). Depressive symptoms and cigarette smoking among teens. *Pediatrics* 106(4):748-755.

Grant, B.F.; Hasin, D.S.; Chou, P.; Stinson, F.S.; Dawson, D.A. (2004). Nicotine dependence and psychiatric disorders in the United States: Results from the national epidemiologic survey on alcohol and related conditions. *Arch Gen Psychiatry* 61(11):1107-1115.

Gupta, P.C.; Hamner, J.E.; Murti, P.R. (1992). *Control of Tobacco-Related Cancers and Other Diseases; Proceedings of an International Symposium*. Bombay, India: Tata Institute of Fundamental Research, Oxford University Press.

Harris, J.E. (2004). Incomplete compensation does not imply reduced harm: Yields of 40 smoke toxicants per milligram nicotine in regular filter versus low-tar cigarettes in the 1999 Massachusetts Benchmark Study. *Nicotine Tob Res* 6(5):797-808.

Harris, J.E.; Thun, M.J.; Mondul, A.M.; Calle, E.E. (2004). Cigarette tar yields in relation to mortality from lung cancer in the Cancer Prevention Study II prospective cohort, 1982-8. *BMJ* 328(7431):72.

Heatherton, T.F.; Kozlowski, L.T.; Frecker, R.C.; Fagerstrom, K.O. (1991). The Fagerstrom Test for Nicotine Dependence: A revision of the Fagerstrom Tolerance Questionnaire. *Br J Addict* 86(9):1119-1127.

Hecht, S.S. (1999). Tobacco smoke carcinogens and lung cancer. *J Natl Cancer Inst* 91(14):1194-1210.

Henley, S.J.; Thun, M.J.; Chao, A.; Calle, E.E. (2004). Association between exclusive pipe smoking and mortality from cancer and other diseases. *J Natl Cancer Inst* 96(11):853-861.

Henningfield, J.E.; Fant, R.V.; Radzius, A.; Frost, S. (1999). Nicotine concentration, smoke pH and whole tobacco aqueous pH of some cigar brands and types popular in the United States. *Nicotine Tob Res* 1(2):163-168.

Herman, G.; Cullman, J.; Mintz, M.; Ubell, E. (1971). *Transcript: Face the Nation*. January 3. Bates No. 1002605545-1002605564.

Higgins, S. (2002). Smoking in pregnancy. *Curr Opin Obstet Gynecol* 14(2):145-151.

Hoffman, D.; Hoffman, I. (1998). Chemistry and Toxicology. In: National Cancer Institute, Smoking and Tobacco Control Monograph No. 9, NIH publication 98-4302, *Cigars: Health Effects and Trends*. Bethesda, MD: U.S. Department of Health and Human Services, Public Health Service.

Hughes, J.R.; Gust, S.W.; Pachecek, T.F. (1987). Prevalence of tobacco dependence and withdrawal. *Am J Psychiatry* 144(2):205-208.

Hurt, R.D.; Offord, K.P.; Croghan, I.T.; Gomez-Dahl, L.; Kottke, T.E.; Morse, R.M.; Melton, M.J. (1996). Mortality following inpatient addictions treatment. *JAMA* 275(14):1097-1103.

Johnson, L.C.; Letzel, H.W. (1984). Measuring passive smoking: Methods, problems, and perspectives. *Prev Med* 13(6):705-716.

Knight-Lozano, C.A.; Young, C.G.; Burow, D.L.; Hu, Z.Y.; Uyeminami, D.; Pinkerton, K.E.; Ischiropoulos, H., Ballinger, S.W. (2002). Cigarette smoke exposure and hypercholesterolemia increase mitochondrial damage in cardiovascular tissues. *Circulation* 105(7):849-854.

Knoke, J.D.; Shanks, T.G.; Vaughn, J.W.; Thun, M.J.; Burns, D.M. (2004). Lung cancer mortality is related to age in addition to duration and intensity of cigarette smoking: An analysis of CPS-I data. *Cancer Epidemiol Biomarkers Prev* 13(6): 949-957.

Kozlowski, L.T.; Mehta, N.Y.; Sweeney, C.T.; Schwartz, S.S.; Vogler, G.P.; Jarvis, M.J.; West, R.J. (1998). Filter ventilation and nicotine content of tobacco in cigarettes from Canada, the United Kingdom and the United States. *Tob Control* 7:369-375.

Kozlowski, L.T.; O'Connor, R.J. (2002). Cigarette filter ventilation is a defective design because of misleading taste, bigger puffs, and blocked vents. *Tob Control* 11(Suppl 1):I40-I50.

Kwitny, J. (1972). Defending the weed. *The Wall Street Journal.* January 24. Bates No. 500324162-500324164.

Lasser, K.; Wesley, B.J.; Woolhandler, S.; Himmestein, D.U.; McCormick, D.; Bor, D.H. (2000). Smoking and mental illness: A population-based prevalence study. *JAMA* 284:2606-2610.

Law, M.R.; Morris, J.K.; Wald, N.J. (1997). Environmental tobacco smoke exposure and ischemic heart disease: An evaluation of the evidence. *BMJ* 315:973-980.

Law, M.R.; Morris, J.K.; Watt, H.C.; Wald, N.J. (1997). The dose-response relationship between cigarette consumption and biochemical markers and risk of lung cancer. *Br J Cancer* 75(11):1690-1693.

Law, M.R.; Wald, N.J. (2003). Environmental tobacco smoke and ischemic heart disease. *Prog Cardiovasc Dis* 46:31-38.

Levy, D.T.; Mumford, E.A.; Cummings, K.M.; Gilpin, E.A.; Giovino, G.; Hyland, A.; Sweanor, D.; Warner, K.E. (2004). The relative risks of a low-nitrosamine smokeless tobacco product compared with smoking cigarettes: Estimates of a panel of experts. *Cancer Epidemiol Biomarkers Prev* 13(12):2035-2042.

Lopez, A.D.; Collishaw, N.E.; Piha, T. (1994). A Descriptive Model of the Cigarette Epidemic in Developed Countries. *Tob Control* 3:242-247.

Malson, J.L.; Lee, E.M.; Murty, R.; Moolchan, E.T.; Pickworth, W.B. (2003). Clove cigarette smoking: Biochemical, physiological, and subjective effects. *Pharmacol Biochem Behav* 74(3):739-745.

Malson, J.; Sims, K.; Murty, R. (2001). Comparison of the nicotine content of tobacco used in bidis and conventional cigarettes. *Tob Control* 10(2):181-183.

Martin, J.; Dunn, W.L. (1967). *A Study of the Effect of Air Hole Blockage on Gross Puff Volume in Air Diluted Cigarettes*. Philip Morris; Bates No. 1001892505.

McGinnis, J.M.; Foege, W.H. (1993). Actual causes of death in the United States. *JAMA* 270(18):2207-2212.

McNeill, A.; Bedi, R.; Islam, S.; Alkhatib, M.N.; West, R. (2006). Levels of toxins in oral tobacco products in the UK. *Tob Control* 15(1):64-67.

National Cancer Institute (1996). Smoking and Tobacco Control Monograph No. 7, *The FTC Cigarette Test Method for Determining Tar, Nicotine and Carbonmonoxide Yields of US Cigarettes*. Bethesda, MD: NCI.

National Cancer Institute (1998). Smoking and Tobacco Control Monograph No. 9, NIH publication 98-4302, *Cigars: Health Effects and Trends*. Bethesda, MD: U.S. Department of Health and Human Services, Public Health Service.

National Cancer Institute (1999). Smoking and Tobacco Control Monograph 10, *Health Effects of Exposure to Environmental Tobacco Smoke*. Bethesda, MD: NCI. Retrieved October 16, 2005 from http://cancercontrol.cancer.gov/tcrb/monographs/10/index.html.

Nusselder, W.J.; Looman, C.W.; Marang-van de Mheen, P.J.; Van e Mheen, H.; Mackenbach, J.P. (2000). Smoking and the compression of morbidity. *J Epidemiol Community Health* 54(8):566-574.

Nyman, A.L.; Taylor, T.M.; Biener, L. (2002). Trends in cigar smoking and perceptions of health risks among Massachusetts adults. *Tob Control* 11(Suppl 2):ii25-ii28.

Ockene, J.K.; Pechacek, T.F.; Vogt, T.; Svendsen, K. (1987). Does switching from cigarettes to pipes or cigars reduce tobacco smoke exposure? *Am J Public Health* 77(11):1412-1416.

O'Loughlin, J.; Tarasuk, J.; Difranza, J.; Paradis, G. (2002). Reliability of selected measures of nicotine dependence among adolescents. *Ann Epidemiol* 12(5):353-362.

Pakhale, S.S.; Maru, G.B. (1998). Distribution of major and minor alkaloids in tobacco, mainstream and sidestream smoke of popular Indian smoking products. *Food Chem Toxicol* 36(12):1131-1138.

Pauly, J.L.; Mepani, A.B.; Lesses, J.D.; Cummings, K.M.; Streck, R.J. (2002). Cigarettes with defective filters marketed for 40 years: What Philip Morris never told smokers. *Tob Control* 11(Suppl 1):I51-I61.

Peto, R.; Darby, S.; Deo, H.; Silcocks, P.; Whitley, E.; Doll, R. (2000). Smoking, smoking cessation, and lung cancer in the UK since 1950: Combination of national statistics with two case-control studies. *BMJ* 321(7257):323-329.

Peto, R.; Lopez, A.D.; Boreham, J.; Thun, M.; Clark, H. (1994). *Mortality from Smoking in Developed Countries 1950-2000*. Oxford: Oxford University Press.

Powell, J.T. (1998). Vascular damage from smoking: Disease mechanisms at the arterial wall. *Vascular Medicine* 3(1):21-28.

Pryor, W.A.; Stone, K. (1993). Oxidants in cigarette smoke: Radicals, hydrogen peroxide, peroxynitrate, and peroxynitrite. *Ann NY Acad Sci* 686:12-28.

Royal College of Physicians (2000). *Nicotine Addiction in Britain*. A report of the tobacco advisory group of the Royal College of Physicians. London.

Royal College of Physicians of London (1962). *Smoking and Health.* Summary and report on smoking in relation to cancer of the lung and other diseases. New York: Pitman Publishing.

Sargent, R.P.; Shephard, R.M.; Glantz, S.A. (2004). Reduced incidence of admissions for myocardial infarction associated with public smoking ban: Before and after study. *BMJ* 328(7446):977-980.

Scanlon, P.D.; Connett, J.E.; Waller, L.A.; Altose, M.D.; Bailey, W.C.; Buist, A.S. (2000). Smoking cessation and lung function in mild-to-moderate chronic obstructive pulmonary disease. *Am J Respir Crit Care Med* 161(2 Pt 1):381-390.

Shaper, A.G.; Wannamethee, S.G.; Walker, M. (2003). Pipe and cigar smoking and major cardiovascular events, cancer incidence and all-cause mortality in middle-aged British men. *Int J Epidemiol* 32(5):802-808.

Shaw, M.; Mitchell, R.; Dorling, D. (2000). Time for a smoke? One cigarette reduces your life by 11 minutes. *BMJ* 320(7226):53.

Stampfer, M.J.; Hu, F.B.; Manson, J.E.; Rimm, E.B.; Willett, W.C. (2000). Primary prevention of coronary heart disease in women through diet and lifestyle. *N Engl J Med* 342(1):16-22.

Stepanov, I.; Hecht, S.S.; Ramakrishnan, S.; Gupta, P.C. (2005). Tobacco-specific nitrosamines smokeless tobacco products marketed in India. *Int J Cancer* 116(1):16-19.

Stroup, T.S.; Gilmore, J.H.; Jarskog, L.F. (2000). Management of medical illness in persons with schizophrenia. *Psych Annals* 30(1):35-40.

Thun, M.J.; Apicalla, L.F.; Henley, S.J. (2000). Smoking vs. other risk factors as the cause smoking-attributable deaths: Confounding in the courtroom. *JAMA* 284: 706-712.

Thun, M.J.; Myers, D.G.; Day-Lally, C.; Namboodiri, M.M.; Calle, E.E.; Flanders, W.D.; Adams, S.L.; Heath, C.W. (1997). Age and exposure-response relationships between cigarette smoking and premature death in Cancer Prevention Study II. In: Shopland, D.R.; Burns, D.M.; Garfinkel, L.; Samet, J.M. (Eds.), Smoking and Tobacco Control Monograph No. 8, NIH publication number 97-4213, *Changes in Cigarette-Related Disease Risks and Their Implications for Prevention and Control.* Bethesda, MD: DHSS, National Cancer Institute.

Tobacco Industry Research Committee (1954). *A Frank Statement to Cigarette Smokers.* Bates No. 500849398-500849399.

U.S. Department of Health and Human Services (1988). *The Health Consequences of Smoking: Nicotine Addiction.* Washington, DC: U.S. Government Printing Office.

U.S. Department of Health and Human Services (1990). *The Health Benefits of Smoking Cessation.* Washington, DC: CDC Office on Smoking and Health.

U.S. Department of Health and Human Services (2004). *The Consequences of Smoking: A Report of the Surgeon General.* Washington, DC: U.S. Department of Health and Human Services, Centers for Disease Control and Prevention, National Center for Chronic Disease Prevention and Health Promotion, Office on Smoking and Health.

U.S. Department of Health, Education and Welfare, Public Health Service (1964). *Smoking and Health Report of the Advisory Committee to the Surgeon General of the Public Health Service.* PHS Publication No.1103.

Valkonen, M.; Kuusi, T. (1998). Passive smoking induces atherogenic changes in low-density lipoprotein. *Circulation* 97:2012-2016.

Wallenfeldt, K.; Hulthe, J.; Bokemark, L.; Wikstrand, J.; Fagerberg, B. (2001). Carotid and femoral atherosclerosis, cardiovascular risk factors and C-reactive protein in relation to smokeless tobacco use or smoking in 58-year-old men. *J Intern Med* 250(6):492-501.

Webb, D.A.; Boyd. N.R.; Messina, D.; Windsor, R.A. (2003). The discrepancy between self-reported smoking status and urine continine levels among women enrolled in prenatal care at four publicly funded clinical sites. *J Public Health Manag Pract* 9(4):322-325.

Wellman, R.J.; DiFranza, J.R.; Savageau, J.A.; Godiwala, S.; Friedman, K.: Hazelton, J. (2005). Measuring adults' loss of autonomy over nicotine use: The Hooked on Nicotine Checklist. *Nicotine Tob Res* 7(1):157-161.

White, J.L.; Conner, B.T.; Perfetti, T.A.; Bombick, B.R.; Avalos, J.T.; Fowler, K.W.; Smith, Cl.J.; Doolittle, D.J. (2001). Effect of pyrolysis temperature on the mutagenicity of tobacco smoke condensate. *Food Chem Toxicol* 39(5):499-505.

World Health Organization (1992). *International Statistical Classification of Diseases and Related Health Problems,* 10th revision. Geneva: WHO.

World Health Organization (1997). *Tobacco or Health: A Global Status Report.* Geneva: WHO.

Wynder, E.L.; Graham, E.A. (1950) Tobacco smoking as a possible etiologic factor in bronchogenic carcinoma. *JAMA* 143:329-336.

Yeaman, A. (1963). Implications of Battelle Hippo I & II and the Griffith Filter. July 17, 1963. Bates Bo. 1802.05. http://legacy.library.ucsf.edu/tid/xrc72d00.

Chapter 14

Medical Consequences of the Use of Hallucinogens: LSD, Mescaline, PCP, and MDMA ("Ecstasy")

Timothy Wiegand
Dung Thai
Neal Benowitz

INTRODUCTION AND OVERVIEW

Hallucinogens are a class of drugs that cause alterations in cognition and perception. They can be obtained from both natural and synthetic sources. Their history dates as far back as 3,000 years during which time indigenous cacti and plants were used in religious practices. More recently, a number of synthetic analogs have become popular among recreational users and as part of experimental psychotherapy. This chapter covers the medical consequences of four of the more commonly used hallucinogens: lysergic acid diethylamide (LSD), phencyclidine (PCP), mescaline, and 3, 4-methylenedioxymethamphetamine (MDMA). The structures of these hallucinogens is presented in Figure 14.1.

LYSERGIC ACID DIETHYLAMIDE (LSD)

Overview

LSD is a synthetic ergoline which contains 2 stereocenters thus providing four possible optical isomers. Only d-LSD possesses hallucinogenic properties. A number of proposed pharmacological mechanisms help to

Handbook of the Medical Consequences of Alcohol and Drug Abuse
© 2008 by The Haworth Press, Taylor & Francis Group. All rights reserved.
doi:10.1300/6039_14

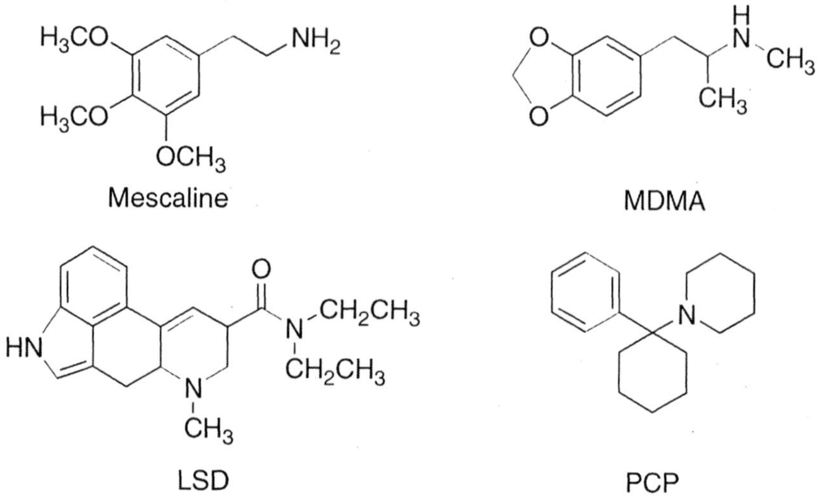

FIGURE 14.1. Chemical structure of mescaline, MDMA, LSD, and PCP. *Source:* Figures created in ChemDraw, from CambridgeSoft® by Dung Thai, MD, PhD.

explain its physiologic and psychedelic properties. LSD is thought to act in the serotonin (5-HT) system which contains a number of receptor subtypes. Boakes et al. have blocked 5-HT excitatory effects by applying LSD by iontophoresis into cat brain stem cells (Boakes et al., 1970). In addition, the specific 5-HT2A antagonist, pirenperone, blocks LSD's effects in rats (Mokler, Stoudt, and Rech, 1985). The hallucinogenic properties of LSD are believed to be mediated through binding to an excitatory postsynaptic receptor 5-HT2A in the forebrain of the cortex.

Although LSD's hallucinogenic effects are related to its activity in the 5-HT pathway, it also exhibits sympathetic and parasympathetic properties. An excellent review on the biochemical pharmacology of LSD was written by Caldwell and Sever (Caldwell and Sever, 1974). The psychological and physical effects are dose-related. Hallucinatory psychosis usually occurs at a dose of 1 mcg/kg of body weight. The lethal dose of LSD is estimated at 14 mg. Morbidity and mortality is mostly related to erratic and dangerous behavior during a "bad trip."

History

LSD was first synthesized by the Swiss chemist Albert Hofmann, at Sandoz Pharmaceuticals in 1938. Five years later, Hofmann accidentally absorbed a small amount of LSD through his finger and experienced the first human "trip," which he described as "an uninterrupted stream of fantastic pictures, extraordinary shapes with intense, kaleidoscope-like play of color." In the early 1950s, Charles Savage published the first human study of LSD used to treat depression. During this same time, the United States Central Intelligence Agency began funding human experiments of this drug. The popularity of LSD was catapulted by Harvard University's Timothy Leary who promoted it as a part of the psychedelic cultural movement. LSD became a Schedule I drug in 1970. Despite its popularity among recreational users, the vast majority of literature regarding the physiologic and toxicologic properties is scarce after the 1970s.

Psychologic Effects

The most well-documented experiences with LSD are those related to the "acid trip." It can produce changes in mood, perception, consciousness, and thought. Perceptual distortions usually begin within 60 minutes of ingestion. Many sensory modalities are intensified. Colors may appear more vivid, and smells may have greater pungency. Users may experience visual hallucinations though they are usually aware that these hallucinations are not real. These hallucinations are often distortions of perceived sensory cues. Interestingly, users often report a fusion of sensory modalities or synesthesia wherein the real information of one sense is accompanied by a perception in another sense such as smelling colors. In addition, they report an overlapping of prior and present images to produce the equivalent of photographic double exposure.

One time or chronic users of LSD may experience flashbacks (Shick and Smith, 1970). These episodes are spontaneous recurrences of the psychedelic experience similar to the acute LSD episode but they occur long after drug cessation. Although flashbacks can occur after a single use of LSD, they tend to be more frequent with prolonged or increased use. Shick and Smith divide these flashbacks into three distinct categories: perceptual, somatic, and emotional (Shick and Smith, 1970). Perceptual flashbacks are the most commonly reported among users and range from minor visual changes to frank hallucinations. Examples of perceptual flashbacks include greater intensity of color, faces changing shape, and insects crawling. Somatic flashbacks, which occur after a bad trip, are described as transient recurrent states of altered bodily sensation such as paresthesias or pain. Emotional flashbacks are considered the most dangerous because they tend to bring up disturbing emotions such as loneliness or depression. These emotions become so intense that some individuals attempt suicide. Abraham reported a study of 133 individuals with prior history of LSD use compared with 40 controls (Abraham, 1983). Over 50 percent of LSD users admitted to visual disturbances labelled as "flashbacks" one week or more after last exposure to the drug. Geometric pseudohallucinations, perceptions in the peripheral field, flashes of color, and intensification of colors were most commonly described. Control subjects reported significantly fewer symptoms. Flashbacks have occurred as great as five years after discontinuation of LSD. Benzodiazepines have been suggested as a treatment to reduce these episodes.

A number of psychiatric disturbances have been attributed to the use of LSD. Prolonged abuse has been associated with four distinct psychiatric conditions: (1) prolonged psychosis, (2) depression, (3) personality disruption, and (4) post-hallucinogen perceptual disorder. Although not life-threatening in itself, LSD can also cause acute panic episodes often labeled as the "bad trip" (Ungerleider, Fisher, and Fuller, 1966; Ungerleider et al., 1968). These may occur after just one use. The reaction manifests as frightening illusions and hallucinations, overwhelming anxiety, destructive behavior such as jumping out a window, depression and suicidality, and paranoid delusions. There have been studies evaluating the link between LSD use and the development of schizophrenia or affective disorders. Hensala evaluated users and nonusers in an inpatient psychiatric setting and concluded that LSD was not responsible for the development of psychiatric disorder (Hensala, Epstein, and Blacker, 1967). Bowers failed to find differences in age of symptom onset or hospitalization in schizophrenics using LSD versus nonusers (Bowers, 1977). Vardy and Kay reported that patients who presented with a schizophrenic picture within two weeks of LSD use were similar to nonuser schizophrenics in terms of genealogy, phenomenology, and course of illness (Vardy and Kay, 1983). Taken together, there appears to be no relation between LSD use and the induction of schizophrenia, though it could precipitate or accelerate pre-existing psychiatric illness.

Genetic

There is some debate over the potential chromosomal and teratogenic effects of LSD use. In vitro studies in leukocytes revealed LSD-induced chromosomal damage (Cohen, Marinello, and Back, 1967). However, a similar rate of chromosomal breakage was observed in drug and nondrug situations (Gilmour et al., 1971). Furthermore, no clear relationship between the chromosomal damage and increased rate of birth defects has been demonstrated. In 1972, Dishotsky et al. published an article in *Science* titled "LSD and Genetic Damage—Is LSD Chromosome Damaging, Carcinogenic, Mutagenic, or Teratogenic?" The publication evaluated 68 studies and case reports between 1967 and 1972 and concluded that there was no link between moderate LSD use and in vivo chromosomal damage or detectable genetic damage (Dishotsky et al., 1972).

Adverse Effects of LSD

Cardiovascular

At typical recreational doses of 1 to 6 μg/kg, LSD exerts minimal cardiovascular effects. Controlled observational studies of schizophrenic patients dosed with LSD have shown mild elevation of blood pressure and heart rate (Forrer and Goldner, 1951). These changes occur approximately one to two hours after oral dosing. Rinkel et al. reported similar findings (Rinkel et al., 1955). Even with LSD overdose, cardiovascular parameters are not significantly compromised. Eight patients treated at San Francisco General Hospital for massive LSD overdose presented to the emergency with sinus tachycardia and transient hypertension both of which resolved. All subjects survived the event (Klock, Boerner, and Becker, 1973).

Neurologic

A number of interesting observations have been reported after LSD use. Flushing and salivation are common features of acute LSD intoxication. The appearance of salivation appears to be correlated to the dose (higher doses cause more salivation). Ophthalmic signs include pupillary dilatation, lacrimation, and conjunctival injection at higher doses. Almost all individuals exhibit pupillary dilatation. This reaction is also dose-related and occurs after oral but not topical application. These autonomic nervous system signs peak at two to three hours post dosing (Forrer and Goldner, 1951). Other notable features of LSD intoxication include hyperreflexia with a dose-dependent relationship to a knee jerk reflex test and gait instability. At every high doses, subjects can become comatose (Klock, Boerner, and Becker, 1973).

Respiratory

The effects of LSD on the respiratory system are minimal unless very high doses are taken. Forrer and Goldner's studies of LSD at a dose of 1 to 6 μg/kg show no change in respiratory status (Forrer and Goldner, 1951). With massive overdoses, respiratory arrest requiring intubation was seen in half of the patients. Aspiration was also reported in a few of these patients. All intubated subjects were eventually extubated and survived the overdose (Klock, Boerner, and Becker, 1973).

Hematologic

Two major hematologic parameters which appear to be altered by LSD are white blood cell (WBC) counts and platelet function. Platelet activity is mediated in part by serotonin receptor activity (Michael, 1969). Inhibition of this system can lead to prolonged bleeding. In the cases of massive LSD overdose, coagulopathy related to platelet dysfunction was observed in all patients (Klock, Boerner, and Becker, 1973). Blood specimens obtained in the emergency room showed an absence of clot retraction. Generalized bleeding in the form of hematuria, guaiac positive stools and emesis, and post-venipuncture oozing was also seen. No alteration in WBC count was reported. At a lower dose of 1 µg/kg, WBC counts increased. After six weeks, both WBC count and hemoglobin were similar to baseline.

PHENCYCLIDINE (PCP)

Overview

Phencyclidine (PCP, 1-(1-phenylcyclohexyl) piperidine) is an arylcyclohexylamine hallucinogen that possesses stimulant, depressant, and analgesic properties. It acts at both central and peripheral sites to produce a myriad of effects. The hallmark signs and symptoms of PCP intoxication are hallucinations, nystagmus, violent behavior, and sensory anesthesia. PCP has been shown to inhibit the GABA system to deregulate dopaminergic tracts (Shepherd and Jagoda, 1990). It binds to cortical and limbic NDMA-type glutamate receptors which are implicated in ischemic neuronal cell death (O'Brien, 2001). This understanding has lead to the development of PCP analogs that block NDMA receptors and may have therapeutic value as a protective agent in post-stroke ischemia/reperfusion injury. In addition, PCP stimulates the adrenergic system potentiating the pressor response to norepinephrine, epinephrine, and serotonin leading to profound cardiovascular instability (Litovitz, 1998). Pressor effects appear to be related to PCP's alpha-adrenergic receptor stimulation and direct blood vessel vasospastic properties (Shepherd and Jagoda, 1990).

History

PCP was first synthesized in 1926 and was introduced as a human anesthetic in the mid-1950s. Also during this time, it was evaluated as a treatment for schizophrenia. It enjoyed a short-lived two-year stint as a surgical analgesic and anesthetic but was withdrawn because of a number of psychological side effects. PCP then emerged as a tranquilizer and anesthetic in animals and at the same time appeared as a street drug under the names "angel dust," "hog," and "super-weed." Between the early and late 1970s, it was placed in Schedule III of the Controlled Substance Act and is currently a Schedule I drug. Its use peaked in the late 1970s and declined in the 1980s. There has been some resurgence in PCP's illicit use in the 1990s. In some parts of the country PCP is added to marijuana "joints" and smoked as a mixture called "fry." Data from drug monitoring sources indicate that use of PCP in this manner may be increasing in frequency (Peters et al., 2005).

Psychologic Effects

Like many other hallucinogens, the psychological effects of PCP are dose-dependent. Reports are available from both formal clinical studies and toxicology case reports. Studies in healthy volunteers are abundant owing to early human investigation of PCP as an anesthetic. There is some variability in response among healthy subjects. Intravenous administration of doses between 5 and 15 mg in healthy volunteers produced apathy and altered proprioception as well as depression, altered body image, and hostility (Luby et al., 1959). Six of twelve normal volunteers who received 0.075 mg/kg to 0.10 mg/kg intravenously had nausea and vomiting (Davies and Beech, 1960). Other studies in healthy subjects have reported delirium, mental confusion, hallucinations, apathy, and feelings of isolation at 10 mg (Domino, 1964). At intravenous doses of 0.275 to 0.44 mg/kg, anesthesia could be produced lasting approximately 30 minutes. However, the authors also observed postoperative confusion and hallucinations (Gool and Clarke, 1964). Violent and manic behavior was reported in a few patients.

The presentation of an acutely poisoned PCP patient or a PCP overdose can be quite different from those obtained during moderate dosing. Its popularity as a drug of abuse owes to its euphoric properties. A study of PCP smokers revealed that it caused body image distortion, dizziness, apathy, and double vision, accompanied by feelings of either talkativeness or detachment (Lundberg, Gupta, and Montgomery, 1976). The acute mental state as described by Luisada et al. recounts an epidemic in Washington, DC, involving multiple mental health facility admissions for PCP-related psychosis (Luisada, 1977). These acute psychotic reactions were characterized by several days of confusion, paranoid ideation, insomnia, and intermittent restlessness. Abusers are prone to both risky and violent behavior.

> Family members generally described the pre-admission periods as characterized by continuous insomnia, tension, hyperactivity, and intermittent unexpected aggressive behavior, bizarre paranoid delusions, ideas of reference, delusion of being controlled by others, grandiosity, but no fixed or systematized delusional system. (Luisada, 1977 in Peterson R.C.; and Stillman, S.C.)

Long-term use of PCP may lead to memory gaps, disorientation, visual disturbances, and difficulty with speech (Cohen, 1977). Tolerance and dependence can also develop with long-term exposure. Fearfulness, tremors, and facial twitches follow abrupt withdrawal in monkeys. In humans, this can lead to anxiety, nervousness, and antisocial behavior (Peterson and Stillman, 1978).

Adverse Effects of PCP

Cardiovascular

The cardiovascular consequences of PCP abuse are related to its potentiation of noradrenergic and adrenergic activity as well as direct sympathomimetic action on the alpha-adrenergic receptor. Hypertension is seen in nearly two-thirds of patients taking PCP with a mean systolic increase of 26 mg Hg and a mean diastolic increase of 19 mg Hg (Aniline and Pitts, 1982). Hypertensive crises after high doses have also been reported with consequent intracerebral hemorrhage found at autopsy (Bessen, 1982; Eastman and Cohen, 1975; McCarron et al., 1981). Accompanying tachycardia is noted among these patients. The mechanism of these effects is multiple as described in previous text and includes both direct vasospastic as well as dopaminergic activities. Cardiovascular complications are usually seen at doses above 20 mg. Cardiac arrest is rare among PCP abusers though it does provoke negative, chronotropic, and inotropic effects in isolated myocardial cells (Ilett et al., 1966). Cholinergic muscarinic interaction appears to explain this myocardial effect (Fosset et al., 1979).

Neurologic

The neurologic manifestations of PCP intoxication and overdose are responsible for much of the significant morbidity and mortality seen with this drug. At low doses (<5 mg), signs and symptoms include catatonic rigidity, nystagmus, hyperacousis, and loss of pinprick response. At moderate doses

(5-10 mg), coma or stupor, myoclonus and repetitive motor movements, muscle rigidity upon stimulation, and decreased peripheral sensation are observed. At high doses (>10 mg), prolonged coma lasting 12 hours to days, decerebrate posturing, muscle rigidity, tonic-clonic seizures, diminished gag and corneal reflexes are encountered (Aronow and Done, 1978). Pupillary dilatation may be present during mild to moderate coma though mydriasis is not common and its absence among PCP users distinguishes them from those using other hallucinogens (Bailey, 1979; McCarron et al., 1981). Diaphoresis, flushing, hypersalivation, and miosis often observed at moderate to high doses are related to the cholinergic stimulation. Death from direct intoxication usually results from seizures or from violent behavior, and may include sudden death during physical restraint (e.g., in police custody) (Crosley and Binet, 1979; Fauman and Fauman, 1979; Kessler et al., 1974).

Respiratory

The anesthesiology literature provides valuable information regarding the effects of PCP on respiratory function. Minimal changes in both respiratory rate and tidal volume have been reported with high doses (0.25 mg/kg) (Bakker and Amini, 1961; Greifenstein et al., 1958). Massive doses (500 mg) can lead to hypoventilation and respiratory arrest. Respiratory failure may also be secondary to aspiration pneumonia (McCarron et al., 1981). Strap and masseter muscle spasm helps maintain airway patency though care should be taken to avoid laryngeal and pharyngeal spasm during suctioning and intubation (McCarron et al., 1981).

Renal

PCP abuse has been associated with acute renal failure. The two major mechanisms responsible for renal impairment include increased muscle activity and hyperthermia. Both predispose patients to rhabdomyolysis, which is the breakdown of muscle fibers leading to the release of myoglobin into the blood. The myoglobin is toxic to the proximal tubules leading to acute tubular necrosis. A diagnosis of rhabdomyolysis is established by the presence of elevated plasma creatine kinase (CPK) and urinary and plasma myoglobin. The incidence of rhabdomyolysis in PCP intoxicated patients seen in the emergency room is estimated at 1 percent to 2.5 percent. Peak CPK levels are usually between 180,000 and 200,000 (Cogen et al., 1978). Of those who do present with rhabdomyolysis, two-thirds are oliguric or anuric and half require dialysis (Patel and Connor, 1985-86). Akmal et al. reported a 40 percent incidence of renal failure and a 30 percent incidence of renal impairment in patients with rhabdomyolysis (Akmal et al., 1981). Increased muscle activity resulting from tonic-clonic seizures as well as muscle rigidity and isometric contractions contributes to elevated levels of CPK (Goode and Meltzer, 1975). Studies in rats have shown that restraints increased CPK levels in PCP-treated animals and that denervation eliminated these effects (Konel and Meltzer, 1974). Interestingly, a majority of patients with PCP-induced rhabdomyolysis had been restrained during the acute intoxication. In addition, paralysis with pancuronium leads to a rapid reduction in CPK levels (Cogen et al., 1978). Hyperthermia is a second mechanism of CPK elevation among PCP users. Muscle breakdown secondary to malignant hyperthermia has been reported in the literature (Rowland and Penn, 1972). McCarron reports an incidence rate for PCP-associated hyperthermia of 2.6 percent with temperatures as high as 108°F. (McCarron et al., 1981). Treatments for PCP-induced rhabdomyolysis include intravenous hydration, close monitoring of CPK levels and renal function, paralysis in severe cases, and dialysis if renal function is profoundly impaired.

MESCALINE AND PEYOTE

Overview

The peyote plant, *Lophophora williamsii,* is a member of the Cactaceae family and represents one of the oldest known hallucinogenic drugs. The cactus is orally ingested as buttons and has been used in rituals among North American Indians dating back several thousand years. Its main active ingredient, mescaline, is a trimethoxy-substituted phenethylamine, which is structurally analogous to epinephrine. Since the elucidation of its chemical structure, a number of structural analogs have been synthesized and studied, and their psychological properties described (Shulgin, 1979; Shulgin and Shulgin, 2000). Mescaline's mechanism of action is not completely understood though it is thought that the drug affects serotonergic, noradrenergic, and dopaminergic systems (Buchanan and Brown, 1988). Like other hallucinogens, mescaline's psychedelic properties are mediated through interaction with the 5HT2a serotonin receptor. Its close structural analogy to catecholamines may contribute to some of its sympathomimetic properties.

History

Archeological evidence dates human peyote use as far back as 3,000 years. Peyote use was widespread among many different Indian groups including the Aztec, Apache, and Pima for religious, ceremonial, and medicinal purposes (Schaefer, 1997; Schaefer and Bauml, 1997). During the age of Spanish colonization, peyote was demonized as a diabolical root by clergymen who tried to suppress its consumption. A description of peyote's history is detailed by several authors (Kapadia and Fayez, 1970).

Mescaline was first isolated by Hefter in 1896 but it was not until Spath's chemical synthesis in 1919 that its chemical structure was confirmed (Heffter, 1897; Spath, 1919). Human mescaline experiments were discovered within the Nazi Dachau concentration camp records in the late 1940s, and around the same time the U.S. Navy also began conducting human studies. In the 1960s, mescaline became a popular hallucinogen during the psychedelic movement. Over 250 chemical analogs of mescaline were prepared and self-tested by Shulgin between the 1960s and 1990s (Shulgin and Shulgin, 2000). In 1970, mescaline along with other hallucinogens was placed in Schedule I of the Controlled Substance Act. Related chemical derivatives were included in this scheduling. Despite mescaline's Schedule I status, peyote and mescaline use, as part of a religious ceremony within the Native American Church, is exempt from prosecution.

Psychologic Effects of Mescaline

Perhaps, the best descriptions of mescaline's hallucinogenic effects are provided by Shulgin based mostly on personal experimentation (Shulgin and Shulgin, 2000). The usual dose of the sulfate salt is between 300 and 500 mg orally. The psychedelic experience can last up to 12 hours.

> During the next two to three hours, there is the development of a sensory responsiveness, largely expressed by color enhancement and imagery of many sorts. A benign attitude is taken towards nature with the user experiencing feelings of benevolent and comfortable acceptance of sounds, images, animals and inanimate objects. Imagery can be fanciful and visual interpretations can assume profound significance. From the fifth to the eighth hour, there is a gentle recovery that allows personal integration of these stimuli into a peaceful and restful state of mind. There is rarely any sleep disturbance or any tiredness the following day. (Shulgin, 1979, p. 355)

This description is similar to that of Aldous Huxley's in *The Door of Perception*. Sensory alterations in the form of visual hallucinations are normally experienced a few hours after ingestion. Color, geometric imagery, and altered color and texture perception are described. Although Shulgin recounts a generally peaceful experience after mescaline use, some individuals may feel anxiety, paranoia, and emotional lability though this is a rare event (Zevin and Benowitz, 1998). Unlike LSD, mescaline use is not accompanied by late flashbacks, psychosis, or other delayed psychological effects.

Adverse Effects of Mescaline

Cardiovascular

Mescaline's effects on blood pressure and heart rate are dose and species dependent. In cats and dogs, dose-related hypotension is seen while in rats, a pressor response occurs (Orzechowski and Goldstein, 1973). In rabbits, mescaline produces bradycardia. The human response to mescaline is also variable. At low doses (4 mg/kg), very little change in cardiovascular parameters is observed (Speck, 1957). At doses seen among mescaline users, autonomic adrenergic stimulation results in elevated systolic blood pressure and mild tachycardia (Leikin et al., 1989). High doses produce hypotension, bradycardia, and respiratory depression (Grace, 1934). Cardiovascular collapse, or respiratory failure, resulting in death has not been reported with mescaline use.

Neurologic

Similar to other hallucinogens, mescaline possesses autonomic sympathomimetic properties. Users present with mydriasis, diaphoresis, and hyperreflexia. Photophobia secondary to pupillary dilatation along with ataxia, nystagmus, tremors, and hyperreflexia may also be seen (Shulgin, 1979).

Gastrointestinal

When ingested in large quantities, mescaline often causes nausea, vomiting, and abdominal pain (Teitelbaum and Wingeleth, 1977). The abdominal pain can last several days and may mimic acute gastroenteritis, pancreatitis, or an acute abdomen. Abdominal pain is often described as, "crampy" and can be accompanied by diarrhea. Fortunately, the condition is self-limiting and requires mainly supportive care. Nausea and vomiting may also occur and usually do so within the first hour of ingestion when blood levels are the highest. This may explain the low incidence of true mescaline overdose as much of it is expelled prior to absorption into systemic circulation. Strategies for avoiding these effects include ingesting peyote buttons individually over the course of several hours and thus avoiding a high peak level of mescaline in the plasma. The extracts are also been ground, diluted into a tea, and sipped over the course of 30 minutes or more.

Pregnancy

Mescaline use has been linked to both low postpartum birth weights and teratogenicity in animals but the evidence in humans is less clear. Geber and Schramm have shown that pups of mescaline treated mothers are similar in weight to controls at birth but lose weight as the growth period continues (Geber and Schramm, 1974). Pregnant hamsters administered mescaline on the seventh through tenth days of gestation demonstrated a dose-dependent decrease in reproductive success, resulting in diminished litter size (Hirsch and Fritz, 1981). Delay in ossification of the skull, sternum, and metatarsals has also been noted in mescaline treated groups. Despite these findings, there has been no definitive evidence of mescaline-associated teratogenicity or increased rate of birth defects in humans. Dorrance et al. compared the lymphocyte chromosomal abnormalities of 57 Huichol Indians who were regular users of peyote with nonuser Huichol Indian controls located in a different area of Mexico (Dorrance, Janiger, and Teplitz, 1975). No difference in the frequency of chromosomal breaks or abnormalities was reported between the two groups. The report also mentioned that the physician caring for these Huichol Indians had observed pregnant women using peyote on a regular basis without an apparent increase in the rate of congenital defects. The peyote alkaloids can find their way into breast milk. It has been reported that colicky babies become happy and begin to grab at invisible things in the air after being breast fed by mothers who used peyote alkaloids.

METHYLENEDIOXYMETHAMPHETAMINE (MDMA)

Overview

MDMA is a ring-substituted amphetamine derivative. In its pure form, it is a white crystalline powder. MDMA is similar in structure to methamphetamine with the addition of the methylenedioxy ($-O-CH_2-O-$) group attached to positions 3 and 4 of the aromatic ring of the methamphetamine molecule. MDMA exists as two enantiomers, both the R and S (d- and l-) forms. It has been suggested that the S enantiomer contributes to "amphetamine-like" effects while the R enantiomer gives more hallucinogenic and empathogenic qualities to the experience. These suggestions are based on dose-response curves for changes in serotonergic and other monoamine functions. In vitro studies indicate that MDMA releases CNS monoamine neurotransmitters via "calcium-independent release" while also inhibiting the reuptake of monoamines: dopamine, norepinephrine and, particularly, serotonin (5-HT). Despite this effect on multiple neurotransmitter systems the centrally mediated hallucinogenic or empathogenic effects are thought to be mediated mainly by altered 5-HT neurotransmission (Kalant, 2001; Shulgin, 1986). Compared with the hallucinogenic phenethylamine, mescaline, and LSD which exert their effects on the postsynaptic 5-HT receptors, MDMA causes presynaptic release of 5-HT while also inhibiting its reuptake. Radioisotope studies have shown that MDMA may enter the presynaptic terminal via the same receptor that selective serotonin reuptake inhibitors (SSRIs) block. Accordingly, there are case reports in which patients have had the effects of MDMA attenuated while taking SSRIs (Liechti et al., 2000).

History

MDMA was originally synthesized in 1912 and patented by Merck Pharmaceuticals in 1914 for use as a precursor from which to synthesize other research chemicals, ultimately with the goal of finding an efficacious and marketable appetite suppressant (Henry, 1992). Although MDMA never gained commercial interest in this respect it became popular for other reasons. In 1978, in a report called *The Psychopharmacology of Hallucinogens,* Shulgin and Nichols reported that ingestion of MDMA caused heightened emotional awareness with significant "sensual overtones" (Shulgin and Nichols, 1978). Subsequently, it was suggested that MDMA may have use as an adjuvant to psychotherapy. Through the 1970s into the 1980s MDMA was used by psychiatrists as well as therapists for a variety of indications including treatment of alcohol dependence, marriage counseling, and chronic depression. The popularity of MDMA spread and recreational use surfaced in the 1980s. MDMA's recreational popularity coincided with the development of a rave "dance-club" culture that grew in popularity through the 1980s and 1990s. During a "rave" MDMA is ingested to fuel all-night marathon dance sessions in which special effects such as lights and laser shows coincide with fast paced "techno" music. MDMA became commonly referred to as Ecstasy, X, E, XTC, Adam, and multiple other "street" or slang terms. As recreational use increased, the Drug Enforcement Administration (DEA) issued an emergency scheduling and in April 1985 MDMA became a Schedule I drug—similar to heroin, PCP, and LSD. Drugs placed under Schedule I are thought to have a strong potential for abuse and dependence and no medical utility. MDMA was the first drug scheduled under this emergency scheduling act. The decision to place MDMA under Schedule I restrictions was partly based on research with the MDMA congener, the N-demethylated analog, methylenedioxyamphetamine (MDA), which Ricaurte demonstrated had toxic effects on brain serotonin neurons in rodents (Ricaurte, Bryan, et al., 1985; Ricaurte, Finnegan, et al., 1985). In addition, there was increasing public exposure to MDMA. Although basic science research suggested neurotoxicity the popular media published articles which generally recounted favorable MDMA experiences. A 1985 article in *Newsweek* magazine reported, "This was the drug LSD was supposed to be, coming 20 years too late to save the world" (referring to the idea that MDMA would promote peace, tranquillity, and facilitate communication among those who used it). Also, at this time the first emergency department visits for adverse effects of MDMA ingestion were being reported.

Since this ruling, however, the FDA has allowed limited human research studies with MDMA to proceed. Ongoing research with MDMA involves its use as an adjunctive agent to palliative care in terminally ill cancer and HIV patients. Though classified by U.S. law as a hallucinogen MDMA is part of a newer class of synthetic amphetamine derivatives in which, while hallucinations may be present, feelings of empathy and euphoria predominate; the terms "empathogens" and "enactogens" (to touch within) are used to describe MDMA and similar drugs (e.g., MDA).

Despite claims that MDMA use is "epidemic" there is limited data on longitudinal use patterns. In 1999 the Monitoring the Future Survey (MTF, from the U.S. National Institute on Drug Abuse) found that 5.6 percent of high school seniors had used MDMA at least once. In addition, while overall use of illicit drugs had declined since 1999 in all age groups, the use of MDMA had increased. In 1987, Peroutka studied a randomly selected group of 369 U.S. college undergraduates. Thirty-nine percent of them reported use of MDMA at least once (range from 1 to 38 times) (Peroutka, 1987). Although data from the Drug Abuse Warning Network (DAWN), MTF, and the National Household Survey on Drug Abuse (NHSDA) note increased use of MDMA, its prevalence is significantly less than other drugs of abuse (Yacoubian, 2003).

MDMA is available in capsule form, in pressed pills, or as loose powder. The current (2005) average cost ranges from $10 to $30 (U.S.) per dose (www.erowid.com and www.bluelight.nu/vb/home/php). Cost has decreased over the past five years as purity has diminished and other substituted amphetamines have gained popularity. MDMA is most commonly taken orally; however, it is absorbed across any mucous membrane, and there are reports of intranasal, rectal, intravaginal as well as intravenous use.

Physiologic Effects of MDMA

When MDMA is taken by mouth effects manifest in approximately 30 to 45 minutes; while snorting or injecting results in much quicker onset of effects. The primary effects usually reach a plateau at two to three hours post ingestion and diminish in intensity over the next three to four hours. In the peripheral nervous system MDMA releases norepinephrine (NE). Tachycardia, hypertension, sweating, mydriasis, and other signs of sympathetic autonomic stimulation are typical. The physical effects of usual doses (75-150 mg) of MDMA are subtle and variable: some users report dryness of mouth, jaw clenching, teeth grinding (trismus), nystagmus, sweating, or nausea. Others report feelings of profound physical relaxation. Users generally describe a ceiling effect for the desired "empathogenic" response to MDMA. At higher doses the physical effects of MDMA resemble those of amphetamines: fast or pounding heartbeat, sweating, dizziness, restlessness, etc. Pharmacodynamic tolerance may develop and some users ingest increasingly higher doses subsequently causing sympathetic stimulation to predominate.

Two prospective studies in the literature describe the physiologic as well as behavioral effects of MDMA. The first study, by Downing, assessed the cardiovascular, biochemical, and neurobehavioral effects of the single dose administration of MDMA. Twenty-one healthy volunteers with previous MDMA experience received a dose ranging between 1.75 and 4.18 mg/kg of body weight (average dose of 2.5 mg/kg or 175 mg for a 70 kg individual). Acute effects (time of ingestion to three hours post ingestion) included: euphoria, increased feelings of energy, emotional stimulation, increased sensual awareness, and anorexia. The majority of patients in this study experienced trismus, increased deep tendon reflexes and gait instability. No residual effects were documented in this group (Downing, 1986).

In another study involving 29 separate clinical sessions volunteers were given between 75 and 150 mg of MDMA. This dose was given after a six hour fast. After the effects of the first dose began to subside a second dose of 50 to 75 mg was offered. This study was part of "couple's therapy" and all individuals involved in these sessions reported increased closeness and facilitation of communication with their partner. The other 8 sessions were part of a "psychotherapeutic adjunct" to a clinical session. All 29 patients reported positive emotional changes and 22 of 29 reported "cognitive benefits" including: "an expanded mental perspective, insight into personal patterns or problems, improved self-examination or intrapsychic communication skills or issue resolution." All patients reported some adverse effects associated with MDMA use: 28 had symptoms of anorexia, 22 had trismus or bruxism, 9 described nausea, 8 complained of muscle aches or stiffness and 3 had ataxia. Twenty-three complained of fatigue of varying duration and 11 had subsequent insomnia. One patient, with a remote history of panic attacks, had recurrence of intermittent episodes of panic after this MDMA session

(Greer and Tolbert, 1986). To place the study doses mentioned previously in context, a usual "recreational" dose of MDMA generally ranges from 75 to 150 milligrams (orally) (Kalant, 2001).

Adverse Effects of MDMA

Psychologic

Most MDMA users describe feelings of closeness with others and empathy. They also claim that it increases the desire to move (e.g., dance). Most of the psychotropic effects are attributed to MDMA's action at the 5-HT synapses. Physical dependence has not been reported with MDMA; however psychological dependence (as seen with methamphetamine and cocaine) may lead to compulsive use. Tolerance develops with repeated use of MDMA and chronic users report diminished effects even after periods of abstinence. Reports of adverse neuropsychiatric effects include: anxiety, insomnia, and panic attacks. Depression is a common finding in the days following MDMA use as well as anxiety and irritability (Curran and Travill, 1997; Parrott et al., 2002). This has been commonly referred to as the "Tuesday Blues"—after MDMA use on a Friday or Saturday night. It is postulated that certain populations may be at increased risk for neuropsychiatric complications from MDMA particularly those taking repeatedly high doses of MDMA as well as users with underlying psychiatric disorders and those using multiple psychotropic substances.

Cardiovascular

The cardiovascular effects of MDMA were assessed in a double-blind placebo controlled trial. Patients received either oral MDMA or placebo one hour prior to echocardiographic assessment and serial vital sign measurement. The patients had previously received a dobutamine echocardiogram. A dose of 1.5 mg/kg MDMA increased mean heart rate by 28 beats/minute, systolic blood pressure by 25 mm Hg, diastolic blood pressure by 7 mm Hg, and cardiac output by 2 liters/minute. These effects were comparable to 20 and 40 mcg/kg per minute of dobutamine in this group of subjects (Lester et al., 2000).

Cardiac abnormalities reported after emergency department presentation following MDMA use are rare but have included arrhythmias and asystole (Dowling, McDonough, and Bost, 1987; Henry, Jeffreys, and Dawling, 1992) as well as cardiorespiratory arrest (Suarez and Riemersma, 1988). In one series describing drug-related deaths attributed to MDMA, in 81 percent of 71 deaths the patients were found with asystole at the scene (Patel et al., 2004). Atrial fibrillation in a previously healthy adolescent was reported after ingestion of MDMA (Madhok, Boxer, and Chowdhury, 2003). Myocardial hypertrophy is a well-recognized complication of cocaine and methamphetamine abuse and is a strong, independent risk factor for sudden death, myocardial infarction, and congestive heart failure. A recent retrospective case-control series found significant increases in heart size in MDMA-positive deaths compared with matched MDMA-negative controls. This study suggested that MDMA users might also be at risk for cardiac toxicity from MDMA, similar to other stimulants. The etiology of cardiotoxicity associated with MDMA may be mediated by a sustained high level of catecholamines. However, other factors, like the direct toxic effects of MDMA and its metabolites on cardiac myocytes, remain to be investigated (Patel et al., 2005).

Neurologic

There is experimental evidence that MDMA administered in large doses and/or repeatedly causes partial loss of serotonergic neurons in laboratory animals. It is uncertain is whether this loss is permanent, reversible, or clinically important. In a study by Ricuarte, nonhuman primates were dosed with MDMA and their brains were examined for morphological changes. Ricaurte found that there was no effect after 2.5 mg/kg oral doses given every two weeks, for a total of eight doses. However, after a single oral dose of 5 mg/kg, he observed a 20 percent reduction in serotonin and its metabolite 5-HIAA, but only in the thalamus and hypothalamus. There appeared to be some regrowth of neurons over time, although not necessarily complete, and also some "collateral sprouting" growth of other types of neurons in the reduced serotonin areas (Ricaurte, 1989). Confounding and clouding research on the neurotoxicity of MDMA, however, are retractions of some of Ricaurte's experiments in which he reported irreversible damage and disappearance of dopaminergic axons and neurons from MDMA administration. It was discovered that he had used methamphetamine rather than MDMA as was originally reported in his experiments (Ricaurte et al., 2002, 2003).

The clinical relevance of MDMA's effect on 5-HT neurons remains unclear. In animal studies, even when there are quite large serotonin system reductions (up to 90 percent in high MDMA dose rat studies), behavioral deficits attributable to the reduction in serotonergic neurons have not been observed. One mechanism of action for the purported neurotoxicity of MDMA is via an increase in free radical production as evidenced by lipid peroxidation (a marker for free radical damage) on autopsy. Direct evidence that MDMA produces free radicals in the brain was provided by Colado and colleagues (Colado et al., 1997). Colado's group inserted a microdialysis probe into the hippocampus which was perfused with salicylic acid. MDMA was subsequently given peripherally and salicylate was converted to 2, 3-dihydroxybenzoic acid, a reaction only occurring in the presence of free radicals (Colado et al., 1997). Recently, there has been increased interest in positron emission tomography PET scans for studying the effects of various drugs on the CNS. In 14 previous MDMA users who were matched with 15 controls (who had never used MDMA) PET imaging conducted with a radiolabeled carbon-11 isotope (a selective binding ligand for the 5-HT transporter) demonstrated differences in binding characteristics between the previous MDMA users and controls. The MDMA users had diminished global and regional 5-HT transporter binding. The extent of decrease in 5-HT transporter binding correlated with extent of previous MDMA use. The clinical significance of this, however, remains unknown (McCann et al., 1998). Despite the reported effects of MDMA on serotonergic neurotransmission in both animals and man, its long-term effect on the human brain is unknown.

Fatal neurologic events or cases of permanent neurological injury after MDMA use are relatively uncommon but have been reported. These include subarachnoid hemorrhage, intracranial hemorrhage, cerebral infarction, and cerebral venous sinus thrombosis (Auer et al., 2002). Whether these complications are from transient hypertension, cerebral angiitis, dehydration, or are multifactorial remains to be elucidated (Green et al., 2003).

Seizures have been reported with MDMA ingestion. In one case a 14-month-old toddler accidentally ingested a portion of an MDMA pill. Forty-five minutes after ingestion the child suffered a generalized tonic-clonic seizure. Additional findings included hyperthermia, tachycardia, and other signs of autonomic stimulation, including mydriasis, hypertension, and diaphoresis (Melian et al., 2004). In a retrospective review of 32 MDMA ingestions three patients were admitted to the hospital after seizures. The amount of MDMA ingested was reported: "from 1 to 3 tabs of 150 mg MDMA." In addition to seizures these three patients also had hyponatremia, metabolic acidosis, rhabdomyolysis and impaired liver and renal function. All three recovered with supportive care (Ben-Abraham et al., 2003). Animal studies demonstrate that high doses of MDMA cause seizures in rats, dogs, and monkeys.

Multiple cases of cerebral edema have been reported after MDMA ingestion and unrestricted water intake. The etiology of the cerebral edema is thought to be secondary to MDMA-induced syndrome of inappropriate antidiuretic hormone secretion SIADH concomitant with excess free water intake. Hyponatremia ensues and serum osmolality falls thus leaving CNS cells susceptible to fluid shifts and swelling (Matthai et al., 1996).

Hyperthermia and MDMA

Hyperthermia is a serious adverse effect associated with MDMA ingestion. In rodents, primates, and humans MDMA produces dose-dependent hyperthermia which is potentially fatal. The mechanism for MDMA-induced hyperthermia is thought to be multifactorial including sympathetic stimulation as well as derangements in serotonin regulation (which is important in thermoregulation). Hyperpyrexia is often aggravated by extreme exertion (e.g., marathon dance sessions) in locations with high ambient temperatures, close proximity to multitudes of people, and decreased water intake (Green et al., 2003). Users may not initially be aware of pyrexia as MDMA may block or attenuate noxious or unpleasant stimuli.

Under normal ambient conditions MDMA administration in rats produces a hyperthermic response of approximately 1 to 2°C with a peak temperature increase 40 to 60 minutes after injection (Nash, 1988). Various other studies have found that ambient temperature plays a crucial role in thermoregulation with both hypothermic and hyperthermic responses depending on the ambient temperature. When MDMA was given to rats at a temperature of 30°C the MDMA-treated rats had an evaporative water loss of 275 percent above control rats. Rectal temperature increased in these study animals as ambient temperature was changed from 10 to 20°C and finally to 30°C. Animals dosed at 10°C had a change of −2°C, whereas there was no change between MDMA and saline-treated animals at 20°C, and at 30°C a hyperthermic response of +2°C was observed (Gordon and Fogelson, 1994; Gordon, Watkinson et al., 1991; Green et al., 2003). An exaggerated hyperthermic response was noted when water deprivation and a change in cage construction to diminish evaporative heat loss were combined in animal models. These studies were designed to mimic conditions at dance parties or "raves" (Dafters, 1995; Gordon and Fogelson, 1994).

Hyperthermia often leads to secondary complications such as rhabdomyolysis, disseminated intravascular coagulation and multiorgan system failure.

Endocrine

Hyponatremia has been reported after MDMA ingestion, postulated to be secondary to a SIADH and unrestricted free water intake. Deaths have been reported. In isolated hypothalamic tissue in vitro studies, MDMA has been shown to stimulate release of both oxytoxcin and vasopressin, in a dose-dependent fashion (Forsling et al., 2001, 2002; Green et al., 2003). In a retrospective review of MDMA ingestion admitted to a London hospital, 17 patients, aged 15 to 26 years, were identified with hyponatremia. Ten of these patients were reported to have polydipsia prior to becoming ill. Serum sodium levels ranged between 107 mmol/l and 128 mmol/l. SIADH was identified as the etiology of hyponatremia in six of the patients based on urine and serum chemistries. Eleven of these 17 patients had seizures and altered mental status persisted for up to three days in some patients. Two patients ultimately died (Hartung et al., 2002). Budisavljevic reviewed the literature for MDMA-associated hyponatremia fatalities and found that young, premenopausal women were at highest risk for severe, symptomatic hypo-natremia from MDMA (Budisavljevic et al., 2003). Treatment of MDMA-associated hyponatremia depends on whether or not the patient is symp-tomatic. Hypertonic saline is recommended for symptomatic hyponatremia (seizures, altered mental status). In the review by Budisavljevic no patient treated with hypertonic saline died (Budisavljevic et al., 2003).

Gastrointestinal

Recurrent acute hepatitis has been reported after repeated use of MDMA. A 27-year-old was reported to have had an idiosyncratic reaction to MDMA (or a contaminant of the drug) based on symptoms and histological findings in association with two episodes of jaundice and hepatitis eight to ten days after ingestion of MDMA (Shearman et al., 1992). Henry and Jeffreys re-ported seven cases of hepatotoxicity, described as idiosyncratic toxic hepa-titis (Henry, Jeffreys, and Dawling, 1992). In a review of eight patients with MDMA-associated hepatotoxicity, histological examination showed wide-spread microvesicular fatty change in two patients, massive lobular col-lapse in four, and lobular hepatitis with cholestasis in two. Four of these patients died (Ellis et al., 1996).

Renal

Acute renal failure has been associated with severe MDMA intoxication. As described in previous text, the etiology is multifactorial—intravascular volume depletion from dehydration, rhabdomyolysis, and hyperthermia. Other abnormalities have also been reported. Kwon reported a case of tran-sient proximal tubular renal injury following MDMA ingestion (Kwon, Zaritsky, and Dharnidharka, 2003).

Drug Interactions and MDMA

Deaths have been reported when MDMA has been ingested along with monoamine oxidase inhibitors (MAOIs)—both as prescription agents and as part of a recreational "cocktail" (e.g., drugs with MAOI properties). The serotonin syndrome and drug-induced hyperthermia have been implicated as causes of death. There are case reports of hypertensive crisis from this interaction (Copeland, Dillon, and Gascoigne, 2006; Smilkstein, Smolinske, and Rumack, 1987).

SSRIs interact with MDMA in that they are thought to block the action of MDMA if ingested prior to MDMA by inhibiting its neuronal uptake at the presynaptic 5-HT receptor. Users describe decreased effects of MDMA when taken after or in conjunction with their SSRI (e.g., citalopram, fluoxetine, and sertraline) (Green et al., 2003; Liechti et al., 2000; and Stein, 1999).

MDMA often contains adulterants or is misrepresented and replaced with another substance entirely. Common adulterants include: methamphetamine, amphetamine, caffeine, dextromethorphan, ketamine, ephedrine, pseudoephedrine, and prior to the FDA banning of its sale, phenylpropanolamine. PMA (paramethoxyamphetamine) has been sold as MDMA and several deaths due to hyperthermia and subsequent multiorgan system failure after ingestion of PMA have been reported (Dams et al., 2003; Martin, 2001).

Pharmacokinetics of MDMA

The half-life of MDMA is from six to eight hours with metabolism occurring mainly in the liver. After oral administration MDMA achieves peak plasma concentration in about two hours (Kalant, 2001). MDMA is metabolized by the cytochrome P450 system. Although CYP2D6 has been reported to be responsible for most of the metabolism of MDMA (via demethylation) other P450 isozymes have the capacity to contribute to the oxidative metabolism of MDMA (important for individuals genetically deficient in functional CYP2D6) and create a potential source for increased toxicity of MDMA via drug interaction by interruption of its metabolism. N-dealkylation, deamination, and oxidation to the corresponding benzoic acid derivatives subsequently conjugated with glycine are the other pathways for MDMA metabolism (de la Torre et al., 2004; Kreth et al., 2000). MDMA is metabolized by CYP2D6 by demethylation to 3, 4-dihydroxymethamphetamine (HHMA). HHMA is subsequently 0-methylated by catechol-o-methyltransferase (COMT) mainly to 4-hydroxy-3-methoxy-methamphetamine (HMA). These metabolites are then conjugated with glucuronic acid and excreted in the urine as the glucuronide or sulfate metabolites. In a pharmacokinetic study using patients phenotyped for CYP2D6 activity and classified as "extensive metabolizers" volunteers showed increases in MDMA concentration out of proportion to the increase in dose (50, 100, and finally 150 mg doses). The area under the curve (AUC) for MDMA was ten times that expected for a linear increase going from the 50 to 150 mg dose. This implies that relatively small increases in the dose of MDMA ingested may give rise to disproportionate rises in MDMA plasma concentrations and thus lead to increased risk for acute toxicity (de la Torre et al., 2000; Kalant, 2001).

Treatment of Hallucinogen and MDMA Associated Toxicity

Early recognition and understanding of possible complications is essential for treating the intoxicated patient. Care is supportive with respect to hallucinogen or MDMA-associated toxicity. Often these patients may present an agitated state. Benzodiazepines are the agent of first choice in an agitated patient with hallucinogen or MDMA ingestion. Benzodiazepines not only help reduce agitation, but they also often lower blood pressure and heart rate. Patients unable to protect their airway or at risk for aspiration should be intubated and mechanically ventilated. Blood pressure and cardiac monitoring should be regularly assessed. Hypertension can be treated with labetolol, vasodilating agents (e.g., nitroprusside), or direct alpha-adrenergic antagonists (phentolamine). Rapid determination of temperature and early treatment of hyperthermia are essential in preventing significant morbidity and mortality. Patients should receive adequate volume resuscitation (if they show signs of dehydration—pale skin, absence of sweating, elevated blood urea nitrogen and creatine) with normal saline. Evaporative cooling is the most effective means of reducing the temperature in these patients. Clothing should be removed and a fine mist sprayed over the patient with fans blowing across the body. If the patient shows signs of increased muscle tone such as tremor or rigidity, paralysis should be considered if treatment with benzodiazepines does not ameliorate the increased tone. Seizures should be treated with benzodiazepines. Lorazepam is an excellent agent for use in this situation. Seizures refractory to large doses of benzodiazepines should be treated with barbiturates (phenobarbital) or propofol. Propofol has shown promise in stopping seizures related to status epilepticus from refractory alcohol withdrawal and has been used successfully in gamma-hydroxybutyrate (GHB) withdrawal refractory to large doses of benzodiazepines (Wiegand, Smith, and Zvosec, 2005). Hyponatremia must be recognized early and correction of serum sodium at a rate of 1 to 2 mmol/hour is appropriate, unless the patient has seizures related to hyponatremia which necessitates more rapid correction. Hypertonic saline should be used for the symptomatic patient with

MDMA-associated hyponatremia. Rhabdomyolysis and acute renal failure will often respond to intravenous crystalloids (e.g., normal saline). Bicarbonate has been advocated for facilitating the clearance of myoglobin in these situations and often 2 to 3 amps of NaHCO3 are added to each liter of normal saline. The volume status of the patient, the serum sodium, and blood gas should be monitored closely in this situation.

SUMMARY AND CONCLUSIONS

The incidence of serious acute adverse events related to hallucinogen or MDMA ingestion is low. However, the unpredictability of these adverse events and the risk of mortality and substantial morbidity make the health consequences of these drugs a public health concern. In addition, the high prevalence of contaminants and adulterants (many of which have significant toxicity in and of themselves, e.g., paramethoxyamphetamine [PMA]) sold as MDMA contributes to the risk of recreational use of MDMA.

REFERENCES

Abraham, H.D. (1983). Visual phenomonology of the LSD flashback. *Arch Gen Psychiatry* 40: 884-889.

Akmal, M.; Valdin, J.R.; McCarron, M.M.; Massry, S.G. (1981). Rhabdomyolysis with and without acute renal failure in patients with phencyclidine intoxication. *Am J Nephrol* 1: 91-96.

Aniline, O.; Pitts, F.N. (1982). Phencyclidine (PCP): A review and perspectives. *CRC Crit Rev Toxicol* 10: 145-177.

Aronow, R.; Done, A.K. (1978). Phencyclidine overdose: An emerging concept of management. *JACEP* 7(2): 33-36.

Auer, J.; Berent, R.; Weber, T.; Lassnig, F.; Eber, B. (2002). Subarachnoid hemorrhage with "Ecstasy" abuse in a young adult. *Neurologic Sciences* 23(4): 199-201.

Bailey, D.N. (1979). Phencyclidine abuse: Clinical findings and concentrations in biological fluids after nonfatal intoxication. *Am J Clin Pathol* 72: 795-799.

Bakker, C.B.; Amini, F.B. (1961). Observations on the psychotomimetic effects of Sernyl. *Compr Psychiatry* 2: 269-180.

Ben-Abraham, R.; Szold, O.; Rudnick, V.; Weinbroum, A.A. (2003). "Ecstasy" intoxication: Life-threatening manifestations and resuscitative measures in the intensive care setting. *Eur J Emerg Med* 4: 309-313.

Bessen, H.A. (1982). Intracranial hemorrhage associated with phencyclidine abuse. *JAMA* 248(5): 585-586.

Boakes, R.J.; Bradley, P.B.; Briggs, I.; Dray, A. (1970). Antagonists of 5-hydroxytryptamine by LSD-25 in the central nervous system: A possible neuronal basis for the actions of LSD-25. *Br J Pharmacol* 40: 202-218.

Bowers, M.B., Jr. (1977). Psychoses precipitated by psychotomimetic drugs. A follow-up study. *Arch Gen Psychiatry* 34(7): 832-835.

Buchanan, J.F.; Brown, C.R. (1988). 'Designer drugs'. A problem in clinical toxicology. *Med Toxicol Adverse Drug Exp* 3: 1-17.

Budisavljevic, M.N.; Stewart, L.; Sahn, S.A.; Ploth, D.W. (2003). Hyponatremia associated with 3, 4-methylenedioxymethamphetamine ("Ecstasy") use. *Am J Med Sci* 326(2): 89-93.

Caldwell, J.; Sever, P.S. (1974). The biochemical pharmacology of abused drugs. I. Amphetamines, cocaine, and LSD. *Clin Pharmacol Ther* 16(4): 625-638.

Cogen, F.C.; Rigg, G.; Simmons, J.L.; Domino, F.F. (1978). Phencyclidine-associated acute rhabdomyolysis. *Ann Intern Med* 88: 210-212.

Cohen, M.M.; Marinello, M.J.; Back, N. (1967). Chromosomal damage in human leukocytes induced by lysergic acid diethylamine. *Science* 155: 1417-1419.

Cohen, S. (1977). Angel dust. *JAMA* 238(6): 515-516.

Colado, M.I.; O'shea, E.; Granados, R.; Murray, T.K.; Green, A.R. (1997). In vivo evidence for free radical involvement in the degeneration of rat brain 5-HT following administration of MDMA ("Ecstasy") and p-chloroamphetamine but not the degeneration following fenfluramine. *Br J Pharmacol* 121(5): 889-900.

Copeland, J.; Dillon, P.; Gascoigne, M. (2006). Ecstasy and the concomitant use of pharmaceuticals. *Addict Behav* 31: 367-370.

Crosley, C.J.; Binet, E.F. (1979). Cerebrovascular complications in phencyclidine intoxication. *J Pediatr* 94: 316-318.

Curran, H.V.; Travill, R.A. (1997). Mood and cognitive effects of +/−3, 4-methylenedioxymethamphetamine (MDMA, "Ecstasy"): Week-end "high" followed by mid-week low. *Addiction* 92(7): 821-831.

Dafters, R.I. (1995). Hyperthermia following MDMA administration in rats: Effects of ambient temperature, water consumption and chronic dosing. *Physiol Behav* 58: 877-882.

Dams, R.; De Letter, F.A.; Mortier, K.A.; Cordonnier, J.A.; Lambert, W.F.; Piette, M.H.; Van Calenbergh, S.; De Leenheer, A.P. (2003). Fatality due to combined use of the designer drugs MDMA and PMA: A distribution study. *J Anal Toxicol* 27(5): 318-322.

Davies, B.M.; Beech, H.R. (1960). The effect of 1-arylcyclohexylamine (Sernyl) on twelve normal volunteers. *J Ment Sci* 106: 912-924.

de la Torre, R.; Farre, M.; Ortuno, J.; Mas, M.; Brenniesen, R.; Roset, P.N.; Segura, J.; Cami, J. (2000). Non-linear pharmacokinetics of MDMA ("Ecstasy") in humans. *Br J Clin Pharmacol* 49: 104-109.

de la Torre, R.; Farre, M.; Roset, P.N.; Pizarro, N.; Abanedes, S.; Segura, M.; Segura, J.; Cami, J. (2004). Human pharmacology of MDMA: Pharmacokinetics, metabolism and disposition. *Ther Drug Monit* 26(2): 137-144.

Dishotsky, N.I.; Loughman, W.D.; Mogar, R.F.; Lipscomb, W.R. (1972). LSD and genetic damage—Is LSD chromosome damaging, carcinogenic, mutagenic, or taratogenic? *Science* 172(3982): 431-440.

Domino, E.F. (1964). Neurobiology of phencyclidine (Sernyl), a drug with an unusual spectrum of pharmacological activity. *Int Rev Neurobiol* 6: 303-347.

Dorrance, D.L.; Janiger, O.; Teplitz, R.L. (1975). Effect of peyote on human chromosomes. Cytogenetic study of the Huichol Indians on northern Mexico. *JAMA* 234(3): 299-302.

Dowling, G.P.; McDonough, E.T., 3rd; Bost, R.O. (1987). "Eve" and "Ecstasy." A report of five deaths associated with the use of MDEA and MDMA. *JAMA* 257(12): 1615-1617.

Downing, J. (1986). The psychological and physiological effects of MDMA on normal volunteers. *J Psychoactive Drugs* 18: 335-340.

Eastman, J.W.; Cohen, S.N. (1975). Hypertensive crisis and death associated with phencyclidine poisoning. *JAMA* 231: 1270-1271.

Ellis, A.J.; Wendon, J.A.; Portmann, B.; Williams, R. (1996). Acute liver damage and ecstasy ingestion. *Gut* 38(3): 454-458.

Fauman, M.A.; Fauman, B.J. (1979). Violence associated with phencyclidine abuse. *Am J Psychiatry* 136(12): 1584-1586.

Forrer, G.R.; Goldner, R.D. (1951). Experimental physiological studies with lysergic acid diethylamide (LSD-25). *AMA Arch Neurol Psychiatry* 65: 581-588.

Forsling, M.; Fallon, J.K.; Kicman, A.T.; Hutt, A.J.; Cowan, D.A.; Henry, J.A. (2001). Arginine vasopressin release in response to the administration of 3, 4-methylenedioxymethamphetamine ("Ecstasy"): Is metabolism a contributory factor? *J Pharm Pharmacol* 53: 1357-1363.

Forsling, M.L.; Fallon, J.K.; Shah, D.; Tilbrook, G.S.; Cowan, D.A.; Kicman, A.T.; Hutt, A.J. (2002). The effect of 3,4-methylenedioxymethamphetamine (MDMA, "Ecstasy") and its metabolites on neurohypophysial horomone release from the isolated rat hypothalamus. *Br J Pharmacol* 135: 649-656.

Fosset, M.; Renaud, J.F.; Lenoir, M.C.; Kamenka, J.M.; Geneste, P.; Lazdunski, M. (1979). Interaction of molecules of the phencyclidine series with cardiac cells. Association with the muscarinic receptor. *FEBS Letters* 103(1): 133-137.

Geber, W.F.; Schramm, L.C. (1974). Postpartum weight alteration in hamster offspring from females injected during pregnancy with heroin, methadone, a composite drug mixture, or mescaline. *Am J Obstet Gynecol* 120(8): 1105-1111.

Gilmour, D.G.; Bloom, A.D.; Lele, K.P.; Robbins, E.S.; Maximilian, C. (1971). Chromosomal aberration in users of psychoactive drugs. *Arch Gen Psychiatry* 24: 268-272.

Goode, D.J.; Meltzer, H.Y. (1975). The role of isometric muscle tension in the production of muscle toxicity by phencyclidine and restraint stress. *Psychopharmacologia* 42: 105-108.

Gool, R.Y.; Clarke, H.L. (1964). Anesthesia for under-doctor areas. *Anesthesia* 18: 265-270.

Gordon, C.J.; Fogelson, L. (1994). Metabolic and thermoregulatory responses of the rat maintained in acrylic or wire-screen cages; implications for pharmacological studies. *Physiol Behav* 56: 73-79.

Gordon, C.J.; Watkinson, W.P.; O'Callaghan, J.P.; Miller, D.B. (1991). Effects of 3,4-methylenedioxymethamphetamine on autonomic thermoregulatory responses of the rat. *Pharmacol Biochem Behav* 39: 359-372.

Grace, G.S. (1934). The action of mescaline and related compounds. *J Pharmacol Exp Ther* 50: 359.

Green, R.A.; Mechan, A.O.; Elliott, J.M.; O'Shea, E.; Colado, M.I. (2003). The pharmacology and clinical pharmacology of 3, 4-methylenedioxymethamphetamine (MDMA, "Ecstasy"). *Pharmacol Rev* 55: 463-508.

Greer, G.; Tolbert, R. (1986). Subjective reports of the effects of MDMA in a clinical setting. *Journal of Psychoactive Drugs* 18: 319-27.

Greifenstein, F.E.; DeVault, M.; Yoshitake, J.; Gajewski, J.E. (1958). 1-Arylcyclohexylamine for anesthesia. *Curr Res Anesth Analg* 37: 283-294.

Hartung, T.K.; Schofield, E.; Short, A.I.; Parr, M.J.; Henry, J.A. (2002). Hyponatraemic states following 3, 4-methylenedioxymethamphetamine (MDMA, "Ecstasy") ingestion. *QJM* 95(7): 431-437.

Heffter, A. (1897). Ueber pellote. *Arch Exp Pathol Pharmakol* 40: 418-425.

Henry, J.A. (1992). Ecstasy and the dance of death. *BMJ* 305: 5-6.

Henry, J.A.; Jeffreys, K.J.; Dawling, S. (1992). Toxicity and deaths from 3,4-methylenedioxymethamphetamine ("Ecstasy"). *Lancet* 340: 384-387.

Hensala, J.D.; Epstein, L.J.; Blacker, K.H. (1967). LSD and psychiatric inpatients. *Arch Gen Psychiatry* 16(5): 554-559.

Hirsch, K.S.; Fritz, H.I. (1981). Teratogenic effects of mescaline, epinephrine, and norepinephrine in the hamster. *Teratology* 23: 287-291.

Ilett, K.F.; Jarrott, B.; O'Donnell, S.R.; Wanstall, J.C. (1966). Mechanism of cardiovascular actions of 1-(1-phenylcyclohexyl) piperidine hydrochloride (phencyclidine). *Br J Pharmacol Chemother* 28: 73-83.

Kalant, H. (2001). The pharmacology and toxicology of "Ecstasy" (MDMA) and related drugs. *Can Med Assoc J* 165(7): 917-928.

Kapadia, G.J.; Fayez, M.B.E. (1970). Peyote constituents: Chemistry, biogenesis, and biological effects. *J Pharm Sci* 59(12): 1699-1727.

Kessler, G.F., Jr.; Demers, L.M.; Berlin, C.; Brennan, R.W. (1974). Phencyclidine and fatal status epilepticus. *N Eng J Med* 291(18): 979.

Klock, J.C.; Boerner, U.; Becker, C.E. (1973). Coma, hyperthermia, and bleeding associated with massive LSD overdose—A report of eight cases. *West J Med* 120: 183-188.

Konel, R.W.; Meltzer, H.Y. (1974). Pathological effect of phencyclidine and restraint on rat skeletal muscle structure: Prevention by prior denervation. *Expl Neurol* 45: 387-402.

Kreth, K.; Kovar, K.; Schwab, M.; Zanger, U.M. (2000). Identification of the human cytochromes P450 involved in the oxidative metabolism of "Ecstasy" related designer drugs. *Biochem Pharmacol* 59: 1563-1571.

Kwon, C.; Zaritsky, A.; Dharnidharka, V.R. (2003). Transient proximal tubular renal injury following Ecstasy ingestion. *Pediatr Nephrol* 18(8): 820-822.

Leikin, J.B.; Krantz, A.J.; Zell-Kanter, M.; Barkin, R.L.; Hryhorczuk, D.O. (1989). Clinical features and management of intoxication due to hallucinogenic drugs. *Med Toxicol Adverse Drug Exp* 4: 324-350.

Lester, S.J.; Baggott, M.; Welm, S.; Schiller, N.B.; Jones, R.T.; Foster, E.; Mendelson, J. (2000). Cardiovascular effects of 3,4-methylenedioxymetham-phetamine. *Ann Intern Med* 133(12): 969-973.

Liechti, M.E.; Baumann, C.; Gamma, A.; Vollenweider, F.X. (2000). Acute psychological effects of 3-4, methylenedioxymethamphetamine (MDMA, "Ecstasy") are attenuated by the serotonin uptake inhibitor citalopram. *Neuropsychopharmacology* 5: 513-521.

Litovitz, T.L. (1998). Phencyclidine (PCP). In: L.M. Haddad; J.F. Winchester (Eds.), *Clinical Management of Poisoning and Drug Overdose* (pp. 448-455). Philadelphia: W.B. Saunders Company.

Luby, E.D.; Cohen, B.D.; Rosenbaum, G.; Gottlieb, J.S.; Kelley, R. (1959). Study of a new schizophrenomimetic drug—Sernyl. *AMA Arch Neurol Psychiatry* 81: 363-369.

Luisada, P.V. (1977). The PCP psychosis: A hidden epidemic. *VI World Congress of Psychiatry,* Honolulu, Hawaii. 245.

Lundberg, G.D.; Gupta, R.C.; Montgomery, S.H. (1976). Phencyclidine: Patterns seen in street drug analysis. *Clin Toxicol* 9: 4.

Madhok, A.; Boxer, R.; Chowdhury, D. (2003). Atrial fibrillation in an adolescent—The agony of Ecstasy. *Pediatr Emerg Care* 19(5): 348-349.

Martin, T.L. (2001). Three case of fatal paramethoxyamphetamine overdose. *J Anal Toxicol* 7: 649-651.

Matthai, S.M.; Davidson, D.C.; Sills, J.A.; Alexandrou, D. (1996). Cerebral oedema after ingestion of MDMA ("Ecstasy") and unrestricted intake of water. *Br Med J* 312(7042): 1359.

McCann, U.D.; Szabo, Z.; Sheffel, U.; Dannals, R.F.; Ricaurte, G.A. (1998). Positron emission tomographic evidence of toxic effect of MDMA ("Ecstasy") on brain serotonin neurons in human beings. *The Lancet* 352: 1433-1437.

McCarron, M.M.; Schulze, B.W.; Thompson, G.A.; Conder, M.C.; Goetz, W.A. (1981). Acute phencyclidine intoxication: Incidence of clinical findings in 1000 cases. *Ann Emerg Med* 10(5): 237-242.

Melian, A.M.; Barillo-Putze, G.; Campo, C.G.; Padron, A.G.; Ramos, C.O. (2004). Accidental ecstasy poisoning in a toddler. *Pediatr Emerg Care* 8: 534-535.

Michael, F. (1969). D-receptor for serotonin on blood platelets. *Nature* 221: 1253-1254.

Mokler, D.J.; Stoudt, K.W.; Rech, R.H. (1985). The 5HT2 antagonist pirenperone reverses disruption of FR-40 by hallucinogenic drugs. *Pharmacol Biochem Behav* 22: 677-682.

Nash, J.F. (1988). Elevation of serum prolactin and corticosterone concentrations in the rat after the administration of 3,4-methylenedioxymethamphetamine. *J Pharmacol Exp Ther* 245: 873-879.

O'Brien, C.P. (2001). Drug addiction and drug abuse. In: J.G. Hardman; L.E. Limbird (Eds.), *Goodman and Gilman's Pharmacological Basis of Therapeutics* (pp. 621-642). New York: McGraw-Hill.

Orzechowski, R.F.; Goldstein, F.J. (1973). Species variation in blood pressure responses to mescaline: Evidence of histamine release. *Toxicol Appl Pharmacol* 25: 525-533.

Parrott, A.C.; Buchanan, T.; Scholey, A.B.; Heffeman, T.; Ling, J.; Rogers, J. (2002). Ecstasy/MDMA attributed problems reported by novice, moderate and heavy recreational users. *Hum Psychopharmacol* 17(6): 309-312.

Patel, M.M.; Belson, M.G.; Wright, D.; Lu, H.; Heninger, M.; Miller, M.A. (2005). Methylenedioxymethamphetamine (Ecstasy)-related myocardial hypertrophy: An autopsy study. *Resuscitation* 66(2): 197-202.

Patel, M.M.; Wright, D.W.; Ratcliffe, J.J.; Miller, M.A. (2004). Shedding new light on the "safe" club drugs: Methylenedioxymethamphetamine (Ecstasy)-related fatalities. *Acad Emerg Med* 11(2): 208-210.

Patel, R.; Connor, G. (1985-86). A review of thirty cases of rhabdomyolysis-associated acute renal failure among phencyclidine users. *Clin Toxicol* 23: 547-556.

Peroutka, S.J. (1987). Incidence of recreational use of 3, 4-methylenedioxymethamphetamine (MDMA, "Ecstasy") on an undergraduate campus. *N Engl J Med* 317: 1542-1543.

Peters, R.J., Jr.; Kelder, S.H.; Meshak, A.; Yacoubian, G.S.; Jr.; McCrimmons, D.; Ellis, A. (2005). Beliefs and social norms about cigarettes or marijuana sticks laced with embalming fluid and phencyclidine (PCP): Why youth use "fry." *Subst Use Misuse* 40(4): 563-571.

Peterson, R.C.; Stillman, S.C. (1978). Phencyclidine (PCP) abuse: An appraisal. *NIDA Research Monograph Number,* 21. 245.

Ricaurte, G.A. (1989). Studies of MDMA-induced neurotoxicity in nonhuman primates: A basis for evaluating long-term effects in humans. *NIDA Research Monograph* 94: 306-322.

Ricaurte, G.A.; Bryan, G.; Strauss, L.; Seiden, L.; Schuster, C. (1985). Hallucinogenic amphetamine selectively destroys brain serotonin nerve terminals. *Science* 229(4717): 986-988.

Ricaurte, G.A.; Finnegan, K.F.; Nichols, D.E.; DeLanney, L.E.; Irwin, I.; Langston, J.W. (1985). 3,4-Methylenedioxyethylamphetamine (MDE), a novel analogue of MDMA, produces long-lasting depletion of serotonin in the rat brain. *Eur J Pharmacol* 137(2-3): 265-268.

Ricaurte, G.A.; Yuan, J.; Hatzidimitriou, G.; Cord, B.J.; McCann, U.D. (2002). Severe dopaminergic neurotoxicity in primates after a common recreational dose regimen of MDMA "Ecstasy." *Science* 297(5590): 2260-2263.

Ricaurte, G.A.; Yuan, J.; Hatzidimitriou, G.; Cord, B.J.; McCann, U.D. (2003). Retraction. *Science* 301(5639): 1479.

Rinkel, M.; Hyde, R.W.; Solomon H.C.; Hoagland, H. (1955). Experimental psychiatry II. Clinical and physio-chemical observations in experimental psychosis. *Am J Psychiatry* 111: 881-895.

Rowland, L.P.; Penn, A.S. (1972). Myoglobinuria. *Med Clin North Am* 56: 1233-1256.

Schaefer, S.B. (1997). Pregnancy and peyote among the Huichol Indians of Mexico: A preliminary report. In: C. Rätsch; J. Baker (Eds.), *Yearbook for Ethnomedicine and the Study of Consciousness.* Berlin, Germany.

Schaefer, S.B.; Bauml, J.A. (1997). Peyote: Status report on an endangered sacrament. *49th International Congress of Americanists,* Quito, Equador.

Shearman, J.D.; Chapman, R.W.; Satsangi, J.; Ryley, N.G.; Weatherhead, S. (1992). Misuse of Ecstasy. *Br Med J* 305(6848): 309.

Shepherd, S.M.; Jagoda, A.S. (1990). Phencyclidine and the hallucinogens. In: W.B. Sanders; L.M. Haddad (Eds.), *Clinical Management of Poisoning and Drug Overdose* (pp. 749-769). Philadelphia: WB Saunders.

Shick, J.F.E.; Smith, D.E. (1970). Analysis of the LSD flashback. *J Psychedelic Drugs* 3(1): 13-19.

Shulgin, A. (1979). Profiles of psychedelic drugs. *J Psychedelic Drugs* 11(4): 355.

Shulgin, A.; Shulgin, A. (2000). *PIHKAL: A Chemical Love Story.* Berkeley, CA: Transform Press.

Shulgin, A.T. (1986). The background and chemistry of MDMA. *J Psychoactive Drugs* 18: 291-304.

Shulgin, A.T.; Nichols, D.E. (1978). Characterization of three new psychotomimetics. In: R.C. Stillman; R.E. Willette (Eds.), *The Psychopharmacology of Hallucinogens* (pp. 74-83). New York: Pergamom Press.

Smilkstein, M.J.; Smolinske, S.C.; Rumack, B.H. (1987). A case of MAO inhibitor/MDMA interaction: Agony after Ecstasy. *J Toxicol Clin Toxicol* 25(1-2): 149-159.

Spath, E. (1919). Uber die Anhalonium-Alkaloide. 1. Anhalin und Mezcalin. *Monatsh Chem* 40: 129-154.

Speck, L.B. (1957). Toxicity and effects of increasing doses of mescaline. *J Pharmacol Exp Ther* 119: 78.

Steele, T.D.; McCann, U.D.; Ricaurte, G.A. (1994). 3, 4-Methylenedioxymethamphetamine (MDMA, "Ecstasy"): Pharmacology and toxicology in animals and humans. *Addiction* 18: 539-551.

Stein, D.J.; Rink, J. (1999). Effects of "Ecstasy" blocked by serotonin reuptake inhibitors. *J Clin Psychiatry* 60(7): 485.

Suarez, R.V.; Riemersma, R. (1988). "Ecstasy" and sudden cardiac death. *Am J Forensic Med Pathol* 9(4): 339-341.

Teitelbaum, D.T.; Wingeleth, D.C. (1977). Diagnosis and management of recreational mescaline self poisoning. *J Anal Toxicol* 1: 36-37.

Ungerleider, J.T.; Fisher, D.D.; Fuller, M. (1966). The dangers of LSD. *JAMA* 197: 109-112.

Ungerleider, J.T.; Fisher, D.D.; Fuller, M.; Caldwell, A. (1968). The "bad trip"—The etiology of the adverse LSD reaction. *Am J Psychiatry* 124(11): 1483-1490.

Vardy, M.M.; Kay, S.R. (1983). LSD psychosis or LSD-induced schizophrenia? A multimethod inquiry. *Arch Gen Psychiatry* 40(8): 877-883.

Wiegand, T.J.; Smith, S.W.; Zvosec, D.L. (2005). Use of propofol for severe GHB withdrawal: Two cases. *J Toxicol Clin Toxicol* 43(6): 665.

Yacoubian, G. (2003). Tracking ecstasy trends in the United States with data from three drug surveillance systems. *J Drug Educ* 33(3): 245-258.

Zevin, S.; Benowitz, N.L. (1998). Drug-related syndromes. In: S.B. Karch (Ed.), *Drug Abuse Handbook* (pp. 542-567). Boca Raton, FL: CRC Press.

Chapter 15

Medical Consequences
of Over-the-Counter (OTC)
Substance Abuse

Karen E. Simone

INTRODUCTION AND OVERVIEW

Abuse of over-the-counter (OTC) products is common for many reasons including easy access, relatively low cost, and the perception that OTC medications are safe. Abuse is especially prevalent in adolescents who do not always have easy access to other substances of abuse. For example, the purchase of OTC cough syrups containing dextromethorphan is not limited to age, as is purchase of alcohol or cigarettes. Neither a drug dealer nor a prescriber is necessary. Moreover, the detection and intervention of OTC abuse can be delayed because therapeutic use is expected, so abuse may not be obvious to family members, teachers, law enforcement, or health care professionals, at least during initial use.

For many of the reasons mentioned, the medical and other consequences of long-term OTC abuse are not well studied in comparison with other drugs, which are abused more frequently and are more easily detected. Many of the better-known effects of OTC are limited to acute intoxication involving single case studies or studies involving a relatively small number of subjects. In this chapter, three broad types of medications common to many OTC medications will be discussed: antihistamines, dextromethorphan, ephedrine, and related stimulant decongestants. Where appropriate, the interaction between these common OTCs and other popular drugs will be discussed.

OTC medications are frequently misused. In a survey regarding OTC misuse, 86 Scotland pharmacists were questioned about their experiences

Handbook of the Medical Consequences of Alcohol and Drug Abuse
© 2008 by The Haworth Press, Taylor & Francis Group. All rights reserved.
doi:10.1300/6039_15

with OTC misuse. Fifty-eight percent indicated misuse is occasional; 31 percent indicated that it is frequent. The frequency was greater in urban areas than in rural ones. The estimated mean number of patients per week suspected of misusing OTC medications was six. The medications most commonly involved were sleeping preparations, laxatives, analgesics, cough syrups, and other products containing pseudoephedrine, caffeine, codeine, and dextromethorphan (MacFadyen, Eadie, and McGowan, 2001).

Chung et al. (2004) discussed substance abuse in Korea, which is growing. There, noncontrolled drugs like dextromethorphan account for 10 percent of the total substance abuse problem. The drug is especially attractive to young people due to easy access and noncontrolled status. Large doses are taken for hallucinogenic effects. Of the nearly 100 drug-related deaths reported in Korea since the mid-1980s, dextromethorphan is responsible for 10. The decedents ranged from 19 to 42 years of age, were female more often than male, and used the drug for either recreational purposes or suicide. Causes of death included ingestion of a large amount, fall, suicide, "death on road," and others (Chung et al., 2004).

United States health care professionals interviewed adolescents aged 13 to 25 years who presented to the Adolescent Substance Abuse Program at Children's Hospital (Boston, MA) or the Emergency Department at the UMASS–Memorial Medical Center (Worcester, MA), and who indicated that they used the Internet to obtain psychoactive drug information. The interviews took place in 2002 and 2003. Twelve subjects participated. One-third of the respondents sought information about dextromethorphan, an OTC medication. One subject increased use as a result, because he felt use was safe. According to him, it was safe because it was a "real drug" and he "couldn't find a reason not to use it" based on what he read on the Internet (Boyer, Shannon, and Hibberd, 2005).

The Utah Poison Control Center reported on substance abuse of OTC medications in Utah over a ten-year period from 1990 to 1999. Substance abuse in children and teens aged 6 to 19 years was evaluated. The study reported 332,049 poisonings; 43,558 (13.1 percent) involved children and teens. (4,141) Of all poisonings, 1.25 percent involved substance abuse; 2,214 (53.5 percent) of these involved children and teens. OTC medications were involved in 844 (38.1 percent) of child and teen substance abuse poisonings. Most of these occurred in those who were 13 to 17 years of age. Two or more substances were involved in 129 (15.3 percent of cases). The OTC medications involved were as follows (in ranked order): anticholinergics (30 percent), caffeine (23 percent), cough and cold products containing dextromethorphan (13 percent), ephedrine (8 percent), cough and cold products not containing dextromethorphan (5 percent), analgesics

(5 percent), gastrointestinal (3 percent), and others (3 percent). Anticholinergics were chiefly antihistamines used for allergy relief, sleep, nausea, or motion sickness. The remaining 10 percent involved prescription, illicit and other substances taken concomitantly with the OTC medications abused. Sixty-five percent of abuse occurred at a residence; 10 percent occurred at school. Sixty-eight percent were treated at a health care facility. Twenty-six percent of cases with known outcomes had more than minor effects as a result of the substance abuse (Crouch, Caravati, and Booth, 2004).

ANTIHISTAMINES

Antihistamines have been available both by prescription and over the counter. The American Association of Poison Control Centers (AAPCC) cited antihistamine products 3,000 times in cases of abuse/misuse in 2005; more than half of these cases involved diphenhydramine. Cough and cold product citings of abuse/misuse in the same year totaled 7,897. Many of these are products containing multiple ingredients, one of which may be an antihistamine. AAPCC data are derived from calls voluntarily placed to poison centers throughout the United States, Puerto Rico, and the District of Columbia, and are only a subset of all poisonings within the region (Toxic Exposure Surveillance System data from the American Association of Poison Control Centers, search run April 18, 2006).

Antihistamines are also a problem in other countries. A survey of 297 addicts in treatment in the United Kingdom showed 29 percent used diphenhydramine. Twenty percent took it for something a physician did not recommend. Thirteen percent purchased it on the street; 15 percent said it was prescribed by a physician. Fifty-one percent claimed that they took it "for sleep," and 12 percent took it to "get high." Thirty-five percent liked the effects. Twenty percent thought they needed it, 1 percent felt addicted and 8 percent felt they might become addicted. The survey showed that of this 18 percent used chlorpheniramine. Eight percent took it for something a physician did not recommend. Eight percent purchased it on the street; 28 percent said it was prescribed by a physician. Seventeen percent claimed that they took it "for sleep," 4 percent took it to "get high." Thirty-two percent liked the effects. Nineteen percent thought they needed it, none felt addicted or that they might become addicted (Jaffe, Bloor, and Crome, 2004).

The dosage form may enhance abuse liability. Pharmacists in Glasgow reported requests for excessive quantities of diphenhydramine sold in a soft gel liquid capsule formulation within three months after it became available over the counter. The product was reportedly being abused as an injectable "downer." It was thought that the desired effect was euphoria, hallucinations, and perhaps stimulation. Used with opiates, antihistamine effects are described as a "rush" followed by stimulation and hallucination (Roberts, Gruer, and Gilhooly, 1999).

Young adults sometimes take large numbers of dimenhydrinate for a "high" when other more desirable drugs, such as lysergic acid diethylamide (LSD) or marijuana, are unavailable. The following effects are described: elation and a feeling of floating, seeing smoke and patterns of colored lights on the wall or in the sky, seeing trails after movement, music sounding better than normal, a feeling of bugs or rats crawling on the skin, and imagining a mermaid on the beach (Malcolm and Miller, 1972).

Adolescents taking antihistamines for a "high" may develop mood disorders as a result. Three adolescent patients were referred for psychiatric evaluation of depression and other mood disorders that may have been due to abuse of excessive quantities of dimenhydrinate. The patients described a "cheap high," and that it was used by "lots of kids," and by "mostly everybody I know." A reason given for use was that it was perceived as permissible because it was not illegal (Gardner and Kutcher, 1993).

Schizophrenics are another group prone to antihistamine abuse. They initially use antihistamines to treat symptoms, then continue because they like the way the antihistamines make them feel. Several examples of abuse in this population are reported in the literature.

A 34-year-old male ingested up to 5,000 mg of diphenhydramine liquid weekly for five months for a "knock-out" effect (Cox, Ahmed, and McBride, 2001).

A 33-year-old schizophrenic taking multiple medications reportedly ingested up to 3,000 mg of diphenhydramine daily for six months to relieve aggressive feelings. He described a pleasant feeling in his head, then abdomen, a calming effect, feeling "stupefied," and "more likely to stare out into space than ordinarily you would" (Barsoum et al., 2000, p. 847).

A 52-year-old schizophrenic reportedly abused 5,000 mg of dimenhydrinate daily for a euphoric effect. She abused the drug for ten years. She exhibited craving, prostituted herself to pay for the habit, used multiple pharmacies to buy the drug, resisted intervention, and experienced withdrawal when abstinent (Bartlik, Galanter, and Angrist, 1989).

A 34-year-old schizophrenic reportedly abused diphenhydramine for six months to assist with insomnia. He also noticed sedation and euphoria. He was referred for inpatient care for rapid tapering of the diphenhydramine. At that time, he had been taking 800 mg twice daily for a month (Feldman and Behar, 1986).

A 38-year-old schizophrenic patient reportedly abused diphenhydramine for a "relaxing" effect over a ten-month period. She had increased her dose to 2,500 mg daily, then tapered to 1,250 mg daily over the previous four weeks. She presented to an emergency department confused and refusing to take any medications two days after discontinuing diphenhydramine as well as her prescribed medications (Shiuh and Wax, 2001).

A female schizophrenic patient began ingesting up to 5,000 mg of dimenhydrinate at a time while in the hospital "to get high" and get through the day when she was 29 years old. A male schizophrenic patient abused up to 3,000 mg of dimenhydrinate at a time because it was a cheaper alternative to cocaine. He claimed that it made him "musical" and "creative." Both were able to decrease craving and the dose of dimenhydrinate abused with clozapine therapy (Prost and Millson, 2004).

A 32-year-old schizophrenic resorted to harassment of other patients at a mental health center for money to buy diphenhydramine, and theft of diphenhydramine, to support his habit. Another sold household items for money to buy the drug. Both exhibited withdrawal when diphenhydramine was abruptly discontinued (De Nesnera, 1996).

Other patients report desirable effects. A 26-year-old patient with anorexia and bulimia took up to 2,500 mg of dimenhydrinate daily for anorexic and sedative effects. Dose-related vomiting was desirable, but did not persist. Another patient took the drug in doses up to 600 mg for the dose-related sedative effect (Young, Boyd, and Kreeft, 1988). Yet another patient described a dimenhydrinate high as follows: "puts you in a mood you don't understand . . . high but not high . . . don't know who you are or where you're going . . . pleasant but confusing" (Craig and Mellor, 1990, p. 971).

Mechanisms of Action

Antihistamines block histamine-1 receptors, resulting in bronchodilation and vasoconstriction. The older generation antihistamines, such as diphenhydramine, dimenhydrinate, chlorphiramine and others, also block muscarinic receptors, causing anticholinergic effects. Anticholinergic effects include tachycardia, dry skin and mouth, constipation, urinary retention, flushing, elevated temperature, dilated pupils, hallucinations or delirium, and perhaps antinausea effects. Central nervous system effects include both stimulation and depression. Depression, or sedation, is common with normal doses of first generation antihistamines such as ethanolamines (e.g., diphenhydramine). Excitation, including seizures and hallucinations, is either an uncommon reaction to normal doses or a toxic reaction to excessive doses (Hardman, Limbird, and Gilman, 2001).

Many of the reported deleterious effects of antihistamines are from first generation antihistamines including ethanolamines (e.g., diphenhydramine). Unlike older H1 antagonists, the newer (post 1980s) second generation drugs have fewer central nervous system effects, including greatly reduced effects on driving an automobile (Moskowitz and Wilkinson, 2004). As many of these newer antihistamines including alkylamines (e.g., Acrivastine) and piperazines (e.g., Cetirizine hydrochloride, Loratadine, and fexofenadine) are "nonsedating," they have become popular in allergy medications (Hardman, Limbird, and Gilman, 2001).

Medical Consequences of Abuse

Cardiac

Possible cardiac effects include tachycardia, hypertension, symptomatic postural hypotension (Brown and Sigmundson, 1969; Cox, Ahmed, and McBride, 2001; Feldman and Behar, 1986). Injection of 200 mg of diphenhydramine capsules, 4 × 50 mg capsules, caused tachycardia to 220 beats per minute, hypotension (70/30 mm Hg supine), a widened QRS (110 ms which later normalized to 80 ms), right bundle branch block, anterior ST-T wave changes, and inverted T waves. The patient also developed pulmonary hypertension (central venous pressure of 12 mm Hg), right ventricular hypertension (right ventricular systolic pressure of 56 mm Hg), and dilation (right ventricular end diastolic dimension of 24.4 mm Hg) (Sundararaghavan and Suarez, 2004).

Pulmonary

In a case of oral capsules injected through a central line, labored breathing with a respiratory rate increased to 60 breaths per minute occurred. The patient also developed pulmonary hypertension (Sundararaghavan and Suarez, 2004). Respiratory depression may also occur, secondary to central nervous system depression.

Neurologic

Antihistamines such as diphenhydramine or dimenhydrinate produce intoxication with doses of 600 to 5,000 mg daily (Barsoum et al., 2000; Bartlik, Galanter, and Angrist, 1989; Cox, Ahmed, and McBride, 2001; Feldman and Behar, 1986; Prost and Millson, 2004; Shiuh and Wax, 2001; Young, Boyd, and Kreeft, 1988). Lethargy and sleepiness is reported with 800 mg doses of dimenhydrinate (Malcolm and Miller, 1972). After ingestion of 5,000 mg of dimenhydrinate daily a patient exhibited drowsiness, ataxia, and slurred speech. Already present tardive dyskinesia was exacerbated both by abuse and withdrawal (Bartlik, Galanter, and Angrist, 1989). Psychomotor agitation, choreoathetoid movements, disorientation, fidgety behavior, and tremors have been reported with excessive use of injectable diphenhydramine by hematology/oncology pediatric and adolescent patients (Dinndorf, McCabe, and Frierdich, 1998). Difficulty in swallowing and speaking, possibly due to dystonia, may also occur. In one patient, administration of benztropine seemed to help (Brown and Sigmundson, 1969), but it is important to consider the additive anticholinergic effects of benztropine with antihistamines as anticholinergic toxicity may result. Reported ingestions of 5,000 mg of dimenhydrinate caused generalized seizures in a schizophrenic patient (Prost and Millson, 2004).

Gastric

Dry mouth has been reported with diphenhydramine and dimenhydrinate (Barsoum et al., 2000; Brown and Sigmundson, 1969; Dinndorf, McCabe, and Frierdich, 1998; Malcolm and Miller, 1972). Vomiting may occur with doses up to 500 to 2,500 mg of dimenhydrinate (Young, Boyd, and Kreeft, 1988).

Hepatic

A chemotherapy patient who injected capsules of diphenhydramine centrally developed elevated liver enzymes (ALT 117 U/l, AST 30 U/l, GGT 87 U/l, alkaline phosphatase 88 U/l, total bilirubin 1.4 mg/dl, albumin 3.1 g/dl, total protein 4.4 g/dl) (Sundararaghavan and Suarez, 2004).

Genitourinary

Urinary difficulty and retention were reported with excessive use of injectable diphenhydramine by hematology/oncology pediatric and adolescent patients (Dinndorf, McCabe, and Frierdich, 1998).

Hematologic

After injecting diphenhydramine centrally, hemoglobin dropped from 10.9 to 7.5 g/dl in one day. Platelets were unaffected (Sundararaghavan and Suarez, 2004).

Ears, Eyes, Nose, and Throat

Pupils may be dilated (Brown and Sigmundson, 1969; Cox, Ahmed, and McBride, 2001). Vision may be blurry (Barsoum et al., 2000).

Dermal

Skin may be flushed with excessive antihistamine dose (Brown and Sigmundson, 1969).

Psychiatric

Some antihistamines produce euphoria, elation, and floating sensation (Bartlik, Galanter, and Angrist, 1989; Malcolm and Miller, 1972) as well as changes in perception of vision, sound, and sensation (Brown and Sigmundson, 1969; Malcolm and Miller, 1972). Formication (sensation of bugs crawling on the skin) is described (Malcolm and Miller, 1972). Confusion, inattentiveness, inability to think clearly and difficulty socializing can occur with doses of 600 to 2,500 mg of dimenhydrinate. In one case report, an acute abuse of 900 to 1,250 mg of dimenhydrinate caused an 18-year-old male to become incoherent, emotionally labile, violent, out of touch with his environment, and fearful. He also hallucinated, seeing smoke coming out of others' ears and noses (Brown and Sigmundson, 1969). Paranoia may occur (Malcolm and Miller, 1972). In another case report, a schizophrenic patient who abused 5 grams at a time was loud, aggressive, and exhibiting poor self-care during abuse (Prost and Millson, 2004). Long-term abuse of single doses as high as 250 to 750 mg may cause depression that can be refractory to treatment. Specific effects described include anhedonia, lethargy, amotivation, irritability, low mood, hypersomnolence, poor concentration, and low appetite/weight loss (Gardner and Kutcher, 1993). Psychiatric effects of medications, including OTCs must be interpreted cautiously in psychiatric patients for obvious reasons. In one case, these effects improved within a week when discontinued on different occasions (Gardner and Kutcher, 1993). Use of up to 3,000 mg daily for six months was described as calming, causing a patient to feel "stupefied," and "stare out into space" (Barsoum et al., 2000). Again, caution must be exercised in generalizing effects from this population, particularly when relying upon single subject case reports.

Withdrawal/Dependence

Five hematology/oncology patients receiving intravenous diphenhydramine exhibited drug-seeking behavior. An 11-year-old admitted requesting doses due to supposed itching but in actuality requested doses for the sedative effect. An eight-year-old became distressed and inconsolable when diphenhydramine was discontinued due to related adverse effects. A 20-year-old stole parenteral diphenhydramine from a medication cart and locked herself in a bathroom to inject it. A 16-year-old boy demanded bolus injections of diphenhydramine from hospital staff, insisted on injecting it himself, and was found by his mother to have a "stash" of injectable diphenhydramine in his bedroom at home. A 12-year-old boy injected himself with 50 mg of diphenhydramine every two waking hours (Dinndorf, McCabe, and Frierdich, 1998).

Craving, a feeling of helplessness, and tremor may occur with doses up to 5,000 mg weekly upon withdrawal (Cox, Ahmed, and McBride, 2001).

Discontinuation of 5,000 grams of dimenhydrinate daily caused agitation, pacing, hostility, panic, clumsiness, and a sensation of mouth and face swelling within hours of abstinence. The effects lasted for several days. Fecal incontinence may also occur (Bartlik, Galanter, and Angrist, 1989).

Rapid tapering over nine days of a daily dose of 1,600 mg of diphenhydramine caused return of the insomnia, which was the initial reason for the use of diphenhydramine, as well as restlessness, irritability, excessive blinking, and increased defecation (Feldman and Behar, 1986).

A schizophrenic patient developed confusion, disorientation, and tachycardia within two days of abrupt discontinuation of up to 2,500 mg of diphenhydramine daily for 18 months. Her mental status was improved by day three, but anorexia, nausea, and anxiety developed after discontinuation. On day four, she developed diarrhea, abdominal cramping, and episodes of flushing (Shiuh and Wax, 2001).

Abrupt discontinuation of 1,000 to 2,500 mg of diphenhydramine daily for four months to one year in two schizophrenic patients caused diarrhea, abdominal cramping, sweating, excessive drooling, tachycardia, hypertension, and increased respiratory rate. One patient was anxious and aggressive. A diphenhydramine taper induced resolution in one patient. The other patient's symptoms improved in three days (De Nesnera, 1996).

Discontinuation of 500 to 2,500 mg of dimenhydrinate daily caused withdrawal. Increased excitability, increased heart rate and blood pressure, and mydriasis was reported after discontinuation of 2,500 mg daily. Malaise has also been reported (Young, 1988).

Patients abusing up from 1,250 up to 3,750 mg of dimenhydrinate daily developed anorexia, nausea, vomiting, diarrhea, dehydration, weight loss, depersonalization, hallucinations, shakiness, and weakness. Symptoms resolve in seven to ten days (Craig and Mellor, 1990).

Fetal/Newborn Exposure

A newborn developed tremors and diarrhea five days after birth. Her mother had been treated with 150 mg of diphenhydramine daily for a rash during her pregnancy for an undetermined amount of time. The amount of diphenhydramine measured in the blood was still at a toxic level five days after birth. Phenobarbital appeared to cause partial improvement of the tremor over three days. However, some tremor was still present at ten days (Parkin, 1974).

Other

Elevated temperature may occur with abuse of large amounts of antihistamines (Brown and Sigmundson, 1969). A patient who injected diphenhydramine capsules through a central line was found in shock, cool with clammy extremities. She also developed acidosis (Sundararaghavan and Suarez, 2004).

Antihistamine/Decongestant Combinations

A 27-year-old bipolar patient stabilized on lithium developed paranoia, unlike effects experienced in the past, after increasing abuse of pseudoephedrine with triprolidine (Actifed) from "one to two bottles" on weekends to two bottles daily. He described body vibrations and hearing a third person commentary. The effects developed within two weeks of increasing his dose and reportedly resolved within a day of discontinuation. Users describe that sounds seem louder and colors more vivid (Leighton, 1982).

A 21-year-old patient with depression took 300-1,800 mg of pseudoephedrine with 12.5 to 75 mg of triprolidine daily because it "gave her a lift." Psychotic symptoms including visual and auditory hallucinations and feelings of passivity developed one year later and were fluctuating in nature. Negative effects associated with schizophrenia were not present (Pugh and Howie, 1986).

Antihistamine and Opioid Combinations

Use of butorphanol with intravenous diphenhydramine in a 1:1 mixture is described to cause an "unusual sensation" in the abdomen followed by confusion, clouded sensorium, inability to communicate, and stupor. Doses used are typically 75 mg of Benadryl with 3 mg of butorphanol. The dose is repeated until the desired effect is achieved. Initially, 150 to 225 mg of diphenhydramine is needed. Over time, tolerance requires doses as high as

450 to 750 mg of diphenhydramine. Adverse effects reported include: sedation, drowsiness, impairment of mental and physical performance, cloudy thinking, mood changes, dizziness, nausea, vomiting, respiratory depression, irregular breathing, and death from respiratory failure. Withdrawal effects are described, and include irritability, agitation, dysphoria, difficulty concentrating and sleeping, and emotional lability (Smith and Davis, 1984).

CAFFEINE

Caffeine is available in liquid form through coffee, tea, and soft drinks; through dietary supplements such as guarana; and through OTC medications including NoDoz, Vivarin, 357 HR Magnum, and Molie. Caffeine use is very widespread and caffeine abuse is common. The AAPCC cites caffeine-containing products 1,556 times in abuse/misuse cases during 2005. AAPCC data are derived from calls voluntarily placed to poison centers throughout the United States, Puerto Rico, and the District of Columbia, and are only a subset of all poisonings within the region (Toxic Exposure Surveillance System data from the American Association of Poison Control Centers, search run April 18, 2006).

Anorexic patients sometimes take caffeine in excessive amounts to enhance weight loss and control appetite (Shaul, Farrell, and Maloney, 1984). Patients with a history of abuse report using excessive amounts of caffeine, 800 to 1,600 mg per day, sometimes in combination with large volumes of coffee. One patient initially used caffeine when cocaine was unavailable, but then continued and increased usage. Another used caffeine to increase energy and productivity. He noted increased excitement (Russ, 1988). Others use caffeine in order to remain awake and alert on the job, increase to excessive doses due to tolerance, then have difficulty discontinuing the drug (Adams, Ditzler, and Haning, 1993).

A 22-year-old male ingested 15 to 20 of 225 milligram caffeine capsules to get "high." He suffered abdominal pain and vomiting within 30 minutes. His heart rate was 150 beats per minute; blood pressure 90/60 mm Hg. His serum caffeine level was 74.6 µg/ml and he felt anxious. A 21-year-old male ingested 40 "hits of speed," in the form of caffeine capsules. He also experienced abdominal cramping and vomiting, tachycardia (95 beats per minute), but had slightly elevated blood pressure (130/90 mm Hg). In addition to being anxious, he was also combative and hostile. His serum level was 42 µg/ml (May et al., 1981).

A 30-year-old female with bipolar affective illness with hypomanic behavior and hallucinations reportedly took 24,000 mg of caffeine in the form of tablets over several days. She was found acting bizarrely. At the hospital, she was awake but unable to communicate. She vomited coffee-ground, guaiac-positive emesis. Her heart rate was 192, blood pressure 80/60 mm Hg, and respiration 32 per minute. The electrocardiogram showed Wenckebach's atrioventricular nodal block. Pupils were dilated and reactive. The white blood cell count and glucose were elevated, while potassium was low. She had a metabolic acidosis with an anion gap of 20. Glucose and ketones were found in her urine. After three days of supportive care, the patient became more responsive. Her admission blood level was 200 µg/ml. Norepinephrine and epinephrine levels were 2,000 (normal of 218 ± 59) and 900 (normal of 20 ± 6) picograms per ml, respectively (Benowitz et al., 1982).

Mechanism of Action

Caffeine is a mild central nervous system stimulant that increases secretion of norepinephrine, a stimulating neurotransmitter, and enhances neural activity in several areas of the brain. This can cause increases in heart rate, blood pressure, alertness, tremor and seizures in excessive doses. It also antagonizes adenosine, which can cause bronchodilation, and inhibits phosphodiesterase at very a high level, further increasing stimulation (Goldfrank et al., 2002; Hardman, Limbird, and Gilman, 2001).

Medical Consequences of Caffeine

Cardiac

As a stimulant, it is not surprising that caffeine produces tachycardia and hypertension but it may also produce hypotension (Benowitz et al., 1982; May et al., 1981). Wenckebach atrioventricular block (repetitive cycle with progressive slowing of atrioventricular conduction until a beat is dropped) may occur (Benowitz et al., 1982). Electrocardiogram changes consistent with hypokalemia (prolonged QT and T wave changes) occurred with borderline hypokalemia (3.5 mEq/l) after ingestion of 4,800 mg of caffeine to lose weight (Shaul, Farrell, and Maloney, 1984). Although tachycardia is expected, one case of bradycardia with a rate of 60 beats per minute was reported after ingestion of a product that also contained ammonium chloride (Shaul, Farrell, and Maloney, 1984). Patients may note "arrhythmias."

Neurologic

Caffeine produces dizziness, tremor, restlessness, confusion, insomnia, fatigue, combativeness, and lethargy which are reported after a large single dose (May et al., 1981; Shaul, Farrell, and Maloney, 1984). "Shakes" and twitching are also reported (Russ, 1988).

Gastric

Abdominal pain and vomiting may occur with large acute doses (May et al., 1981). Gastrointestinal bleeding is reported (Benowitz et al., 1982). Excessive thirst may occur with chronic use of large doses (Russ, 1988). Abdominal pain and diarrhea may occur (Siegel, 1980).

Genitourinary

Increased diuresis may occur (Russ, 1988).

Fluid/Electrolyte

Hypokalemia may occur with large doses of caffeine (Benowitz, et al., 1982; Shaul, Farrell, and Maloney, 1984). Electrocardiogram changes consistent with hypokalemia (prolonged QT and T wave changes) occurred with borderline hypokalemia (3.5 mEq/l) after ingestion of 4,800 mg of caffeine (in a product that also contained ammonium chloride) to lose weight (Shaul, Farrell, and Maloney, 1984).

Acid-Base/Endocrine

Anion gap metabolic acidosis and ketonuria may occur when caffeine is ingested in large amounts with or without ammonium chloride (Benowitz et al., 1982; Shaul, Farrell, and Maloney, 1984). Elevated glucose and glucosuria was reported after massive subacute dosing (Benowitz et al., 1982). Norepinephrine and epinephrine levels may be dramatically increased by caffeine (Benowitz et al., 1982).

Hematologic

Elevated white blood cell count may occur with large doses of caffeine (Benowitz et al., 1982).

Dermal

Facial flushing may occur in some instances (Russ, 1988).

Psychiatric

Anxiety (May et al., 1981; Russ, 1988; Shaul, Farrell, and Maloney, 1984), hostility (May et al., 1981), bizarre behavior, inability to communicate (Benowitz et al., 1982), fear, distraction, visual hallucinations, disorientation, and emotional lability were described after a large dose of caffeine (Shaul, Farrell, and Maloney, 1984). Rambling flow of thought and speech and periods of inexhaustibility were reported (Russ, 1988). Irritability is also reported after chronic high doses of caffeine (Adams, Ditzler, and Haning, 1993).

Withdrawal/Dependence

A 29-year-old patient developed headache, anxiety, a trapped feeling, fatigue, daytime somnolence, and sleep disturbances after discontinuation of daily doses up to 2,000 mg of caffeine. Symptoms resolved within six days after discontinuation (Adams, Ditzler, and Haning, 1993).

DEXTROMETHORPHAN (DXM)

Dextromethorphan is a cough suppressant chemically related to opioids, but without significant opioid-like effects. It is especially popular because it is available over the counter. If unable to pay, some shoplift the drug (Boyer, 2004). Reasons suggested for the choice to abuse DXM follow:

1. Availability: licit OTC is more likely than illicit or prescription drug abuse.
2. Approval: cough syrup is more socially acceptable than other substances.
3. Ignorance: less is known about the negative effects possible.
4. Fear: cough syrup is less intimidating than powders, pills, or needles. (Darboe, 1996)

The AAPCC cited DXM-containing products 6,034 times in cases of DXM abuse/misuse in 2005. AAPCC data are derived from calls voluntarily placed to poison centers throughout the United States, Puerto Rico, and the District of Columbia, and are only a subset of all poisonings within the region (Toxic Exposure Surveillance System data from the American Association of Poison Control Centers, search run April 18, 2006).

When DXM is taken in large amounts, the major metabolite—dextrorphan, provides a phencyclidine (PCP)-like out-of-body experience. For years, large doses of DXM-containing cough syrup have been ingested. As Robitussin is a common brand name, this is sometimes called "Robo-tripping." As early as 1997, when a new product with DXM in tablet form became available, many teens and young adults began abusing that product, Coricidin HBP Cough & Cold. This is referred to as "Triple C," "Skittles," or "Red Devils" due to the three "C"s on the shiny, round, red tablets (see Figure 15.1) (Boyer, 2004; http://www.streetdrugs.org/dxm.htm, accessed June 28, 2007). Some describe the ingestion of large amounts of DXM to be easier to take, and less nauseating, in the Coricidin tablet form than the thick cough syrup form (Simone and Bond, 2002).

Unfortunately, the Coricidin product contains an antihistamine, chlorpheniramine, which increases the toxicity of DXM abuse and causes unpleasant effects. Poison centers receive many calls as teens using Coricidin for a "high" present to emergency departments sick and frightened. Cases of Coricidin-related poisoning in patients aged 6 to 20 years reported to the AAPCC from 1997 to 2000 more than doubled each year, ultimately numbering nearly 2,500 cases per year (Simone and Bond, 2002). Thirty-nine of

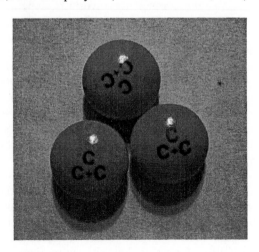

FIGURE 15.1. Coricidin HBP Cough & Cold tablets, "Triple C," which contain DXM and chlorpheniramine.

44 DXM substance abuse-related poisonings reported to an Ohio poison center over a four-month period in 2000 involved Coricidin abuse. The dose was 6 to 23 tablets (average of 13) taken at once. Each tablet contains 30 mg of DXM and 4 mg of chlorpheniramine. Three of the 39 abused Coricidin on a daily basis. These individuals reported using 24 to 56 (average of 51) tablets daily. Patients' ages ranged from 13 to 21 years. Most were 15- to 17-years-old. The most common effects reported were (in rank order) drowsiness, tachycardia, other (numbness, tremor, and pallor), mydriasis, hypertension, and ataxia. Effects lasted no more than eight hours in 60 percent, no more than 24 hours in 33 percent, and no more than three days in 7 percent of those with effects of known duration (Simone et al., 2000).

In another study of 92 cases of Coricidin use/abuse reported to the California poison centers during a nine-month period in 2000, most were 13 to 17 years of age and most ingested 8 to 16 tablets (range of 2 to 60) of Coricidin HBP Cough & Cold. The most common effects (in rank order) were altered mental status, tachycardia, lethargy, hypertension, mydriasis, ataxia/dizziness, confusion, vomiting, elevated temperature, dry mouth, agitation, slurred speech, and hallucinations (Banerji and Anderson, 2001).

Yet another study was done involving cases of intentional use/abuse of Coricidin products in those ten years or older reported to the Texas poison centers during 1998 and 1999. Seventy-eight cases were found. Most involved adolescents 13 to 17 years of age. The most commonly reported effects were (in rank order) tachycardia, somnolence, mydriasis, hypertension, agitation, disorientation, slurred speech, ataxia, vomiting, dry mouth, hallucinations, tremor, headache, dizziness, syncope, seizure, chest pain, and nystagmus (Baker and Borys, 2002).

DXM is available in many forms, including liquid cough syrup, tablets, and powder (Fleming, 1986; Nordt, 1998; Simone et al., 2000). The tablet forms, and sometimes the syrups, often contain other ingredients, such as antihistamines, decongestants, guaifenesin and acetaminophen. Choosing the "wrong" Coricidin is cause for additional concern. Some Coricidin products also contain acetaminophen, which can be hepatotoxic (Kirages, Sule, and Mycyk, 2003).

Much information about DXM is obtained through friends, the Internet or news programs (Boyer, 2004; Boyer, Shannon, and Hibberd, 2005; Iaboni and Aronomitz, 1995). The Vaults of Erowid is a site known to substance abusers (Boyer, Shannon, and Hibberd, 2005). It provides information that appears scientific and promotes "safe" abuse of various drugs, plants, and chemicals (The Vaults of Erowid Web site: http://www.erowid.org/, accessed June 28, 2007). It has links to other sites that provide information about the "plateaus" of DXM high. The First Plateau (1.5 to 2.5 mg/kg

DXM) is described as a low dose that is similar to drinking alcohol or smoking marijuana, and will alter perception of sights and sounds. The Second Plateau (2.5 to 7.5 mg/kg of DXM) is described as one causing visual hallucinations that are not quite like LSD or psychedelic mushrooms, and will cause double vision and staggering. The Third Plateau (7.5 to 15 mg/kg of DXM) reportedly provides hallucinations and an altered state of consciousness, but also delusions and disorientation. The user may not be able to ambulate. The Web site recommends a sitter to prevent harm to self or others. The Fourth Plateau (15 to 30 mg/kg DXM) is the level that disassociates mind from body, may cause vomiting, and renders the user helpless. A sitter is recommended to monitor for choking on vomit, seizures, or other medical emergencies. The user may see God, aliens, or a strange world.

Psychiatric patients also abuse DXM. In one case, a schizophrenic male ingested 240 ml of DXM syrup twice weekly because he was curious about it and it helped him abstain from using alcohol. He described a five- to six-hour high during which he had deep, pleasurable thoughts, heightened awareness of environmental stimuli, thought broadcasting, and altered time perception, as well as a newfound willingness toward previously unpleasant activities. He sought assistance when tolerance to the euphoria developed and side effects became prevalent and unpleasant (Iaboni and Aronomitz, 1995). In another case, a bulimic deliberately took large doses of DXM after purging or fasting to maximize the high (Marsh, Key, and Spratt, 1997).

Mechanism of Action

Dextromethorphan is chemically like an opioid derived from codeine, but does not stimulate opioid receptors at normal doses. It works centrally to suppress coughing by elevating the cough threshold (Hardman, Limbird, and Gilman, 2001). High doses can lead to stimulation of the opioid receptors, causing central nervous system depression and pinpoint pupils. When doses are high enough for the metabolite, dextrorphan, to build up, dissociative effects can occur (Goldfrank et al., 2002). Dextrorphan is chemically similar to phencyclidine, a dissociative analgesic anesthetic that stimulates the glutamate-N-methyl-D-aspartate receptor complex (Schadel and Sellers, 1992).

Medical Consequences of DXM

Cardiac

DXM. Tachycardia and hypertension were reported with abuse (Nordt, 1998).

DXM with Chlorpheniramine. Tachycardia and hypertension were reported (Baker and Borys, 2002; Banerji and Anderson, 2001; Kirages, Sule, and Mycyk, 2003; Simone et al., 2000). Syncope and chest pain were reported (Baker and Borys, 2002).

Neurologic

DXM. Somnolence, drowsiness, easy distractibility, disorientation, confusion, ataxia, slurred speech, exhaustion, and agitation are reported with acute large doses of DXM (Nordt, 1998; Wolfe and Caravati, 1995). Unstable gait/lack of coordination (Nordt, 1998), slurred speech, shivering and tremors, restlessness and insomnia are reported with chronic abuse of large doses, three or four bottles daily, of DXM cough syrup (Wolfe and Caravati, 1995). Insomnia and vertigo are reported with large chronic doses of DXM (Iaboni and Aronomitz, 1995). Restlessness was followed by dizziness and tiredness after snorting 250 mg of DXM "powder" (Fleming, 1986). Cognitive impairment affecting recent memory and problem-solving ability were noted in a case of chronic, frequent ingestion of 1,500 mg of DXM (Hinsberger, Sharma, and Mazmanian, 1994). Blackouts were reported after several consecutive nights of ingestion of 237 mls of DXM cough syrup. Poor concentration was also reported (Marsh, Key, and Spratt, 1997).

DXM with Chlorpheniramine. Altered mental status, lethargy, somnolence, or drowsiness (Baker and Borys, 2002; Banerji and Anderson, 2001; Simone et al., 2000), confusion (Boyer, 2004), ataxia (Banerji and Anderson, 2001; Simone et al., 2000), slurred speech (Banerji and Anderson, 2001), and dizziness (Baker and Borys, 2002; Banerji and Anderson, 2001) were reported. Tremor (Baker and Borys, 2002; Simone et al., 2000), numbness (Simone et al., 2000), and agitation may occur (Baker and Borys, 2002; Banerji and Anderson, 2001). Headache, seizure, and disorientation were also reported (Baker and Borys, 2002).

Gastric

DXM. Nausea (McCarthy, 1971) and vomiting were reported with large doses of DXM cough syrup (Wolfe and Caravati, 1995). Nausea, vomiting, and diarrhea were reported with 240 ml of DXM taken twice weekly (Iaboni and Aronomitz, 1995). Nausea following a high from snorting 250 mg of DXM has been reported (Fleming, 1986) as well as dysphagia with chronic use of DXM-containing liquid taken in large doses chronically (McCarthy, 1971).

DXM with Chlorpheniramine. Dry mouth/oral mucosa, nausea, vomiting, and hypoactive bowel sounds are reported with abuse of large doses

(Baker and Borys, 2002; Banerji and Anderson, 2001; Boyer, 2004; Kirages, Sule, and Mycyk, 2003).

Hepatic

DXM with Chlorpheniramine. Ingestion of a large amount of acetaminophen in a Coricidin product which contained acetaminophen in addition to DXM and chlorpheniramine caused hepatotoxicity (ALT 9000 IU/l, AST 8001 IU/l, PT 42.6 seconds, INR 4.6) in a 16-year-old female (Kirages, Sule, and Mycyk, 2003).

Genitourinary

DXM. Erectile dysfunction was reported with chronic use of large doses of DXM (Iaboni and Aronomitz, 1995; McCarthy, 1971). Serum creatinine was elevated (1.6 mg/dl) in a patient acutely toxic after abusing DXM chronically (Wolfe and Caravati, 1995).

DXM with Chlorpheniramine. A distended bladder and urinary retention occurred in a 16-year-old who abused 50 tablets of Coricidin containing DXM, chlorpheniramine, and acetaminophen (Kirages, Sule, and Mycyk, 2003).

Ears, Eyes, Nose, and Throat

DXM. Mydriasis is reported with abuse (Nordt, 1998). Miosis may occur (Goldfrank et al., 2002). Blurred vision is reported with chronic use of large doses, three to four bottles of DXM cough syrup daily. Horizontal and vertical nystagmus occurred in the same patient with acute use (Wolfe and Caravati, 1995). Bilateral, incomplete, intermittent, recoverable hearing loss was reported in a patient dependent on DXM. Sounds were less loud and less sharp, television and conversation were difficult, and others noticed the difficulty. Hearing was completely recovered within days of cessation of use. This is a self-report (Iqbal, 2002).

DXM with Chlorpheniramine. Mydriasis (Baker and Borys, 2002; Banerji and Anderson, 2001; Simone et al., 2000) and horizontal nystagmus are reported (Boyer, 2004; Kirages, Sule, and Mycyk, 2003).

Dermal

DXM. Diaphoresis is reported with acute abuse and large chronic doses of DXM (Iaboni and Aronomitz, 1995; Nordt, 1998).

DXM with Chlorpheniramine. Facial flushing (Boyer, 2004) and pallor (Simone et al., 2000) are reported.

Psychiatric

DXM. Twenty patients interviewed indicated euphoria, enhanced visual and auditory sensations, altered time perception (time slowing), floating and feeling "distant," tactile hallucinations (hand and finger swelling), visual distortion and hallucinations involving people and animals, and paranoia. The high was occasionally followed by depression (McCarthy, 1971). Visual and auditory hallucinations, floating and flying sensations, "numb" sensation, increased perception intensity, and dysphoria are reported with chronic use of large doses, three to four bottles of DXM cough syrup daily (Wolfe and Caravati, 1995). A patient reported deep, pleasurable thoughts, heightened awareness of environmental stimuli, though broadcasting and altered time perception, as well as newfound willingness toward previously unpleasant activities with twice weekly doses of 240 ml of DXM (Iaboni and Aronomitz, 1995). Another reported feeling "high," "out of my head," and "on top of the world" after snorting 250 mg of pure DXM powder, then depressed after the high was over (Fleming, 1986). Manic-like psychosis was followed by depression and suicidal ideation, and insomnia after acute on chronic episodes of DXM abuse (Hinsberger, Sharma, and Mazmanian, 1994). Hallucinations and blackout were reported after several consecutive nights of ingestion of 237 ml of DXM by a bulimic patient (Marsh, Key, and Spratt, 1997).

DXM with Chlorpheniramine. Inappropriate laughing (Boyer, 2004) and hallucinations (Baker and Borys, 2002; Banerji and Anderson, 2001) are reported.

Withdrawal/Dependence

DXM. Withdrawal craving is reported after chronic use of large doses of DXM cough syrup (Fleming, 1986; Iaboni and Aronomitz, 1995; Marsh, Key, and Spratt, 1997; Wolfe and Caravati, 1995). Increased sensitivity to environmental allergens is reported after withdrawal of large, chronic doses (Iaboni and Aronomitz, 1995).

Other

DXM. Creatinine phosphokinase was elevated (244 IU/l) in an acutely toxic patient abusing large amounts of DXM chronically (Wolfe and Caravati, 1995).

DXM with Chlorpheniramine. Elevated temperature may occur (Banerji and Anderson, 2001).

Laboratory

Excessive doses of DXM may cause a false positive for PCP when measured by high-pressure liquid chromatography. This letter to the editor was based on history only. No further confirmatory laboratory evaluation was reported (Budai and Iskandar, 2002). Gas chromatography/mass spectrophotometry confirmation is suggested to distinguish between PCP and DXM.

EPHEDRINE, PSEUDOEPHEDRINE, AND PROPYLHEXEDRINE

Introduction

Ephedrine and pseudoephedrine are stimulants that are abused as sole ingredients, abused along with other stimulants such as caffeine, and used to manufacture methamphetamine in clandestine laboratories. Propylhexedrine is an inhaled decongestant that is sometimes swallowed or extracted from a cotton pledget and injected for a stimulant effect.

Methamphetamine Laboratories

In addition to use in larger than normal doses for a stimulant effect, ephedrine is a methamphetamine precursor. The source of most of the methamphetamine available in the United States for abuse was thought to be clandestine laboratories (Cunningham and Liu, 2005). Currently as "a result of law enforcement pressure, public awareness campaigns, and increased regulation of sale and use of precursor and essential chemicals," more methamphetamine is coming from Mexico. California and Mexico are now the chief sources of methamphetamine in the United States (U.S. Drug Enforcement Agency Web site: http://www.usdoj.gov/dea/concern/18862/meth.htm, accessed June 28, 2007). The main ingredients for cooking methamphetamine are a decongestant (ephedrine, pseudoepedrine, or phenylpropanolamine) and anhydrous ammonia (Colker, 2005). The phenylpropanolamine actually makes amphetamine, which is sometimes then sold as methamphetamines Closer monitoring of ephedrine due to use in clandestine methamphetamine labs led to the use of pseudoephedrine in the labs (Cunningham and Liu, 2003). Nearly half of the states in the United States restrict the sale of pseudoephedrine as a result; most are West and Midwest states, where the problem is most significant (Colker, 2005). Cunningham and Liu evaluated the impact of methamphetamine precursor regulations on hospital admissions due to methamphetamine abuse complications. Sale and distribution of bulk ephedrine and pseudoephedrine was regulated, then sale of ephedrine-only tablets, and the sale of pseudoephedrine (with or without other active ingredients) tablets. Each time one of these new regulations was enforced, methamphetamine hospital admissions dropped significantly. However, admissions would then increase again within 6 to 24 months, when new methods or supplies replaced the old. Although the overall trend due to increased regulations was a decrease in methamphetamine hospital visits, given time manufacturers were able to find ways around the regulations. Such work-arounds included finding supplies in Canada. It is evident that while regulations regarding sale and distribution are probably helpful in decreasing supply, at least temporarily, the demand side must still be addressed in order to succeed in preventing abuse (Cunningham and Liu, 2003). The recent decrease in availability of ephedrine in dietary supplements may lead to an increase in pseudoephedrine abuse for stimulant effect. However, ephedrine is still available over the counter, and displayed behind the counter at gas stations and other convenience stores. It is in a form that includes guaifenesin, probably due to initial regulations monitoring distribution of products that contain ephedrine as the sole active ingredient. Regulations now also cover ephedrine in combination with other ingredients, although it is unlikely to be used to make methamphetamine.

Look-Alikes and Cocaine Substitutes

"Look-alikes" are OTC medications manufactured to look like and/or have "street names" like controlled drugs. The stimulant look-alikes are tablets and capsules that have effects similar to amphetamine, methamphetamine, and cocaine. Look-alikes usually contain caffeine, ephedrine, or pseudoephedrine. Before it was removed from the market due to association with stroke, phenylpropanolamine was also an ingredient. The drugs may be sold "on the street" as amphetamine or other illicit drugs or purchased legally at stores, from magazines and over the Internet. One common look-alike is the "white cross," a double-scored white tablet that often contains ephedrine, but is meant to look like methamphetamine (see Figure 15.2). At one time, it was estimated that 80-95 percent of stimulants sold on the street as amphetamine were actually look-alikes. The OTC stimulants were initially sold in truck stops in the southeastern United States to fatigued truck drivers in the early 1970s. Most were caffeine with or without other OTC stimulant medications. By 1980, most contained caffeine, ephedrine, and phenylpropanolamine. The age of the average user ranged mostly from elementary school to college. Most were then ordered from magazines. When the Food

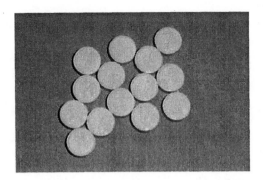

FIGURE 15.2. "White cross" look-alike tablets that may contain ephedrine and are meant to look like methamphetamine.

and Drug Administration (FDA) determined they could seize look-alikes using counterfeiting regulations, manufacturers skirted the law by changing the appearance so that look-alikes no longer looked like amphetamines. Then the United States Postal Service refused to deliver products containing caffeine, ephedrine, and phenylpropanolamine because the claims of safety were misrepresentative. In 1982, the FDA banned sale of the three drugs, and then just caffeine and PPA together, unless a new license for the combination was obtained (Lake and Quirk, 1984). During the 1990s, dietary supplements containing ephedra (ephedrine and pseudoephedrine) with guarana, cola nut, green tea, and/or other plant sources of caffeine largely replaced look-alikes. The new products were offered over the Internet and through magazines such as *High Times*. Although most states have banned the manufacture and marketing of look-alike drugs, and the FDA has taken action against some manufacturers (Quackery targets teens, 1988), look-alikes are still available.

Cocaine substitutes were sold through magazines and in stores in the 1970s. Many contained caffeine, although other ingredients were also used. Other ingredients included nicotine, ephedra (ephedrine and pseudoephedrine), and yohimbe (yohimbine). Users claimed the products caused excitement, stimulation, mental alertness, and euphoria. Adverse effects from caffeine-containing products included abdominal cramping and diarrhea (Siegel, 1980).

Ephedrine Restrictions

Ephedrine-only products were restricted by the FDA in 1994. As a result, manufacturers made a product containing ephedrine with guaifenesin available for OTC treatment of asthma (Whelan and Schwartz, 2004). The products contain 12.5 to 25 mg of ephedrine and 200 to 400 mg of guaifenesin per tablet. For a substance abuser seeking a stimulant ephedrine "high," the guaifenesin would not cause effects significant enough to alter the desired effects.

Mechanisms of Action

Ephedrine is a potent central nervous stimulant that directly stimulates alpha and beta adrenergic receptors and indirectly causes stimulation through release of norepinephrine. It increases heart rate and blood pressure, and causes bronchodilation. Pseudoephedrine is a nasal decongestant isomer of ephedrine with less potent central nervous system and cardiovascular effects (Bruno, Nolte, and Chapin, 1993; Hardman, Limbird, and Gilman, 2001). Propylhexedrine is an alpha-adrenergic sympathomimetic with one-twelfth the central nervous system stimulant effects of amphetamine (Garriott, 1975).

MEDICAL CONSEQUENCES OF EPHEDRINE

Cardiac

A 25-year-old male suffered a myocardial infarction after injecting white ephedrine powder that he thought was amphetamine. Tachycardia, myocardial infarction, and severe left ventricular dysfunction occurred after injection of ephedrine powder. The associated electrocardiogram (ECG) showed widespread ST-segment depression with T-wave inversion. Follow-up ECG one month later showed nonspecific T-wave and ST-segment changes (Cockings and Brown, 1997).

Pulmonary

Tachypnea, cyanosis, and pulmonary edema developed with myocardial infarction after injection of powdered ephedrine. The blood gas showed respiratory alkalosis, hypoxia, and hypercapnea (Cockings and Brown, 1997).

Neurologic

Three adults suffered either ischemic or hemorrhagic stroke after use of ephedrine. Proposed causes include vasculitis and vasoconstriction. A 37-year-old male developed right-sided numbness associated with a left-thalamic infarct after ingestion of ten "white cross" tablets daily (15.3 mg per tablet, 153 mg ingested daily) purchased as street "speed" for diet. A 42-year-old male with a history of hypertension was found dead after ingesting 10 to 20 "white cross" tablets daily for 23 years presumably to get "high." He was suffering from hypertensive cerebral vasculopathy, which would predispose him to stroke. Ephedrine was found in the blood of an 84-year-old female with right subarachnoid hemorrhage and subdural hemorrhage. She was predisposed to stroke due to a berry aneurysm, which ruptured (Bruno, Nolte, and Chapin, 1993).

Genitourinary

A 22-year-old male developed two renal calculi, 4 and 8 millimeters in size, secondary to ingesting 6 to 12 "speed" tablets containing 12.5 mg of ephedrine and 200 mg of guaifenesin daily. The stones were composed of beta-(2-methoxyphenoxy)-lactic acid, a metabolite of guaifenesin (Whelan and Schwartz, 2004). Use of 40 to 120 ephedrine 25 mg tablets (1,000 to 3,000 mg daily) for several years for "stimulation" caused kidney stones in a 24-year-old male. It is not clear whether guaifenesin was also an ingredient or whether the metabolite of guaifenesin was found in the urine (Blau, 1998).

Hematologic

Leukocytosis occurred with myocardial infarction after injection of powdered ephedrine, probably due to physiologic stress (Cockings and Brown, 1997).

PSEUDOEPHEDRINE

See also Antihistamine/Decongestant Medical Consequences of Combinations under Antihistamines in previous text.

A 13-year-old female with a familial history predisposing her to affective disorders became psychotic after ingesting eight 60 mg pseudoephedrine tablets over several hours. Initially she felt "light-headed and giddy," then had psychomotor agitation, became argumentative and confused, laughed and cried, and failed to sleep that night, pacing and talking to herself. The hospital noted insomnia, fatigue, dysphoria, anorexia, auditory hallucinations, pressured speech, psychomotor agitation, difficulty concentrating and extreme distractibility, flight of ideas and elation, thoughts of death, grandiosity, and worthlessness. The patient improved with discontinuation and administration of an antipsychotic, then had similar symptoms several months later when no pseudoephedrine or other medications were known to have been taken. She was diagnosed with mixed bipolar disorder, treated for 18 months, and suffered no further effects during the next year (Dalton, 1990).

A 37-year-old female took 3,000 to 4,500 mg of pseudoephedrine daily for mild euphoria as well as to combat fatigue, apathy, and depression. She increased her usual therapeutic dose over a period of five years, then had difficulty discontinuing without assistance, citing fatigue, depression, and visual hallucinations and illusions as difficulties. Prior to discontinuation, she was hypertensive and tachycardic. She also had slowed speech and general psychomotor retardation, as well as lethargy, insomnia, and some problems with recent memory, and a flat affect. She was tapered to 200 to 300 mg daily until 700 mg, then more slowly, to 90 mg daily, due to onset of depression. She had no difficulties for a two-week observation period after discontinuation (Diaz, Wise, and Semchyshyn, 1979).

Cardiac

Tachycardia and hypertension are reported with excessive daily use (Diaz, Wise, and Semchyshyn, 1979).

Neurologic

Excessive chronic use may cause slowed speech, psychomotor retardation, and disturbance of recent memory (Diaz, Wise, and Semchyshyn, 1979).

Psychiatric

Blunted affect is described after excessive chronic use (Diaz, Wise, and Semchyshyn, 1979).

Withdrawal/Dependence

Discontinuation of excessive chronic use may cause fatigue, depression, and visual hallucinations and illusions (Diaz, Wise, and Semchyshyn, 1979).

PROPYLHEXEDRINE (BENZEDREX NASAL INHALER): USE AND MEDICAL CONSEQUENCES

Most abuse of propylhexedrine involves injection to obtain a "rush" or "high." One patient dissolved the contents in coffee, with lots of sugar to overcome the bitter taste, to relieve fatigue and tension, and to increase alertness. He found that two inhalers daily gave similar but gentler and shorter methamphetamine-like highs (Anderson, 1970).

Propylhexedrine is available in an OTC decongestant inhaler (see Figure 15.3). It is a cotton wick containing 250 mg of propylhexedrine, 4.5 mg of menthol, and other aromatic compounds. It is extracted to make "homemade crank." Extraction involves removing the cotton wick, soaking it in hydrochloric acid, squeezing out the liquid, and heating the liquid at just below boiling point to evaporate the liquid until nearly dry, then allowing it to dry to a powder overnight (Mancusi-Ungaro et al., 1983-1984; Perez, Burton, and McGirr, 1994). Although this process eliminates aromatic compounds in the product, some fine fibers from the cotton wick remain (Mancusi-Ungaro et al., 1983-1984). Another reported method involves soaking the cotton in warm water, then injecting the solution that results (Garriott, 1975). Other street names for the product are "stove-top speed," "bathtub crystal," "peanut butter meth," "bathtub crank," and "bathtub speed." The mixture can be corrosive if not neutralized. The irritation caused by the homemade product is probably responsible for the common choice of neck over peripheral injec-

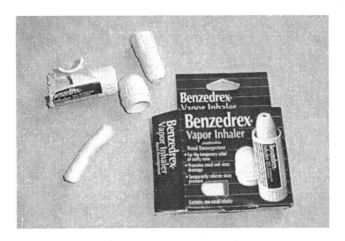

FIGURE 15.3. Propylhexedrine (Benzedrex) inhaler shown with cotton pledget removed.

tion sites, although a better "rush" may also contribute (Fornazzari, Carlen, and Kapur, 1986; Perez, Burton, and McGirr, 1994).

Twelve sudden deaths in Texas were associated with chronic intravenous use of propylhexedrine. The cause was thought to be cardiac arrhythmias in combination with pulmonary hypertension and right ventricular hypertrophy. Most of the cases involved young, black males, and occasionally females (Anderson et al., 1979; White and DiMaio, 1977). Chronic injection of propylhexedrine was associated with left ventricular failure in four patients, three of whom also had right ventricular dilation, and two of whom had pulmonary hypertension. Their ages were 26 to 36 years (Croft, Firth, and Hillis, 1982).

Several hours after swallowing one Benzedrex nasal inhaler, a 22-year-old male developed palpitations, chest pain, and headache. Upon arrival at the emergency department, the patient was cold, diaphoretic, breathless, and had dilated pupils. Initially tachycardic and hypotensive, the patient developed ventricular arrhythmias and became hypotensive. He developed pulmonary edema, and had a myocardial infarction. His course was complicated by pericardial effusion and surgical emphysema (Marsden and Sheldon, 1972).

Cardiovascular

A patient became tachycardic and hypertensive after injecting the right internal jugular vein with propylhexedrine. The patient suffered cardiopulmonary arrest and died two days later (Perez, Burton, and McGirr, 1994). Oral ingestion of one cotton pledget of propylhexedrine initially caused palpitations and severe chest pain, then tachycardia and hypertension occurred initially. This was followed by hypotension with ventricular arrhythmias, anterior myocardial infarct, and pericardial effusion. Prior to this episode, the 22-year-old patient was healthy (Marsden and Sheldon, 1972). Chronic use may lead to arrhythmias, pulmonary hypertension, right and/or left ventricular hypertrophy or dilation. Arrhythmias may occur acutely in chronic users, especially with stress or excitement (Anderson et al., 1979; Croft, Firth, and Hillis, 1982; White and DiMaio, 1977).

Pulmonary

A patient became tachypneic and developed respiratory distress and inspiratory stridor after injecting the right internal jugular vein with propylhexedrine. The patient suffered cardiopulmonary arrest and died two days later (Perez, Burton, and McGirr, 1994). Oral ingestion of one cotton pledget of propylhexedrine resulted in breathlessness, pulmonary edema, and surgical emphysema in an otherwise healthy 22-year-old male. After initial improvement, acute respiratory distress syndrome followed (Marsden and Sheldon, 1972). Diffuse fibrosis, pulmonary hypertension, pulmonary edema, and foreign body granulomas may result from chronic use (Anderson et al., 1979; Croft, Firth, and Hillis, 1982; White and DiMaio, 1977).

Neurological

Generalized headache, diplopia and numbness, and decreased sense of pain and temperature, of half of the face occurred after injection of a neck vein. Neurologic dysfunction when it occurs may be permanent. In two such cases, it is thought that damage to the medial longitudinal fasciculus and brainstem were the cause. In cases of temporary neurologic dysfunction, cranial nerves are affected (Fornazzari, Carlen, and Kapur, 1986; Marsden and Sheldon, 1972).

Gastrointestinal

Dysphagia is reported after injection of the neck veins (Fornazzari, Carlen, and Kapur, 1986).

Hepatic

Liver function markers such as AST, ALT, and GGPT as well as alkaline phosphatase may be elevated after central injection of the neck (Fornazzari, Carlen, and Kapur, 1986).

Hematologic

White blood cell count was elevated in a patient who injected propyl-hexedrine centrally (Covey, Nossaman, and Albright, 1988; Perez, Burton, and McGirr, 1994).

Ears, Eyes, Nose, and Throat

Horizontal and vertical diplopia, horizontal nystagmus, asymmetric pupils, and ophthalmoplegia are reported, as is hemiparesis of the tongue after injection of neck veins (Fornazzari, Carlen, and Kapur, 1986). Mydriasis occurred after ingestion of one cotton pledget (Marsden, 1972).

Dermal and Soft Tissue

A patient developed massive edema and extensive tissue necrosis after injecting his right internal jugular vein with propylhexedrine (Perez, Burton, and McGirr, 1994). Skin ulcers and cellulitis of limbs, and induration of veins in the neck may be present after injection at these sites (Fornazzari, Carlen, and Kapur, 1986). Injection and infiltration of veins in hands and feet may cause pain and cellulitis. Injection of veins and arteries in arms can lead to loss of feeling or numbness, paresthesias, coldness, tenderness, tenseness, cyanosis, ecchymosis, petechiae, abscess, poor capillary filling at the injection site and/or downstream. If significant necrosis results, amputation of fingers may be necessary. Based on evaluation of the effect in animals, the cause for injury is a combination of vasospasm, local vasoconstriction, extravasation, inflammation, infection, and necrosis (Mancusi-Ungaro et al., 1983-1984). Pain, swelling, erythema, mottling, cyanosis, hypesthesia and poor capillary refill, and necrosis necessitating amputation of fingers occurred after injection of the radial aspect of the left wrist (Covey, Nossaman, and Albright, 1988). Ingestion of one cotton pledget resulted in diaphoresis (Marsden and Sheldon, 1972).

Psychiatric

Psychosis developed after ingestions of propylhexedrine with coffee. Symptoms cleared within 24 hours of discontinuation (Anderson, 1970). A 30-year-old schizophrenic exacerbated his underlying disorder several times by chewing propylhexedrine inhalers. The effects reported during exacerbations included acute delusional mood and paranoid delusions (Johnson, Johnson, and Robins, 1972).

Other

Shaking, chills, and fever may occur after injection of propylhexedrine centrally or peripherally (Mancusi-Ungaro et al., 1983-1984; Perez, Burton, and McGirr, 1994). Sepsis is reported (Fornazzari, Carlen, and Kapur, 1986).

NICOTINE REPLACEMENT PRODUCTS

Use of nicotine replacement products sometimes leads to transference of the initial tobacco products addiction to nicotine replacement products addiction. A case of nasal spray misuse and a survey assessing nicotine gum misuse follow. Both involve patients unable to discontinue nicotine replacement therapy.

A 54-year-old male with major depression, alcohol dependence in remission, and a recent tobacco habit requested assistance when unable to discontinue use of 10 mg/ml homemade nicotine nasal spray that he had been using for one year. In the nine months prior to seeking assistance, he increased use to two sprays per nostril every waking hour. Although he was able to quit tobacco, attempts to discontinue the nasal spray caused withdrawal, which manifested as intense craving, irritability, and instability of mood. A daily dose of 2,400 mg of gabapentin allowed the patient to discontinue the nicotine spray more comfortably (Myrick et al., 2001).

One article suggested that 0.7 to 1.4 percent of nicotine gum users develop dependence, defined by an inability to satisfactorily control drug use. A set of telephone surveys interviewed 266 nicotine gum users, and 100 nicotine gum users who felt they were addicted to the gum. In the first group, 84 percent used the gum to discontinue smoking, 9 percent to maintain abstinence, 6 percent to reduce smoking and 1 percent to avoid smoking restrictions. Almost half, 46 percent, were using the nicotine gum longer than the recommended three-month period, much higher than previously reported ranges of 5-10 percent. Twenty percent volunteered that they were "addicted." Those who used the gum for at least 90 days averaged 242 days. Those who used the gum for less than 90 days averaged 23 days. The amount for both was 15-16 mg per day with a standard deviation of 11. Thirty-five percent smoked and chewed gum on the same day. Of these, most (91 percent) were able to reduce the number of cigarettes smoked. Of the 100 "addicted" nicotine gum users, the median duration of gum use was 32 months. The mean daily dose was 30 mg. The 80 percent who attempted to decrease gum usage reported craving for gum (90 percent), restlessness (86 percent), anxiety (84 percent), irritability (80 percent), difficulty concentrating (64 percent), and craving for cigarettes (58 percent). Sixty-one percent indicated gum discontinuation was "extremely difficult." Two-thirds to three-quarters of the self-proclaimed addicted patients met criteria for dependence, based on the *Diagnostic and Statistical Manual of Mental Disorders,* Fourth Edition, Text Revision (DSM-IV-TR), and the *International Classification of Diseases,* Tenth Revision (ICD-10), criteria, respectively (Hughes et al., 2004).

SUMMARY AND CONCLUSIONS

Abuse of over-the-counter (OTC) medications is common. Abusers are often adolescents, due to easy access, and psychiatric patients, who may use OTCs to self-treat psychiatric conditions, then escalate the doses after euphoric or other desirable effects are noted. Although attempts to decrease abuse by controlling access are helpful, at least initially, suppliers and users often find ways to work around laws and regulations. In order to successfully curb abuse of these products, not only supply, but also demand must be addressed. Abuse of OTCs often leads to significant physical and psychiatric effects, some of which are potentially life-threatening, and while others interfere with the long-term health of abusers, including psychiatric well-being. As noted, much of the literature regarding OTC abuse involves single case reports, small samples, or may involve subjects who are part of a special population (e.g., psychiatric patients). Although it is important to understand the possible medical and other consequences of OTC abuse, it is equally important to realize that not all people react to these medications in the same way. Most people experience relatively minor side effects from these medications when taken in therapeutic doses, whereas more severe effects may occur in individuals who abuse OTCs in larger-than-normal doses in an effort to obtain a desired altered state (e.g., intoxication). It is equally important to note that although many OTCs are commonly used and legal, they nevertheless can be harmful and may produce both dependence and withdrawal. Health care professionals need to be aware of the potential for abuse of OTC medications and the associated consequences.

REFERENCES

Adams, D.; Ditzler, T.; Haning, W.F. (1993). Primary caffeine dependence: A case report. *Hawaii Medical Journal* 52(7):190-191, 194.

Anderson, E.D. (1970). Propylhexedrine (Benzedrex) psychosis. *New Zealand Medical Journal* 71(456):302.

Anderson, R.J.; Garza, H.R.; Garriott, J.C.; DiMaio, V. (1979). Intravenous propyl-hexedrine (Benzedrex®) abuse and sudden death. *The American Journal of Medicine* 67(1):15-20.

Baker, S.D.; Borys, D.J. (2002). A possible trend suggesting increased abuse from Coricidin® exposures reported to the Texas Poison Network: Comparing 1998 to 1999. *Veterinary and Human Toxicology* 44(3):169-171.

Banerji, S.; Anderson, I.B. (2001). Abuse of Coricidin HBP cough & cold tablets: Episodes recorded by a poison center. *American Journal of Health-System Pharmacy* 58(19):1811-1814.

Barsoum, A.; Kolivakis, T.T.; Margolese, H.C.; Chouinard, G. (2000). Diphenhydramine (Unisom), a central anticholinergic and antihistaminic: Abuse with massive ingestion in a patient with schizophrenia. *Canadian Journal of Psychiatry* 45(9):846-847.

Bartlik, B.; Galanter, M.; Angrist, B. (1989). Dimenhydrinate addiction in a schizophrenic woman. *Journal of Clinical Psychiatry* 50(12):476.

Benowitz, N.L.; Osterloh, J.; Goldschlager, N.; Kaysen, G.; Pond, S.; Forhan, S. (1982). Massive catecholamine release from caffeine poisoning. *The Journal of the American Medical Association* 248(9):1097-1098.

Blau, J.J. (1998). Ephedrine nephrolithiasis associated with chronic ephedrine abuse. *The Journal of Urology* 160(3 Pt 1):825-826.

Boyer, E.W. (2004). Dextromethorphan abuse. *Pediatric Emergency Care* 20(12): 858-863.

Boyer, E.W.; Shannon, M.; Hibberd P.L. (2005). The Internet and psychoactive substance use among innovative drug users. *Pediatrics* 115(2):302-305.

Brown, J.H.; Sigmundson, H.K. (1969). Delirium from misuse of dimenhydrinate. *Canadian Medical Association Journal* 101(12):49-50.

Bruno, A.; Nolte, K.B.; Chapin, J. (1993). Stroke associated with ephedrine use. *Neurology* 43(7):1313-1316.

Budai, B.; Iskandar, H. (2002). Dextromethorphan can produce false positive phencyclidine testing with HPLC. *American Journal of Emergency Medicine* 20(1):61-62.

Chung, H.; Park, M.; Hahn, E.; Choi, H.; Choi, H.; Lim, M. (2004). Recent trends of drug abuse and drug-associated deaths in Korea. *Annals of the New York Academy of Sciences* 1025:458-464.

Cockings, J.G.L.; Brown, M.A. (1997). Ephedrine abuse causing acute myocardial infarction. *Medical Journal of Australia* 167(4):199-200.

Colker, A.C. (2005). Restricting the sale of pseudoephedrine to prevent methamphetamine production. *National Conference of State Legislatures Legisbrief* 13(7):1-2.

Covey, D.C.; Nossaman, B.D.; Albright, J.A. (1988). Ischemic injury of the hand from intra-arterial propylhexedrine injection. *The Journal of Hand Surgery* 13A(1):58-61.

Cox, D.; Ahmed, Z.; McBride, A.J. (2001). Diphenhydramine dependence. *Addiction* 96(3):516-517.

Craig, D.F.; Mellor, C.S. (1990). Dimenhydrinate dependence and withdrawal. *Canadian Medical Association Journal* 142(9):970-973.

Croft, C.H.; Firth, B.G.; Hillis, L.D. (1982). Propylhexedrine-induced left ventricular dysfunction. *Annals of Internal Medicine* 97(4):560-561.

Crouch, B.I.; Caravati, E.M.; Booth, J. (2004). Trends in child and teen nonprescription drug abuse reported to a regional poison control center. *American Journal of Health-System Pharmacy* 61(12):1252-1257.

Cunningham, J.K.; Liu, L.M. (2003). Impacts of federal ephedrine and pseudoephedrine regulations on methamphetamine-related hospital admissions. *Addiction* 98(9):1229-1237.

Cunningham, J.K.; Liu, L.M. (2005). Impacts of federal precursor chemical regulations on methamphetamine arrests. *Addiction* 100(4):479-488.

Dalton, R. (1990). Mixed bipolar disorder precipitated by pseudoephedrine hydrochloride. *Southern Medical Journal* 83(1):64-65.

Darboe, M.N. (1996). Abuse of dextromethorphan-based cough syrup as a substitute for licit an illicit drugs: A theoretical framework. *Adolescence* 31(121):239-245.

De Nesnera, A.P. (1996). Diphenhydramine dependence: A need for awareness. *Journal of Clinical Psychiatry* 57(3):136-137.

Diaz, M.A.; Wise, T.N.; Semchyshyn, G.O. (1979). Self-medication with pseudoephedrine in a chronically depressed patient. *The American Journal of Psychiatry* 136(9):1217-1218.

Dinndorf, P.A.; McCabe, M.A.; Frierdich, S. (1998). Risk of abuse of diphenhydramine in children and adolescents with chronic illnesses. *The Journal of Pediatrics* 133(2):293-295.

Feldman, M.D.; Behar, M. (1986). A case of massive diphenhydramine abuse and withdrawal from use of the drug. *Journal of the American Medical Association* 255(22):3119-3120.

Fleming, P.M. (1986). Dependence on dextromethorphan hydrobromide. *British Medical Journal (Clinical Research Edition)* 293(6547):597.

Fornazzari, L.; Carlen, P.L.; Kapur, B.M. (1986). Intravenous abuse of propylhexedrine (Benzedrex®) and the risk of brainstem dysfunction in young adults. *The Canadian Journal of Neurological Sciences* 13(4):337-339.

Gardner, D.M.; Kutcher, S. (1993). Dimenhydrinate abuse among adolescents. *Canadian Journal of Psychiatry* 38(2):113-116.

Garriott, J.C. (1975). Propylhexadrine—A new dangerous drug? *Clinical Toxicology* 8(6):665-666.

Goldfrank, L.R.; Flomenbaum, N.E.; Lewin, N.A.; Howland, M.A.; Hoffman, R.S.; Nelson, L.S. (2002). *Goldfrank's Toxicologic Emergencies,* Seventh Edition. New York: McGraw-Hill.

Hardman, J.G.; Limbird, L.E.; Gilman A.G. (2001). *Goodman and Gilman's The Pharmacological Basis of Therapeutics,* Tenth Edition. New York: McGraw-Hill.

Hinsberger, A.; Sharma, V.; Mazmanian, D. (1994). Cognitive deterioration from long-term abuse of dextromethorphan: A case report. *Journal of Psychiatry and Neuroscience* 19(5):375-377.

Hughes, J.R.; Pillitteri, J.L.; Callas, P.W.; Callahan, R.; Kenny, M. (2004). Misuse of and dependence on over-the-counter nicotine gum in a volunteer sample. *Nicotine & Tobacco Research* 6(1):79-84.

Iaboni, R.P.; Aronowitz, J.S. (1995). Dextromethorphan abuse in a dually diagnosed patient. *The Journal of Nervous and Mental Disease* 183(5):341-342.

Iqbal, N. (2002). Recoverable hearing loss with amphetamines and other drugs. *Journal of Psychoactive Drugs* 36(2):285-288.

Jaffe, J.H.; Bloor, R.; Crome, I. (2004). A postmarketing study of relative abuse liability of hypnotic sedative drugs. *Addiction* 99(2):165-173.

Johnson, J.; Johnson, D.A.W.; Robins, A.J. (1972). Propylhexedrine chewing and psychosis. *British Medical Journal* 3(825):529-530.

Kirages, T.J.; Sule, H.P.; Mycyk, M.B. (2003). Severe manifestations of Coricidin intoxication. *American Journal of Emergency Medicine* 21(6):473-475.

Lake, C.R.; Quirk, R.S. (1984). CNS stimulants and look-alike drugs. *Psychiatric Clinics of North America* 7(4):689-701.

Leighton, K.M. (1982). Paranoid psychosis after abuse of Actifed. *British Medical Journal* 284(6318):789-790.

MacFadyen, L.; Eadie, D.; McGowan, T. (2001). Community pharmacists' experience of over-the-counter medicine misuse in Scotland. *The Journal of the Royal Society for the Promotion of Health* 121(3):185-192.

Malcolm, R.; Miller, W.C. (1972). Dimenhydrinate (Dramamine) abuse: Hallucinogenic experiences with a proprietary antihistamine. *The American Journal of Psychiatry* 128(8):126-127.

Mancusi-Ungaro, H.R., Jr.; Decker, W.J.; Forshan, V.R.; Blackwell, S.J.; Lewis, S.R. (1983-1984). Tissue injuries associated with parenteral propylhexedrine abuse. *Clinical Toxicology* 21(3):359-372.

Marsden, P.; Sheldon, J. (1972). Acute poisoning by propylhexedrine. *British Medical Journal* 1(5802):730.

Marsh, L.D.; Key, J.D.; Spratt, E. (1997). Bulimia and dextromethorphan abuse. A case study. *Journal of Substance Abuse Treatment* 14(4):373-376.

May, D.C.; Long, T.; Madden, R.; Hurst, H.E.; Jarboe, C.H. (1981). Caffeine toxicity secondary to street drug ingestion. *Annals of Emergency Medicine* 10(10): 549.

McCarthy, J.P. (1971). Some less familiar drugs of abuse. *The Medical Journal of Australia* 2(21):1078-1081.

Moskowitz, H.; Wilkinson, C.J. (2004). Antihistamines and driving-related behavior: A review of the evidence for impairment. Report No. DOT HS 809 714. Washington, DC: U.S. Department of Transportation.

Myrick, H.; Malcolm, R.; Henderson, S.; McCormick, K. (2001). Gabapentin for misuse of homemade nicotine nasal spray. *American Journal of Psychiatry* 158(3):498.

Nordt, S.P. (1998). "DXM": A new drug of abuse? *Annals of Emergency Medicine* 31(6):794-795.

Parkin, D.E. (1974). Probable Benadryl withdrawal manifestations in a newborn infant. *The Journal of Pediatrics* 85(4):580.

Perez, J.; Burton, B.T.; McGirr, J.G. (1994). Airway compromise and delayed death following attempted central vein injection of propylhexedrine. *The Journal of Emergency Medicine* 12(6):795-797.

Prost, E.; Millson, R.C. (2004). Clozapine treatment of dimenhydrinate abuse. *American Journal of Psychiatry* 161(8):1500.

Pugh, C.R.; Howie, S.M. (1986). Dependence on pseudoephedrine. *The British Journal of Psychiatry* 149:798.

Quackery targets teens (1988, updated 1990). DHHS Publication No. (FDA) 90-1147, accessed through the FDA Web site: http://www.cfsan.fda.gov/~dms/wh-teen2 .html.

Roberts, K.; Gruer, L.; Gilhooly, T. (1999). Misuse of diphenhydramine soft gel capsules (Sleepia®): A cautionary tale from Glasgow. *Addiction* 94(10): 1575-1578.

Russ, N.W. (1988). Abuse of caffeine in substance abusers. *The Journal of Clinical Psychiatry* 49(11):457.

Schadel, M.; Sellers, E.M. (1992). Psychosis with Vicks Formula 44-D abuse. *Canadian Medical Association Journal* 147(6)843-844.

Shaul, P.W.; Farrell, M.K.; Maloney, M.J. (1984). Caffeine toxicity as a cause of acute psychosis in anorexia nervosa. *The Journal of Pediatrics* 105(3):493-495.

Shiuh, T.; Wax, P. (2001). Diphenhydramine abuse and withdrawal in a patient with a history of a 2.5 gram/day dependency (abstract). *Journal of Toxicology Clinical Toxicology* 39(5):543-544.

Siegel, R.K. (1980). Cocaine substitutes. *The New England Journal of Medicine* 302(14):817-818.

Simone, K.E.; Bond, G.R. (2002). Detection of unusual abuse patterns using broad searching of the Toxic Exposure Surveillance System (abstract). *Journal of Toxicology Clinical Toxicology* 40(5):657-658.

Simone, K.E.; Bottei, E.M.; Siegel, E.S.; Tsipis, G.B. (2000). Coricidin abuse in Ohio teens and young adults (abstract). *Journal of Toxicology Clinical Toxicology* 38(5):532.

Smith, S.G.; Davis, W.M. (1984). Nonmedical use of butorphanol and diphenhydramine. *Journal of the American Medical Association* 252(8):1010.

Sundararaghavan, S.; Suarez, W.A. (2004). Oral Benadryl and central venous catheter abuse—A potentially "lethal combination." *Pediatric Emergency Care* 20(9): 604-606.

Whelan, C.; Schwartz, B.F. (2004). Bilateral guaifenesin ureteral calculi. *Urology* 63(1):175-176.

White, L.; DiMaio, V.J.M. (1977). Intravenous propylhexedrine and sudden death. *The New England Journal of Medicine* 297(19):1071.

Wolfe, T.R.; Caravati, E.M. (1995). Massive dextromethorphan ingestion and abuse. *American Journal of Emergency Medicine* 13(2):174-176.

Young, G.B.; Boyd, D.; Kreeft, J. (1988). Dimenhydrinate: Evidence for dependence and tolerance. *Canadian Medical Association Journal* 138(5):437-438.

Chapter 16

Interaction of Alcohol with Medications and Other Drugs

John Brick
Mark C. Wallen
William J. Lorman

INTRODUCTION AND OVERVIEW

This chapter reviews the interaction between alcohol (ethanol, unless otherwise specified) and therapeutic medications used during the course of treatment for alcohol dependence, or in patients being treated for mental illness who continue to drink alcohol. The interaction between alcohol and other drugs, particularly those commonly used and most likely to be encountered during the clinical evaluation of a multidrug abuser is also reviewed. The focus on alcohol as the common denominator is due to the fact that alcohol is the most widely encountered drug of abuse. The widespread use and social acceptance of alcohol in society, coupled with the extensive medical consequences and overwhelming representation of alcohol in accidental and other injuries, hospital emergency department visits and admissions justifies the need and focus of this review. Even a brief summary of all other drug interactions would go well beyond the scope of this chapter, but an understanding of the mechanisms by which drug interactions occur will allow reasonable predictions about many of the interactions between classes of drugs not covered in this review.

Here, the term "drug" may refer to both licit or illicit drugs, whereas the term "medication" will refer specifically to therapeutic medications. The study of alcohol-drug interactions in a laboratory environment allows investigators to carefully define and control dependent and independent vari-

Handbook of the Medical Consequences of Alcohol and Drug Abuse
© 2008 by The Haworth Press, Taylor & Francis Group. All rights reserved.
doi:10.1300/6039_16

ables. The biobehavioral efforts of the drug interactions discussed are based upon reported research. However, potential alcohol-drug interactions outside of the laboratory are complicated by real-world variations in dose and drug potency, duration and frequency of use, concomitant use of other drugs, and individual characteristics of the user, including physiological factors such as tolerance, metabolic state, diseases, and anthropometrics.

Understanding Alcohol

Alcohol generally acts as a central nervous system depressant, although under some conditions, alcohol increases locomotor activity, loquaciousness, and other behaviors leading to the perception that alcohol is also a stimulant. The perceived stimulating properties of alcohol are related more to the decrease in inhibitions produced by this drug rather than actual stimulant effects, at least in humans. Pharmacologically, alcohol acts much more like a central nervous system (CNS) depressant or anxiolytic. The chemistry and specific CNS depressant and other effects of alcohol are discussed elsewhere in this book. As discussed in Chapters 1, 2, 3, and 5, the pharmacology of alcohol is complex and its biobehavioral effects quite broad, probably because alcohol is capable of altering receptors, ion transport, cell membranes, and most cellular mechanisms critical to neurophysiology and ultimately a range of behaviors. Alcohol also has the ability to alter the pharmacokinetics and pharmacodynamics of other drugs. Changes in bioavailability and efficacy of drugs in the presence of alcohol, or in patients with a history of alcohol dependence, have important implications for diagnoses, treatment, and outcome and should be part of a complete clinical evaluation.

Why Do People Use Multiple Drugs?

We live in a society in which the use and abuse of drugs, including alcohol, is common. In an age when people live longer and are treated for multiple illnesses using multiple medications over the course of their lifetimes, the risk for drug interactions is probably greater than at any previous point in history. Moreover, the risk for harmful drug interactions is still greater when those drugs are not prescribed and their use not monitored, such as in the case of illicit drugs, or when commonly used and available drugs such as alcohol are used in combination with psychoactive medications. Most persons trained in neuropharmacology, toxicology, or medicine are aware of the pernicious effects of some of the more commonly used drugs and inherent dangers of combining drugs. Public education about the dangers of drug use has been mainstream for decades, yet multiple drug ingestion is relatively common in our society. Clearly we can do more. Graduate and medical school curricula need to emphasize further the consequences of drug interactions and public education about this problem must continue. Although the biopsychosocial factors of drug use and drug interactions are complex and not fully identified, the following explanations may be helpful in understanding multidrug use.

Common Reasons for Drug Use

1. To feel good, relieve stress, temporarily escape
2. Peer pressure, rite of passage, influence by media glamorization
3. Enhanced performance (e.g., stimulants to stay awake to meet a deadline or enhance sexual performance/pleasure, or steroid use to enhance athletic performance)

Common Reasons for Multidrug Use

1. *Increase the primary drug effect.* Many drug effects are increased when another drug is added, thereby increasing the intensity of the "high" or, when used clinically, increasing the effectiveness of treatment.
2. *Decrease the undesirable side effects of the primary drug.* Some therapeutic cancer treatments cause decreased appetite and nausea as a side effect. The use of "medical marijuana" reduces these symptoms (although marijuana has its own side effects). Similarly, alcohol or some other depressant may be used to alleviate the edgy feeling many people experience after the desired effects of a stimulant wear off.
3. *Short supply of the primary drug.* Sometimes when the availability of the drug of choice is limited, another drug with similar properties will be substituted. Heroin addicts, for example, often drink large amounts of alcohol or use other depressants to reduce or delay the opioid withdrawal syndrome or until additional narcotics can be procured.
4. *Sensation seeking.* Some individuals will often take any combination of drugs without regard for safety, and without any particular rationale other than the desire to become intoxicated. This form of drug use can be particularly dangerous.
5. *Medical management.* In the course of medical treatment, it is not uncommon to prescribe drugs that may interact with therapeutic or nontherapeutic drugs. Physicians must recognize the potential for these interactions as in addition to a prescription medication, their patients may ingest other drugs (e.g., alcohol, being the most common), and advise patients accordingly.

PHARMACOLOGICAL BASIS
OF ALCOHOL-DRUG INTERACTIONS

Drug interactions can produce alterations in physiology and ultimately behavior through two broad but interrelated mechanisms: changes in pharmacokinetics, or changes in pharmacodynamics. Pharmacokinetic mechanisms account for drug interactions when the presence of one drug affects the bioavailability of another drug. Pharmacodynamic interactions account for drug interactions when drugs interact at the receptor level.

Pharmacokinetic Interactions

Pharmacokinetic interactions alter the bioavailability of the drug. The greater the availability of a drug to interact with receptors or other cellular components, the greater the effect will be whether it is desirable or undesirable. Pharmacokinetic interactions can occur through changes in drug absorption, distribution, metabolism, and excretion.

Absorption

Delays or acceleration in absorption can alter the amount of drug that enters the circulation. The most common site for such an interaction would be through the gastrointestinal system. For example, alcohol increases the absorption rate of some sedatives such as benzodiazepine, so that more drug will enter the circulation than if the drug were taken without alcohol in the stomach.

Distribution

Once a drug is absorbed from the gastrointestinal tract into the circulation, it is for all practical purposes distributed throughout the watery portions of the body. Although the mechanisms for changes in distribution are often not well understood, changes by one drug in the volume of distribution of another drug will alter the effectiveness of that drug. For example, alcohol increases the volume of distribution of cocaine, which may decrease the concentration of cocaine in the circulation.

Metabolism

Once a drug has been administered, it is subject to biotransformation at different sites in the body and via different physiological mechanisms. Studies of the cytochrome P450 and their substrates can be helpful in predicting drug interactions. The P450 isoenzymes are located primarily in the endoplasmic reticulum of hepatocytes and play an important role in the oxidative metabolism of many drugs, including alcohol. Isosymes are classified into different groups or families based upon their amino acid sequence. The nomenclature is as follows: prefix CYP is followed by the family (Arabic number), the subfamily (upper case number), followed by the individual isoenzyme (Arabic number). The major isoenzymes involved in drug metabolism are CYP3A4, CYP2D6, CYP1A2, CYP2E1, and the subfamily of CYP2C (Michalets, 1998).

Many drugs share enzyme systems (e.g., cytochrome P450, alcohol dehydrogenase, aldehyde dehydrogenase) in their biotransformation. When two drugs share the same metabolic pathway, the presence of one drug can alter the metabolism (and thus the bioavailability) of the other drug. For example, beverage alcohol alters the metabolism of methanol by competing for the enzyme that transforms methanol to toxic metabolites. As the metabolism of a drug is an important factor in its bioavailability, changes in drug half-life (the time it takes for the concentration of a drug in circulation to decrease 50 percent) can have significant consequences on the efficacy and toxicity of one or more drugs. Table 16.1 illustrates the amount of drug present with each remaining half-life. If the half-life is increased or decreased by a pharmacokinetic interaction, the amount of drug remaining in the circulation to produce some physiological or psychological change will be proportionally increased or decreased.

Excretion

Drugs are eliminated from the body through the lungs, kidneys, and less important routes, such as through sweat, saliva, or tears. With the exception

TABLE 16.1. How drug half-life affects drug concentration in the circulation.

Number of half-lives	Eliminated (%)	Remaining (%)
0	0	100
1	50	50
2	75	25
3	87.5	12.50
4	93.75	6.250
5	96.875	3.125
6	98.437	1.563
7	99.2470	0.753

of the pulmonary system, excretory organs eliminate drugs based upon their electrical charge (e.g., polar compounds leave the body more easily than lipid soluble drugs). Therefore, changes in the pH of the urine produced by a physiological condition such as respiratory or metabolic acidosis or alkalosis, or by a drug, can drastically alter drug elimination. For example, there is maximum excretion of drugs that are weak acids (such as salicylate and phenobarbital) when the urine is alkaline. On the other hand, renal excretion of alkaline drugs (such as amphetamines and phencylidine) is enhanced when the urine is acidic. Thus, shifts in acid-base physiology may alter drug bioavailability (Ellenhorn and Barceloux, 1988).

Pharmacodynamic Interactions

Pharmacodynamics is the study of the physiological and biochemical effects of drugs and their mechanism of action. For most psychoactive drugs, the mechanism of their action is the alteration of the functional activity of receptors or endogenous ligands (i.e., neurotransmitters and hormones) in the brain. Many other drugs exert similar effects outside the central nervous system (e.g., cardiac beta-receptor antagonists). Changes in the pharmacodynamics or functional activity of neurons that modulate cognitive and psychomotor effects, for example, will alter physiology and behavior. The four major types of pharmacodynamic drug interactions are shown in Figure 16.1.

Additive

When the combination of two drugs is equal to the sum of the effect of each drug (e.g., $2 + 2 = 4$). For example, the CNS depressant effects of many benzodiazepines and alcohol are additive, as are the effects of many barbi-

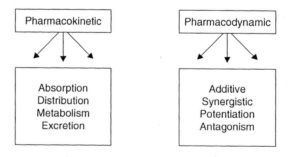

FIGURE 16.1. Pharmacological bases of drug interactions.

turates with alcohol (see the section titled Alcohol and Sedative Hypnotics in this chapter).

Synergistic

The combination of two drugs produces an effect that is greater than the effect of either drug combined (e.g., 2 + 2 = 6). Synergistic interactions produce effects far greater than would be predicted from the sum of either drug. For example, alcohol and carbon tetrachloride, a cleaning fluid, are toxic to the liver. However, the combination of the two produces much more liver damage than would be predicted from the sum of their individual effects. Similarly in some cases alcohol synergistically enhances the sedative effect of barbiturates and some effects of opiates (see the section titled Alcohol and Opiates, this chapter).

Potentiation

Potentiated drug effects are similar to synergistic effects but usually describe an increase in the toxic effect of a drug when combined with a nontoxic drug (e.g., 0 + 1 = 2). Histamine$_2$ (H$_2$) antagonists such as cimetadine can be considered to potentiate the toxic effects of alcohol by increasing alcohol bioavailability (see the section titled Alcohol and Histamines, this chapter).

Antagonism

An antagonist is a drug that blocks the effect of another drug (e.g., 2 + 2 = 1 or 2 + 2 = 0). Antagonists are very specific. For example, Naloxone has a much higher affinity for opiate receptors than heroin. Administering Naloxone to someone who has overdosed on heroin will produce a rapid reversal of the respiratory depression produced by the heroin. Similarly, many antipsychotics reduce symptoms of schizophrenia because they are dopamine receptor antagonists. Dispositional antagonism occurs when the absorption, metabolism, distribution, or excretion of one drug is affected by another drug. For example, alcohol increases the absorption rates of some benzodiazepines (see the section on Alcohol and Anxiolytics, this chapter).

SPECIFIC ALCOHOL-DRUG INTERACTIONS

With a basic understanding of the pharmacological mechanisms by which alcohol-drug interactions may occur, let us examine specific alcohol-drug interactions.

Alcohol and Acetaminophen

The over-the-counter (OTC) medication acetaminophen (Tylenol) is one of the most commonly consumed medications in the United States because of its effective analgesic and antipyretic properties. Acetaminophen is metabolized by the CYP2E1 isozyme to a toxic intermediate, N-acetyl-p-benzoquinone imine (NAPQI), which is detoxified by the antioxidant glutathione (Kuffner, 2001). Chronic alcohol use reduces the amount of the glutathione produced in the liver cell mitochondria. When a person ingests large amounts of acetaminophen and/or has reduced glutathione levels resulting from chronic alcohol use, the amount of NAPQI produced overwhelms the detoxification system of the liver. The resulting hepatotoxicity may progress to the point of fulminant hepatic failure and death.

There is some controversy in the medical community as to the amount of alcohol consumed and/or the amount of acetaminophen necessary to cause this toxic effect to occur. Older studies indicated that liver damage can occur in individuals consuming alcohol even when acetaminophen is consumed in therapeutic dosage amounts (Black, 1984; Girre et al., 1993; Seeff et al., 1986). A more recent study indicated that there was no increase in liver toxicity among alcoholics given the maximal therapeutic dose (4 g/day) of acetaminophen (Kuffner and Dart, 2001). They concluded that there was no clinical evidence of increased risk for these patients when acetaminophen is used within recommended doses. As a result of these findings, people who are consuming alcohol in mild to moderate amounts should be cautioned against exceeding the recommended daily dose of acetaminophen. Individuals who are heavy consumers of alcohol, are active alcoholics, or individuals with any type of liver damage should probably be advised to avoid acetaminophen use totally.

Alcohol and Antibiotics

Antibiotics are used to treat infectious diseases. In combination with acute alcohol consumption, some antibiotics may cause nausea, vomiting, headache, and possibly convulsions. Among these antibiotics are furazolidone, griseofulvin, metronidazole, and the antimalarial quinacrine.

Isoniazid and rifampin are used together to treat tuberculosis, a disease especially problematic among the elderly in nursing homes and among homeless alcoholics. Although the incidence of tuberculosis has declined dramatically during the last century, pockets of the disease among the indigent alcoholic population have been a major factor in preventing its eradication in this country. Treatment of this population has been problematic, mainly because of patients' lack of cooperation with their therapy, including failure to take prescribed medications. This noncompliant behavior in alcohol and other drug-abusing populations is mainly responsible for the recent occurrence of multidrug-resistant tuberculosis. Thus, overall, the effectiveness of the antituberculosis medications is greatly reduced. In addition, acute alcohol consumption decreases the bioavailability of isoniazid in the bloodstream, whereas chronic alcohol use decreases the bioavailability of rifampin. Consequently, the pharmacokinetic interaction between alcohol and these antibiotics may reduce their effectiveness (Jacobson, 1992).

The antibiotic erythromycin accelerates gastric emptying and may reduce first-pass metabolism of alcohol in the stomach resulting in increased absorption in the intestines and higher blood alcohol levels. Conversely, many aerobic bacteria in the colon are capable of metabolizing alcohol because they possess alcohol dehydrogenase (ADH) activity. In rats, treatment with the antibiotic ciprofloxacin totally eliminated the colonic metabolism of alcohol resulting in increased blood alcohol concentrations (Nosova et al., 1999).

Although controversial, patients drinking alcohol while taking metronidazole or ketoconazole may suffer from symptoms similar to those found with disulfiram (Antabuse): abdominal distress, nausea, vomiting, and headache (Cina, Russell, and Conradi, 1996). Similarly, cefoperazone (Cefobid), griseofulvin (Fulvicin, Grisactin), isoniazide (INH), metronidazole (Flagyl), nitrofurantoin (Furadantin, Macrodantin), and sulfamethoxazole (Bactrim, Septra) inhibit aldehyde dehydrogenase and may also produce a disulfiram-like reaction.

Alcohol and Anticoagulant Medications

Warfarin (Coumadin) is prescribed to reduce the ability of the blood to clot and is commonly used to treat patients with irregular heart rhythms, artificial heart valves, and following open heart surgery. Warfarin is metabolized by the cytochrome P450 enzyme system in the liver. The anticlotting effect of warfarin may be increased above the desired therapeutic effect if a person ingests a few drinks or more while taking warfarin. This increased bioavailability of warfarin is due to alcohol-related inhibition of warfarin metabolism by the cytochrome P450 enzyme system (Lieber, 1994). This could result in the emergence of potentially life-threatening hemorrhages. However, in people who drink alcohol regularly, and especially in some alcoholics, the chronic consumption of alcohol will result in induction of the cytochrome P450 enzyme system. The result of this will be an increased rate of metabolism of warfarin which will interfere with the effectiveness of warfarin in reducing blood clotting (Lieber, 1992). Such individuals will often need larger doses of warfarin to achieve the desired therapeutic effect.

Owing to the potential severity of the consequences of drinking alcohol while taking warfarin, anyone taking this medication should be advised not to drink. Acute alcohol may decrease, whereas chronic alcohol may increase the degradation of warfarin (Hoyumpa, 1983). People who have been consuming alcohol on a regular basis prior to starting warfarin should make sure their physicians are aware of this, and physicians should recommend to patients prescribed warfarin that they should avoid alcohol.

Alcohol and Anticonvulsants

These medications are prescribed for the treatment of seizures and bipolar disorder and are increasingly used for their impulse control properties. Since 1993, eight new anticonvulsant drugs have become available in the United States: felbamate, gabapentin, lamotrigine, topiramate, tiagabine, levetiracetam, oxcarbazepine, and zonisamide. Of the older anticonvulsants, six continue to be widely used: phenobarbital, phenytoin, primidone, ethosuximide, carbamazepine, and valproate. A more favorable pharmacokinetic profile is observed in the majority of the newer drugs in comparison with the classic agents. Good absorption, linear kinetics, and minimal potential for interaction with other drugs make these medications easier to use. The newer anticonvulsants are eliminated through different combinations of liver metabolism and direct renal excretion, thus providing a wider variety of choices in patients with failure of one of these organs.

Depending on its chronicity of use, alcohol will have totally different pharmacokinetic effects with the older anticonvulsants. Acute alcohol consumption increases the availability of phenytoin and the risk of drug-related side effects. Chronic drinking may decrease phenytoin bioavailability, significantly reducing the patient's protection against seizures, even during a period of abstinence (Greenspan and Smith, 1991).

Alcohol and Antidepressants

There is a robust literature on the correlation between alcoholism and depression (Hesselbrock, Meyer, and Keener, 1985). The relationship between alcohol dependence and depression has been attributed to many causes including self-medication of depressive symptoms with alcohol, a view that many patients believe. As symptoms of major depression often continue during periods of abstinence, it suggests that there is a comorbid depressive disorder in alcoholics that typically requires specific pharmacological treatment. Many active alcoholics are prescribed antidepressants leading to a high potential for alcohol-antidepressant interactions. Several classes of antidepressants are available and are defined by how they affect the neurotransmitter system. Some antidepressants cause varying degrees of sedating activity but these drugs should not be described as depressants or sedatives. Nevertheless, alcohol increases the sedative and other effects of tricyclic antidepressants such as amitriptyline (Elavil) (Dorian et al., 1983). In addition, alcohol-induced liver disease further impairs antidepressant metabolism and causes significantly increased levels of active medication in the body (Weathermon, 1999). In a study of alcoholics, the disposition of imipramine in alcoholic and nonalcoholic patients with depression varied significantly. Oral imipramine clearance was more than two times greater in alcoholic patients than controls (Ciraulo et al., 1982). Interestingly in a similar study of recently detoxified men with alcohol dependence, the elimination half-life for imipramine was more than doubled in alcoholics after intravenous infusion. Plasma concentrations of imipramine were also significantly lower in the alcoholics, resulting in the suggestion that standard doses of some antidepressants may fail to produce adequate therapeutic changes in alcoholics. For imipramine, the doses may have to be doubled (Ciraulo et al., 1988).

Serotonin reuptake inhibitors (SSRIs) such as fluoxetine (Prozac), sertraline (Zoloft), paroxetine (Paxil), and citalopram (Celexa) have the best safety profile of all antidepressants, even when combined in large quantities with alcohol. No serious interactions seem to occur when these agents are consumed with moderate doses of alcohol (Matilla, 1990). In addition, neither fluoxetine nor alcohol alters the pharmacokinetics or psychomotor effects of the other, although alcohol impairs performance of most subjects on psychomotor tests (Allen, Lader, and Curran, 1988; Lemberger et al., 1985). As many SSRIs are metabolized by cytochrome P450, the lack of any significant pharmacokinetic interaction is probably because the metabolism of these drugs is through different isozymes. Although cytochrome P450 studies can be useful in identifying drug interactions, some of those interactions have no clinical significance in the case of SSRIs such as fluoxetine.

Concurrent use of the monoamine oxidase inhibitors (MAOIs) with alcohol will potentially precipitate a hypertensive crisis and may also enhance sedation. The mechanism for this reaction has been attributed to increased concentrations of the amino acid tyramine (Simpson and Gratz, 1992), which is present in many alcoholic beverages (e.g., wines) and foods (e.g., cheeses, bananas). Tyramine is a potent hypertensive agent. Although most dietary tyramine is destroyed by MAO in the intestines and liver, tyramine will enter the circulation in patients treated with MAOIs and may produce hypertension. Although rare, the hypertensive effect of this amino acid can result in sudden death (Blackwell et al., 1967). Therefore, alcohol use should be avoided in patients prescribed MAOIs.

Atypical antidepressants generally do not seem to have any problematic interactions with alcohol. However, mirtazapine (Remeron), when combined with alcohol, causes impaired cognition and decreased motor performance (Sitsen, 1995).

Alcohol and Antidiabetic Medications

The oral hypoglycemic agents are commonly prescribed for the treatment of diabetes mellitus in patients not requiring insulin. As previously noted, chlorpropamide (Diabinase), glyburide (Diabeta, Micronase), and tolbutamide (Orinase) inhibit aldehyde dehydrogenase and can cause disulfiramlike reactions following alcohol consumption. Metformin (Glucophage) may increase lactic acid levels in the blood following alcohol ingestion that could result in acute lactic acidosis with potentially lethal results. Alcohol consumption by patients taking many of these medications could increase the risk of causing lower than normal blood sugar levels due to impairment of gluconeogenesis in the liver. This generally occurs in the fasting state when the diabetic's blood sugar is already low and the body depends on the production of new glucose molecules to maintain sufficient blood glucose levels (Weathermon et al., 1999). If these patients choose to consume alcohol, they should be advised to drink only with or shortly after meals. Some additional potential medical complications of consuming alcohol while taking these medications include tachycardia, sudden changes in blood pressure, convulsions, and coma (NIAAA, 2003).

Alcohol and Antihistamines (H₁-Antagonists)

Antihistamines (H_1-antagonists) are the mainstay of symptomatic therapy for allergic disorders. Drugs such as diphenhydramine (Benadryl and others) are available without prescription to treat allergic symptoms. Others, such as hydroxyzine (Vistaril, Atarax), are used to treat anxiety and require a prescription. Many antihistamines cause drowsiness, which make them useful to treat insomnia, but potentially dangerous because they can impair skills necessary for safe motor vehicle operation or other complex divided attention tasks. Alcohol can substantially enhance the sedating effects of these agents and may further impair the ability to drive or operate other types of machinery (Ridout et al., 2003). Many common sedative antihistamines, such as chlorpheniramine and diphenhydramine, significantly impair psychomotor performance and significantly increase the deleterious effects of alcohol on reaction time, coordination, and related psychophysical tests (Burns, 1989; Burns and Mostowitz, 1980; Franks et al., 1979).

Newer antihistamines such as fexofenadine, loratadine, and cetirizine have been developed to minimize drowsiness and sedation while still providing effective therapeutic value. However, these newer medications may still be associated with an increased risk of hypotension and fall-down injuries among the elderly, particularly when combined with alcohol (Weathermon and Crabb, 1999). As reviewed in Chapter 2, the relative risk for a fall-down injury is significantly elevated by alcohol alone. This may be especially problematic in older patients or alcohol abusers who may also have osteopenia. Therefore, the interaction of alcohol and antihistamines in geriatric populations is of significant interest.

The deleterious interaction between alcohol and most sedative antihistamines is well documented. Antihistamines can produce significant drowsiness which is worsened by the use of an additional depressant, alcohol. When an interaction occurs, it appears to be due to the combined or additive central nervous depressant effects of both the alcohol and the antihistamine. The effects of many of the antihistamines with alcohol have not been formally studied, but it seems more probable than not that the combined use of these drugs will result in increased drowsiness and increased driving risks (Roehrs, Zwyghuizen-Doorenbos, and Roth, 1993). This has been further clarified by Zimatkin and Anichtchik (1999) who has found that histamine receptor antagonism can affect alcohol metabolism and change the sensitivity to the hypnotic effects of alcohol.

Alcohol and Antipsychotics

Many antipsychotics produce sedation and psychomotor impairment. Acute alcohol consumption increases the sedative effect of these drugs, resulting in further impaired coordination and potentially fatal respiratory depression. This effect appears to be additive, but the mechanisms of this interaction are uncertain. The low potency conventional antipsychotics (e.g., chlorpromazine and thioridazine) are much more sedating than the high potency antipsychotics (e.g., haloperidol and fluphenazine) and tend to cause more significant CNS depression. For example, earlier reports revealed that daily 200 mg doses of chlorpromazine and relatively low blood alcohol concentrations (42 mg/dl) produced significant impairment in the performance of skills related to driving and produced subjective complaints of feeling sleepy, lethargic, dull, groggy, and poorly coordinated behavior (Zirkle et al., 1959). A similar effect is observed when lower doses of chlorpromazine (1 mg/kg) were combined with higher (80 mg/dl) blood alcohol concentrations (Millner and Landauer, 1971). Rather less psychomotor impairment was observed when alcohol was combined with flupenthixol (Linnoila, 1973; Linnoila et al., 1975) or thioridazine (Linnoila, 1973; Linnoila et al., 1975; Millner and Landauer, 1971), but not with haloperidol (Linnoila, 1973; Linnoila et al., 1975). Changing doses, steady-state pharmacokinetics, and type of antipsychotic medication make predictions about the interaction of these drugs with alcohol difficult. More work is needed to understand the nature of this interaction.

Long-term effects of some psychotropic medications present other problems. Patients who are taking high potency antipsychotics concurrently with alcohol are at higher risk for worsening of extrapyramidal symptoms (EPS) associated with long term use of these medications alone. Also, chronic alcohol consumption causes increased metabolism of the antipsychotic medications resulting in lower blood levels and, ultimately, lesser efficacy of the medication. As antipsychotic medications are typically used to treat mental illnesses such as schizophrenia, this may result in a particularly challenging and unpredictable patient. Coupled with the increased risk for hepatitis in patients treated with antipsychotics, the combination of chronic alcohol ingestion and antipsychotic drugs may result in even greater susceptibility for liver damage (Goff and Baldessarini, 1993), as well as a less stable mental status.

Alcohol and Cannabinoids

The medical consequences of alcohol and of cannabinoids are discussed separately elsewhere in this book. Less well studied are the consequences of the combined use of these widely used drugs. As alcohol and tetrahydrocannibinol (THC) which is derived from marijuana are two of the most commonly encountered drugs detected in motor vehicle collisions, the interactive effects of these drugs has received considerable scientific attention. The effects of marijuana on drowsiness, memory, and distortion of space and time are particularly important because of the obvious need for such skills in motor vehicle operation, for example. Two major reviews, primarily on the effects of marijuana on laboratory tests, driving simulators, and other tasks believed to represent those skills necessary for safe driving, concluded that marijuana impairs driving (Moskowitz, 1976, 1985).

In one of the earlier interactive studies on the effects of marijuana and alcohol on driving, Casswell (1977) tested drivers on a 35-minute closed course. While driving the course, drivers were given instructions via headphones, and road signs, brake and accelerator pedal speed and steering were monitored. The authors found that (1) alcohol alone increased speed and impaired steering; (2) marijuana alone reduced speed and slowed response to instruction; and (3) alcohol and marijuana tended to increase speed, impair steering, and increase response times to instructions. More recent studies examined the effects of alcohol and marijuana on road-tracking tests and car following tests (similar to Casswell's 1977 method) and concluded that (1) the effects of THC and alcohol appear to be additive; (2) 100 mg/kg doses of THC combined with 40 mg/dl blood alcohol concentration impairs visual search patterns while driving; and (3) together, marijuana and alcohol increase reaction time (40 mg/dl) more than either drug separately. The authors point out that the effects of alcohol are greater than those of marijuana, noting that the combination of both drugs is particularly dangerous with regard to motor vehicle operation (Lamers and Ramaekers, 2000; Robbe and O'Hanlon, 1999).

Although the overwhelming majority of studies support the conclusion that alcohol and marijuana impair driving, not all investigators found an alcohol-marijuana interaction. For example, Smiley, Ziedman, and Moskowitz (1981) found that after taking marijuana, drivers became more cautious in overtaking tasks. Alcohol (45 or 75 mg/dl) had a slight effect but no interaction between alcohol and marijuana was observed. Using a driving simulator, Stein et al. (1983) found that after alcohol (100 mg/dl), drivers had more "accidents" and "speeding tickets" and slower and less accurate responses to road signs. Marijuana (4 or 8 mg) had "only an occassional effect" and no interaction was observed. Many of these older studies indicate that the primary effects of marijuana are different to those produced by alcohol. Marijuana intoxication results in decreased driving speed and decreased risk-taking behavior under some driving conditions, whereas alcohol has the opposite effect. However, the combination of alcohol and marijuana is believed to be more dangerous than for either drug alone. The nature of any pharmacodynamic interaction is difficult to explain as the neuropharmacological effects of these drugs are complex and diverse.

There is some evidence of a pharmacokinetic interaction between alcohol and marijuana. Lukas et al. (1992) found that smoking marijuana decreases the bioavailability of alcohol, reducing the maximum serum alcohol concentration and delaying the time to peak concentration from 78 mg/dl (50 minutes after drinking) to about 55 mg/dl (105 minutes after drinking). More research on this potential pharmacokinetic interaction is needed.

Alcohol and Cardiovascular Medications

This class of drugs includes a wide variety of medications prescribed to treat disorders of the heart and circulatory system. Acute alcohol consumption interacts with some of these drugs to cause dizziness or fainting upon standing (orthostatic hypotension). These drugs include nitroglycerin, used to treat chest pain (angina), and reserpine, methyldopa (Aldomet), hydralazine (Apresoline), and guanethidine (Ismelin), used to treat high blood pressure (hypertension). Chronic alcohol consumption decreases the availability of propranolol (Inderal), used to treat high blood pressure, potentially reducing its therapeutic effect. Alcohol acts as an osmotic diuretic and also causes hypokalemia. Patients taking loop (e.g., furosemide, ethacrynic acid, and bumetanide) or less potent thiazide (e.g., various sulfonamide derivatives) diuretics are at greater risk for dehydration and hypokalemia, which increases the risk of seizure activity.

Blood alcohol levels can be raised by verapamil and may remain elevated for a much longer period of time. It appears that verapamil inhibits the metabolism of the alcohol by the liver (Bauer et al., 1992). Alcohol may also increase the bioavailability of nifedipine by inhibiting its metabolism (Perez-Reyes, 1992).

Elevated blood pressure is a risk factor for cardiovascular disease, including heart attacks. Alcohol is known to cause a dose-dependent elevation in blood pressure (Beilin, 1995). Consequently, patients who chronically abuse alcohol may be misdiagnosed with primary hypertension and placed inappropriately on antihypertensives (Doyal, Morton, and Crane, 1988). In addition, those patients who consume any alcohol respond less well to antihypertensive treatments than do total abstainers and alcohol may change the pharmacokinetics of those medications that are metabolized by the liver (Beevers, Maheswaran, and Potter, 1990).

The coronary artery dilator isosorbide dinitrate (Isordil, Dilatrate, and Sorbitrate) and nitroglycerin (Nitro-Bid and Nitrostat) inhibit aldehyde dehydrogenase. Therefore, the use of these medications with alcohol may produce a disulfiram-like reaction (e.g., dilation of blood vessels, hypotension, and tachycardia). As discussed in the following text, depending upon the severity of this sympathomimetic reaction, it could be fatal, particularly in patients with preexisting cardiovascular disease.

Alcohol and Disulfiram

Disulfiram (Antabuse) is a medication that has been used in the treatment of alcoholism since the 1950s. Alcohol is metabolized by alcohol dehydrogenase to acetaldehyde, which is metabolized by aldehyde dehydrogenase.

Disulfiram inhibits the enzyme aldehyde dehydrogenase resulting in the accumulation of acetaldehyde in the body. Acetaldehyde is highly toxic and has many sympathomimetic effects. The buildup of acetaldehyde can cause an unpleasant, aversive reaction characterized most commonly by the symptoms of facial flushing, nausea, vomiting, breathing difficulties, and headache. The severity of the reaction usually depends on the amount of alcohol consumed but some people are extremely sensitive to acetaldehyde toxicity. In extreme cases, respiratory depression, cardiovascular collapse, cardiac arrhythmias, unconsciousness and convulsions leading to death can occur.

The use of disulfiram as part of alcoholism treatment is essentially an aversive conditioning treatment approach based on the premise that an individual taking disulfiram will refrain from the use of alcohol in order to avoid experiencing the unpleasant reaction. Adverse drug reactions involving other medications following disulfiram therapy resulting in fatal outcomes are infrequent, with hepatic failure accounting for most of them. Disulfiram is also a cytochrome P450 (CYP2E1) enzyme inhibitor and numerous interactions with several drugs metabolized in the liver by P450 isozymes have been reported. Interactions with drugs such as diazepam (Valium), phenytoin (Dilantin), theophylline (Theodur), and isoniazid (INH) have been described (Paulson et al., 1992). Disulfiram also inhibits the CYP3A4 isoenzyme. Clarithromycin (Biaxin), a macrolide antibiotic commonly used in the treatment of respiratory infections, also inhibits the same isoenzyme. A case of fatal toxic epidermal necrolysis (Lyell disease) and fulminant hepatitis resulting in death has been reported in a patient who was started on this antibiotic while he was receiving disulfiram (Masia et al., 2002).

In the ADH pathway, alcohol is metabolized to its primary metabolite acetaldehyde via alcohol dehydrogenase. Acetaldehyde is metabolized via mitochondrial aldehyde dehydrogenase to acetate, which is then metabolized to water and carbon dioxide.

$$CH_3CH_2OH + NAD^+ \xrightarrow[ADH]{} CH_3CHO + NADH + H^+$$

Alcohol can also be metabolized through a microsomal enzyme oxidizing system (MEOS). It has been suggested that MEOS can be responsible for a significant part of alcohol metabolism in chronic alcoholics (Lieber, 1999).

$$CH_3CH_2OH + NADPH + H^+ + O_2 \xrightarrow[MEOS]{} Ch_3CHO + NADP^+ + 2H_2O$$

There are a number of prescribed medications that also can inhibit aldehyde dehydrogenase and can therefore produce a disulfiram-like reaction in people who consume alcohol while taking them (Lieber, 1992). Medications in this category include, but are not limited to, the antidiabetic oral medications chlorpropamide (Diabinase), glyburide (Micronase, Diabeta), tolazamide, and tolbutamide; a number of antibiotic medications including cefoperazone (Cefobid), griseofulvin (Fulvicin, Grisactin), isoniazide (INH), metronidazole (Flagyl), nitrofurantoin (Furadantin, Macrodantin), and sulfamethoxazole (Bactrim, Septra); the analgesics phenacetin and phenylbutazone; and the coronary artery dilator medications isosorbide dinitrate (Isordil, Dilatrate, and Sorbitrate) and nitroglycerin (Nitro-Bid and Nitrostat). The severity of a disulfiram-like reaction can vary depending upon many factors. In individuals with certain medical conditions (i.e., those with coronary artery disease), the disulfiram-like reaction could be potentially fatal as a result of cardiovascular effects involved in the pathogenesis of the disulfiram-like reaction (dilation of blood vessels, hypotension, and tachycardia). As it is impossible to predict with certainty the severity of the disulfiram-like reaction, individuals taking any of these medications should be advised to refrain from the consumption of alcohol while they are taking the medication.

Alcohol and Herbal Medications

Herbal medications are commonly consumed by many individuals for a wide variety of physical and psychological problems. Some of these substances (including chamomile, echinacea, and valerian) are commonly used as sleep enhancing agents. Alcohol use may increase the sedative effects if consumed along with these agents. Other herbal medications such as kava and yohimbine have been implicated in causing liver damage in some individuals and concomitant consumption of alcohol might further increase the potential for liver damage. Garlic, ginkgo biloba, and ginseng have been associated with problems with blood clotting (Bent and Ko, 2004). This could be a potential danger if a person was to ingest any of these herbal substances along with the anticoagulant medication warfarin. The potential for possible negative effects would be compounded further if the person was also to ingest alcohol because of the possible interactions between alcohol and warfarin as previously noted. As there have not been many medical studies examining the potential interactions between alcohol and herbal substances, individuals should probably be cautious about their consumption of alcohol if they are regularly ingesting amounts of any herbal substance.

Alcohol and Histamines (H₂-Antagonists)

One of the medical consequences of alcohol abuse is gastrointestinal disease, including gastritis, ulcers, and gastroesophageal reflux disorder (GERD). H_2-antagonists such as cimetidine (Tagamet), rantidine (Zantac), and nizatidine (Axid), which reduce the amount of gastric acid produced, have commonly been used to treat these disorders. As these medications also inhibit gastric ADH, an increase in the bioavailability of alcohol might result. It has been estimated that gastric ADH may account for a significant percentage of alcohol metabolism (Baraona, Abittan, and Lieber, 2000). In addition, the first-pass metabolism of alcohol is also reduced by cimetidine due to the effect it may have on increasing the rate of gastric emptying, again resulting in increased blood alcohol levels (Lieber, 1997). In fact, several studies have demonstrated the effect of these H_2-antagonists on first-pass alcohol metabolism (Caballeria, Baraona, Deulofeu et al., 1991; Roine, DiPadova et al., 1990). In many studies, the effect was quite significant—increases of blood alcohol concentrations of about 17 percent to 33 percent by cimetidine and to a much lesser degree by rantidine, if at all (Caballeria, Baraona, Rodamilans et al., 1989; Roine, Gentry et al., 1990). Although these investigators examined this effect through a series of detailed studies and identified dose, drug type, gender, and drinking history to be important variables, the clinical significance of this interaction has been questioned by some researchers (Levitt, 1993). Another H_2-antagonist, famotidine (Pepcid), appears to have no effect on blood alcohol levels. Nevertheless, until fully resolved, patients treated with H_2-antagonists should probably be advised to limit their drinking and be cognizant of any increased response to alcohol.

The use of the H_2-antagonists for the treatment of GERD has largely been supplanted by a newer class of agents that reduce gastric acid secretion, the proton pump inhibitors (PPIs). This group includes such medications as omeprazole (Prilosec), lansoprazole (Prevacid), esomeprazole (Nexium), and rabeprazole (Acidphex). The PPIs do not appear to interact significantly with alcohol. However, it is important to be aware of the fact that alcohol itself can damage the gastric mucosa (Hagel, Melchner, and Kachel, 1987) and can also increase gastric acid secretion if individuals consume alcoholic beverages (i.e., beer, wine) with low alcohol content (Chari, Teyssen, and Singer, 1993). These two effects could certainly reduce the therapeutic effectiveness of any of these medications. As a result of these effects, patients with medical problems requiring the use of any of these medications should be advised of the potential for alcohol to cause damage to the stomach that could negatively impact the therapeutic benefits from their medications.

Alcohol and HIV Medications

Research into possible interactions between alcohol and HIV medications is sparse. Alcohol dehydrogenase and specific isozymes of the P450 system play an important role in the metabolism of HIV medications. Inducement of these enzymes with chronic alcohol use could change the bioavailability of HIV medications and present dosing difficulties for drugs with narrow therapeutic ranges (Kresina et al., 2002). Alcohol use has been shown to increase the plasma concentration of the reverse transcriptase inhibitor abacavir (Ziagen) following a single 600 mg dose of abacavir (McDowell et al., 2000). This could certainly be a clinically significant issue, as about 3 percent of patients prescribed abacavir develop a hypersensitivity reaction to it characterized by fever, rash, nausea, vomiting, or malaise. In rare instances this reaction can result in death.

Alcohol and Lipid Reducing Medications

Medications used in the treatment of elevated lipids and cholesterol are formally described as 3-hydroxy-3-methylglutaryl coenzyme A (HMG-CoA) reductase inhibitors but are more commonly known as statins. Most of the statins are metabolized through the cytochrome P450 enzyme system. Atorvastatin (Lipitor), simvastatin (Zocor), and lovastatin (Mevacor, Altocor) are metabolized through the CYP3A4 isoenzyme. CYP3A4 is involved in the metabolism of alcohol and a number of other medications that bind more strongly to the enzyme than these statins bind to it. When alcohol or any of these substances block the statin from binding to the CYP3A4 enzyme, the metabolism of the statin is reduced, resulting in increased statin levels that can cause an increase in the potential for statin-related toxicity (Farmer and Torre-Amione, 2000; Igel, Sudhop, and von Bergmann, 2001; Paoletti, Corsini, and Bellosta, 2002; Worz and Bottorff, 2001). The major toxic reactions of concern include myotoxicity (myalgia, myopathy, and rhabdomyolysis) and hepatotoxicity. Milder cases are often reversible without serious sequelae with substance discontinuation, but severe cases although rare, may be potentially fatal. As a result of these potential interactions, people utilizing these medications should be advised to abstain from the use of alcohol.

Alcohol and Methanol

Alcoholics may drink other forms of alcohol when beverage alcohol (ethanol) is not available. One such alcohol, methanol (methyl alcohol), is highly toxic and may result in metabolic acidosis, blindness, and death. The interaction between ethanol and methanol is critical in averting methanol poisoning. Methanol is metabolized by the enzyme ADH to formaldehyde and then to formic acid, a highly toxic compound. Even when relatively small doses of methanol (several ounces) are consumed, these metabolites may cause metabolic acidosis, blindness, and cardiovascular instability and death. It is noteworthy that methanol poisoning can be prevented by the administration of ethyl alcohol because ethanol (alcohol) is preferentially metabolized by ADH, thereby decreasing the formation of toxic metabolites. The decrease in methanol metabolism allows methanol to be excreted unchanged and before toxic metabolites are formed. Patients admitted for acute intoxication or detoxification should be screened for methanol use so that appropriate prophylactic treatment (e.g., hemodialysis, ADH inhibitors, and ethanol administration) can be initiated.

Alcohol and Nicotine

Anyone working in the alcohol treatment field is keenly aware of the apparent relationship between alcohol and nicotine dependence and that the combined use of these drugs creates medical consequences that are greater than smoking alone, for example (Bien and Burge, 1990). Empirical research has pointed to various neurobiological interactions between these drugs in terms of pharmacokinetics, pharmacodynamics, and psychological effects, much of which suggest that alcohol potentiates the reinforcing or rewarding effects of nicotine. The hepatic metabolism of alcohol and nicotine may be altered by changes in cytochrome oxidases when exposure is long-term, but these interactions are not understood (Littleton and Little, 2002).

An additive pharmacodynamic interaction may exist between alcohol and nicotine as both drugs facilitate dopamine release in the nucleus accumbens, the anatomical region believed to be part of the brain's reward mechanisms. Littleton and Little (2002) and Crews (2004) have pointed out that in addition to the reinforcing effects of alcohol on dopamine, serotonin, $GABA_A$, and glutamate receptors, alcohol also affects nicotinic receptors that involve reward. Interestingly, chronic alcohol use may alter nicotinic receptors involved in reward, but that chronic nicotine has little or minor effects on the reinforcing effects of alcohol. However, it has been suggested that alcohol abusers may benefit from using nicotine because nicotine offsets the hangover produced by alcohol (Hughes, Rose, and Callas, 2000). Alcohol also seems to increase cigarette craving (Sayette, 2002). Although there is apparently an alcohol-nicotine interaction at different levels, the neurobiological substrates of this interaction are not well understood. An understanding of this interaction may have beneficial health outcomes by designing smoking cessation drugs.

Alcohol and Nonnarcotic Pain Relievers (ASA and NSAIDs)

Aspirin (acetylsalicylic acid [ASA]) and other nonsteroidal anti-inflammatory drugs (NSAIDs) are the most frequently employed drugs for relieving mild to moderate pain of varied origin (e.g., headache and musculoskeletal pain). Many of these drugs can cause gastric bleeding and inhibit blood from clotting. Alcohol can exacerbate these effects by enhancing the ability of these medications to damage the gastric mucosa (Adams, 1995; Kaufman et al., 1999). Older persons who mix alcoholic beverages with large doses of aspirin to self-medicate for pain are therefore at particularly high risk for episodes of gastric bleeding (Dufour, Archer, and Gordis, 1992).

Aspirin has been found to decrease the activity of gastric ADH, thus increasing the bioavailability of ingested alcohol, and heightening the effects of a given dose of alcohol (Roine Gentry et al., 1990). However, the anxiolytic effects of alcohol have been found to be attenuated with the use of aspirin (LaBuda and Fuchs, 2000). There are a number of other nonnarcotic pain relievers including phenacetin, an acetaminophen precursor (and often found in other drugs including acetaminophen, aspirin, caffeine, codeine, and propoxyphene), and phenylbutazone (Butasolidin), both of which inhibit aldehyde dehydrogenase. Therefore, the use of these drugs with alcohol may result in an aversive disulfiram-like reaction.

Alcohol and Opiates

Opiate medications are most commonly prescribed for the treatment of moderate to severe pain. Included are medications such as codeine, morphine preparations, propoxyphene (Darvon), oxycodone preparations (Percocet, Oxycontin), hydromorphone (Dilaudid), hydrocodone (Vicodin, Lortab), meperidine (Demerol), and fentanyl. Alcohol enhances the depressant effect of these agents on the CNS that can result in decreased motor skills, respiratory problems, drowsiness, and sedation. A single dose of alcohol can increase the bioavailability of propoxyphene, potentially increasing its sedative effect (Girre et al., 1991). All patients receiving narcotic prescriptions should be cautioned about the potential for increased drowsiness and impaired motor skills if they consume alcohol.

Overdoses from alcohol and opiates are potentially lethal due to a direct synergistic depressant effect in the brain's respiratory center when they are consumed together. In addition, the cough reflex is diminished and people are at risk for getting foods, fluids, or other objects stuck in their airways resulting in breathing difficulties. A number of opiate medications (i.e., codeine, propoxyphene, and oxycodone) are manufactured as combination products with the nonopiate analgesic acetaminophen. When people who consume alcohol take any of these combined products, they are also susceptible to interactions between alcohol and the acetaminophen as well as the opiate. As previously noted, the accumulation of toxic breakdown products form an acetaminophen/alcohol interaction and can be potentially dangerous resulting in liver damage or failure. Patients who are prescribed any of the opiate/acetaminophen combination preparations should be cautioned about consuming any additional amounts of acetaminophen.

Methadone is a synthetic opioid with a relatively long half-life which is widely used in clinical settings to reduce heroin use in opiate dependent patients. Methadone and heroin share similar receptor sites (e.g., both are μ-agonists) and both drugs are psychoactive. New patients or patients receiving a significant increase in their daily oral dose of methadone may present with symptoms of mild psychomotor and cognitive impairment. However, unlike many other opioids, prolonged methadone use, even at relatively high doses, does not impair cognitive or psychomotor performance (Zacny, 1995), including driving (Byas-Smith et al., 2005; Galski, Williams, and Ehle, 2000; Zacny, 1996). However, the combination of alcohol and opiates does increase respiratory depression. It is generally advisable not to drink while taking methadone for a variety of reasons related to recovery, but the interaction between these drugs is limited. Opiate and other drug interactions are discussed in Chapter 9.

Alcohol and Sedative Hypnotics

Barbiturates have been used therapeutically as sedative hypnotics for many years but have been replaced by safer medications such as benzodiazepines, which will be discussed later. Much like alcohol, the depressant effects of barbiturates range from mild sedation to general anesthesia. The interaction between these drugs is additive probably due to both pharmacokinetic and pharmacodynamic mechanisms. Alcohol appears to inhibit the hepatic metabolism of barbiturates (Mezey and Robles, 1974; Rubin and Lieber, 1970) which would increase their bioavailability and effectivness. Both alcohol and barbiturates derive some pharmacodynamic properties through the $GABA_A$ receptor which is responsible for most of the rapid inhibitory neurotransmissions in the brain. Barbiturates enhance the binding of GABA to $GABA_A$ receptors. Alcohol also shares the ability to increase GABA-mediated synaptic inhibition and chloride ion flux. Although other mechanisms are involved in the psychoactive effects of both drugs, the combination of alcohol and barbiturates will result in greater psychomotor and other impairments than either drug alone, including CNS depression, coma or fatal respiratory depression.

Benzodiazepines are one of the most widely prescribed drugs in the United States. This class of anxiolytics has a significantly greater safety margin than barbiturates and has largely replaced barbiturates in the treatment of anxiety, insomnia, and related disorders. Even so, the sedative side effects of these drugs is well known and fatal poisoning due to the combination of alcohol and benzodiazepines is still relatively common (Tanaka, 2002). As with the interaction between alcohol and other drugs, this problem has enhanced the range of acute and chronic drinking patterns that affect alcohol pharmacokinetics. In spite of adverse publicity and a problematic public image, the most widely prescribed psychiatric medication in the United States over the past few years is the benzodiazepine alprazolam (Stahl, 2002). Tolerance develops to many of the CNS depressant effects of benzodiazepines after prolonged use but varies greatly based upon the drug and the dependent measure of tolerance being studied. More rapidly eliminated benzodiazepines, such as alprazolam, are associated with hyperexcitability (rebound anxiety, disinhibiton, panic attacks, and mania) (Vgontzas, Kales, and Bixler, 1995), which could complicate the diagnosis and treatment of alcohol withdrawal syndrome.

Alcohol and many benzodiazepines share similar pharmacokinetic and pharmacodynamic mechanisms (see Chapter 5), so it is not surprising that the combination of alcohol and benzodiazepines is associated with drug-induced deaths, drug overdoses, and traffic accidents or fatalities (Girre and Schuckit, 1988; Girre et al., 1988). Regardless of the mechanisms, the interaction between alcohol and benzodiazepines can be dangerous and potentially impair cognitive, psychomotor and related skills.

In addition to pharmacodynamic interactions, a pharmacokinetic interaction between alcohol and benzodiazepines exists. There is a decline in the efficiency of the metabolism of the benzodiazepines as a result of increasing age or liver disease. In the elderly, there is a 50 percent decrease in clearance, with a four- to ninefold increase in half-life, and a two- to fourfold increase in the volume of distribution (Peppers, 1996).

Sellers and Busto (1982) point out that acute alcohol abuse impairs the metabolism of diazepam, desmethyldiazepam, chlordiazepoxide, clobazam, and temazepam. However, they also point out that many studies lack precision of instrumentation and understanding of the pharmacokinetics of alcohol and benzodiazepines. The authors conclude that the importance of this interaction has been overemphasized and is probably less important than the effect of alcohol alone or in combination with other drugs, such as cannabinoids, neuroleptics, stimulants, and antidepressants (Sellers and Busto, 1982).

Alprazolam (Xanax) produces relatively long-lasting impairments on tests of psychomotor tasks, information processing, and memory, effects that are similar to those produced by relatively low concentrations of alcohol. When alcohol (less than 70 mg/dl) is combined with 2 mg doses of alprazolam, there is an additive interaction on performance decrements on verbal word tests, suggesting information processing is vulnerable to the combination of these two drugs. Although alcohol impaired psychomotor and cognitive performance as did diazepam, but to a lesser extent, there was no significant interaction between drugs with regard to impaired performance on tests such as tracking and verbal information processing (Linnoilla et al., 1990).

Despite possible complexities, more recent reviews have confirmed and further identified the pharmacokinetic interaction between these drugs (Tanaka, 2000). The pharmacokinetic interaction between acute alcohol and benzodiazepine use is probably due to the inhibition of a benzodiazepine-enzyme complex. When alcohol concentrations are high as is often the case in alcoholics, alcohol is metabolized through ADH and CYP2E1 which results in the competitive inhibition of benzodiazepine metabolism. However, at lower alcohol concentrations in social drinkers, alcohol metabolism is primarily through ADH and minimally through the CYP2E1 isozyme (Tanaka, 2000).

Chronic alcohol use increases the elimination of diazepam during alcohol-free periods, probably because in humans, the CYP2E1 enzyme is induced so that drugs that are metabolized by demethylation (e.g., diazepam) and hydroxylation are eliminated more rapidly (Hollister, 1990). Therefore, in the chronic alcoholic, for example, diazepam pharmacokinetics will vary diversely depending upon whether the person is actively drinking or recently abstinent.

There are potentially serious additive pharmacodynamic effects when benzodiazepines are combined with alcohol (van Steveninck et al., 1996). This is the result of different mechanisms. Principal among these are the effects of alcohol on multiple neurotransmitter systems, which adapt in different ways to the acute and/or chronic presence of ethanol. For example, both basic and clinical research studies suggest a role for catecholamines in the acute intoxicating effects of, and the development of tolerance to, alcohol (Pohorecky and Brick, 1988). The role of the noradrenergic system in benzodiazepine tolerance and withdrawal has been suggested by many studies (see Vgontzas, Kales, and Bixler, 1995, for a review), further suggesting that variations in the balance of CNS neurotransmitter systems may undermine the therapeutic response to sedative hypnotics. This pharmacologic interaction is discussed, in detail, elsewhere in this textbook. Alcohol also modifies the clearance and disposition of metabolites of some sedative hypnotics and interferes with their clinical effectiveness. Neurotransmitter responses may additionally be manifested clinically by rebound phenomena, akin to a subsyndromal withdrawal, which affects sleep and precipitates anxiety and mood symptoms. Recent alcohol use may also alter the subjective interpretation of the patient's "internal milieu," causing confusion and eliciting reactive psychopathology (Castaneda et al., 1996). Alcohol is not bound to plasma proteins extensively enough to modify drug distribution. However, serum albumin levels in chronic alcoholics may be abnormally low so that some drugs (e.g., diazepam) have an increased volume of distribution (Linnoila, Mattila, and Kitchell, 1979). Linnoila also found that low doses of flurazepam (Dalmane) interact with low doses of alcohol to impair driving ability, even when alcohol is ingested the morning after taking Dalmane, which, along with many other benzodiazepines, is still present in appreciable amounts the next day (Betts and Birtle, 1982). As alcoholics often suffer from anxiety and insomnia, and many of them drink in the morning, this interaction may be dangerous.

Alprazolam (Xanax), a benzodiazepine analog, is often used in the treatment of anxiety disorders and is currently the most prescribed medication in the United States. Although there is no synergistic action between these drugs, an additive interaction between alprazolam and alcohol has been reported on certain psychomotor and cognitive tasks. Alprazolam produced long lasting impairments on tests of tracking, information processing, and memory. Although alcohol demonstrated additive performance decrements in the performance of some tasks, no synergistic interaction was observed (Linnoila et al., 1990). The combination of these drugs also produces increases in self-reported drowsiness (Linnoila et al., 1990). Hindmarch (1983) also examined the effects of alprazolam and alcohol on psychomotor skills. A clear dose-related effect of alprazolam was observed but no significant interaction between alprazolam and alcohol was reported (Hindmarch, 1983).

Some nonbenzodiazepine anxiolytics, such as buspirone, do not appear to interact with alcohol to potentiate cognitive or motor performance impairment. Unlike some benzodiazepine-based anxiolytics, buspirone has been found to have no significant effect on body sway, coordination skills, tracking skills, or nystagmus even when combined with alcohol (Mattila, Aranko, and Seppala, 1982).

As a result of the potentially serious consequences of consuming alcohol with sedative/hypnotic medications, individuals taking these medications should be advised to abstain from the use of alcohol.

Alcohol and Stimulants

Amphetamines and other CNS stimulants decrease fatigue and reaction time while causing an increase in arousal, body temperature, heart rate, blood pressure, and other changes (decreased sleep). Although there is some evidence that stimulants may decrease some of the depressant effects of alcohol (e.g., sleepiness), the combination of a stimulant and a depressant is often erroneously assumed by laypersons to result in a neutralizing or balancing-out of these two opposite effects. For example, while some researchers have reported alcohol-amphetamine interactions in humans, the results are inconsistent and often complex. Some studies reported no antagonistic effect of dextroamphetamine on the mental and psychomotor impairment produced by alcohol, whereas others have found improved performance compared with controls (see Kaplan et al., 1966). Perez-Reyes et al. reported the results of a placebo-controlled study of the interaction of two doses of dextroamphetamine (0.09 or 0.18 mg/kg) and one dose of alcohol on multiple measures. The doses of dextroamphetamine (0.09 or 0.18 mg/kg) were similar to therapeutic doses that might be used to treat attention-deficit disorder patients and resulted in peak plasma concentrations of approximately 18.3 and 21.4 ng/ml, respectively. The single dose of alcohol (0.85 g/kg) resulted in peak blood alcohol concentrations of about 100 mg/dl. Alcohol significantly increased the bioavailability of high, but not the low dose of dextroamphetamine (25.5 ng/ml versus 15.7 ng/ml). They found that amphetamine did not significantly alter peak blood alcohol concentrations which were in the 100 mg/dl range. However, alcohol significantly increased the bioavailability of dextroamphetamine (Perez-Reyes et al., 1992). Dextroamphetamine had no effect on ratings of subjective alcohol intoxication but alcohol did increase self-reported ratings of the "high" produced by dextroamphetamine. Although no significant interactive effects on heart rate were noted, the authors reported that dextroamphetamine attenuated alcohol-induced increases in latency and accuracy while performing an eye-hand-foot reaction time task believed to be related to driving abilities. As the effect was greatest about four hours after alcohol administration and when blood alcohol concentrations had dropped from a peak of about 100 mg/dl to about 60 mg/dl, fatigue and dose were probably important factors in the latter finding. The statistical significance of these results probably outweighs their actual value.

Although the interaction between alcohol and amphetamines have been studied, the only clear conclusion is that the interaction is complex and task specific, and that there is no simple antagonism between alcohol and amphetamines.

More is known about the interaction between alcohol and another stimulant, cocaine. Cocaine and alcohol are often co-ingested. The effects of this drug combination are shorter in duration than those of amphetamines and alcohol. One novel consequence of cocaine and alcohol use is that a third compound called cocaethylene is formed (sometimes referred to as ethyl cocaine or cocaine ethyl-ester). Cocaethylene is not a natural alkaloid of the coca plant and is not found in pharmaceutical or street cocaine. In fact, cocaine is metabolized to its ethyl configuration only in the presence of ethanol.

The effects of cocaethylene are similar to, but extend, the euphorogenic and reinforcing effects of cocaine. In humans, the combination of alcohol and cocaine is greater than the effect of either drug alone and is associated with an enhanced subjective euphoria, increased heart rate, and increased plasma cocaine concentrations (McCance et al., 1995; McCance-Katz et al., 1993). Like cocaine, cocaethylene appears to block presynaptic dopamine transporters which increases the functional activity of dopamine by enhancing the availability of neurotransmitters to engage post synaptic receptors.

In humans, cocaethylene has a smaller elimination rate constant (0.42 versus 0.67/h), a longer elimination half-life (1.68 versus 1.07/h), lower ratings of the subjective "high" and smaller changes in heart rate compared with cocaine, even though the concentrations of cocaethylene and cocaine were statistically indistinguishable (Perez-Reyes, 1994). Similar results have been reported by others (Hart et al., 2000).

In bovines, preadministration of alcohol for ten days decreases the plasma half-life, and increases the volume of distribution and clearance rate of cocaine. Alcohol also seems to increase the plasma concentrations of cocaine's metabolite, benzoylecognine (Kambam et al., 1994). It is not clear that a simple pharmacokinetic effect occurs in humans. In humans, insufflation of cocaine before alcohol ingestion does not appear to alter blood alcohol levels or subjective ratings of intoxication of alcohol intoxication. When alcohol is administered prior to cocaine insufflation, there is a significant increase in both cocaine plasma levels (possibly due to an inhibition of hepatic cocaine metabolism produced by alcohol) and an augmentation of cocaine's subjective and heart rate effects (Perez-Reyes and Jeffcoat, 1992; Perez-Reyes et al., 1994).

In another study, combining cocaine and alcohol produced a nonsignificant decrease in subjective feelings of drunkenness, and increase in cocaine-induced euphoria, and a significant improvement in alcohol-related changes in psychomotor performance along with a marked increase in heart rate. Subjects who were administered cocaine and alcohol interpreted the effects as "more pleasant" than compared with alcohol alone (Farre et al., 1993).

Cocaethylene is about one and a half times more lethal than cocaine in animals. Although both drugs produce convulsions in mice, cocaethylene had a greater propensity to cause death. Moreover, the administration of alcohol and cocaine is associated with greater risk for cardiovascular toxicity (e.g., increased systolic and diastolic blood pressure, and heart rate) than alcohol or cocaine alone. Some clinicians believe that cocaethylene is primarily responsible for deaths that occur among cocaine abusers (Bunn and Ginnini, 1992). Although many drugs are metabolized to form other psychoactive compounds, cocaethylene is the only known example of a third psychoactive drug being formed as a result of administering two other psychoactive drugs of abuse. As cocaine-induced deaths have been observed with a wide range of postmortem cocaine concentrations often with presence of low blood alcohol levels, the possibility exists that cocaethylene may be partially responsible for these deaths. Additional research is clearly required in this area.

SUMMARY AND CONCLUSIONS

The interactions between alcohol and therapeutic medications or other drugs are very complex, highly variable events, and dependent upon a number of pharmacodynamic and pharmacokinetic factors. These interactions are further complicated by the potential for alcohol to cause direct physical damage in many organ systems which may alter the effect of a medication even if the patient is not acutely intoxicated by alcohol at the time of the evaluation. In addition, a multitude of other factors can affect alcohol-drug interactions including, but not limited to, the anthropometric characteristics of the patient (age, gender, body weight, and height), medication/drug dosage, and the amount and frequency of alcohol consumption. This is especially important in certain populations (e.g., geriatric) as many of these individuals are on multiple medications and are also more susceptible to negative age-related physiological effects that could increase the potential for more severe interactions. It is also important to note that most empirical research or clinical studies involve relatively small alcohol doses for a variety of practical and ethical reasons. Some effects observed at relatively low blood alcohol concentrations may be very different in highly intoxicated patients. Similarly, the lack of a significant interaction with low doses of a drug do not guarantee the same results when higher doses are used. As a result of all these variables, it is very difficult to recommend a dose of alcohol that can be considered safe when taking most medications.

Alcohol and medication/drug interactions have been extensively studied in individuals who are chronic heavy drinkers. Interactions between alcohol and various drugs, both licit and illicit, as well as interactions in individuals who consume alcohol more moderately or episodically, have been studied much less extensively. Children or others with little or no tolerance to alcohol or other drugs may be more sensitive to these interactions and are an understudied population. As a general rule, the CNS depressant effects of alcohol can be expected to increase the depressant effects of most medications and other drugs with similar CNS effects, but the ultimate nature and degree of that interaction will be drug-specific.

In conclusion, there are well-documented interactions between alcohol and therapeutic medications, as well as between alcohol and various drugs of abuse. Although not all alcohol-drug combinations produce pharmacokinetic or pharmacodynamic interactions, individuals who are taking prescribed or OTC medications should always be advised to read product warning labels (provided by pharmacists with prescriptions or on the products themselves with OTC medications) in order to ascertain if there is a potential interaction with alcohol. Those interactions may increase or decrease the therapeutic effectiveness of a prescribed medication, impair the ability to engage in complex tasks such as operating a motor vehicle, or produce a range of psychic and physiological side effects that may obscure an accurate diagnosis or treatment plan. Unfortunately most individuals consuming illicit drugs are not likely to be concerned about possible interactions with alcohol. Physicians and other medical professionals need to be aware of possible alcohol-drug interactions and advise patients accordingly.

REFERENCES

Adams, W.L. (1995). Interactions between alcohol and other drugs. *International Journal of Addictions* 30:1903-1923.

Allen, D.; Lader, M.; Curran, H.V. (1988). A comparative study of the interactions of alcohol with amitriptyline, fluoxetine and placebo in normal subjects. *Progress in Neuro-Psychopharmacology & Biological Psychiatry* 12:63-80.

Baraona, E.; Abittan, C.S.; Lieber, C.S. (2002) Contribution of gastric oxidation to ethanol first pass metaboism in baboons. *Alcoholism: Clinical and Experimental Research* 24(7):946-951.

Bauer, L.A.; Schumock, G.; Horn, J.;·Opheim, K. (1992). Verapamil inhibits ethanol elimination and prolongs the perception of intoxication. *Clinical Pharmacology and Therapeutics* 52(1):6-10.

Beevers, D.G.; Maheswaran, R.; Potter, J.F. (1990). Alcohol, blood pressure, and
antihypertensive drugs. *Journal of Clinical Pharmacy and Therapeutics* 15(6):
395-397.

Beilin, L.F. (1995). Alcohol and hypertension. *Clinical and Experimental Pharmacology and Physiology* 22:185-188.

Bent, S.; Ko, R. (2004). Commonly used herbal medications in the United States:
A review. *American Journal of Medicine* 116:478-485.

Betts, T.A.; Birtle, J. (1982). Effect of two hypnotic drugs on actual driving performance next morning. *British Medical Journal (Clinical Research Ed.)* 285
(6345):852.

Bien, T.H.; Burge, R. (1990). Smoking and drinking: A review of the literature. *The
International Journal of the Addictions* 25:1429-1454.

Black, M. (1984). Acetaminophen hepatotoxicity. *Annual Review of Medicine*
35:577-593.

Blackwell, B.; Barley, E.; Price, J.; Taylor, D. (1967). Hypertensive interactions
between monoamine oxidase inhibitors and food stuffs. *British Journal of
Psychiatry* 113:349-365.

Bunn, W.H.; Ginnini, A.J. (1992). Cardio vascular complications of cocaine abuse.
American Family Physician 46(3):769-773.

Burns, M. (1989). Alcohol and antihistamines in combination; effects on performance. *Alcoholism: Clinical and Experimental Research* 13:243.

Burns, M.; Mostowitz, H. (1980). Effects of diphenhydramine and alcohol on skills
performance. *European Journal of Clinical Pharmacology* 17:259.

Byas-Smith, M.G. Chapman, S.L. Reed, B. Cotsonis, G. (2005). The effects of
opioids on driving and psychomotor performance in patients with chronic pain
[Comparitive Study. Journal Article. Research Support, Non-U.S. Gov't]. *Clinical Journal of Pain* 21(4):345-52.

Caballeria, J.; Baraona, E.; Deulofeu, R.; Hernandez-Munoz, R.; Rodes, J.; Lieber,
C.S. (1991). Effects of H-2 receptor antagonists on gastric alcohol dehydrogenase activity. *Digestive Digest Sciences* 36:1673-1679.

Caballeria, J.; Baraona, E.; Rodamilans, M.; Liever, C.S. (1989). Effects of cimetidine on gastric alcohol dehydrogenase activity and blood alcohol levels. *Gastroenterology* 96:388-392.

Casswell, S. (1977). *Cannabis and Alcohol: Effects on Closed Course Driving Behaviour.* Paper presented to Seventh International Conference on Alcohol, Drugs
and Traffic Safety, Melbourne.

Castaneda, R.; Sussman, N.; Westreich, L.; Levy, R.; O'Malley, M. (1996). A review of the effects of moderate alcohol intake on the treatment of anxiety and
mood disorders. *Journal of Clinical Psychiatry* 57(5):207-212.

Chari, S.; Teyssen, S.; Singer, M.V. (1993). Alcohol and gastric acid secretion in
humans. *Gut* 34(6):843-847.

Cina, S.J.; Russell, R.A.; Conradi, S.E. (1996). Sudden death due to metronidazole/ethanol interaction. *American Journal of Forensic Medicine and Pathology* 17(4):343-346.

Ciraulo, D.A.; Anderson, L.M.; Chapron, D.J.; Jaffe, J.H.; Bollepalli, S.; Kramer, P.A. (1988). Clinical pharmacokinetics of imipramine and desipramine in alcoholics and normal volunteers. *Journal of Clinical Psychopharmacology* 43:509-518.

Crews, F.T. (2004). Effects of alcohol abuse in the brain. In: Brick, J. (ed.), *Handbook of the Medical Consequences of Alcohol and Drug Abuse* (pp. 85-138). Binghamton, NY: The Haworth Medical Press.

Dorian, P.; Sellers, E.M.; Reed, K.L.; Warsh, J.J.; Hamilton, C.; Kaplan, H.L.; Fan, T. (1983). Amitriptyline and ethanol: Pharmacokinetic and pharmacodynamic interaction. *European Journal of Clinical Pharmacology* 25:325-331.

Doyal, L.E.; Morton, W.A.; Crane, D.F. (1988). Antihypertensive drug therapy in alcohol dependence. *Psychosomatics* 29(3):301-306.

Dufour, M.C.; Archer, L.; Gordis, F. (1992). Alcohol and the elderly. *Clinics in Geriatric Medicine* 8(1):127-141.

Ellenhorn, M.J.; Barceloux, D.G. (1988). *Medical Toxicology: Diagnosis and Treatment of Human Poisoning* (p. 66). New York: Elsevier Press.

Farmer, J.A.; Torre-Amione, G. (2000). Comparative tolerability of the HMG-CoA reductase inhibitors. *Drug Safety* 23:197-213.

Farre, M.; De LaTorre, R.; Llorente, M.; Lamas, X.; Ugena, B.; Segura, J.; Cami, J. (1993). Alcohol and cocaine interactions in humans. *Journal of Pharmacology and Experimental Therapeutics* 266(3):1364-1373.

Franks, H.M.; Hensley, V.R.; Hensley, W.J.; Starmer, G.A.; Teo, R.K.C. (1979). The interaction between ethanol and antihistamines. 2. Clemastine. *The Medical Journal of Australia* 1:185-186.

Galski, T.; Williams, J.B.; Ehle, H.T. (2000). Effects of opioids on driving ability. *Journal of Pain and Symptom Management* 19:200-208.

Girre, C.; Facy, F.; Lagier, G.; Dally, S. (1988). Detection of blood benzodiazepines in injured people. Relationship with alcoholism. *Drug and Alcohol Dependence* 21(1):61-65.

Girre, C.; Hirschhorn, M.; Bertaux, L.; Palombo, S.; Dellatolas, F.; Ngo, R.; Moreno, M.; Fournier, P.E. (1991). Enhancement of propoxyphene bioavailability by ethanol: Relation to psychomotor and cognitive function in healthy volunteers. *European Journal of Clinical Pharmacology* 41(2):147-152.

Girre, C.; Hispard, E.; Palombo, S.; N'Guyen, C.; Daily, S. (1993). Increased metabolism of acetaminophen in chronically alcoholic patients. *Alcoholism: Clinical and Experimental Research* 17(1):170-173.

Girre, C.; Schuckit, M.A.. (1988). Alcohol and drug interactions with antianxiety medications. *The American Journal of Medicine* 82(S5A):27-33.

Goff, D.C.; Baldessarini, R.S. (1993). Drug interactions with antipsychotic agents. *Journal of Clinical Psychopharmacology* 13(1):59-67.

Greenspan, K.; Smith, T.J. (1991). Perspectives on alcohol and medication interactions. *Journal of Alcohol and Drug Education* 36(3):103-107.

Hagel, H.J.; Melchner, M.; Kachel, G. (1987). Gastric mucosal cell loss caused by aspirin and alcohol. *Hepatogastroenterology* 34:262-264.

Harger, R.N. (ed.) (1966). *Alcohol and Traffic Safety* (pp. 215-219). Proceedings of the Fourth International Conference on Alcohol and Traffic Safety. Bloomington, IN: Indiana University Press.

Hart, C.L.; Jatlow, P.; Sevarino, K.A.; McCance-Katz, E.F. (2000). Comparison of intravenous cocaethylene and cocaine in humans. *Psychopharmacology (Berl)* 149(2):153-162.

Hesselbrock, M.H.; Meyer, R.E.; Keener, J.J. (1985). Psychopathology in hospitalized alcoholics. *Archives of General Psychiatry* 42:1050-1055.

Hindmarch, I. (1983) Measuring the side-effects of psychoactive drugs: A pharmacodynamic profile of alprazolam. *Alcohol and Alcoholism* 18(4):361-367.

Hollister, L.E. (1990). Interactions between alcohol and benzodiazepines. *Recent Developments in Alcoholism* 8:233-239.

Hoyumpa, A. (1983). *Alcohol Interactions with Benzodiazepines and Cocaine.* Fourteenth Annual AMSA-RSA Medical-Scientific Conference National Council on Alcoholism Meeting in Houston, Texas, April.

Hughes, J.R.; Rose, G.L.; Callas, P.W. (2000). Nicotine is more reinforcing in smokers with a past history of alcoholism than in smokers with out this history. *Alcoholism: Clinical and Experimental Research* 24:1633-1638.

Igel, M.; Sudhop, T.; von Bergmann, K. (2001). Metabolism and drug interactions of 3-hydroxy-3-methyglutaryl coenzyme A-reductase inhibitors (statins). *European Journal of Clinical Pharmacology* 57:357-364.

Jacobson, J.M. (1992). Alcoholism and tuberculosis. *Alcohol Health and Research World* 16(1):39-45.

Kambam, J.R.; Franks, J.J.; Janicki, P.K.; Mets, B.; Watt, M.; Hickman, R. (1994). Alcohol pretreatment alters the metabolic pattern and accelerates cocaine metabolism in pigs. *Drug and Alcohol Dependence* 36(1):9-13.

Kaplan, H.L.; Forney, R.D.; Richards, A.B.; Hughes, F.W. (1966). Dextro-amphetamine, alcohol and dextro-amphetamine-alcohol combination and mental performance. In: Harger, R.N. (ed.), *Alcohol and Traffic Safety* (pp. 211-214). Proceedings of the Fourth International Conference on Alcohol and Traffic Safety. Bloomington, IN: Indiana University Press.

Kaufman, D.W.; Kelly, J.P.; Wiholm, B.E.; Laszlo, A.; Sheehan, J.E.; Koff, R.S.; Shapiro, S. (1999). Risk of acute major upper gastrointestinal bleeding among users of aspirin and ibuprofen at various levels of alcohol consumption. *American Journal of Gastroenterology* 94(11):3189-3196.

Kresina, T.F.; Flexner, C.W.; Sinclair, J.; Correia, M.A.; Stapleton, J.T.; Adeniyi-Jones, S.; Cargill, V. (2002). Alcohol and HIV therapy. *AIDS Research and Human Retroviruses* 18(11):757-770.

Kuffner, E.K. (2001). New perspectives on acetaminophen and alcohol use. *The American Journal of Managed Care* 7(19):S590-S591.

Kuffner, E.K.; Dart, R.C. (2001). Acetaminophen use in patients who drink alcohol: Current study evidence. *The American Journal of Managed Care* 7(19): S592-S596.

LaBuda, C.J.; Fuchs, P.N. (2000). Aspirin attenuates the anxiolytic actions of ethanol. *Alcohol: An International Biomedical Journal* 21(3):287-290.

Lamers, C.T.J.; Ramaekers, J.G. (2000). *Visual Search and Urban City Driving Under the Influence of Marijuana and Alcohol.* Report DOT HS 809 020. Washington, DC: National Highway Traffic Safety Administration, U.S. Department of
Transportation.

Lemberger, L.; Rowe, H.; Vergstron, R.F.; Farid, K.Z.; Enas, G.G. (1985). Effect of
fluoxetine on psychomotor performance, physiological response and kinetics of
ethanol. *Clinical Pharmacology and Therapeutics* 37:658-664.

Levitt, M.D. (1993). Review article: Lack of clinical significance of the interaction
between H2-receptor antagonists and ethanol. *Alimentary Pharmacology &
Therapeutics* 7:131-138.

Lieber, C.S. (1992). Interaction of ethanol with other drugs. In: Lieber, C.S. (ed.),
*Medical and Nutritional Complications of Alcoholism: Mechanisms and Man-
agement* (pp. 165-183). New York: Plenum Press.

Lieber, C.S. (1992). Interactions of ethanol with other drugs. In: Lieber, C.S. (ed.),
*Medical and Nutritional Complications of Alcoholism: Mechanisms and Man-
agement* (pp. 165-183). New York: Plenum Press.

Lieber, C.S. (1994). Alcohol and the liver: 1994 update. *Gastroenterology* 106:
1085-1105.

Lieber, C.S. (1997). Gastric ethanol metabolism and gastritis: Interactions with
other drugs, *Helicobacter pylori,* and antibiotic therapy. *Alcoholism: Clinical
and Experimental Research* 21:1360-1366.

Lieber, C.S. (1999). Microsomal ethanol-oxidizing system (MEOS): The first 30
years (1968-1998)—A review. *Alcoholism* 23(6):991-1007.

Linnoila, M. (1973). Effects of diazepam, chlordiazepoxide, thioridazine, haloperidol, flupenthixol and alcohol on psychomotor skills relating to driving. *Annales
medicinae experimentalis et biologiae Fenniae* 51:125.

Linnoila, M.; Mattila, M.J.; Kitchell, B.S. (1979). Drug interactions with alcohol.
Drugs 18(4):299-311.

Linnoila, M.; Sarrio, I.; Olkonieme, J.; Liljeqvist, R.; Maki, M. (1975). Effect of
two weeks' treatment with chlordiazepoxide or flupenthixol, alone or in combination with alcohol, on psychomotor skills related to driving. *Arzneim-Forsch
(Drug Res)* 25:1088.

Linnoila, M.; Stapleton, J.M.; Lister, R.; Moss, H.; Lane, E.; Granger, A; Eckardt,
M.J. (1990). Effects of single doses of alprazolam and diazepam alone and in
combination with ethanol, on psychomotor and cognitive performance and on
autonomic nervous system reactivity in healthy volunteers. *Journal of Clinical
Pharmacology* 39:21-38.

Littleton, J.; Little, H. (2002). Interactions between alcohol and nicotine dependence; A summary of potential mechanisms and implications for treatment. *Alcoholism: Clinical and Experimental Research* 26:1922-1924.

Lukas, S.E.; Benedikt, R.; Mendelson, J.H.; Kouri, E.; Sholar, M.; Amass, L.
(1992). Marijuana attenuates the rise in plasma ethanol levels in human subjects.
Neuropsychopharmacology 7:77-81.

Masia, M.; Gutierrez, F.; Jimeno, A.; Navarro, A.; Borras, J.; Mattarredona, J.; Martin-Hidalgo, A. (2002). Fulminant hepatitis and fatal toxic epidermal necrolysis (Lyell disease) coincident with clarithromycin administration in an alcoholic patient receiving disulfiram therapy. *Archives of Internal Medicine* 162(4):474-476.

Matilla, M.J. (1990). Alcohol and drug interactions. *Annals of Medicine* 22:363-369.

Mattila, M.J.; Aranko, K.; Seppala, T. (1982). Acute effects of buspirone and alcohol on psychomotor skills. *Journal of Clinical Psychiatry* 43:56-61.

McCance, E.F.; Price, L.H.; Kosten, T.R.; Jatow, P.I. (1995). Cocaethylene: Pharmacology, physiology and behavioral effects in humans. *Journal of Pharmacology and Experimental Therapeutics* 274(1):215-223.

McCance-Katz, E.F.; Price, L.H.; McDougle, C.J.; Kosten, T.R.; Black, J.E.; Jetlow, P.I. (1993). Concurrent cocaine-ethanol ingestion in humans: Pharmacology, physiology, behavior, and the role of cocaethylene. *Psychopharmacology (Berl)* 111(1):39-46.

McDowell, J.A.; Chittick, G.E.; Pilati-Stevens, C.; Edwards, K.D.; Stein, D.S. (2000). Pharmacokinetic interaction of abacavir (1592U89) and ethanol in human immunodeficiency virus-infected adults. *Antimicrobial Agents and Chemotherapy* 44(6):1686-1690.

Michalets, E.L. (1998). Update: Clinically significant cytochrome P-450 drug interactions. *Journal of Pharmacotherapy* 18(1):84-112.

Millner, G.; Landauer, A.A. (1971). Alcohol, thioridazine and chlorpromazine effects on skills related to driving behaviour. *The British Journal of Psychiatry* 118:351-352.

Moskowitz, H. (1976). Marijuana and driving. *Accident Analysis and Prevention* 8:21-26.

Moskowitz, H. (1985). Marijuana and driving. *Accident Analysis and Prevention* 17:323-346.

National Institute on Alcohol Abuse and Alcoholism (2003). *Special Report to the U.S. Congress on Alcohol and Health.* Washington, DC: U.S. Department of Health and Human Services.

Nosova, T.; Jokelainen, K.; Kaihovaara, P.; Vakevainen, S.; Rautio, M.; Jousimies-Somer, H.; Salaspuro, M. (1999). Ciprofloxacin administration decreases enhanced ethanol elimination in ethanol-fed rats. *Alcohol and Alcoholism* 34(1):48-54.

Paoletti, R.; Corsini, A.; Bellosta, S. (2002). Pharmacological interactions of statins. *Atherosclerosis Supplements* 3:35-40.

Paulson, H.; Loft, S.; Anderson, J.; Anderson, M. (1992). Disulfiram therapy-adverse drug reactions and interactions. *Acta Psychiatrica Scandinavica* 86:59-66.

Peppers, M.P. (1996). Benzodiazepines for alcohol withdrawal in the elderly and in patients with liver disease. *Pharmacotherapy* 16:49-58.

Perez-Reyes, M. (1994). The order of drug administration: It's effects on the interaction between cocaine and ethanol. *Life Sciences* 55(7):541-550.

Perez-Reyes, M.; Jeffcoat, A.R. (1992). Ethanol/cocaine interaction: Cocaine and cocaethylene plasma concentrations and their relationship to subjective and cardiovascular effects. *Life Sciences* 51(8):553-563.

Perez-Reyes, M.; Jeffcoat, A.R.; Myers, M.; Sihler, K.; Cook, C.E. (1994). Comparison in humans of the potency and pharmacokinetics of intravenously injected cocaethylene and cocaine. *Psycopharmacology (Berl)* 116(4):428-432.

Perez-Reyes, M.; White, W.R.; McDonald, S.A.; Hicks, R.E. (1992). Interaction between ethanol and dextroamphetmaines: Effects of psychomotor performance. *Alcoholism: Clinical and Experimental Research* 16:75-81.

Pohorecky, L.; Brick, J. (1988). The pharmacology of alcohol. In: Balfour, D.J.K. (ed.), *International Encyclopedia of Pharmacology and Therapeutics: Psychotropic Drugs of Abuse* (pp. 189-254). New York: Pergamon Press.

Ridout, F.; Shamsi, Z.; Meadows, R.; Johnson, S.; Hindmarch, I. (2003). A single-center, randomized, double-blind, placebo-controlled, crossover investigation of the effects of fexofenadine hydrochloride 180 mg alone and with alcohol, with hydroxyzine hydrochloride 50 mg as a positive internal control, on aspects of cognitive and psychomotor function related to driving a car. *Clinical Therapeutics* 25(5):1518-1538.

Robbe, H.W.J.; O'Hanlon, J.F. (1999). *Marijuana, Alcohol and Actual Driving Performance*. Report DOT HS 808 939, National Highway Traffic Safety Administration, U.S. Department of Transportation.

Roehrs, T.; Zwyghuizen-Doorenbos, A.; Roth, T. (1993). Sedative effects and plasma concentrations following single doses of tiazolam, diphenhydramine, ethanol and placebo. *Sleep* 16(4):301-305.

Roine, R.; DiPadova, C.; Frezza, M.; Merhandez-Munoz, R.; Baraona, E.; Lieber, C.S. (1990). Effects of omeprazole, cimetidine and ranitidine on blood ethanol concentrations. *Gastroenterology* 98:A114.

Roine, R.; Gentry, R.T.; Hernandez-Munoz, R.; Baraona, F.; Lieber, C.S. (1990). Aspirin increases blood alcohol concentrations in humans after ingestion of ethanol. *Journal of the American Medical Association* 264(18):2406-2408.

Rubin, E.; Gang, H.; Misra, P.S.; Lieber, C.S. (1970). Inhibition of drug metabolism by acute ethanol intoxication: A hepatic microsomal mechanism. *The American Journal of Medicine* 49:801.

Sayette, M. (2002). The effects of alcohol on cigarette craving. *Alcoholism: Clinical and Experimental Research* 26(12):1925-1927.

Seeff, L.B.; Cuccherini, B.A.; Zimmerman, H.J.; Adler, E.; Benjamin, S.B. (1986). Acetaminophen hepatotoxicity in alcoholics: A therapeutic misadventure. *Annals of Internal Medicine* 104(3):399-404.

Sellers, E.M.; Busto, U. (1982). Benzodiazepines and ethanol: Assessment of the effects and consequences of psychotropic drug interactions. *Journal of Clinical Psychopharmacology* 2:249-261.

Simpson, G.M.; Gratz, S.S. (1992). Comparison of the pressor effect of tyramine after treatment with phenelzine and moclobemide in healthy male volunteers. *Journal of Clinical Pharmacology and Therapeutics* 52:286-291.

Sitsen, J.M.A.; Zikov, M. (1995). Mirtazapine: Clinical profile. *CNS Drugs* 4(Suppl 1):39-48.

Smiley, A.; Ziedman, K.; Moskowitz, H. (1981). *Pharmacokinetics of Drug Effects on Driving Performance: Driving Simulator Tests of Marijuana Alone and in*

Combination with Alcohol. Report prepared for NIDA and the National Highway Traffic Safety Administration. Contract 271-76-3316. Los Angeles, CA: Southern California Research Institute.

Stahl, S.M. (2002). Don't ask, don't tell, but benzodiazepines are still the leading treatments for anxiety disorder. *Journal of Clinical Psychiatry* 63:756-757.

Stein, A.C.; Allen, R.W.; Cook, M.L.; Karl, R.L. (1983). *A Simulator Study of the Combined Effects of Alcohol and Marijuana on Driving Behavior—Phase II.* Report DOT HS-5-01257. Washington, DC: National Highway Traffic Safety Administration.

Tanaka, E. (2002). Toxicological interactions between alcohol and benzodiazepines. *Journal of Toxicology. Clinical Toxicology* 40(1):69-75.

van Steveninck, A.L.; Gieschke, R.; Schoemaker, R.C.; Roncari, G.; Tuk, B.; Peiters, M.S.; Briemer, D.D.; Cohen, A.F. (1996). Pharmacokinetic and pharmacodynamic interactions of bretazenil and diazepam with alcohol. *British Journal of Clinical Pharmacology* 41:565-73.

Vgontzas, A.N.; Kales, A.; Bixler, E.O. (1995). Benodiazepine side effects: Role of pharmacokinetics and pharmacodynamics. *Pharmacology* 51:202-223.

Weathermon, R.; Crabb, D. (1999). Alcohol and medication interactions. *Alcohol Research & Health* 23(1):40-54.

Worz, C.R.; Bottorff, M. (2001). The role of cytochrome P450-mediated drug-drug interactions in determining the safety of statins. *Expert Opinion on Pharmacotherapy,* 2:1119-1127.

Zacny, J.P. (1995). A review of the effects of opioids on psychomotor and cognitive functioning in humans. *Experimental and Clinical Psychopharmacology* 3:432-466.

Zacny, J.P. (1996). Should people taking opioids for medical reasons be allowed to work and drive. *Addiction* 91:1581-1584.

Zimatkin, S.M.; Anichtchik, O.V. (1999). Alcohol-histamine interaction. *Alcohol and Alcoholism* 34(2):141-147.

Zirkle, G.A.; King, P.D.; McAtee, O.B.; Van Dyke, R. (1959). Effects of chlorpromazine and alcohol on coordination and judgment. *Journal of the American Medical Association* 171:1496-1499.

Chapter 17

The Adverse Effects of Alcohol
and Drug Abuse in the Oral Cavity

Terry D. Rees
Robert A. Levine

INTRODUCTION AND OVERVIEW

It has been said that the mouth is a treasure trove of diagnostic signs and symptoms of systemic diseases (U.S. Department of Health and Human Services, 2000). A similar statement could be made regarding the clinical features of drug abuse. The characteristic physiologic, immunologic, and neuroendocrine changes associated with drug abuse and described throughout this text also manifest in the oral cavity. In this chapter we discuss the oral features most often associated with chemical dependency and the effect in the mouth of the adverse psychologic changes associated with drug abuse. Principles of dental management of individuals who practice substance abuse will be described. Special emphasis will be placed on the role of drug abuse as etiologic risk factors for periodontal diseases and on the potential impact of chemical dependency on therapeutic outcomes.

The oral effects of drugs of abuse have not been studied as extensively as the adverse, mental and general, physiologic changes associated with their use. It is well established, however, that chronic use of mood altering drugs may adversely affect one's compliance with effective oral hygiene practices and routine dental visits. The oral cavity is often the first site of lesions suggestive of HIV infection, diabetes mellitus, venereal diseases, liver disease, and kidney failure, all of which occur at increased frequency among those who abuse drugs or alcohol. Excessive use of illicit drugs may alter host

Handbook of the Medical Consequences of Alcohol and Drug Abuse
© 2008 by The Haworth Press, Taylor & Francis Group. All rights reserved.
doi:10.1300/6039_17

susceptibility to oral infections and delay wound healing. In addition, nutritional deficiencies secondary to drug or alcohol abuse can have a profound effect on oral soft tissues and bone. For example, vitamin B complex (B_1, B_2, B_6, and B_{12}) deficiencies may be associated with a generalized stomatitis, glossitis, gingivitis, and ulcerations with or without manifestations of stomatodynia (burning mouth) (Abrams and Romberg, 1999). Vitamin B_{12} deficiency may also induce abnormalities of oral epithelial cells leading to epithelial thinning and increased mitotic activity, potentially increasing the risk for epithelial dysplasia or malignant transformation (Mitchell et al., 1986; Theaker, Porter, and Fleming, 1989). Vitamin C (ascorbic acid) deficiency may adversely affect periodontal connective tissues, capillary integrity, and wound healing, resulting in increased severity of gingivitis and periodontitis (Bsoul and Terezhalmy, 2004). This is probably the result of altered immune function, increased permeability of gingival sulcular epithelium, increased levels of tissue metalloproteins, and retention of extracellular fluid as a result of altered capillary permeability. Prolonged ascorbic acid deficiency (scurvy) may result in severe periodontal pathoses including increased tooth mobility, destruction of the periodontal ligament, osseous abnormalities, and, ultimately, exfoliation of the dentition (Leggott et al., 1991; Touyz, 1997). It should be noted that there is no evidence that mild ascorbic acid deficiency initiates periodontitis. However, Nishida et al. (2000) identified a small but statistically significant increase in periodontitis among current and past smokers and smoking may be ubiquitous among those who abuse drugs.

Xerostomia (mouth dryness) is a common effect of the use of opiates, stimulants, sedatives, hallucinogens, cannabis, and alcohol (Atkinson, Grisius, and Massey, 2005; Colon, 1972; Friedlander et al., 2003; Scheutz, 1983; Shaner, 2002). This dryness may affect the effectiveness of oral hygiene procedures and predispose drug users to an increased susceptibility to dental caries and periodontal diseases (Khocht et al., 2003; Hutchinson, 1990). In addition, individuals with excessive mouth dryness are more likely to experience traumatic injuries to mouth soft tissues, burning oral discomfort (burning mouth syndrome), and delays in wound healing (Chimenos-Kuster and Marques-Soares, 2002; Drage and Rogers, 2003).

Several authors have reported an increase in dental caries among alcoholics and drug addicts (Angelillo et al., 1991; Araujo et al., 2004; Driscoll, 2003; Du et al., 2001; Shaner, 2002; Zador, Lyons Wall, and Webster, 1996). This relates in part to failure to maintain adequate oral health habits but it also has been reported that addicted individuals may crave refined carbohydrates, and refined sugar is reported to be often used to dilute injected drugs (Scheutz, 1986). An increase in dental hypersensitivity to heat, cold, and certain foods has also been suggested. This may relate to the erosive nature of some drugs of abuse but is more likely to be associated with caries and bruxism. (Pallasch and Joseph, 1987). Excessive tooth wear (abrasion) has been reported as a frequent oral finding in association with increased jaw clinching and grinding among individuals who use illicit drugs (Colon, 1972; McGrath and Chan, 2005; Milosevic et al., 1999; Winocur et al., 2001, 2003). Dental erosion may be a common problem among abusers who experience an increased incidence of gastric reflux, nausea, and vomiting (Couper, Thatcher, and Logan, 2004; Frenia and Schauben, 1993; Kolecki, 1998; Yahchouchy, Debet, and Fingerhut, 2002).

ORAL EFFECTS OF ALCOHOL ABUSE

The adverse systemic effects of excessive use of alcohol are well known and alcohol is the most commonly used potentially addictive substance among polydrug abusers. In conjunction with smoking, alcohol abuse is considered to represent a major risk factor for oral cancer (squamous cell carcinoma) (Llewellyn, Johnson, and Warnakulasuriya, 2004). The exact mechanism for carcinogenesis is not yet fully understood but evidence suggests that the effects of alcohol on oral epithelial surfaces may alter absorption of carcinogenic agents from tobacco, marijuana, or crack cocaine and increase the risk for oncogenic changes (Banoczy et al., 2003; Howie et al., 2001; Squier, Kremer, and Wertz, 2003; Rodriquez et al., 2003). In addition, acetaldehyde, a metabolite of ethyl alcohol has been demonstrated to damage oral soft tissue DNA and alter keratinizing cell gene expression (Friedlander et al., 2003). Other cofactors include immunosuppression, human papillomavirus infection, iron deficiency, pernicious anemia, and oncogene and tumor suppressor gene dysregulation (Fowler, 1999; Herrero, 2003; Li et al., 2004).

Subtle effects of alcohol abuse that occur in the oral cavity and perioral area may enable the dentist to detect alcohol abuse long before it is suspected by family or friends. Alcohol induced parotid sialosis (enlargement) is relatively common in severe alcoholism due to fatty degeneration of the salivary glands (Carda et al., 2004). Skin conditions such as spider angiomata (netlike prominence of blood capillaries) and acne rosacea (facial flushing with or without acnelike skin lesions) may suggest excessive alcohol ingestion while an early sign of severe liver disease may be a yellow or dirty gray skin pigmentation (biliary melanderma), yellow sclera, and a yellowish cast to oral mucosa, especially the soft palate (Larato, 1972; Shellow, 1983). In alcohol abuse, oral tissues become dry and often assume an unusual magenta hue. This may or may not be associated with underlying nutritional deficiencies. Heavy drinkers who smoke have been reported to occasionally develop splotchy areas of depigmentation surrounded by hyperpigmentation on the oral mucosa and gingiva (Natali et al., 1991). Involuntary tongue tremor has been described and oral candidiasis and fungal induced angular cheilitis (perleche) is very common. The cheilitis may also be related to nutritional deficiency induced by alcoholism. Alcohol abusers are particularly prone to dental caries and periodontal disease due to lack of attention to oral hygiene and failure to request dental appointments (Araujo et al., 2004; Khocht et al., 2003; Nishida et al., 2004; Pitiphat et al., 2003; Tezal et al., 2004). Finally, those who abuse alcohol and other mood altering drugs may develop increased tolerance to local anesthetics and to drugs used to achieve conscious sedation. This may have an important impact on the ability of the dentist to provide treatment for dental diseases (Friedlander et al., 2003).

ORAL EFFECTS OF COCAINE

Owing to the harmful effects associated with nasal insufflation of cocaine, the agent is apparently being applied more frequently to the oral soft tissues. This practice has been shown by case reports and case series to induce epithelial desquamation, gingival leukoplakia, erythema, and ulceration Necrotizing gingivitis and periodontitis may be evident and extensive loss of alveolar bone may occur in sites where the drug is applied (Dello Russo and Temple, 1982; Garguilio, Toto, and Garguilo, 1985; Kapila and Kashani, 1997; Morgan and Hillman, 1996; Parry et al., 1996; Yukna, 1991). It is proposed that these effects are the result of ischemic necrosis caused by acute vasoconstriction associated with tissue contact with cocaine. As the changes just described are not characteristic of known oral soft tissue diseases, the dentist may be the first to suspect possible cocaine abuse in afflicted patients. Dental erosion and abrasion is common and cervical caries may occur in conjunction with use of a cocaine/sugar mixture (Parry et al., 1996). Smoking of crack cocaine may be associated with physical burns of the oral soft tissues, ulcerations (especially midpalatal), nodular erythematous lesions, and severe xerostomia. Mixed red and white tissue changes have been reported in the soft and hard palate giving an appearance similar to nicotinic stomatitis found in heavy smokers. It is assumed that these lesions are related to the increased heat associated with smoking crack cocaine as compared with tobacco as well as possible chemical injury (Mitchell-Lewis et al., 1994).

ORAL EFFECTS OF AMPHETAMINES, METHAMPHETAMINES (SPEED), AND MDMA (ECSTASY)

Abuse of amphetamines, methamphetamines, and MDMA (Ecstasy) has reached epidemic proportions (Teter and Guthrie, 2001). Therapeutic medications such as appetite suppressants (phenylpropanolamine and ephedrine) are readily available and can be "cooked" into potent forms of "designer" drugs (Colker, 2005). The stimulant effects of these drugs are similar to cocaine and they may be administered orally, intravenously, by inhalation or insufflation. The solid form, d-methamphetamine (ice and crystal), can be smoked (Rees, 1992; Schneir and Manoguerra, 2004). The drug effects are prolonged (up to 24 hours) and a number of dental and oral problems have been associated with their use. These drugs are often components of poly-drug use and oral signs and symptoms may be similar to those previously discussed (Mendelson et al., 1995). Severe xerostomia is an almost universal complaint and users may spasmodically chew, grind, or clench their teeth, leading to excessive wear, pain in the muscles of mastication, and temporomandibular joint discomfort. Rampant caries is a hallmark of methamphetamine abuse possibly due to excessive plaque accumulation associated with xerostomia. In addition there appears to be a marked increase in the consumption of sugar containing soft drinks among these individuals. Anorexia and nausea are common and afflicted individuals appear to devote minimal attention to oral hygiene while under the influence of the drugs. Abusers also tend to be noncompliant with dental treatment recommendations (Lee, Heffez, and Mohammadi, 1992; McGrath and Chan, 2005; Shaner, 2002; Wynn, 1997). Although these drugs do not appear to induce cardiovascular risks equal to cocaine abuse, multiple body organs are affected and concomitant use of some therapeutic dental drugs may induce intoxication or even sudden death.

ORAL EFFECTS OF CANNABIS

To date, the adverse intraoral and perioral effects of cannabis have not been adequately studied under controlled experimental conditions. However, numerous case reports have described xerostomia, nicotinic stomatitis, gingival and mucosal burns, erythematous enlargement of the uvula, leukoedema, traumatic ulcers, leukoplakia (white patches), overgrowth of gingival soft tissues, increased severity of gingivitis, and oral cancer (Arendorf, 1993; Baddour, Audemorte, and Layman, 1984; Baddour et al., 1984; Colon, 1972; Darling, 2003; Donald, 1986; Layman, 1978).

These effects appear to be dose related, and, except for leukoplakia, dysplasia, and squamous cell carcinoma, the lesions may be reversible if the use of cannabis is discontinued (Darling, 2003). Cannabis is sometimes used for medical purposes in the form of delta-9-tetrahydrocannabinol (THC). The drug is legally prescribed in some states for the management of a variety of conditions in individuals with terminal cancer and AIDS and to reduce ocular pressure in glaucoma. THC is taken orally and its absorption rate is slower than smoked cannabis (Attal et al., 2004). To date, there are no reports in the dental literature describing the adverse oral effects of medically prescribed cannabis.

Considerable evidence indicates that chronic, heavy cannabis smoking may represent a risk factor for oral squamous cell carcinoma (Firth, 1997). The various forms of the drug contain more potential carcinogenic agents than tobacco and it may be capable of altering the epithelial integrity of the oral mucous membranes. It has been suggested that more tar is ingested during inhalation of cannabis smoke and retained longer (Goldenberg et al., 2004; Hashibe, Ford, and Zhang, 2002). Despite this, there is little direct evidence that cannabis smoking is a risk factor for oral carcinoma (Rosenblatt et al., 2004). In part, this is because most cannabis users are also exposed to confounding etiologic factors such as tobacco and alcohol. Numerous case reports and some case series, however, implicate cannabis abuse in development of oral cancer in young individuals (Almadori et al., 1990; Caplan and Brigham, 1990; Donald, 1986).

DENTAL MANAGEMENT OF THE PATIENT WHO ABUSES ALCOHOL OR DRUGS

Individuals who abuse prescription drugs (codeine, morphine, oxycodone, etc.) may present to the dental office complaining of unexplained pain or discomfort. In addition, addicted individuals may deliberately inflict oral injury to entice the dentist to prescribe a narcotic pain medication. Other addicts may retain periodontally hopeless, deeply carious, or abscessed teeth in order to achieve an apparently forthright reason to request narcotic pain medication. Oxycodone (a semisynthetic opioid) is frequently prescribed in dental practice to control postoperative pain and discomfort. This drug is available in a more potent controlled release form (OxyContin) that is one of the most frequently abused prescription drugs (Anonymous, 2001; Cone et al., 2004). Dental practitioners should be especially cautious in prescribing narcotics for individuals who insist that only a specific narcotic agent is effective in controlling his or her pain. It is imperative that only a limited quantity of narcotic is provided at any one time and non-narcotic analgesic agents are preferable for individuals with unexplained pain or untreated dental disease (Huynh and Yagiela, 2003).

The dental practitioner must remain alert for signs and symptoms suggestive of drug or alcohol abuse (Saitz, 2005). Any dental patient who displays rhinorrhea, increased lacrimal flow, and dilated pupils should be questioned carefully about the possible use of opiates, while excessive thirst may be the first warning sign of chronic use of Ecstasy or other "designer" drug stimulants. Dental patients who exhibit bizarre behavior, inordinate excitement, or panic attacks may require careful medical evaluation to rule out use of stimulant drugs that are harmful, yet do not induce a physiologic addiction (Wilson et al., 2004). Facial acneiform dermatosis may also be an early sign of excessive use of stimulant agents. The oral features of cannabis abuse have been described in previously and one should be alert for evidence suggestive of a heavy cannabis habit.

Some dental treatment procedures (injection of local anesthetics, use of retraction cord containing epinephrine, and use of other agents that contain epinephrine) may induce tachycardia and peripheral vasodilation. This has prompted some authors to recommend that dental patients who are known to be frequent users of cannabis be advised to discontinue the practice for at least one week before dental treatment (Darling, 2003). From the discussion in the previous text, it is apparent that drugs and alcohol can seriously impact the safety and efficacy of dental care for afflicted individuals. However, with careful attention to detail, the dental practitioner can often detect the afflicted patient and provide necessary dental treatment safely and comfortably for the patient. Obviously, it is important to identify the substances being abused early in treatment and to refer drug abusers for counseling and detoxification whenever possible (Kosten and O'Connor, 2003; Legrand, Iacono, and McGue, 2005).

Standard operating procedure in the dental office should include a written health questionnaire that allows the patient the opportunity to identify existing or past drug-related problems. The questionnaire should query patients regarding alcohol and the frequency and quantity of its use. It should also ask whether the patient does or ever did use drugs of abuse. Although patients may not respond honestly to these questions, many individuals recognize the importance of informing the dentist about such issues. The medical history questionnaire should always be followed by a verbal interview with the patient to elicit additional information regarding any responses noted. It is certainly appropriate to query the patient in detail if signs or symptoms suggestive of abuse are evident. If the patient acknowledges past or current drug abuse, he or she should be questioned regarding the specific substance or substances used, whether or not the use is current, any known adverse physical effects the patient may have experienced as the result of the drug(s), and whether or not the patient is still under the influence of the drug. It is relatively common for anxious individuals who abuse drugs to use their drug of preference prior to a dental appointment to allay apprehension and induce euphoria during the dental procedure. Consequently, one should be aware of the signs and symptoms associated with drug intoxication and avoid treatment procedures that have the potential for inducing a medical emergency. Local anesthetics containing a vasoconstrictor such as epinephrine should be used with caution and use of materials such as a retraction cord containing a vasoconstrictor should be avoided. This may be of special concern in patients suspected of using cocaine or related substances. If emergency dental treatment is required for an individual suspected of cocaine intoxication, benzodiazepine conscious sedation may be appropriate as diazepines are commonly used in the management of cocaine toxicity (Rees, 1992).

Under most circumstances, elective dental treatment should be avoided until medical evaluation can be performed. Screening blood tests may be appropriate for individuals suspected of alcohol abuse to identify possible bleeding abnormalities and avoid postsurgical infection or delayed wound healing. Appropriate screening tests include a complete blood count with differential, platelet count, prothrombin time, partial thromboplastin time, and bleeding time. If liver disease is suspected, additional tests may be appropriate to include total serum protein, serum albumin, and liver transaminases such as AST, ALT, and GGT. Individuals with abnormal screening test results should be referred to their physician for evaluation prior to extensive periodontal or oral surgical procedures. However, laboratory testing has not been found to be a reliable method of detecting individuals who misuse alcohol. Careful questioning of the patient and possibly the patient's family may be more beneficial, but, to date, no consistently accurate diagnostic method exists for confirming suspected alcohol abuse.

Current or past users of drugs of abuse may suffer from unwanted effects such as gastrointestinal disorders, liver dysfunction, blood dyscrasias, renal disease, or cardiovascular disease. If this is the case, aspirin, acetaminophen or nonsteroidal anti-inflammatory drugs may be contraindicated. This often creates a dilemma in management of dental pain. Use of a mild narcotic agent may be necessary, but the medication should be prescribed in the minimal strength and quantity necessary to minimize the painful experience. The use of narcotic medications should be closely monitored by a family member or responsible friend. Intravenous conscious sedation and nitrous oxide/oxygen sedation should be used carefully as they may induce significant depression of respiratory and cardiovascular function.

The use of mouth rinses containing alcohol by abusers of alcohol or drugs is controversial. It is at least theoretically possible that the alcohol contained in the mouth rinse might trigger a relapse in abstaining alcoholic individuals. In addition, these mouth rinses may accentuate drug-induced xerostomia leading to the associated complications described previously. Nonalcoholic antimicrobial mouth rinses are now readily available. Not all alcohol-free mouth rinses have been confirmed to have acceptable antimicrobial properties but others, such as chlorhexidine in water or cetylpyridinium chloride in water have been demonstrated to be effective in controlled studies (Arweiler, Netuschil, and Reich, 2001; Leyes Borrajo et al., 2002; Witt et al., 2005).

Xerostomia is probably the most common adverse oral effect of drug or alcohol abuse. In order to minimize oral dryness, affected individuals should be instructed to avoid use of substances that contain caffeine (coffee, colas, and tea). Chewing sugarless gum (preferably containing xylitol) and firm healthy foods such as raw carrots and celery can stimulate natural salivary flow (Stewart et al., 1998). In most instances the individual should be encouraged to consume copious quantities of water daily. There is some evidence that ice water is more soothing than room temperature water in allaying oral discomfort. Artificial saliva substitutes are of some but limited benefit. Two systemic prescription drugs, pilocarpine and cevimeline HCL, will increase salivary gland output in some individuals. These drugs should only be prescribed after careful evaluation of the patient's overall health status. The prescribing dentist must also be aware of other medications the patient may be taking and their potential for creating an adverse drug interaction.

Parenteral drug users are at markedly increased risk for contracting infectious diseases such as HIV, hepatitis B, hepatitis C, and opportunistic infections such as candidiasis. It is imperative to employ appropriate infection control measures as required by the Centers for Disease Control to ensure safe management of these patients as well as to provide protection for the dental staff and other patients.

SUMMARY AND CONCLUSIONS

It is clear that the dental practitioner of today is very likely to encounter patients who abuse alcohol or other drugs. In some instances, the patient's status is known, but it is imperative that the dentist be alert for the signs and symptoms of alcohol and drug abuse. In most instances, it is possible to provide safe and effective dental care for patients who abuse drugs using the principles described previously. Close medical/dental coordination is imperative and it may be necessary to limit elective periodontal or surgical procedures. The goals of therapy should be to assist patients who abuse drugs in maintaining a high level of personal oral hygiene and oral health.

REFERENCES

Abrams, RG.; Romberg, E. (1999). Gingivitis in children with malnutrition. *J Clin Periodontol,* 23:189-194.

Almadori, G.; Paludetti, G.; Cerullo, M.; Ottaviani, F.; D'Alatri, L. (1990). Marijuana smoking as a possible cause of tongue carcinoma in young patients. *J Laryngol Otol,* 104:896-899.

Angelillo, I.F.; Grasso, G.M.; Sagliocco, G.; Villari, P.; D'Errico, M.M. (1991). Dental health in a group of drug addicts in Italy. *Community Dent Oral Epidemiol,* 19:336-337.

Anonymous (2001). Oxycodone and oxycontin. *Med Lett,* 43:80-81.

Araujo, M.W.; Dermen, K.; Connors, G.; Ciancio, S. (2004). Oral and dental health among inpatients in treatment for alcohol use disorders: A pilot study. *J Int Acad Periodontol,* 6:125-130.

Arendorf, T.M. (1993). Effects of cannabis smoking on oral soft tissues. *Community Dent Oral Epidemiol,* 21:78-81.

Arweiler, N.B.; Netuschil, L.; Reich, E. (2001). Alcohol-free mouthrinse solutions to reduce supragingival plaque regrowth and vitality. A controlled clinical study. *J Clin Periodontol,* 28:168-174.

Atkinson, J.C.; Grisius, M.; Massey, W. (2005). Salivary hypofunction and xerostomia: Diagnosis and treatment. *Dent Clin North Am,* 49:309-326.

Attal, N.; Brasseur, L.; Guirimand, D.; Clermond-Gnamien, S.; Atlami, S.; Bouhassira, D. (2004). Are oral cannabinoids safe and effective in refractory neuropathic pain? *European J Pain,* 8:173-177.

Baddour, H.M.; Audemorte, T.B.; Layman, F.D. (1984). The occurrence of diffuse gingival hyperplasia in a patient using marijuana. *J Tenn Dent Assoc,* 64:39-43.

Banoczy, J.; Squier, C.A.; Kermer, M.; Wertz, P.W.; Kovesi, G.; Szende, B.; Dom, C. (2003). The permeability of oral leukoplakia. *Eur J Oral Sci,* 111:312-314.

Bsoul, S.A.; Terezhalmy, G.T. (2004). Vitamin C in health and disease. *J Contemp Dent Pract,* 15:1-13.

Caplan, G.A.; Brigham, B.Q. (1990). Marijuana smoking and carcinoma of the tongue. Is there an association? *Cancer,* 66:1005-1006.

Carda, C.; Gomez de Ferraris, M.E.; Arriaga, A.; Carranza, M.; Peydro, A. (2004). Alcoholic parotid sialosis: A structural and ultrastructural study. *Med Oral,* 9:24-32.

Chimenos-Kuster, E.; Marques-Soares, M.S. (2002). Burning mouth and saliva. *Med Oral*, 7:244-253.

Colker, A.C. (2005). Restricting the sale of pseudoephedrine to prevent methamphetamine production. *NCSL Legisbrief*, 13:1-2.

Colon, P.G., Jr. (1972). Dental disease in the narcotic addict. *Oral Surg Oral Med Oral Pathol*, 33:905-910.

Cone, E.J.; Fant, R.V.; Rohay, J.M.; Caplan, Y.H.; Ballina, M.; Reder, R.F.; Haddo, J.D. (2004). Oxycodone involvement in drug abuse deaths. II. Evidence for toxic multiple drug-drug interactions. *J Anal Toxicol*, 28:616-624.

Couper, F.J.; Thatcher, J.E.; Logan, B.K. (2004). Suspected GHB overdoses in the emergency department. *J Anal Toxicol*, 28:481-484.

Darling, M.R. (2003). Cannabis abuse and oral health care: Review and suggestions for management. *SADJ*, 58:189-190.

Dello Russo, N.M.; Temple, H.V. (1982). Cocaine effects on gingiva. *J Am Dent Assoc*, 104:13.

Donald, P.J. (1986). Possible cause of head and neck carcinoma in young patients. *Otolaryngol Head Neck Surg*, 94:517-521.

Drage, L.A.; Rogers, R.S. 3rd. (2003). Burning mouth syndrome. *Dermatol Clin*, 21:135-145.

Driscoll, S.E. (2003). A pattern of erosive carious lesions from cocaine use. *J Mass Dent Soc*, 52:12-14.

Du, M.; Bedi, R.; Guo, L.; Champion, J.; Fan, M.; Holt, R. (2001). Oral health status of heroin users in a rehabilitation centre in Hubei province, China. *Community Dent Health*, 18:94-98.

Firth, N.A. (1997). Marijuana use and oral cancer: A review. *Oral Oncol*, 33:398-401.

Fowler, C.B. (1999). Benign and malignant neoplasms of the periodontium. *Periodontol 2000*, 21:33-83.

Frenia, M.L.; Schauben, J.L. (1993). Methanol inhalation toxicity. *Ann Emerg Med*, 22:1919-1923.

Friedlander, A.H.; Marder, S.R.; Pisegna, J.R.; Yagiela, J.A. (2003). Alcohol abuse and dependence: Psychopathology, medical management and dental implications. *J Am Dent Assoc*, 134:731-740.

Garguilo, A.V., Jr.; Toto, P.D.; Garguilo, A.W. (1985). Cocaine-induced gingival necrosis. *Periodontal Case Rep*, 7:44-45.

Goldenberg, D.; Lee, J.; Koch, W.M.; Kim, M.M.; Trink, B.; Sidransky, D.; Moon, C-S. (2004). Habitual risk factors for head and neck cancer. *Orolaryngol Head Neck Surg*, 131:986-993.

Hashibe, M.; Ford, D.E.; Zhang, Z.F. (2002). Marijuana smoking and head and neck cancer. *J Clin Periodontol*, 42(11 Suppl):103S-107S.

Herrero, R. (2003). Chapter 7: Human papillomavirus and cancer of the upper aerodigestive tract. *J Natl Cancer Inst Monogr*, 31:47-51.

Howie, N.M.; Trigkas, T.K.; Cruchley, A.T.; Wertz, P.W.; Squier, C.A.; Williams, D.M. (2001). Short-term exposure to alcohol increases the permeability of human oral mucosa. *Oral Dis*, 7:349-354.

Hutchinson, S. (1990). Methadone and caries. *Br Dent J*, 168:430.

Huynh, M.P.; Yagiela, J.A. (2003). Current concepts in acute pain management. *J Calif Dent Assoc,* 31:419-427.

Kapila, Y.L.; Kashani, H. (1997). Cocaine-associated rapid gingival recession and dental erosion. A case report. *J Periodontol,* 68:485-488.

Khocht, A.; Janal, M.; Schleifer, S.; Keller, S. (2003). The influence of gingival margin recession on loss of clinical attachment in alcohol-dependent patients without medical disorders. *J Periodontol,* 74:485-493.

Kolecki, P. (1998). Inadvertent methamphetamine poisoning in pediatric patients. *Pediatr Emerg Care,* 14:385-387.

Kosten, T.R.; O'Connor, P.G. (2003). Management of drug and alcohol withdrawal. *N Engl J Med,* 348:1786-1795.

Larato, D.C. (1972). Oral tissue changes in the chronic alcoholic. *J Periodontol,* 43:772-773.

Layman, F.D. (1978). Marijuana: Harmful or not? *Tex Dent J,* 96:6-8.

Lee, C. Y.; Heffez, L.B.; Mohammadi, H. (1992). Crystal methamphetamine abuse: A concern to oral and maxillofacial surgeons. *J Oral Maxillofac Surg,* 50:1052-1054.

Leggott, P.; Robertson, P.B.; Jacob, R.A.; Zambon, J.J.; Walshm Armitage, G.C. (1991). Effects of ascorbic acid depletion and supplementation on periodontal health and subgingival microflora in humans. *J Dent Res,* 70:1531-1536.

Legrand, L.N.; Iacono, W.G.; McGue, M. (2005). Predicting addiction. *Am Sci,* 93:140-147.

Leyes Borrajo, J.L.; Garcia, V.L.; Lopex, C.G.; Rodriquez-Nunez, I.M.; Garcia, F.M.; Gallas, T.M. (2002). Efficacy of chlorhexidine mouthrinses with and without alcohol: A clinical study. *J Periodontol,* 73:317-321.

Li, G.; Sturgis, E.M.; Wand, L.E.; Chamberlain, R.M.; Amos, C.I.; Spitz, M.R.; El-Naggar, A.K.; Hong, W.K.; Wei, Q. (2004). Association of a p73 exon 2 G4C14-toA4T14 polymorphism with risk of squamous cell carcinoma of the head and neck. *Carcinogenesis,* 25:1911-1916.

Llewellyn, C.D.; Johnson, N.W.; Warnakulasuriya, K.A. (2004). Risk factors for oral cancer in newly diagnosed patients aged 45 years and younger: A case-control study in Southern England. *J Oral Pathol Med,* 33:525-532.

McGrath, C.; Chan, B. (2005). Oral health sensations associated with illicit drug abuse. *Br Dent J,* 198:159-162.

Mendelson, J.; Jones, R.T.; Upton, R.; Jacob, P., 3rd (1995). Methamphetamine and ethanol interactions in humans. *Clin Pharmacol Ther,* 57:559-568.

Milosevic, A.; Agrawal, N.; Redfearn, P.; Mair, L. (1999). The occurrence of tooth wear in users of Ecstasy (3,4-methylenedioxymethamphetamine). *Community Dent Oral Epidemiol,* 27:283-287.

Mitchell, K.; Ferguson, M.; Lucie, N.; MacDonald, D. (1986). Epithelial dysplasia in the oral mucosa associated with pernicious anemia. *Br Dent J,* 161:259-260.

Mitchell-Lewis, D.A.; Phelan, J.A.; Kelly, R.B.; Bradley, J.J.; Lamster, I.B. (1994). Identifying oral lesions associated with crack cocaine use. *J Am Dent Assoc,* 125:1104-1108, 1110.

Morgan, G.; Hillman, L. (1996). Oral cocaine use. *Br Dent J,* 181:241.

Natali, C.; Curtis, J.L.; Suarez, L.; Millman, E.J. (1991). Oral mucosa pigment changes in heavy drinkers and smokers. *J Natl Med Assoc,* 83:434-438.

Nishida, M.; Grossi, S.G.; Dunford, R.G., Ho, A.W., Genco, R.J. (2000). Dietary vitamin C and the risk for periodontal disease. *J Periodontol,* 71:1215-1223.

Nishida, N.; Tanaka, M.; Hayashi, N.; Nagata, H.; Takeshita, T.; Nakayama, K.; Morimoto, K.; Shizukuishi, S. (2004). Association of ALDH(2) genotypes and alcohol consumption with periodontitis. *J Dent Res,* 83:161-165.

Pallasch, T.J.; Joseph, C.E. (1987). Oral manifestations of drug abuse. *J Psychoactive Drugs,* 19:375-377.

Parry, J.; Porter, S.; Scully, C.; Flint, S.; Parry, M.G. (1996). Mucosal lesions due to oral cocaine use. *Br Dent J,* 180:462-464.

Pitiphat, W.; Merchant, A.T.; Rimm, E.B.; Joshipura, K.J. (2003). Alcohol consumption increases periodontitis risk. *J Dent Res,* 82:509-513.

Rees, T.D. (1992). Oral effects of drug abuse. *Crit Rev Oral Biol Med,* 3:163-184.

Rodriquez, T.; Altieri, A.; Chatenoud, L.; Gallus, S.; Bosetti, C.; Negri, E.; Franceschi, S.; Levi, F.; Talamini, R.; La Vecchia, C. (2003). Risk factors for oral and pharyngeal cancer in young adults. *Oral Oncol,* 40:207-213.

Rosenblatt, K.A.; Daling, J.R.; Chen, C.; Sherman, K.J.; Schwartz, S.M. (2004). Marijuana use and risk of oral squamous cell carcinoma. *Cancer Res,* 64:4049-4054.

Saitz, R. (2005). Unhealthy alcohol use. *N Engl J Med,* 352:596-607.

Scheutz, F. (1983). Saliva secretion rate in a group of drug addicts (short communication). *Scand J Dent Res,* 91(6):496-498.

Scheutz, F. (1986). Drug addiction and viral hepatitis in the dental patient. *Dan Med Bul,* 33:228-249.

Schneir, A.; Manoguerra, A.S. (2004). Chapter 8: Medical consequences of the use of cocaine and other stimulants. In: Brick, J. (ed.), *Handbook of the Medical Consequences of Alcohol and Drug Abuse* (pp. 257-279). Binghamton, NY: The Haworth Medical Press.

Shaner, J.W. (2002). Caries associated with methamphetamine abuse. *J Mich Dent Assoc,* 84:42-47.

Shellow, W.V.R. (1983). The skin in alcoholism. *Int J Dermatol,* 22:506-510.

Squier, C.A.; Kremer, M.J.; Wertz, P.W. (2003). Effect of ethanol on lipid metabolism and epithelial permeability barrier of skin and oral mucosa in the rat. *J Oral Pathol Med,* 32:595-599.

Stewart, C.M.; Jones, A.C.; Bates, R.E.; Sandow, P.; Pink, F.; Stillwell, J. (1998). Comparison between saliva stimulants and a saliva substitute in patients with xerostomia and hyposalivation. *Spec Care Dentist,* 18:142-148.

Teter, C.J.; Guthrie, S.K. (2001). A comprehensive review of MDMA and GHB: Two common club drugs. *Pharmacotherapy,* 21:1486-1453.

Tezal, M.; Grossi, S.G.; Ho, A.W.; Genco, R.J. (2004). Alcohol consumption and periodontal disease. The Third National Health and Nutrition Examination Survey. *J Clin Periodontol,* 31:484-488.

Theaker, J.; Porter, S.; Fleming, K. (1989). Oral epithelial dysplasia in vitamin B$_{12}$ deficiencies. *Oral Surg Oral Med Oral Pathol,* 67:81-83.

Touyz, L.Z. (1997). Oral scurvy and periodontal disease. *J Can Dent Assoc,* 63: 837-845.

U.S. Dept of Health and Human Services (2000). *Oral Health in America: A Report of the Surgeon General. Executive Summary.* Rockville, MD: U.S. Department of Health and Human Services, National Institute of Dental and Craniofacial Research, National Institutes of Health.

Wilson, C.R.; Sherritt, L.; Gates, E.; Knight, J.R. (2004). Are clinical impressions of adolescent substance use accurate? *Pediatrics,* 114:536-540.

Winocur, E.; Gavish, A.; Voikovitch, M.; Emodi-Perlman, A.; Eli, I. (2003). Drugs and bruxism: A critical review. *J Orofac Pain,* 17:99-111.

Winocur, E.; Gavish, A.; Volfin, G.; Halachmi, M.; Gazit, E. (2001). Oral motor parafunctions among heavy drug addicts and their effects on signs and symptoms of temporomandibular disorders. *J Orofac Pain,* 15:56-63.

Witt, J.; Ramji, N.; Gibb, R.; Dunavent, J.; Flood, J.; Barnes, J. (2005). Antibacterial and antiplaque effects of a novel, alcohol-free oral rinse with cetylpyridinium chloride. *J Contemp Dent Prac,* 15:1-9.

Wynn, R.L. (1997). Dental considerations of patients taking appetite suppressants. *Gen Dent,* 45:324-328, 330-331.

Yahchouchy, E.; Debet, A.; Fingerhut, A. (2002). Crack cocaine-related prepyloric perforation treated laparoscopically. *Surg Endosc,* 16:220.

Yukna, R.A. (1991). Cocaine periodontitis. *Int J Periodontics Restorative Dent,* 11:73-79.

Zador, D.; Lyons Wall, P.M.; Webster, I. (1996). High sugar intake in a group of women on methadone maintenance in south western Sydney, Australia. *Addiction,* 91:1053-1061.

Chapter 18

Special Issues in Patients with Comorbid Psychiatric and Chemical Dependency Disorders

Mark C. Wallen
William J. Lorman

INTRODUCTION AND OVERVIEW

Individuals with comorbid mental health and chemical dependency disorders present many challenges for treatment professionals. In the past, this grouping of patients has been identified by a number of other titles including, among others: the mentally ill chemical abuser (MICA) population, the mentally ill substance abuser (MISA) population, chemically abusing mentally ill (CAMI) population, the dual diagnosis (DD) patient population, and most recently, patients with co-occurring mental health and addiction (CMHA) problems. From a formal perspective, these patients must meet *Diagnostic and Statistical Manual of Mental Disorders,* Fourth Edition (DSM-IV; American Psychiatric Association, 1994), diagnostic criteria for a psychiatric disorder and simultaneously meet criteria for a separate and distinct chemical dependency disorder. This patient population often experiences the multiple negative consequences of their comorbid disorders including but not limited to social, familial, educational, occupational, legal, medical, interpersonal, financial, and psychological problems. In most instances comorbidity has a significant negative impact on the course, prognosis, and outcomes of both types of disorders (Gonzales and Insel, 2004). This is a very heterogeneous group of patients depending upon the type, severity, and interactions between the disorders and as a result, no one single treatment approach can be utilized to treat all patients with comorbid disorders. It is clear however, that if comorbid disorders exist, it is critical to iden-

Handbook of the Medical Consequences of Alcohol and Drug Abuse
© 2008 by The Haworth Press, Taylor & Francis Group. All rights reserved.
doi:10.1300/6039_18
579

tify and treat both problems on a long-term simultaneous basis. Unfortunately, the vast majority of patients with comorbid disorders do not receive effective treatment for both of their disorders in a comprehensive integrated fashion. In addition, patients with comorbid disorders have to deal with not just one but two societal stigmas as a result of having both mental health and chemical dependency problems.

This chapter will focus on special issues as they relate to patients with comorbid psychiatric and chemical dependency disorders. We start off by looking at the magnitude of the problem by providing statistics regarding the prevalence of patients with comorbid disorders and we will review the complex relationships between psychiatric disorders and chemical dependency disorders. We will then move into the area of assessing patients for comorbid disorders including the utilization of various screening and assessment tools to evaluate patients for the presence of psychiatric disorders, chemical dependency disorders, and comorbid disorders. We will then discuss the so-called post–acute withdrawal syndrome (PAWS) that frequently includes psychiatric symptoms resulting from the effects of addicting substances on the brain that persist beyond the acute withdrawal phase and frequently result in the misdiagnosis of a separate psychiatric disorder. We will then move into the area of the treatment of comorbid disorders including various treatment models, treatment settings, general treatment principles, and will conclude with descriptions in greater detail of specific treatment components. We then will move into the area of the utilization of psychotropic medications to treat psychiatric disorders in comorbid patients. We will review the appropriate utilization of antidepressant medications, mood stabilizers, and anxiolytic medications including some comments concerning the use of potentially addicting medications with this population. We will look at the use in comorbid patients of medications prescribed as adjuncts in the treatment of alcoholism. This will then be followed by a review of one of the leading causes of death in the comorbid patient population, namely suicide. A review of comorbid disorders and their interrelationship with HIV disease and hepatitis C will follow. We will conclude the chapter with a brief summary of our recommendations for effective assessment and treatment of patients with comorbid psychiatric and chemical dependency disorders.

PREVALENCE AND STATISTICS

Prevalence

The National Survey on Drug Use and Health (NSDUH) reported on the prevalence of persons who met the criteria for both serious mental illness and substance dependence and abuse in 2002 (Office of Applied Studies, 2003). The NSDUH defined serious mental illness as having at some time during the past year a diagnosable mental, behavioral, or emotional disorder that met the criteria specified in the DSM-IV (American Psychiatric Association, 1994) and resulted in functional impairment that substantially interfered with or limited one or more major life activities. Data from the survey indicate that serious mental illness is highly correlated with substance dependence or abuse. Among adults with serious mental illness in 2002, 23.2 percent were dependent on or abused alcohol or illicit drugs, while the rate among adults without a psychiatric disorder was only 8.2 percent. Among adults with substance dependence or abuse, 20.4 percent had a serious mental illness while the rate of serious mental illness was 7 percent among adults who were not dependent on or abusing a substance. Flynn et al. (1996) analyzed data from a series of studies that demonstrated that rates of mental disorders increase as the number of substance use disorders increases. For example, the rate of major depressive disorder in persons dependent on heroin alone was found to be 7 percent; in persons dependent on both heroin and alcohol, the rate increased to 13.2 percent. The rate was 17.1 percent in persons dependent on heroin, alcohol, and cocaine.

Psychiatric Symptoms from Substance Usage

Substance-related disorders cause a variety of symptoms that are characteristic of other mental disorders. As these presentations are so frequently encountered in mental health, substance treatment, and primary care settings, a substance-related disorder must be considered in every differential diagnosis. These disorders are among the most frequently missed in clinical practice. In DSM-IV (American Psychiatric Association, 1994) the term "substance-related" refers to disorders associated with drugs of abuse, the side effects of medication, and toxin-induced states. There are two types of substance-related diagnoses: the substance use disorders, which describe a pattern of problematic substance use (substance dependence and substance abuse); and the substance-induced disorders, which describe behavioral syndromes that are caused by a direct effect of the substance on the central nervous system. The recognized list of substance-induced disorders includes delirium, persisting dementia, persisting amnestic disorder, psychotic disorder, mood disorder, anxiety disorder, sexual dysfunction, sleep disorder, and hallucinogen persisting perception disorder (flashbacks). These behavioral syndromes with their associated signs and symptoms are indistinguishable from primary psychiatric disorders.

Relationships Between Chemical Dependency and Psychiatric Illness

There are many possible relationships between chemical dependency and psychiatric illness (see Daley and Moss, 2002). Several of these relationships are now described.

Chemical dependency increases the risk of developing a psychiatric illness. The "two hit hypothesis" describes how a person has a genetic predisposition toward mental illness (the first hit) but it is not manifest until a significant stressor/trauma occurs (the second hit). In this case, the severe consequences of the chemical dependency may constitute the "second hit" for those persons who already have the genetic predisposition.

Psychiatric illness increases the risk of developing a chemical dependency. People give a variety of reasons for using the drugs they do: to feel different, to fit in, it's enjoyable, they feel better when they use it and feel bad when they don't. A popular idea is that of the "self-medication theory" of addictive disorders. This theory suggests that people use the substances to treat their psychological needs pharmacologically; they chemically treat something that they lack or replace something they are missing. It has been difficult to test this theory (Regier et al., 1990) and there has been conflicting evidence that substance use actually reduces psychiatric symptoms. However, as long as some individuals have the expectancy or belief that it will, they will continue to use it to self-medicate (LeFauve et al., 2004). Unfortunately, the reason people start using a substance and the reason they continue may differ dramatically. At some point, the individual may feel compelled to continue its use because drugs cause changes in the nervous system that make their use self-perpetuating and take much of the volitional aspect away.

Psychiatric symptoms may arise as a direct result of chronic substance use (intoxication and withdrawal). These are the substance-induced disorders. Numerous case studies report the phenomena of substance-induced disorders but not the epidemiology. However, there are some estimates of prevalence of alcohol-induced anxiety and depressive disorders. Brown and Schuckit (1988) reported that 42 percent of male alcoholics they studied displayed depressive symptoms in a range comparable to that seen in individuals hospitalized for mood disorders. The symptoms abated rapidly over the first two weeks of abstinence. Anxiety symptoms show similar changes over the early sobriety phase. Schuckit and Hesselbrock (1994) reported high rates of anxiety symptoms among alcoholics in withdrawal, with 80 percent of the male subjects experiencing repeated panic attacks during withdrawal.

The findings of Schuckit et al. (1997) supported three hypotheses related to substance-induced depression. First, there is more substance-induced depression than major depressive disorders; second, those with substance-induced depression have more severe alcohol and drug histories; and third, those with independent depression have more first-degree relatives with mood disorders than the substance-induced group. These proven hypotheses act as a helpful guide when making a diagnosis.

Psychiatric symptoms may arise as a consequence of chemical dependency (adjustment disorders resulting from job loss, dysfunctional family dynamics, etc.). In this case, the identification and resolution of the external stressors should eliminate or greatly reduce the maladaptive response. It is often difficult, in the early stages of treatment, to tease out the various components of the presenting symptomatology as many patients provide a history full of complexities such as a family history of mental illness, multiple severe consequences of substance use, and a description of psychiatric symptoms that became evident long after the substance use became a problem. These patients are usually given a "not otherwise specified" (NOS) diagnosis until clearer definitions, time frames, and criteria can be evaluated.

Psychiatric symptoms/disorders can develop independently from chemical dependency (true co-occurring disorders). There are many variables concerning accurate diagnoses of comorbid substance use and psychiatric disorders. A period of abstinence is optimal for diagnosis, but the necessary minimum time frame is likely to differ for each diagnosis and can be highly individualized. A family history of mental illness, clear onset of psychiatric symptoms before onset of the substance use disorder, and the presence of sustained psychiatric symptoms during lengthy periods of abstinence improve the accuracy of a comorbid diagnosis.

ASSESSMENT OF COMORBID DISORDERS

Introduction

The complexity of dealing with this patient population is complicated by the difficulties a clinician has in accurately making diagnoses when initially presented with a patient who exhibits both psychiatric symptoms and substance usage. Are the patients' symptoms due to their substance usage (substance induced), are they due to a separate and distinct psychiatric disorder, or are they due to a combination of both problems (substance induced symptoms superimposed upon a coexisting psychiatric disorder)? This requires that clinicians in both the mental health and chemical dependency fields develop the skills necessary to comprehensively screen and assess patients for both psychiatric disorders and chemical dependency disorders while at the same time being aware of the potential complicating factor that substance usage can have on being able to accurately make psychiatric diagnoses. This requires that patient diagnoses be reviewed, and changed if indicated, on a longitudinal basis as a patient is able to maintain abstinence from substance usage and continues in ongoing treatment. It is also important to keep in mind that we are dealing with two types of medical illnesses that individually have suffered historically from social stigmatization.

Initial assessment requires evaluating patients for both chemical dependency and psychiatric disorders involving the completion of a comprehensive clinical history, substance use history, and mental status examination. A number of screening/assessment tools, as delineated in the following text, have been formulated to assist clinicians in evaluating patients for addiction and mental health disorders. Psychiatric symptoms such as depression, mood swings, agitation, anxiety, concentration/attention problems, memory problems, and even psychotic symptoms are frequently associated with substance use and withdrawal. When any of these symptoms are identified from the patient's clinical history or mental status examination, the temporal relationship between the presence of the symptom and substance use needs to be ascertained. The initial task is to try and distinguish between a substance-induced psychiatric disorder, likely to remit with abstinence and treatment, and an independent psychiatric disorder that would often require psychopharmacological intervention. The time frame following cessation of substance use required to ascertain whether psychiatric symptoms are independent from substance use can be highly variable, depending on the type of substance used, the duration of substance use, and whether any type of toxic, irreversible brain damage has occurred from the use of the substance. Work by Brown, Inaba, and Gillin (1995) has shown that a minimum of three weeks of complete abstinence is required for the resolution of depressive symptoms caused by alcohol intoxication and withdrawal, which has led to the recommendation in the DSM-IV (American Psychiatric Association, 1994) of at least one month of abstinence before making a diagnosis of a mood disorder in alcoholics with depression. In early recovery, psychiatric diagnoses should, in most cases, be identified as being either substance-induced or should be identified as being NOS diagnoses with rule outs for substance-induced disorders and/or specific psychiatric disorders.

A number of factors have been identified that may be predictive of a greater probability of a patient having a comorbid mental health problem. The presence of psychiatric symptoms consistent with a psychiatric disorder prior to the onset of substance use or during a period of complete abstinence from substance use for at least several months might be suggestive of a separate psychiatric disorder. Similar to addictive disorders, many major psychiatric disorders tend to run in families as a result of increased genetic vulnerability. A family history of a major psychiatric disorder might therefore put patients at greater risk of developing a similar disorder themselves. However, if a family history of a psychiatric disorder is identified in a biological relative, it is also important to ascertain whether that relative also had a history of substance use, as the relative may have been misdiagnosed with a psychiatric disorder that was in reality substance related or induced. Even if a patient falls into any of the categories noted in previous text suggestive of a higher probability of a separate psychiatric diagnosis, it is important to keep in mind that this should not, in itself, be viewed as diagnostic.

Over the years, a variety of assessment instruments have been developed to identify psychiatric syndromes. These can either be in the form of *direct interviews,* which are person-to-person interactions, or *indirect surveys,* which use a structured self-report form. The indirect survey method lacks the clinical judgment of an experienced clinician that may be necessary in certain circumstances. The most common assessment approach, however, is an interview format, which may be *structured* (there is a standard list of questions which are asked of every subject) or *unstructured* (the clinician utilizes his or her own clinical judgment in selecting the appropriate questions). An effective assessment instrument must be reliable and valid. *Reliability* refers to the degree to which the conclusions can be replicated when the instrument is used by different examiners (inter-rater reliability) or on different occasions (test-retest reliability). *Validity* refers to whether the instrument measures what it is supposed to measure.

Assessment instruments must also be sensitive and specific. *Sensitivity* refers to the degree the instrument is able to detect the thing being evaluated (e.g., to diagnose a disorder when it is present). If a disorder is detected that is not, in fact, present, the result is called a *false positive. Specificity* refers to the degree an instrument does not detect those things not being evaluated. For example, an instrument with a high degree of specificity is able to determine the absence of a disorder in a person who does not have the disorder. This is called a *true negative.* If the instrument reports the presence of a disorder that is not, in fact, present, this is called a *false negative.*

Chemical Dependency Screening/Assessment Tools

A large number of screening/assessment tools have been formulated to aid clinicians in evaluating patients for chemical dependency disorders.

These tools should be viewed as components of a comprehensive comorbid assessment and should not be utilized alone as diagnostic instruments. Although a comprehensive review of specific instruments is beyond the scope of this chapter, it is useful to be aware of some of the most commonly utilized tools. Probably the most widely utilized screening tool for alcohol problems, due to its ease of application, is the CAGE Questionnaire (Ewing, 1984). It also has been modified to assess for drug abuse screening as the CAGE-AID (Brown and Rounds, 1995). Some additional screening tools include the Michigan Alcoholism Screening Test (MAST) (Selzer, 1971) and the Short MAST (SMAST) (Selzer, Vinokur, and Van Rooijen, 1975). The Michigan Alcoholism Screening Test–Geriatric Version (MAST-G) (Blow et al., 1992) has been validated for use with older adults. The Tolerance, Worried friends/relatives, Eye opener, Amnesia when drinking, Kut down (TWEAK) Questionnaire (Russel, 1994) appears to be more sensitive in screening women, especially pregnant women, for alcohol problems. The Problem Oriented Screening Instrument for Teenagers (POSIT) (Rahdert, 1991) can be useful in the screening and assessment of young people. The Alcohol Use Disorders Identification Test (AUDIT) is a ten-item questionnaire developed by the World Health Organization to identify persons with potentially harmful or hazardous alcohol consumption (Babor et al., 2002; Saunders et al., 1993). The University of Rhode Island Change Assessment (URICA) is an instrument designed to measure patient status in relation to the following four stages of change: precontemplation, contemplation, action, and maintenance (DiClemente and Prochaska, 1998). This tool can also be used longitudinally in treatment to assess patients' status regarding their acceptance to effectively address their addiction problems.

Psychiatric Disorder Screening/Assessment Tools

There are hundreds of screening and assessment tools available to assist in diagnosing psychiatric conditions. Unfortunately, these tools may accurately identify the presence of psychiatric syndromes, but they do not identify the cause of the syndrome. For instance, substances can mimic symptoms of mental disorders—hallucinogens may produce psychotic symptoms and cocaine withdrawal commonly produces a depressed state. Thus, many well-tested instruments will produce false positive results (a low degree of sensitivity).

The most commonly used tools for the assessment of depression are the Beck Depression Inventory–II (BDI-II) (Beck, Steer, and Brown, 1996) and the Hamilton Rating Scale for Depression (HAM-D) (Hedlung and Vieweg, 1979). Similarly, the most common tools for assessment of anxiety are the

Beck Anxiety Inventory (BAI) (Beck et al., 1988) and the Hamilton Anxiety Scale (HAM-A) (Hamilton, 1959). Although a well-validated and reliable tool, the Minnesota Multiphasic Personality Inventory–2 (MMPI-2) (Butcher et al., 2001) is quite lengthy (over 500 items) and requires specific training to administer and evaluate. This tool measures multiple traits and is useful in identifying characterological pathology.

Often, instruments are shortened when true positives correlate with specific items on the original instrument. For example, the Brief Symptom Inventory–18 (BSI-18) is an 18-item questionnaire that provides subscales for anxiety, depression and somatization. This instrument was derived from the 53-item Brief Symptom Inventory, which was derived from the Symptom Checklist–90–Revised (SCL-90-R) (Derogatis, 1975).

Unfortunately, most screening and assessment instruments are proprietary and the clinician must pay a fee to use the tool. However, there are many public domain instruments available. In addition to the Hamilton scales identified in the previous text, the Internet can be a source of a variety of instruments, such as the Montgomery-Asberg Depression Rating Scale (MADRS); Inventory of Depressive Symptomatology (IDS-C); Young Mania Rating Scale (YMRS); Clinical Global Impression–Bipolar (CGI-BP); and Mood Disorder Questionnaire (MDQ). The name of the instrument generally defines the syndrome being evaluated.

Cormorbid Disorder Screening/Assessment Tools

Several screening/assessment tools have been found to be useful in the evaluation of patients with comorbid disorders. The Addiction Severity Index (ASI) (McLellan et al., 1992), which includes domains related to the severity of both mental health and addiction problems, has been shown to be a valid and reliable instrument for mentally ill substance abusers (Appleby et al., 1997; Carey, Cocco, and Correia, 1997). The Dartmouth Assessment of Lifestyle Instrument (DALI) has been designed to screen for substance use disorders among patients hospitalized for psychiatric illnesses (Rosenberg et al., 1998). The Drug Abuse Screening Test (DAST-10) has been shown to be reliable and valid for assessing problems associated with drug use in psychiatric outpatient populations (Cocco and Carey, 1998; Maisto et al., 2000). The Problems Assessment for Substance Using Psychiatric Patients (PASUPP) is a valid and reliable instrument for assessing the range of negative consequences experienced by patients with comorbid disorders (Carey et al., 2004). Brems, Johnson, and Namyniuk, (2002) have developed an intake form protocol, which was designed to be utilized by clinicians of all disciplines, to gather information from comorbid patients with the goals of making appropriate diagnoses and setting the stage for initial treatment planning. The form includes gathering information related to substance use history and mental status examination, along with associated clinical data, in an objective format utilizing checklists and Likert scales wherever available to decrease inter-assessor differences and errors.

POST–ACUTE WITHDRAWAL SYNDROME

The chronic use of alcohol and/or drugs can have complex negative effects on brain cell membranes, receptor sites, and on intracellular metabolism and processes. As a result of this, upon cessation of substance usage, many patients will experience a wide array of psychiatric and physical symptoms that may persist for weeks to months (or longer) beyond the acute withdrawal phase (Trevisan et al., 1998). These symptoms have been identified as the so-called post–acute withdrawal syndrome (PAWS). Other terms that have been utilized to identify these symptoms include the protracted or prolonged withdrawal/abstinence syndrome and the post–withdrawal abstinence syndrome. Frequent symptoms of PAWS include anxiety, depressive symptoms, tremors, sleep disruption, and increased autonomic symptoms including breathing rate, body temperature, blood pressure, and pulse (Alling et al., 1982; Schuckit et al., 1991). Mood instability, substance craving, decreased energy, lassitude, decreased overall metabolism may also be seen (Satel et al., 1993). Attention, concentration, and memory problems also frequently occur. Clinically, these symptoms are important because patients frequently cite them as relapse triggers.

Post–acute withdrawal syndrome symptoms tend to exhibit a highly variable course. They tend to come and go and are generally mild to moderate in intensity. There is a high degree of individual patient variability as well with some patients experiencing only a few of these symptoms while other patients experience a much larger number of them. Almost all patients have at least some of them. Symptom severity can also be highly variable. It is critical that all patients be made aware of this syndrome. Patients in early recovery tend to be extremely sensitive in their reaction to these symptoms and may misinterpret their etiology and meaning. They tend to equate any physical/emotional discomfort they may have to the physical and emotional dysphoria they experienced in between episodes of acute substance usage during their active addiction. Although these symptoms are not pleasant to have, patients need to be made aware that they are normal and are an expected component of the recovery process. Patients generally are able to tolerate the symptoms better if they are aware of their source, rather than perceive that something is going wrong for them as they attempt to establish and maintain ongoing recovery.

As previously identified, a number of the symptoms typical of PAWS tend to be psychiatric in nature. This can often result in clinicians making a premature and often erroneous diagnosis of a coexisting psychiatric disorder that is independent from the patient's substance usage. This can have tragic consequences if the focus of treatment shifts primarily to the treatment of the misdiagnosed psychiatric disorder with a decreased focus on the chemical addiction problem, often resulting in relapse. On the other hand, if the patient's symptoms continue to persist or progressively worsen over time with ongoing abstinence, then there is a higher likelihood, though not a certainty, that the symptoms may in fact be due to a separate and distinct psychiatric disorder that will need to be treated concurrently with the chemical addiction problem.

Specific treatment for PAWS has not been extensively investigated or delineated due to a lack of agreement on the distinctive signs and symptoms and the duration of the syndrome. Many patients can effectively deal with their PAWS symptoms just by being made aware of their existence and developing an awareness that they are normal, are expected to occur, and will diminish with time as the patient maintains his or her recovery from substance usage. Supportive and directive counseling, relapse prevention counseling, returning to appropriate diet and exercise, and various adjunctive therapies such as relaxation training can be helpful in addressing many of the symptoms. Certain medications including naltrexone and acamprosate, discussed in greater detail later in the chapter, may be useful in addressing cravings for alcohol. If the symptoms do not respond to these modalities, or are of sufficient severity to place a patient at potential risk for relapse, then psychopharmacological intervention would be indicated utilizing nonaddicting medications to address specific target symptoms. Specific medication regimens will be discussed later in this chapter to address the frequently experienced PAWS symptoms of affective instability, anxiety, and sleep problems. As the PAWS symptoms generally tend to be self-limited in duration, medications usually only have to be prescribed for relatively short periods of time, often ranging from just a few days to up to several months. Further research is needed to explore the nature and treatment of the PAWS syndrome.

TREATMENT OF COMORBID DISORDERS

Treatment Models

Following initial assessment and evaluation, comorbid patients need to become involved in comprehensive treatment to address their dual disorders. Historically, many patients had been involved in a sequential treatment model approach where they received treatment for one disorder followed by treatment of the other. Unfortunately, it became evident that this approach was largely ineffective, with patients often failing in treatment for the first disorder being treated because the other disorder was largely ignored, if even identified. As previously indicated, a major caveat for successful treatment of comorbid patients is long-term simultaneous treatment of both disorders. From a psychiatric perspective patients must be initially stabilized so that their level of acute psychiatric symptoms (psychosis, mania, depressive regression, suicidal ideations, etc.) are reduced to the point where they are able to participate in addiction treatment. Similarly, patients with acute physical dependence must first complete detoxification treatment as soon as possible. However, treatment for both disorders needs to be initiated on a simultaneous basis.

In a parallel treatment model approach, patients receive simultaneous treatment for each disorder at separate treatment sites; one dealing with their mental health problem while the other addresses their addiction problem. Unfortunately, unless there is ongoing effective communication between clinicians at both sites, continuity of care is often compromised resulting frequently in less than optimal outcomes. This model can be very stressful for both patients and clinicians as treatment generally involves multiple treatment episodes over an extended time period. In addition, treatment professionals in one system frequently have little training or experience in treatment approaches utilized in the other system. As a result, crisis situations may arise while the patient is in one setting that involves the "other" problem and therefore may not often be appropriately addressed clinically. Patients may even receive contradictory recommendations or directions from one setting regarding what to do about the other problem.

In the integrated treatment model approach, patients receive simultaneous treatment for both problems at the same setting. Clinicians from both the mental health and addictions system work collaboratively together to meet all the patient's treatment needs. This optimally requires clinicians in one system to obtain some education and training regarding the other system along with specific training regarding the treatment of comorbid patients. Clinicians identified as having expertise in both systems can then provide overall direction and supervision of treatment to patients and clinicians. Integrated treatment has many advantages, not the least of which is that it has been shown to be cost-effective (Gravino, Zastowny, and Wilder, 2001; Johnson, 2000).

Despite the availability of effective treatments, most individuals with comorbid disorders are not receiving effective care (Watkins et al., 2001). As the comorbid patient population is a very heterogeneous group of individuals, treatment models looking at standards of care need to focus on the entire spectrum of care for these patients coupled with integrated system planning involving both the mental health and substance abuse treatment fields (Minkoff, 2001). This will require the further development of integrated treatment approaches, integrated program development, and an overall integrated system of care (SAMHSA, 2002). This will require input from and collaboration among many sources including governmental agencies, treatment providers, program evaluation research, payers of service, and patients and their families.

Integrated Treatment Services/Programs

Integrated treatment for comorbid disorders encompasses a wide variety of program components. Critical components include staged interventions, assertive outreach, motivational interventions, risk reduction, tailored mental health and substance abuse treatment, counseling, social support interventions, a longitudinal view of remission and recovery, and cultural sensitivity and competence (Drake et al., 2001; Minkoff, 1991). In addition, case management, behavioral skills training, and continuity of care are extremely important (Reno, 2001). Programs need to clearly define their mission; their clinicians need to be trained and supervised in providing comorbid treatment, and need to disseminate accurate information to patients and their families in order to promote understanding, demand, and advocacy (Drake et al., 2001). At a higher administrative level, policymakers in state and federal mental health and addiction agencies are finally beginning to collaborate to support the development of programs and services to meet the needs of comorbid patients.

A number of comorbid treatment programs have been developed involving patients at different levels of care as well as specific subpopulation types. They all support the perspective that integrated treatment is the most effective treatment approach for comorbid patients. These include acute inpatient programs (Appleby et al., 2001; Ries et al., 2000), outpatient programs (Granholm et al., 2003; Hellerstein, Rosenthal, and Miner, 1995; Primm et al., 2000), and therapeutic communities (De Leon, 1993; Mierlak et al., 1998). The Arkansas Center for Addictions Research, Education, and Services (2002) conducted a study looking at integrated treatment services for women who were pregnant or had children. They found that women who completed the integrated program or continued in the program, as compared with women who dropped out of the program, had a reduced relapse rate, exhibited an increase in employment, had more full-term births, and showed reduced screens for alcohol and drugs at the time of delivery. Integrated treatment has also been shown to be useful in comorbid patients with schizophrenia (Bennet, Bellack, and Gearon, 2001). The experiences gained from all these programs can serve as models for the future development of effective integrated treatment for comorbid patients.

Special Treatment Components/Issues

Owing to the heterogeneity of the comorbid patient population, there is no one single treatment approach and/or level of care that is applicable to all patients. Patients with low severity of both mental health and addiction problems may effectively be treated on an integrated outpatient basis. Patients with more severe mental health and/or addiction problems may initially require inpatient treatment followed by long-term integrated outpatient treatment. The American Society of Addiction Medicine (Mee-Lee, 2001) has developed patient placement criteria to help clinicians match patients to the appropriate level of care taking into consideration both their addiction and mental health problems. Comorbid treatment involves an adaptive integration of the treatment components commonly utilized in the mental health and addiction fields. Mental health components include the utilization of psychotropic medications; psychoeducational and psychosocial rehabilitation programs; residential support settings (i.e., halfway houses); and multiple forms of psychotherapy (individual, group, family, behavioral, cognitive behavioral, biofeedback, etc.). Addiction treatment program components commonly include individual, group, and family counseling; addiction education seminars; addiction medication adjuncts; relapse prevention/intervention counseling; and a wide range of psychosocial skills training components. Both fields also commonly utilize community peer/family support groups as adjuncts in the treatment process. Although an extensive review of all possible treatment components useful with comorbid patients is beyond the scope of this chapter, awareness of the following special treatment issues is extremely important when formulating treatment plans for this population.

In the addiction treatment field with its emphasis on total abstinence, it is commonly expected that once patients enter treatment, their substance usage will immediately cease. Patients who are unable to do so are commonly discharged from treatment. With comorbid patients, more specifically those patients with severe and persistent mental illnesses, this expectation is frequently impossible to achieve immediately upon entering treatment. While a target of total abstinence is still the overall goal, initially the focus of treatment with many of these patients will need to be on harm reduction, with reduced usage being viewed and presented as a step toward total abstinence. Continued substance usage needs to be monitored and evaluated as it occurs for the identification of relapse triggers, with patients then working on developing the skills to deal with the triggers without resorting to substance use. Abstinent periods should be supported and verbally reinforced to improve the patient's selfimage and self-esteem and to reinforce the concept that the patient is capable of establishing abstinence.

Patients with comorbid disorders will frequently require psychotherapy to help them deal with their mental health problems. Initially, with most patients, psychotherapy should be supportive in nature, with an avoidance of intensive uncovering/regressive therapies that, if utilized, can often result in the emergence of unpleasant memories/feelings, placing the patient at high risk for relapse. Although many patients may ultimately require this type of psychotherapy to deal effectively with their mental health problem, it is usually most appropriate clinically to avoid this type of therapy in early treatment. Supportive recovery-oriented therapy should be employed until it is felt that the patient has developed the coping skills to deal with dysphoric emotions and feelings without resorting to substance use.

In the field of addiction, the initial focus of treatment often centers around the technique of therapeutic confrontation in an effort to break through the denial system that most patients maintain so that there can be an awareness of their addiction problem. Individual and group counseling approaches are most frequently utilized to break through a patient's denial system. Confrontational techniques, however, often result in the emergence of anxiety that can unfortunately result in a worsening of a patient's psychiatric symptoms or may cause the reemergence of psychiatric symptoms if the patient has reached a state of psychiatric remission. Although the elicitation of anxiety may be necessary to break through a patient's denial system, clinicians still need to monitor the patient's anxiety levels closely and need to reduce the intensity of their confrontations if the patient appears to be overwhelmed or is showing signs or symptoms of psychiatric decompensation.

Educational sessions are a very important component in integrated comorbid treatment. Patients need to be educated about their specific mental health and addiction disorders, need to develop an understanding of the complex relationships between the two disorders and how it relates to them, and finally, need to develop an understanding and awareness of the need to continue in treatment for both disorders simultaneously on a long-term basis. Medication education groups are very important to help patients develop an awareness of what to expect clinically from their medications, to help them become aware of the importance of compliance in taking their medications as prescribed, and finally, to develop an awareness of potential side effects and potential medication interactions from their medications. The appropriate utilization of psychotropic medications will be reviewed in the next section of this chapter.

Involvement with community peer support groups can be helpful for most comorbid patients. In the addiction field, these include the self-help twelve-step programs of Alcoholics Anonymous (AA), Narcotic Anonymous (NA), and Cocaine Anonymous (CA). Similarly in the mental health field, a number of support groups have emerged for most of the major mental disorders (i.e., major depression, bipolar disorder, obsessive-compulsive disorder, posttraumatic stress disorder, and even schizophrenia). Some of these programs even utilize a twelve-step approach similar to that seen in addictive disorders. Twelve-step program meetings have been shown to be useful for many patients with comorbid disorders (Galanter, 2000; Ouimette et al., 2001). For comorbid patients, specifically, we have seen the emergence of twelve-step oriented community support groups such as Double-Trouble (DT) meetings and Dual Recovery Anonymous (DRA) meetings. These meetings developed as a result of difficulties many comorbid patients experienced when they went to traditional AA, NA, or CA meetings and disclosed that they were taking psychiatric medications. They have at times been confronted by well meaning but misinformed twelve-step program members who did not feel that it was appropriate for a recovering person to take psychiatric medications because they perceive them as being "mood altering." The comorbid patient might even be told they are not really sober or straight because they are taking the medication and might even be advised to stop taking it. At DT meetings and DRA meetings, patients can speak freely and comfortably about being on psychiatric medications along with speaking about their addiction problems. It should be kept in mind however, that it is the official position of AA, NA, and CA that people should take medications if appropriately prescribed for a diagnosed medical or psychiatric problem. AA has even published a pamphlet, *The AA Member—Medications and Other Drugs* (Alcoholics Anonymous, 1984), which clearly supports this perspective. Nevertheless, comorbid patients should be cautioned about disclosing that they are taking psychiatric medications when they attend addiction-specific twelve-step meetings until they have developed a sense of how it would be received by the members of the twelve-step group they are attending. Fortunately, it appears that this incorrect perception of psychiatric medications is beginning to wane. Meissen et al. (1999) completed a survey of 125 AA members about their beliefs about comorbid patients attending regular AA meetings and taking psychiatric medications. The majority had positive attitudes toward comorbid patients and 93 percent indicated that the patients should continue to take their medications. However, 54 percent still felt that participation in a group especially for persons with a dual diagnosis would be more desirable than attending traditional AA meetings for comorbid patients. Finally it is important for comorbid patients to understand that all these community support groups are an adjunctive part of treatment and should not be utilized as a substitute for, or in lieu of, formal integrated treatment for their mental health and addiction problems.

Family involvement, often neglected in both the mental health and addiction fields, is also very important in the treatment of comorbid patients, especially if patients are residing with family members or will be residing with them in the future. Unfortunately, many families have abandoned the patient, or split up, or are dysfunctional as a result of mental illness or substance abuse in other family members. Family members who are capable of being involved in treatment need to be provided with some basic education about the psychiatric and addiction disorders their loved ones are afflicted with and also need to learn about how they themselves have been victimized as well by the comorbid disorders. Family assessments and family counseling should be utilized if deemed clinically indicated. Many family members would benefit from attending the associated community support of the twelve-step programs of Al-Anon and Nar-Anon to help them deal with the effects of the addiction problem on themselves as a result of the addiction problem within their family system. There are also family support group meetings in many communities to help family members cope with mental illness. Families Anonymous meetings are also available in many areas. Another good resource for family members is the National Alliance for the Mentally Ill (NAMI). Involvement of family members can have a major impact on the effectiveness of the treatment of comorbid patients and therefore is a very important component of integrated treatment.

PSYCHOPHARMACOLOGICAL TREATMENT
OF PSYCHIATRIC DISORDERS
IN COMORBID PATIENTS

Special Medication Issues with Comorbid Disorders

Responsible prescribing practices require an understanding of the development and progression of comorbid disorders. As in the case of mental disorders, chemical dependency is a dynamic process that produces variations in severity, rate of progression, and symptom manifestation over time. These disorders are influenced not only by genetic and environmental factors but also by pharmacologic factors (i.e., some drugs are more likely than others to cause psychiatric or substance use disorder problems). Another important factor is the patient's risk for developing a substance use disorder (or dependency on a second or third substance). High-risk patients include those with both psychiatric and substance use disorders, as well as patients with a psychiatric disorder and a family history of chemical dependency.

The decision to pharmacologically treat the patient is based on the presence of two required factors. The first is an alteration in at least one of the following: behavior, affect, cognition, or physiologic function; the second is the presence of resultant clinical impairment or significant distress. Once the patient begins taking the medication, there are many reasons—other than the obvious—why the patient improves. The obvious reason is the pharmacologic effect of the medication—that is, it is doing exactly what it was intended to do. We refer to this as the efficacy of the medication—it is doing "what they (the drug manufacturers) say it will do." Hopefully, the efficacy and the effectiveness are the same. Effectiveness is "what we see the medication is doing." Sometimes, however, these two descriptors are different and we find the medication is not doing what it was supposed to do.

Another cause for improvement is the placebo effect. This means that the patient's improvement is not due to the pharmacologic effect of the medication at all. Rather, the patient's own belief system (internal stimulus) or the attention the patient is receiving (external stimulus) is the cause of the improvement. A third rationale for the improvement of the patient is the possible remission of the disorder. Many psychiatric syndromes are episodic—there are periods of exacerbation and remission. It is possible that when the patient began taking a specific medication, the disorder itself was in the process of natural remission, coincidentally giving the impression that the medication was the cause of the improvement. Another more surreptitious and conscious cause for improvement is the concurrent use of illicit drugs or alcohol. When treating the dually diagnosed patient, this possibility must always be considered and explored.

There are many factors that influence the choice of medication. At the top of the list is the patient's past history of response. If the patient had a positive response in the past with a specific medication, then there is a good chance a similar response will occur. However, there are reasons for not choosing a specific medication, such as the adverse event profile of the medication. This will be discussed in following text. Also, if the patient is taking any other medication, the potential for drug-drug interactions must be examined. Many drug interactions probably cause subtle effects that are not recognized clinically and most drug interactions are not life-threatening. Nevertheless, some interactions cause side effects that interfere with adherence, or cause a decrease in drug efficacy. If the patient has concurrent medical problems, some medications may be contraindicated. A factor that is not often considered but may significantly affect adherence is the cost of the medication. If the patient does not have a prescription plan or if the plan has a restrictive formulary, the patient will be required to pay for the medication. This should always be explored with the patient and a less expensive generic alternative should be considered. A factor that, at one time, had considerable weight is the familial response to the medication (often referred to as pharmacogenetics). If a close relative with the same disorder had a positive response to a particular medication, then that medication was thought to have a good chance of success with the patient. Today, it is believed that psychiatric syndromes are heterogeneous and even if two family members have the same manifestations of a psychiatric disorder, the cause may be different and therefore, the same medication may not work.

The patient's symptom manifestation should be the primary factor when determining the medication of choice as this is the best way to match putative neurotransmission dysfunction with a medication that works on specific neurotransmitters and receptors. For example, the patient that exhibits obsessive-compulsive features is believed to have serotonin deficiency. A medication that will increase the serotonin available at the receptor sites (a selective serotonin reuptake inhibitor, SSRI) would be the medication of choice.

When selecting medications for their specific therapeutic effects, attention must also be given to adverse responses, such as (1) medication adherence issues, (2) abuse and addiction potential, (3) substance use disorder relapse, and (4) psychiatric disorder relapse (Ries, 1993). For instance, medication side effects that are perceived by the patient as intolerable or noxious might decrease adherence to taking the medication as directed. Some medications may be stimulating, sedating, or euphorigenic and may promote physical dependence and tolerance. Addictive medications also cause compliance problems—patients may use the medication for longer periods and/or at higher doses than prescribed.

Thus, all treatment providers must understand the pharmacological profiles of the medications being prescribed or considered for the patient with co-occurring disorders. For example, most of the medications used to treat depressive and psychotic episodes are not psychoactive or euphorigenic. However, many of the medications used to treat anxiety syndromes, such as the benzodiazepines, are psychoactive, reinforcing, have potential for tolerance and withdrawal, and have an abuse potential, especially for those patients determined to be at high risk for substance use disorders. As psychoactive drugs have a well-defined withdrawal phenomenon after the cessation of chronic use, the high-risk patient is drawn to additional drug use in order to avoid the withdrawal syndrome.

Decisions regarding the selection of medication should be based on a risk-benefit analysis that includes the identification of the risks of prescribing the drug with the therapeutic benefits of resolving the psychiatric and substance use problems. The risks to be considered include the risk of medication abuse, the risk of undertreating a psychiatric problem, the type and severity of the psychiatric problem, and the relationship between the psychiatric disorder and the substance use disorder. For example, the need for acute stabilization of severe presentations of psychiatric illness or substance withdrawal may require the use of psychoactive medications such as benzodiazepines which are often necessary to prevent further deterioration or even death. In contrast, prescribing benzodiazepines to high-risk patients for chronic or less debilitating symptoms involves a substantial risk of promoting or exacerbating a substance use disorder and the use of any psychoactive medication should not be the first line of treatment.

Antidepressant Medications

It is the current belief that the various depressive syndromes are the result of malfunction within the process of chemical neurotransmission within the monoaminergic system. The principal monoamine neurotransmitters in the brain are the catecholamines norepinephrine (NE, also called noradrenaline), and dopamine (DA), and the indoleamine serotonin (5HT). Potential sites of dysfunction include the neurotransmitter, various enzymes, active transport pumps, receptors, and second messengers just to name a few. Medications used to treat depressive disorders target any of the neurotransmitters mentioned in previous text or other areas of dysfunction.

From the 1960s through the 1980s, the tricyclic antidepressants (TCAs) were the mainstay in the pharmacologic treatment of depression. Today, they are rarely used because the dosages required to produce antidepressant effects are so high as to cause intolerable side effects. Their use is now mainly for off-label indications such as pain management and sedation. Owing to their toxic and sometimes fatal interactions with alcohol and other drugs, care should be taken whenever these medications are prescribed for patients with chemical dependency disorders. Common TCAs include amitriptyline (Elavil), desipramine (Norpramin), doxepin (Sinequan), imipramine (Tofranil), and nortriptyline (Pamelor).

The SSRIs represent a significant advance in psychopharmacology. This class of drugs has been referred to as the "clean" class because they selectively increase the available serotonin, have relatively fewer side effects and are rarely toxic. The SSRIs were developed in response to studies that hypothesized that abnormalities in central serotonin function underlie disturbances in mood, anxiety, satiety, cognition, and aggression. These disturbances are frequently manifest in the substance abuser. Owing to their excellent safety profile—even in overdose—the SSRIs are excellent, first-line medications in the treatment of depressive and anxiety syndromes in dually diagnosed patients. Unfortunately, the SSRIs, after a few months' use, may cause emotional blunting (frequently termed "poop-out syndrome") in which the patient reports feeling as if the depression is returning. This could ultimately be a trigger for return to substance use. The SSRIs include citalopram (Celexa), escitalopram (Lexapro), fluoxetine (Prozac), fluvoxamine (Luvox) paroxetine (Paxil), and sertraline (Zoloft).

The so-called novel antidepressants work through various mechanisms of action. For example, increasing available norepinephrine or dopamine or a combination. These medications are becoming more commonly prescribed because they are able to target several different neurotransmitters and mechanisms of action. Examples include bupropion (Wellbutrin), mirtazepine (Remeron), venlafaxine (Effexor), and duloxetine (Cymbalta).

Many patients expect that the antidepressant is a "happy pill" that will maintain the patient in a state of perpetual happiness no matter what happens in their lives. In addition, many patients with co-occurring disorders expect the antidepressant to be a "numbing pill," having the same effects as the illicit substances that they had been previously using and to work just as fast. In all instances, patients must be educated regarding the expected effects of the medication, namely, to normalize the mood state over a period of time. The patient should also understand that the goal is for the mood reaction to be congruent with the external situation: during happy times, the patient will experience happiness; during periods of grief and loss, the patient will experience sadness. The perfect antidepressant is one that lifts the impairing and distressing depressed mood so that the patient can experience feelings congruent with the environment, and the patient does not "feel medicated," that is, does not experience any side effects.

Mood Stabilizers

The mood stabilizers are used to control mood swings such as those found in bipolar disorder. They are also used to reduce violent outbursts and other behaviors that accompany impulse dyscontrol conditions. The gold standard among the mood stabilizers is lithium. However, it has a very narrow therapeutic window and lithium toxicity can occur if blood levels are not monitored. Lithium is elementally close to sodium and when sodium is decreased in the body, lithium is retained—often leading to toxicity. Loss of sodium occurs whenever there is excessive vomiting, diarrhea, sweating, or decreased fluid intake. We often see these symptoms as part of the acute withdrawal syndrome in chemically dependent persons. Thus, use of lithium in this population may not be a first-line medication. The next group of medications used as mood stabilizers are the anticonvulsants. The older drugs also have a narrow therapeutic window and blood levels must be monitored for toxicity. Examples include carbamazepine (Tegretol) and divalproex (Depakote). The second- and third-generation anticonvulsants, on the other hand, are much safer and do not require monitoring blood levels. However, they do have side effect profiles that require regular monitoring, at least during the initial phase of treatment. For example, lamotrigine (Lamictal) can produce a very serious rash that could progress to Stevens-Johnson syndrome which, if untreated, can cause death. Topiramate (Topamax) causes significant cognitive blocking and must be monitored. The latest class of medications to be used as mood stabilizers are the class of drugs referred to as the atypical antipsychotics (more accurately classified as the serotonin-dopamine antagonists). These medications, although they have some side effects, are relatively safe and do not require blood level monitoring. Examples of these medications include olanzapine (Zyprexa), quetiapine (Seroquel), ziprasidone (Geodon), resperidone (Risperdal) and aripiprazole (Abilify). There is a significant amount of literature suggesting that the best outcomes for the treatment of the bipolar patient with comorbid substance use disorder are usually achieved with antiepileptic mood stabilizers and/or atypical antipsychotics, combined with appropriated psychosocial interventions (Albanese and Pies, 2004).

Anxiolytic Medications

The anxiolytic or antianxiety medications are used to reduce and remove symptoms associated with any of the anxiety spectrum disorders such as generalized anxiety disorder, post-traumatic stress disorder (PTSD), panic disorder, the phobias, obsessive-compulsive disorder and substance induced anxiety. Medications used to treat the anxiety spectrum disorders include the benzodiazepines, the nonbenzodiazepine anxiolytics, and the SSRIs. When treating patients suffering from anxiety, it is most important to screen for substance use as the benzodiazepines are cross-tolerant with alcohol, are abusable, and have a high market value as street drugs. Patients with dual diagnoses for whom benzodiazepines were prescribed were more than twice as likely to develop benzodiazepine abuse as those who were not prescribed benzodiazepines (Brunette et al., 2003). Consequently, these medications should only be used as stabilization agents in monitored circumstances, such as alcohol withdrawal or as sedatives in acutely psychoticor manic patients. Examples of benzodiazepines include alprazolam (Xanax), chlordiazepoxide (Librium), clonazepam (Klonopin), diazepam (Valium), Lorazepam (Ativan), and oxazepam (Serax).

The SSRIs variably modulate serotonin and norepinephrine with resultant anxiety-reducing effects. For instance, medications that act as agonists or partial agonists at the serotonin-1A receptor or that block (antagonist) the serotonin-2 receptors will have a calming effect. These medications, however, require a starting dose that is subtherapeutic and is slowly increased to prevent any activating side effects that could cause anxiety.

The nonbenzodiazepine anxiolytics include medications such as propranolol (Inderal) which blocks the effects of norepinephrine, and buspirone (BuSpar) which is a partial agonist at the serotonin-1A receptor. Propranolol works relatively well at controlling anxiety but may cause lowering of blood pressure. Buspirone takes an inordinately long period to be effective and requires high doses. The newest medications—used off-label—to control anxiety (especially in the substance-abusing population) are the atypical antipsychotics. At lower doses, these medications have no antipsychotic effect. Instead, they block serotonin-2 receptors. This class of medications seem to work relatively well and in a short period of time. In fact, quetiapine (Seroquel) at doses of 25-50 mg several times a day, produces anxiolytic effects similar to alprazolam (Xanax) without the abuse potential.

Again, as described in the "antidepressants" in the previous section, the substance abusing patients, while under the influence, are in a state of "numbness" and as the drugs begin to be metabolized, they begin to experience various feeling states—often, anxiety is paramount—which is part of the acute and post–acute withdrawal syndromes. These patients have become somewhat dyslexithymic, that is, they misinterpret their internal stimuli and often describe this feeling as panic. They are unable to tolerate this feeling state and seek immediate relief with anxiolytics, thereby placing themselves at increased risk for relapse. Patients should be prepared for the eventuality of these emotional states. Often, when patients are told about this phenomenon, they are able to tolerate it better. This does not mean that medications should be avoided. To the contrary, patients who have been assessed as experiencing impairing symptoms that prevent them from adequately progressing in treatment should be helped with pharmacological relief. Patients need to be informed that the goal of treatment with the medication is to help them return to a normal level of anxiety, not to make them anxiety free. Nonpharmacological interventions for the treatment of anxiety should also be part of the treatment plan.

Psychostimulants

The psychostimulants, particularly methylphenidate (Ritalin), are the most commonly prescribed and most efficacious medications for both child and adult residual attention-deficit/hyperactivity disorder (ADHD) and have been the first-line treatment for some time (Wilens et al., 1995). There has historically been concern about whether or not the use of such medications in childhood would predispose the child to later substance abuse. Biederman et al.'s (1999) seminal work regarding this has concluded that pharmacotherapy was associated with an 85 percent reduction in risk for a substance use disorder in ADHD youth. They also found that untreated ADHD was a significant risk factor for substance use disorders in adolescence. Unfortunately, many clinicians have misinterpreted the results of this and other studies by assuming that patients with comorbid ADHD and a substance use disorder will benefit from the use of prescribed psychostimulants. These studies did not evaluate the use of psychostimulants in this population.

Current DSM-IV criteria do not permit a diagnosis of ADHD in adults who do not have a history of impairing symptoms before the age of seven. Overdiagnosis of ADHD is common within the population who are dually diagnosed. Levin, Evans, and Sleber (1998) have observed that some individuals with cocaine dependence have impairing ADHD-like symptoms that occur only after a period of regular drug use, but they cannot recall having experienced ADHD symptoms in childhood. When these patients present for psychiatric treatment, they usually neglect to inform the diagnostician that they use cocaine. Another reason for overdiagnosis is that some diagnosticians overlook the criterion that the impairment must be present in at least two different settings. Thus, an individual who is completing difficult projects at home but is unable to finish assigned projects at work may be experiencing job dissatisfaction rather than ADHD. Moreover, the ADHD symptoms need to be impairing, not merely bothersome.

Although stimulants have been shown to be useful in treating patients with adult ADHD, their effect on ADHD symptoms and co-occurring substance use disorders has not been studied in a controlled fashion. Certain precautions are warranted when using stimulants in substance-abusing patients. Persons with ADHD and substance use disorders who are placed on stimulants may abuse the prescribed stimulants or illicit stimulant drugs. Thus, these possibilities should be discussed with the patient before a stimulant is prescribed. Although some clinicians report that the sustained-release form of methylphenidate is less effective than the immediate-release form, it might be preferable because it poses less opportunity for abuse. However, this class of medications should not be considered as first-line treatment.

Other medications that have been studied for the treatment of adult residual ADHD and produced significant reduction in symptoms include desipramine (Norpramin) (Wilens et al., 1996), atomoxetine (Strattera), (Spencer et al., 1998), bupropion (Wellbutrin) (Wilens et al., 2001), and venlafaxine (Effexor) (Wilens, Biederman, and Spencer, 1995). These medications should be considered for first-line treatment in patients with co-occurring disorders as there is no abuse potential.

ALCOHOLISM TREATMENT MEDICATIONS AND COMORBID DISORDERS

Disulfiram

Disulfiram (Antabuse) has been utilized as a medication adjunct in the treatment of alcoholism for over 50 years and is most commonly prescribed in a dosage of 250 mg or 500 mg daily. Disulfiram inhibits the enzyme acetaldehyde dehydrogenase in the liver that leads to increased levels of acetaldehyde in the body if a person were to consume alcohol while taking it. Acetaldehyde is a toxic intermediate in the metabolism of alcohol and increased amounts of it can lead to a wide variety of unpleasant physical symptoms including nausea, vomiting, flushing, headache, sweating, and heart palpitations. In extreme reactions, it can even result in seizures and death. It is basically an aversive conditioning treatment approach in which a person taking disulfiram would not consume alcohol in order to avoid experiencing a physically unpleasant reaction. Research into the efficacy of disulfiram in alcoholism treatment has tended to produce conflicting results. Many studies tended to conclude that disulfiram had negligible effects on abstinence but did decrease the number of days of drinking for patients who relapsed (Fuller and Roth, 1979; Fuller, Roth, and Long, 1983; Fuller, Branchey, and Brightwell, 1986; Garbutt, West, and Carey, 1999). Other research has provided some support for the utilization of disulfiram when its administration is supervised (Carroll et al., 1998; Chick, Gough, and Falkowski, 1992).

Studies of the use of disulfiram in patients with comorbid disorders are relatively few. One major concern about using this medication in severely mentally ill patients (i.e., patients with thought disorders) is that disulfiram also inhibits the brain enzyme dopamine-B-hydroxylase. This can slow the conversion of dopamine to norepinephrine, possibly resulting in the worsening of psychotic symptoms in these patients. Some clinical reports have suggested that disulfiram can worsen psychiatric symptoms, including psychosis, catatonia, confusion, delirium, depression, and mania (Liddon and Satran, 1967; Martensen-Larsen, 1951; Nasrallah, 1979; Poulsen, Loft, and Anderson, 1992). Although the incidence of these psychiatric complications in the general population appears low (Larson, Olincy, and Rummans, 1992), the rate of such complications in patients with severe mental illnesses is unknown. As a result of this, caution should be utilized when prescribing disulfiram in patients with severe mental illnesses with clinicians monitoring such patients very closely for any worsening of their psychiatric symptoms following initiating treatment with disulfiram.

Mueser et al. (2003) reported a retrospective review of 33 patients treated for alcoholism with disulfiram who also suffered from severe mental illness (70 percent schizophrenia or schizoaffective disorder). No significant psychiatric complications were reported. Although 76 percent of patients reported drinking while on disulfiram, only 23 percent experienced negative reactions to alcohol. Sixty-four percent of the patients saw a remission of alcoholism for at least one year during a three-year follow-up, and 30 percent experienced a two-year remission. Disulfiram treatment was associated with decreases in days hospitalized but not with changes in work status. They concluded that disulfiram might be a useful adjunctive medication for the treatment of alcoholism in patients with severe mental illness. Further studies exploring the utilization of disulfiram in patients with comorbid disorders is needed.

Naltrexone

Naltrexone (Revia) was approved by the U.S. Food and Drug Administration (FDA) as an adjunct medication for the treatment of alcohol dependence in 1994. Naltrexone is an opioid receptor blockading agent which was initially approved by the FDA in 1984 for the treatment of opiate dependence under the trade name of Trexan. Research findings have suggested that some nonopioid drugs, including alcohol, may exert some of their effects (i.e., euphoria, craving) through the activation of mu-opioid receptors in the brain's mesolimbic reward system (Herz, 1997; Kreek, 1996). In animal studies, opioid antagonists have been shown to decrease the consumption of alcohol, suggesting that opioid receptors may participate in mediating the reinforcing properties of alcohol (Myers, Borg, and Mossberg, 1986). Naltrexone is usually prescribed in an oral dosage of 50 mg daily. In order to attempt to improve compliance, a long acting parenteral extended release form (with a single injection lasting one month) of naltrexone is being investigated (Garbutt et al., 2005).

Naltrexone approval for alcohol dependence treatment was based upon a relatively small number of research studies (O'Malley et al., 1992; Volpicelli et al., 1992) that showed that it was efficacious in reducing drinking frequency and the likelihood of relapse to heavy drinking in alcoholics. Naltrexone reduced alcohol craving, days of drinking per week, and the rate of relapse among those who drank. From a clinical perspective, it appears that naltrexone reduces, at least in some alcoholic individuals, the level of subjective euphoria that they experience when they consume alcohol. A significant number of controlled studies have subsequently supported efficacy for naltrexone in the treatment of alcohol dependence although some studies have reported no or minimal effectiveness (Bouza et al., 2004; Kranzler and Van, 2001; Kranzler, Modesto-Lowe, and Van, 2000; Krystal et al., 2001; Srisurapanont and Jarusuraisin, 2002; Streeton and Whelan, 2001). Some recent research has indicated that the sensitivity of the mu-opioid receptor to endogenous opioids might be predictive of a patient's response to naltrexone (Ray and Hutchison, 2004). The mu-opioid receptor is encoded by the OPRM1 gene. The A118G polymorphism of the OPRM1 gene binds beta-endorphin three times more strongly than the A variant. Specifically, it has been demonstrated that individuals with the G variant have higher success rates than individuals with the A allele when treated with naltrexone (Oslin et al., 2003).

The number of studies looking at the utilization of naltrexone in comorbid patients with alcoholism are few. Maxwell and Shinderman (2000) reviewed the records of 72 mentally ill outpatients treated with naltrexone for alcohol use disorders at a community mental health center. Psychiatric diagnoses included major depression, schizophrenia, bipolar disorder, schizoaffective disorder, and gender identity disorder. The patients overall showed a good clinical response to naltrexone, with 82 percent reducing their drinking by at least 75 percent with only 17 percent relapsing at eight weeks. The naltrexone was well tolerated with only 11 percent of patients discontinuing the medication because of side effects, primarily nausea. They concluded that naltrexone was useful in the treatment of dually diagnosed patients. Farren and O'Malley (1999) reported on the clinical case of a woman treated with naltrexone for nine months for alcohol dependence who appeared to suffer from mild substance-induced depression at intake and two subsequent episodes of substance-independent depression, both requiring treatment with the antidepressant fluoxetine (Prozac). Naltrexone was effective and well tolerated during the course of treatment and it did not mitigate the effectiveness of the antidepressant. Overall, due to the dearth of studies investigating the use of naltrexone with comorbid patients, its use in such patients as an adjunct for the treatment of alcohol dependence would need to be closely monitored although it does not appear that there are any major contraindications to its utilization in this patient population.

Acamprosate

The most recent (July 2004) and only the third medication approved by the FDA as an adjunct medication in the treatment of alcoholism is acamprosate (Campral). Acamprosate, whose chemical structure is very similar to gamma-aminobutyric acid (GABA), is hypothesized to normalize the dysregulated glutamatergic system during alcohol abstinence and as a result prolong abstinence from alcohol drinking (Littleton et al., 2001). This is believed to be related to the modulation of N-methyl-D-aspartate receptors in the glutamate system. Acamprosate has shown demonstrated efficacy and safety in randomized, double-blind, placebo-controlled trials in alcohol-dependent outpatient volunteers (Garbutt, West, and Carey, 1999; Litten and Allen, 1998; Mason, 2001; Mason and Ownby, 2000; Swift, 1999; Tempesta et al., 2000) as well as in numerous other studies completed in European countries. Most studies have shown higher rates of treatment completion, longer abstinence period to first drink, and higher overall abstinence rates compared with patients treated with placebo (Mason, 2001, 2003).

Acamprosate is absorbed poorly in oral administration and for this reason is prescribed at a dosage of two 333 mg delayed release tablets three times daily. It is not protein bound, nor metabolized by the liver, and is excreted unchanged in the urine. It therefore may be specifically useful in patients with hepatic dysfunction where the utilization of disulfiram or naltrexone is contraindicated due to the potential hepatotoxic properties of these agents. Unfortunately, due to its recent approval, no studies have specifically been completed looking at the utilization of acamprosate with comorbid patients. Further studies are needed in this area.

COMORBID DISORDERS AND SUICIDE

Suicidal behavior and successful suicides, with significant levels of morbidity and mortality, remain as major public health problems in the United States. There are approximately 30,000 deaths annually from successful suicides, and the rate has not varied appreciably over the past three decades. In 2001, suicide was the eleventh leading cause of death in the United States and the third leading cause of death among those aged 15 to 24 (National Center for Health Statistics, 2003). Bertolote et al. (2004) conducted a review for the World Health Organization, of studies of mental disorders in cases of completed suicide with or without admission to mental hospitals. Among all diagnoses, mood disorders accounted for 30.2 percent of suicides, followed by substance use related disorders (17.6 percent), schizophrenia (14.1 percent), and personality disorders (13 percent). A past history of psychiatric illness, past suicide attempts or ideations, and substance abuse are extremely strong predictors of suicide attempts and deaths (Beautrais et al., 1996; Rossow and Lauritzen, 1999; Rossow, Romelsjo, and Leifman, 1999).

Among psychiatric disorders, suicidal behavior has historically been most frequently associated with major depression, bipolar disorder, and schizophrenia. Estimates for successful suicide in schizophrenic patients range from 5 to 13 percent (Bleuler, 1978; Caldwell and Gottesman, 1990; Miles, 1977; Palmer et al., 2005; Tsuang, 1978).

Approximately one-quarter to one-half of patients with bipolar disorder will attempt suicide during their lifetime (Goodwin and Jamison, 1990). Several studies have found that bipolar disorder is especially related to suicidal behavior and successful suicide, even when compared with major depression and other Axis I psychiatric disorders (Ahrens et al., 1995, Chen and Disilver, 1996; Lewinsohn et al., 1995), especially in the adolescent population (Brent et al., 1988; Kelly, Cornelius, and Lynch, 2002). The timing of major depressive episodes in substance abusers also appears to have a relationship to suicide attempts (Aharonovich et al., 2002) and maintenance of abstinence (Hasin et al., 2002). Major depression that occurred before the patient became substance dependent predicted severity of suicidal intent, and major depression that arose during abstinence predicted number of attempts. Patients with a history of major depression prior to lifetime onset of substance dependence had a reduction in the likelihood of remission relative to an absence of such a history. Major depression arising during sustained abstinence predicted substance relapse.

Suicidal ideations and suicide attempts are very common among alcoholics and drug addicts. In fact, depression is a symptom included in many substance withdrawal syndromes. Alcohol dependence and major depression are the most commonly diagnosed psychopathological disorders among people who commit suicide (Anthony, Warner, and Kessler, 1994; Cheng, 1995; Hesselbrock et al., 1988; Henriksson et al., 1993; Weissman, Myers, and Harding, 1980). Roy and Linnoila (1986) estimated that 21 percent of suicides are alcoholics and that about 18 percent of alcoholics subsequently commit suicide. Murphy and Wetzel (1990) estimated that the lifetime risk of suicide in U.S. alcoholics was 2 to 4 percent. Inskip, Harris, and Barraclough (1998) estimated that 7 percent of alcoholics die by suicide, comparable to their estimate of 6 percent lifetime risk associated with affective disorders. A number of risk factors have been identified to predict suicidal behavior in alcoholics including aggression/impulsivity, severe alcoholism, negative affect, and hopelessness (Conner and Duberstein, 2004). In addition, alcoholics who complete suicide are characterized by major depressive episode, suicidal communication, poor social support system, serious medical illness, unemployment, and living alone (Murphy et al., 1992).

Drug-dependent individuals also commonly exhibit suicidal behavior (Dark and Ross, 2002; Harris and Barraclough, 1997). Characteristics of drug addicts who attempt suicide include gender (females), family history of suicidal behavior, childhood trauma, introverted and neurotic personality types, increased comorbidity with alcoholism, history of major depression, and physical health problems (Roy, 2003). Cocaine dependence has also been shown to be a risk factor for suicidal behavior. Marzuk et al. (1992) found that 29 percent of suicide victims in New York aged 21 to 30 tested positive for cocaine. Data from the Epidemiologic Catchment Area survey showed that cocaine abusers had a significantly greater risk of attempting suicide (Petronis et al., 1990).

The presence of comorbid psychiatric disorders and chemical dependency disorders significantly increases the potential for suicidal behavior and successful suicides. Comorbidity of mood disorders with alcohol and other substance use disorders is common among individuals who complete suicide (Beautrais et al., 1996; Conwell et al., 1996). In fact, when looking at individuals who successfully complete suicide, Lesage et al. (1994) came to the conclusion that comorbidity is the rule rather than the exception.

From all of the data presented, it is evident that the presence of either type of disorder is a substantial risk factor for increasing the likelihood of suicidal behavior in the other. This has very significant implications for clinicians working in either field separately or with comorbid patients specifically. All patients need to be thoroughly assessed initially for the presence of suicidal ideations and/or behavior and subsequently need to be monitored during treatment for the emergence of such symptoms. The Chronological Assessment of Suicide Events (CASE Approach) is an interview methodology formulated to aide clinicians of multiple disciplines in eliciting suicidal ideations from patients (Shea, 1998, 2004). When utilized as part of a comprehensive assessment, it can be very helpful in clarifying suicidal intent and immediate danger to the patient. If suicidal symptoms are evident or emerge during the course of treatment, they need to be taken very seriously and need to be aggressively treated.

COMORBID DISORDERS AND HIV/HEPATITIS C

HIV infection is usually acquired through sexual intercourse, exposure to contaminated blood, or perinatal transmission and causes a progressive depletion in CD4 lymphocytes. This marked reduction leads to profound immunosuppression, with the development of the opportunistic infections and neoplasms that constitute AIDS. The number of injection drug users living with AIDS has significantly increased since 1993. This increasing prevalence may indicate that with better pharmacological treatment, these individuals are living longer (Palella et al., 1998). Among U.S. adults with known risk factors who were diagnosed between July 1999 and June 2000, 31 percent reported injection drug use and another 37 percent reported sex with an injection drug user (Centers for Disease Control, 2000). It is important to integrate HIV/AIDS prevention and treatment with substance abuse treatment and mental health services for patients with comorbid disorders because of the association between psychological dysfunction and a tendency to engage in high-risk behaviors (Simpson, Knight, and Ray, 1993). Compared with singly diagnosed persons, dually diagnosed persons were more likely to share a needle, have sex for money or gifts, have sex with an intravenous drug user, and report being raped (Dausey and Desai, 2003). Advances in treatment and improved outcomes have extended the survival of those with HIV/AIDS and comorbid disorders and this will increase the need for continued and integrated mental health and substance abuse services along with medical services. To be successful, this treatment should include an emphasis on treatment adherence. A great deal of emphasis has been placed on identification of impediments to successful adherence. Patients with depression, poor social support, and an active addictive disorder are less likely to adhere to clinical regimens (Mocroft et al., 2000).

Hepatitis C virus (HCV) is transmitted by blood-to-blood contact. It is the most common chronic blood-borne infection in the United States, affecting an estimated 1.8 percent of the population (MMWR, 1998). The most common risk factor for transmission of HCV infection is injection drug use. Approximately 80 percent of injection drug users will develop HCV antibodies after one year of drug use (Garfein et al., 1996). Rates of sexual transmission of HCV are thought to be very low. Chronic hepatitis C and substance abuse (specifically, alcohol abuse) together result in increased severity, more rapid progression of liver disease, and an increased incidence and prevalence of cirrhosis and hepatocellular carcinoma (Bhattacharya and Shuhart, 2003). A diagnosis of hepatitis C often results in a high level of anxiety for the patient. Unfortunately, many of these patients are homeless, indigent, and, frequently, the victims of discrimination and usually lack access to health care (Stephenson, 2001). Even when there is access to health care, compliance with treatment is likely to be poor in patients with active drug or alcohol dependence and/or active psychiatric illness, and this can lead to exacerbation of hepatitis and drug resistance. Antiviral therapy itself has been found to lead to nonadherence because of the possible medication-induced drug cravings and depression that these medications may cause (Sylvestre et al., 2004). The recommendation by the National Institutes of Health (NIH) was against treating such individuals until the addictive disorder is stabilized, that is, six months of abstinence NIH, 1997). This has raised both ethical and public health concerns. Davis and Rodrigue (2001) have disagreed with the NIH guidelines and have modified this recommendation. They contend that treatment should be made available, on an individualized basis, to recent drug injectors who enter treatment for their addictive disorder and who are likely to comply with therapy. In 2002, the NIH changed the guideline with a statement that HCV treatment of active injection drug users should be considered on a case-by-case basis (NIH, 2002).

Injection drug users are exposed to specific and significant risks for HCV and HIV infections from parenteral as well as sexual transmission. They are at risk early in the course of their drug use, and because they typically do not obtain regular medical care, they usually present in the later stages of disease. In order to improve the medical care of these patients, Sullivan and Fiellin (2004) suggest that health care providers need to be aware of these viruses, the appropriate screening, treatment, preventive and referral options, and the intricacies of managing coinfections.

SUMMARY AND CONCLUSIONS

Patients with comorbid mental health and chemical dependency disorders represent a very large and heterogeneous group of individuals in the health care system who unfortunately continue to have difficulty obtaining appropriate clinical care for their dual disorders. It does appear, however, that there is at least a beginning of awareness at many levels in the two fields, ranging from policymakers and administrators down to front line staff, of the importance of developing and implementing the integrated treatment services these patients require. Comprehensive initial assessments for both disorders are critical. As the use of addicting substances can result in a wide variety of psychiatric symptoms, clinicians need to be willing to modify and change diagnoses until it is clear that a genuine comorbid condition exists. Integrated treatment then needs to be implemented as soon as possible to address both disorders. Clinicians working with comorbid patients need to be provided with training to develop an awareness and understanding of the complex relationships between mental health and addictive disorders and need to be supervised in the provision of treatment services to patients. Treatment needs to be tailored to the individual patient in order to ensure that all the patient's biopsychosocial and case management needs are addressed. Except for detoxification and acute psychiatric stabilization, extreme caution should be exercised in the prescription of psychiatric medications with addiction potential to comorbid patients, and then only after nonaddicting medications or alternative treatment approaches have been shown to be ineffective. Treatment needs to be provided on a long-term simultaneous basis utilizing the formal treatment components described in this chapter coupled with the involvement of family members and attendance at community peer self-help support groups. In addition, it is important to integrate HIV and HCV prevention and treatment into the treatment of comorbid patients because of the high association of these severe medical problems with addictive and mental health disorders. It is clear from all of this information that an integrated systems approach is needed in order to meet the complex treatment needs of the comorbid patient population.

REFERENCES

Aharonovich, E.; Liu, X.; Nunes, E.; Hasin, D.S. (2002). Suicide attempts in substance abusers: Effect of major depression in relation to substance use disorders. *Am J Psychiatry* 159:1600-1602.

Ahrens, B.; Berghofer, A.; Wolf, T.; Muller-Oerlinghausen, B. (1995). Suicide attempts, age and duration of illness in recurrent affective disorders. *J Affect Discord* 36:43-49.

Albanese, M.; Pies, R. (2004). The bipolar patient with comorbid substance use disorder: Recognition and management. *CNS Drugs* 18(9):585-596.

Alcoholics Anonymous. (1984). *The AA Member—Medication and Other Drugs.* New York: Alcoholics Anonymous World Press.

Alling, C.; Balldin, J.; Bokstrom, K.; Gottfries, C.G.; Karlsson, I.; Langstrom, G. (1982). Studies on duration of a late recovery period after chronic abuse of ethanol: A cross-sectional study of biochemical and psychiatric indicators. *Acta Psychiatr Scand* 66:384-397.

American Psychiatric Association (1994). *Diagnostic and Statistical Manual of Mental Disorders,* Fourth Edition. Washington, DC: American Psychiatric Association.

Anthony, J.C.; Warner, L.A.; Kessler, R.C. (1994). Comparative epidemiology of dependence on tobacco, alcohol, controlled substances and inhalants: Basic findings from the National Comorbidity Survey. *Exp Clin Psychopharmacol* 2:244-268.

Appleby, L.; Dyson, V.; Altman, E.; Luchins, D.J. (1997). Assessing substance use in multiproblem patients: Reliability and validity of the Addiction Severity Index in a mental hospital population. *J Nerv Ment Dis* 185:159-165.

Appleby, L.; Luchins, D.J.; Dyson, V.; Fanning, T.; Freels, S. (2001). Predischarge linkage and aftercare among dually-diagnosed public psychiatric patients. *J Nerv Ment Dis* 189(4):265-267.

Arkansas Center for Addictions Research, Education, and Services (2002). Integrated services for mothers with dual diagnoses and their children. *Psychiatr Serv* 53(10):1311-1313.

Babor, T.F.; Higgins-Biddle, J.C.; Saunders, J.B.; Monteiro, M. (2002). *AUDIT— The Alcohol Use Disorders Identification Test: Guidelines for Use in Primary Care.* Geneva: World Health Organization.

Beautrais, A.L.; Joyce, P.R.; Mulder, R.T.; Fergusson, D.M.; Deavoll, B.J.; Nightingale, S.K. (1996). Prevalence and comorbidity of mental disorders in persons making serious suicide attempts: A case-control study. *Am J Psychiatry* 153: 1009-1014.

Beck, A.T.; Epstein, N.; Brown, G.; Steer, R.A. (1988). An inventory for measuring clinical anxiety: Psychometric properties. *J Consult Clin Psychol* 56(6):893-897.

Beck, A.T.; Steer, R.A.; Brown, G.K. (1996). *Beck Depression Inventory–II Manual.* San Antonio, TX: The Psychological Corporation.

Bennet, M.E.; Bellack, A.S.; Gearon, J.S. (2001). Treating substance abuse in schizophrenia. *J Subst Abuse Treatment* 20:163-175.

Bertolote, J.; Fleischmann, D.D.L.; Wasserman, D. (2004). Psychiatric diagnoses and suicide: Revisiting the evidence. *Crisis* 25(4):147-155.

Bhattacharya, R.; Shuhart, M. (2003). Hepatitis C and alcohol. *J Clin Gastroenterol* 36(3): 242-252.

Biederman, J.; Wilens, T.; Mick, E.; Spencer, T.; Faraone, S (1999). Pharmaco-therapy of attention-deficit/hyperactivity disorder reduces risk for substance use disorder. *Pediatrics* 104(2):1-5.

Bleuler, M. (1978). *The Schizophrenic Disorders: Long Term Patient and Family Studies.* Clemens, S.M. Trans. New Haven, CT: Yale University Press.

Blow, F.C.; Brower, K.J.; Schulenberg, J.E.; Demo-Dananberg, L.M.; Young, J.P.; Beresford, T.P. (1992). The Michigan Alcoholism Screening Test–Geriatric Version (MAST-G): A new elderly specific screening instrument. *Alcohol Clin Exp Res* 16:372.

Bouza, C.; Magro, A.; Munoz, A.; Amate, J. (2004). Efficacy and safety of naltrexone and acamprosate in the treatment of alcohol dependence: A system-atic review. *Addiction* 99:811-828.

Brems, C.; Johnson, M.E.; Namyniuk, L.L. (2002). Clients with substance abuse and mental health concerns: A guide for conducting intake interviews. *J Behav Health Serv Res* 29(3):327-334.

Brent, D.A.; Perper, J.A.; Goldstein, C.E.; Kolko, D.J.; Allan, D.J.; Allman, C.J.; Zelenak, J.P. (1988). Risk factors for adolescent suicide. A comparison of adoles-cent suicide victims with suicidal inpatients. *Arch Gen Psychiatry* 45:581-588.

Brown, R.L.; Rounds, L.A. (1995). Conjoint screening questionnaires for alcohol and other drug abuse: Criterion validity in a primary care practice. *Wis Med J* 94(3):135-140.

Brown, S.; Inaba, R.; Gillin, J. (1995). Alcoholism and affective disorder: Clinical course of depressive symptoms. *Am J Psychiatry* 152:45-52.

Brown, S.A.; Schuckit, M.A. (1988). Changes in depression among abstinent alco-holics. *J Stud Alcohol* 49:412-417.

Brunette, M.; Noordsy, D.; Xie, H.; Drake, R. (2003). Benzodiazepine use and abuse among patients with severe mental illness and co-occurring substance use disorders. *Psychiatr Serv* 54(10):1395-1401.

Butcher, J.N.; Graham, J.R.; Ben-Porath, Y.S.; Tellegen, A.; Dahlstrom, W.G.; Kaemmer, B. (2001). *Minnesota Multiphasic Personality Inventory–2 (MMPI-2): Manual for Administration, Scoring and Interpretation,* Revised Edition. Minneapolis, MN: University of Minnesota Press.

Caldwell, C.B.; Gottesman II (1990). Schizophrenics kill themselves too: A review of risk factors for suicide. *Schizophr Bull* 16:571-588.

Carey, K.B.; Cocco, K.M.; Correia, C.J. (1997). Reliability and validity of the Addiction Severity Index among outpatients with severe mental illness. *Psychol Assess* 9:422-428.

Carey, K.B.; Roberts, L.J.; Kivlahan, D.R.; Carey, M.P.; Neal, D.J. (2004). Prob-lems assessment for substance using psychiatric patients: Development and initial psychometric evaluation. *Drug Alcohol Depend* 75:67-77.

Carroll, K.M.; Nich, C.; Ball, S.A.; McCance, E.; Rounsavile, B.J. (1998). Treat-ment of cocaine and alcohol dependence with psychotherapy and disulfiram. *Addiction* 93:713-727

Centers for Disease Control and Prevention (CDC) (2000) *HIV/AIDS Surveillance Report* 12(1):1-41.

Chen, Y.W.; Disilver, S.C. (1996). Lifetime rates of suicide attempts among subjects with bipolar and unipolar disorders relative to subjects with other axis I disorders. *Biol Psychiatry* 39:896-899.

Cheng, A.T.A. (1995). Mental illness and suicide: A case-controlled study in East Taiwan. *Arch Gen Psychiatry* 52:594-603.

Chick, J.; Gough, K.; Falkowski, W. (1992). Disulfiram treatment of alcoholism. *Br J Psychiatry* 161:84-89.

Cocco, K.M.; Carey, K.B. (1998). Psychometric properties of the Drug Abuse Screening Test in psychiatric outpatients. *Psychol Assess* 10:408-414.

Conner, K.R.; Duberstein, P.R. (2004). Predisposing and precipitating factors for suicide among alcoholics: Empirical review and conceptual integration. *Alcohol Clin Exp Res* 28(5):6S-17S.

Conwell, Y.; Duberstein, C.; Cox, C.; Herrman, J.H.; Forbes, N.T.; Caine, E.D. (1996). Relationships of age and axis I diagnoses in victims of completed suicide. *Am J Psychiatry* 153:1001-1008.

Cornelius, J.R.; Salloum, I.M.; Day, N.L.; Thase, M.E.; Mann, J.J. (1996). Patterns of suicidality and alcohol use in alcoholics with major depression. *Alcohol Clin Exp Res* 20:1451-1455.

Daley, D.C.; Moss, H.B. (2002). *Dual Disorders—Counseling Clients with Chemical Dependency and Mental Illness,* Third Edition. Minnesota, MN: Hazelden Foundation.

Dark, S.; Ross, J. (2002). Suicide among heroin users: Rates, risk factors, and methods. *Addiction* 97:1383-1394.

Dausey, D.; Desai, R. (2003). Psychiatric comorbidity and the prevalence of HIV infection in a sample of patients in treatment for substance abuse. *J Nerv Ment Dis* 191(1):10-17.

Davis, G.; Rodrigue, J.R. (2001). Treatment of chronic hepatitis C in active drug users. *N Engl J Med* 45:215-217.

De Leon, G. (1993). Modified therapeutic communities for dual disorders. In: Solomon, J., Zimberg, S.; Shollar, E. (Eds.), *Dual Diagnosis: Evaluation, Treatment, Training, and Program Development* (pp. 147-170). New York: Plenum Press.

Derogatis, L.R. (1975). *Symptom Checklist–90–Revised (SCL-90-R)*. Minneapolis, MN: NCS Assessments.

DiClemente, C.C.; Prochaska, J.O. (1998). Toward a comprehensive transtheoretical model of change: Stages of change and addictive behavior. In: Miller, W.R.; Heather, N. (Eds.), *Treating Addictive Behavior,* Second Edition (pp. 3-24). New York: Plenum Press.

Drake, R.E.; Essock, S.M.; Shaner, A.; Carey, K.B.; Minkoff, K.; Kola, L.; Lynde, D.; Osher, F.C.; Clarl, R.E.; Richards, L. (2001). Implementing dual diagnosis services for clients with severe mental illness. *Psychiatr Serv* 52(4):469-476.

Ewing, J.A. (1984). Detecting alcoholism: The CAGE Questionnaire. *JAMA* 252:1905-1907.

Farren, C.K.; O'Malley, S.S. (1999). Occurrence and management of depression in the context of naltrexone treatment of alcoholism (clinical case conference). *Am J Psychiatry* 156(8):1258-1262.

Flynn, P.M.; Craddock, S.G.; Luckey, J.W.; Hubbard, R.L.; Dunteman, G.H. (1996). Cormorbidity of antisocial personality and mood disorders among psychoactive substance-dependent treatment clients. *J Personal Disord* 10(1):56-67.

Fuller, R.K.; Branchey, L.; Brightwell, D.R. (1986). Disulfiram treatment of alcoholism: A Veterans Administration Cooperative Study. *JAMA* 256:1449-1455.

Fuller, R.K.; Roth, H.P. (1979). Disulfiram for the treatment of alcoholism. *Ann Intern Med* 90:901-904.

Fuller, R.; Roth, H.; Long, S. (1983). Compliance with disulfiram treatment of alcoholism. *J Chronic Dis* 36:161-170.

Galanter, M. (2000). Self-help treatment for combined addiction and mental illness. *Psychiatr Serv* 51(8):977-979.

Garbutt, J.C.; Kranzler, H.R.; O'Malley, S.S.; Gastfriend, D.R.; Pettinati, H.M.; Silverman, B.L.; Loewy, J.W.; Ehrich, E.W. (2005). Efficacy and tolerability of long-acting injectable naltrexone for alcohol dependence: A randomized controlled trial. *JAMA* 293(13):1617-1625.

Garbutt, J.C.; West, S.L.; Carey, T.S. (1999). Pharmacological treatment of alcohol dependence: A review of the evidence. *JAMA* 281:1318-1325.

Garfein, R.S.; Vlahov, D.; Galai, N.; Doherty, M.C.; Nelson, K.E. (1996). Viral infections in short-term injection drug users: The prevalence of the hepatitis C, hepatitis B, human immunodeficiency, and human T-lymphotropic viruses. *Am J Public Health* 86:655-661.

Gonzales, J.J.; Insel, T.R. (2004). The conundrum of co-occurring mental health and substance use disorders: Opportunities for research. *Biol Psychiatry* 56:723-725.

Goodwin, F.K.; Jamison, K.R. (1990). *Manic-Depressive Illness.* New York: Oxford University Press.

Granholm, E.; Anthenelli, R.; Monteiro, R.; Sevcik, J.; Stoler, M. (2003). Brief integrated outpatient dual-diagnosis treatment reduces psychiatric hospitalizations. *Am J Addict* 12:306-313.

Gravino, G.; Zastowny, T.; Wilder, A. (2001). Medicaid beneficiaries with a dual diagnosis: System responsibility and costs of care. *Psychiatr Serv* 52(9):1153.

Hamilton, M. (1959). The assessment of anxiety states by rating. *Br J Med Psychol* 32:50-55.

Harris, C.; Barraclough, B. (1997). Suicide as an outcome for mental disorders. *Br J Psychiatry* 170:205-228.

Hasin, D.; Liu, X.; Nunes, E.; McCloud, S.; Samet, S.; Endicott, J. (2002). Effects of major depression on remission and relapse of substance dependence. *Arch Gen Psychiatry* 59:375-380.

Hedlung, J.L.; Vieweg, B.W. (1979). The Hamilton Rating Scale for depression: A comprehensive review. *J Operat Psychiat* 10:149-165.

Hellerstein, D.J.; Rosenthal, R.N.; Miner, C.R. (1995). Prospective study of integrated outpatient treatment for substance abusing schizophrenics. *Am J Addict* 4:33-42.

Henriksson, M.M.; Aro, H.M.; Marttunen, M.J.; Heikkinen, M.E.; Isometsa, E.T.; Kuoppasalmi, K.I.; Lonnqvist, J.K. (1993). Mental disorders and comorbidity in suicide. *Am J Psychiatry* 150:935-940.

Herz, A. (1997). Endogenous opioid systems and alcohol addiction. *Psychopharmacology* 129:99-111.

Hesselbrock, M.; Hesselbrock, V.; Syzmanski, K.; Weidenman, M. (1988). Suicide attempts and alcoholism. *J Stud Alcohol* 49:436-442.

Inskip, H.M.; Harris, E.C.; Barraclough, B. (1998). Lifetime risk of suicide for affective disorder, alcoholism, and schizophrenia. *Br J Psychiatry* 172:35-37.

Johnson, J. (2000). Cost-effectiveness of mental health services for persons with a dual diagnosis. *J Subst Abuse Treat* 18:119-127.

Kelly, T.M.; Cornelius, J.R.; Lynch, K.G. (2002). Psychiatric and substance use disorders as risk factors for attempted suicide among adolescents: A case control study. *Suicide Life Threat Behav* 32:301-312.

Kranzler, H.R.; Modesto-Lowe, V.; Van, K.J. (2000). Naltrexone vs. nefazodone for treatment of alcohol dependence: A placebo-controlled trial. *Neuropsychopharmacology* 22:493-503.

Kranzler, H.R.; Van, K.J. (2002). Efficacy of naltrexone and acamprosate for alcoholism treatment: A meta-analysis. *Alcohol Clin Exp Res* 25:1335-1341.

Kreek, M.J. (1996). Opiates, opioids, and addiction. *Mol Psychiatry* 1:232-235.

Krystal, J.H.; Cramer, J.A.; Krol, W.F.; Kirk, G.F.; Rosenheck, R.A. (2001). Naltrexone in the treatment of alcohol dependence. *N Engl J Med* 345:1734-1739.

Larson, E.W.; Olincy, A.; Rummans, T.A. (1992). Disulfiram treatment of patients with both alcohol dependence and other psychiatric disorders: A review. *Alcohol Clin Exp Res* 16:125-130.

LeFauve, C.E.; Litten, R.Z.; Randall, C.L.; Moak, D.H.; Salloum, I.M.; Green, A.I. (2004). Pharmacological treatment of alcohol abuse/dependence with psychiatric comorbidity. *Alcohol Clin Exp Res* 28(2):302-312.

Lesage, A.D., Boyer, R., Grunberg, F., Vanier, C., Morissette, R., Menard-Buteau, C., Loyer, M. (1994). Suicide and mental disorders: A case-control study of young men. *Am J Psychiatry* 151(7): 1063-8

Levin, F.R.; Evans, S.M.; Sleber, H.D. (1998). Prevalence of adult attention deficit hyperactivity disorder among cocaine abusers seeking treatment. *Drug Alcohol Depend* 52(1):15-25.

Lewinsohn, P.M.; Klein, D.N.; Seeley, J.R. (1995). Bipolar disorders in a community sample of older adolescents: Prevalence, phenomenology, comorbidity, and course. *J Am Acad Child Adolesc Psychiatry* 34:454-463.

Liddon, S.C.; Satran, R. (1967). Disulfiram (antabuse) psychosis. *Am J Psychiatry;* 123:1284-1289.

Litten, R.Z.; Allen, J.P. (1998). Advances in development of medications for alcoholism treatment. *J Psychopharmacol* 139:20-33.

Littleton, J.M.; Lovinger, D.; Liljequist, S.; Ticku, R.; Matsumoto, I.; Barron, S. (2001). Role of polyamines and the NMDA receptors in ethanol dependence and withdrawal. *Alcohol Clin Exp Res* 25:132S-136S.

Maisto, S.A.; Carey, M.P.; Carey, K.B.; Gleason, J.G.; Gordon, C.M. (2000). Use of the AUDIT and DAST-10 to identify alcohol and drug use disorders among adults with a severe and persistent mental illness. *Psychol Assess* 12:186-192.

Martensen-Larsen, O. (1951). Psychotic phenomena provoked by tetra-ethylthiuram disulfide. *Q J Stud Alcohol* 12:206-216.

Marzuk, P.M.; Taediff, K.; Leon, A.C.; Stajic, M.; Morgan, E.B.; Mann, J.J. (1992). Prevalence of cocaine use among residents of New York City who committed suicide during a one-year period. *Am J Psychiatry* 149:371-375.

Mason, B.J. (2001). Treatment of alcohol dependent outpatients with acamprosate: A clinical review. *J Clin Psychiatry* 62 (Suppl 20):42-48.

Mason, B.J. (2003). Acamprosate and naltrexone treatment for alcohol dependence: An evidence-based risk-assessment. *Eur Neuropsychopharmacol* 13(6):469-475.

Mason, B.J.; Ownby, R.I. (2000). Acamprosate for the treatment of alcohol dependence: A review of double-blind, placebo-controlled trials. *CNS Spectr* 5:58-69.

Maxwell, S.; Shinderman, M.S. (2000). Use of naltrexone in the treatment of alcohol use disorders in patients with concomitant major mental illness. *J Addict Dis* 19(3):61-69.

McLellan, A.T.; Kusher, H.; Metzger, D.; Peters, R.; Smith, I.; Grissom, G.; Pettinati, H.; Argeriou, M. (1992). The fifth edition of the Addiction Severity Index. *J Subst Abuse Treat* 9:199-213.

Mee-Lee, D., Ed. (2001). *ASAM Patient Placement Criteria for the Treatment of Substance-Related Disorders,* Second Edition Revised. Chevy Chase, MD: American Society of Addiction Medicine, Inc.

Meissen, G.; Powell, T.J.; Wituk, S.A.; Girrens, K.; Arteaga, S. (1999). Attitudes of AA contact persons toward group participation by persons with a mental illness. *Psychiatr Serv* 50(8):1079-1081.

Mierlak, D.; Galanter, M.; Spivack, N.; Dermatis, H.; Jureewicz, E.; De Leon, G. (1998). Modified therapeutic community treatment for homeless dually diagnosed men. *J Subst Abuse Treatment* 15(2):117-121.

Miles, C.P. (1977). Conditions predisposing to suicide: A review. *J Nerv Ment Dis* 164:231-246.

Minkoff, K. (1991). Program components of a comprehensive integrated care system for serious mentally ill patients with substance disorders. In: Minkof, K.; Drake, R.E. (Eds.), *Dual Diagnosis of Major Mental Illness and Substance Disorders.* San Francisco, CA: Jossey-Bass.

Minkoff, K. (2001). Developing standards of care for individuals with co-occurring psychiatric and substance use disorders. *Psychiatr Serv* 52(5):597-599.

MMWR (1998). Recommendations for prevention and control of hepatitis C virus (HCV) infection and HCV-related chronic disease. *MMWR Morb Mortal Wkly Report* 47(RR-19):1-54.

Mocroft, A.; Katlama, C.; Johnson, A.M.; Pradier, C.; Antunes, F.; Mulcahy, F.; Chiesi, A.; Phillips, A.N.; Kirk, O.; Lundgren, J.D. (2000) AIDS across Europe, 1994-98: The EuroSIDA study. *Lancet* 356(9226):291-296.

Mueser, K.T.; Noordsy, D.L.; Fox, L.; Wolfe, R. (2003). Disulfiram treatment for alcoholism in severe mental illness. *Am J Addict* 12:242-252.

Murphy, G.E.; Wetzel, R.D. (1990). The lifetime risk of suicide in alcoholism. *Arch Gen Psychiatry* 47:383-392.

Murphy, G.E.; Wetzel, R.D.; Robins, E.; McEvoy, L. (1992). Multiple risk factors predict suicide in alcoholism. *Arch Gen Psychiatry* 49(6):459-63.

Myers, R.D.; Borg, S.; Mossberg, R. (1986). Antagonism by naltrexone of voluntary alcohol selection in the chronically drinking macaque monkey. *Alcohol* 3(6):383-388.

Nasrallah, N.A. (1979). Vulnerability to disulfiram psychosis. *West J Med* 130: 575-577.

National Center for Health Statistics (2003). *National Vital Statistics Records*, Vol. 52, No. 3. Washington, DC: U.S. Department of Health and Human Services. Available at: http:www.cdc.gov/nchs/data/nvsr/nvsr52/nvsr52_03.pdf.

National Institutes of Health (NIH) (1997). NIH Consensus Development Conference Panel statement: Management of hepatitis C. *Hepatology* 26:2S-10S.

National Institutes of Health (NIH) (2002). National Institutes of Health Consensus Development Conference Panel statement: Management of hepatitis C. Available at: http://consensus.nih.gov/2002/2002 HepatitisC2002116html.htm.

Office of Applied Studies (2003). *Results from the 2002 National Survey on Drug Use and Health: National Findings.* NHSDA Series H-22. DHHS Publication No. (SMA) 03-3836. Rockville, MD: Substance Abuse and Mental Health Services Administration.

O'Malley, S.S.; Jaffe, A.J.; Chang, G.; Schottenfeld, R.S.; Meyer, R.E.; Rounsaville, B. (1992). Naltrexone and coping skills therapy for alcohol dependence. A controlled study. *Arch Gen Psychiatry* 49(11):881-887.

Oslin, D.W.; Berrettini, W.; Kranzler, H.R.; Pettinati, H.; Gelernter, J.; Volpicelli, J.R.; O'Brian, C.P. (2003). A functional polymorphism of the mu-opioid receptor gene is associated with naltrexone response in alcohol-dependent patients. *Neuropsychopharmacology* 28:1546-1552.

Ouimette, P.; Humphreys, K.; Moos, R.H.; Finney, J.W.; Cronkite, R.; Federman, B. (2001). Self-help group participation among substance use disorder patients with posttraumatic stress disorder. *J Subst Abuse Treat* 20:25-32.

Palella, F.J., Jr.; Delaney, K.M.; Moorman, A.C.; Loveless, M.O.; Fuhrer, J.; Satten, G.A.; Aschman, D.J.; Holmberg, S.D. (1998). Declining morbidity and mortality among patients with advanced human immunodeficiency virus infection. HIV outpatient study investigators. *N Engl J Med* 338:853-860.

Palmer, B.A.; Pankraz, V.S.; Bostwick, J.M. (2005). The lifetime risk of suicide in schizophrenia. *Arch Gen Psychiatry* 62:247-253.

Petronis, K.; Samuels, J.; Moscicki, E.; Anthony, J. (1990). An epidemiologic investigation of potential risk factors for suicide attempts. *Soc Psychiatry Psychiatr Epidemiol* 25:193-199.

Poulsen, E.; Loft, S.; Anderson, J.R. (1992). Disulfiram therapy-adverse drug reactions and interactions. *Acta Psychiatr Scand* 86:59-66.

Primm, A.B.; Gomez, M.B.; Tzolova-Iontchev, I.; Perry, W.; Thi Vu, H.; Crum, R.M. (2000). Mental health verses substance abuse treatment programs for dually diagnosed patients. *J Subst Abuse Treat* 19:285-290.

Rahdert, E., Ed. (1991). *The Adolescent Assessment/Referral System Manual.* DHHS Pub. No. (ADM) 91-1735. Rockville, MD: National Institute on Drug Abuse.

Ray, L.A.; Hutchison, K.E. (2004). A polymorphism of the mu-opioid receptor gene (OPRM1) and sensitivity to the effects of alcohol in humans. *Alcohol Clin Exp Res* 28(12):1789-1795.

Regier, D.A.; Farmer, M.E.; Rae, D.S.; Locke, B.Z.; Keith, S.J.; Judd, L.L.; Goodwin, F.K. (1990). Comorbidity of mental disorders with alcohol and other drugs abuse: Results from the Epidemiological Catchment Area study. *J Am Med Assoc* 264(19):2511-2518.

Reno, R. (2001). Maintaining quality of care in a comprehensive dual diagnosis treatment program. *Psychiatr Serv* 52(5):673-675.

Ries, R.K. (1993). The dually diagnosed patient with psychotic symptoms. *J Addict Dis* 12(3):103-122.

Ries, R.K.; Russo, J.; Wingerson, D.; Snowden, M.; Comtois, K.A.; Srebnik, D.; Roy-Byrne, P. (2000). Shorter hospital stays and more rapid improvement among patients with schizophrenia and substance disorders. *Psychiatr Serv* 51(2):210-215.

Rosenberg, S.D.; Drake, R.E.; Wolford, G.L.; Mueser, K.T.; Oxman, T.E.; Vidaver, R.M.; Carrieri, K.L.; Luckoor, R. (1998). Dartmouth Assessment of Lifestyle Instrument (DALI): A substance use disorder screen for people with severe mental illness. *Am J Psychiatry* 155:232-238.

Rossow, I.; Lauritzen, G. (1999). Balancing on the edge of death: Suicide attempts and life-threatening overdoses among drug addicts. *Addiction* 94:209-219.

Rossow, I.; Romelsjo, A.; Leifman, H. (1999). Alcohol abuse and suicidal behavior in young and middle aged men: Differentiating between attempted and completed suicide. *Addiction* 94:1199-1207.

Roy, A. (2003). Characteristics of drug addicts who commit suicide. *Psychiatry Res* 121:99-103.

Roy, A.; Linnoila, M. (1986). Alcoholism and suicide. *Suicide Life Threat Behav* 16:244-273.

Russel, M. (1994). New assessment tools for risk drinking during pregnancy: T-ACE, TWEAK, and others. *Alcohol Health Res World* 18(1):55-61.

SAMHSA (2002). Report to Congress on the prevention and treatment of co-occurring substance abuse disorders and mental disorders. Available at: http://www.samhsa.gov/reports/congress2002/index.html.

Satel, S.L.; Kosten, T.R.; Schuckit, M.A.; Fischman, M.W. (1993). Should protracted withdrawal from drugs be included in the DSM-IV? *Am J Psychiatry* 150:695-704.

Saunders, J.B.; Aasland, O.G.; Babor, T.F.; de la Fluente, J.R.; Grant, M. (1993). Development of the Alcohol Use Disorders Identification Test (AUDIT): WHO collaborative project on early detection of persons with harmful alcohol consumption-II. *Addiction* 88:791-804.

Schuckit, M.A.; Helzer, J.; Crowley, T.; Nathan, P.; Woody, G.; Davis, W. (1991). Substance use disorders. *Hosp and Community Psychiatry* 42:471-473.

Schuckit, M.A.; Hesselbrock, V. (1994). Alcohol dependence and anxiety disorders: What is the relationship? *Am J Psychiatry* 151:1723-1734.

Schuckit, M.A.; Tipp, J.E.; Bergman, M.; Reich, W.; Hesselbrock, V.M.; Smith, T.L. (1997). Comparison of induced and independent major depressive disorders in 2,943 alcoholics. *Am J Psychiatry* 154:948-957.

Selzer, M.L. (1971). The Michigan Alcoholism Screening Test: The quest for a new diagnostic instrument. *Am J Psychiatry* 127:1653-1658.

Selzer, M.L.; Vinokur, A.; Van Rooijen, L. (1975). A self-administered Short Michigan Alcoholism Screening Test (SMAST). *J Stud Alcohol* 36:117-126.

Shea, S.C. (1998). The chronological assessment of suicide events: A practical interviewing strategy for the elicitation of suicidal ideations. *J Clin Psychiatry* 50 (Suppl 20):58-72.

Shea, S.C. (2004). The delicate art of eliciting suicidal ideation. *Psychiatr Ann* 34(5):387-400.

Simpson, D.D.; Knight, K.; Ray, S. (1993). Psychosocial correlates of AIDS-risk drug use and sexual behaviors. *AIDS Educ Prev* 5(2):121-130.

Spencer, T.; Biederman, J.; Wilens, T.; Prince, J.; Hatch, M.; Jones, J.; Harding, M.; Faraone, S.V.; Seidman, L. (1998). Effectiveness and tolerability of tomoxetine in adults with attention deficit hyperactivity disorder. *Am J Psychiatry* 155(5): 693-695.

Srisurapanont, M.; Jarusuraisin, N. (2002). Opioid antagonists for alcohol dependence. *Cochrane Database Syst Rev* 2:CD0018676.

Stephenson, J. (2001). Former addicts face barriers to treatment for HCV. *JAMA* 285:1003-1005.

Streeton, C.; Whelan, G. (2001). Naltrexone, a relapse prevention maintenance treatment of alcohol dependence: A meta-analysis of random controlled trials. *Alcohol and Alcoholism* 36:544-552.

Sullivan, L.E.; Fiellin, D.A. (2004). Hepatitis C and HIV infections: Implications for clinical care in injection drug users. *Am J Addict* 13:1-20.

Swift, R.M. (1999). Drug therapy for alcohol dependence. *N Engl J Med* 340: 1482-1490.

Sylvestre, D.L.; Loftis, J.M.; Hauser, P.; Genser, S.; Cesari, H.; Borek, N.; Kresina, T.F.; Seeff, L.; Francis, H. (2004). Co-occurring hepatitis C, substance use, and psychiatric illness: Treatment issues and developing integrated models of care. *J Urban Health* 81(4):719-734.

Tempesta, E.; Janiri, L.; Bignamini, A.; Chabac, S.; Potgieter, A. (2000). Acamprosate and relapse prevention in the treatment of alcohol dependence: A placebo-controlled study. *Alcohol and Alcoholism* 35(2):202-209.

Trevisan, L.A.; Boutros, N.; Petrakis, I.L.; Krystal. J.H. (1998). Complications of alcohol withdrawal: Pathophysiological insights. *Alcohol Health Res World* 22 1:61-66.

Tsuang, M.T. (1978). Suicide in schizophrenics, manics, depressives, and surgical controls: A comparison with general population suicide mortality. *Arch Gen Psychiatry* 35:153-155.

Volpicelli, J.R.; Alterman, A.I.; Hayashida, M.; O'Brian, C.P. (1992). Naltrexone in the treatment of alcohol dependence. *Arch Gen Psychiatry* 49(11):876-880.

Watkins, K.E.; Burnam, A.; Kung, F.; Paddock, S. (2001). A national survey of care for persons with co-occurring mental and substance use disorders. *Psychiatr Serv* 52(8):1062-1068.

Weissman, M.M.; Myers, J.K.; Harding, P.S. (1980). Prevalence and psychiatric heterogeneity of alcoholism in a United States urban community. *J Stud Alcohol* 41:672-681.

Wilens, T.E.; Biederman, J.; Spencer, T.J. (1995). Venlafaxine for adult ADHD. *Am J Psychiatry* 152(7):1099-1100.

Wilens, T.E.; Biederman, J.; Prince, J.; Spencer, T.J.; Faraone, S.V.; Warburton, R.; Schleifer, D.; Harding, M.; Linehan, C.; Geller, D. (1996). Six-week, double-blind, placebo-controlled study of desipramine for adult attention deficit hyper-activity disorder. *Am J Psychiatry* 153:1147-1153.

Wilens, T.E.; Biederman, J.; Spencer, T.J.; Prince, J. (1995). Pharmacotherapy of adult attention deficit disorder: A review. *J Clin Psychopharmacol* 15:270-279.

Wilens, T.E.; Spencer, T.J.; Biederman, J.; Girard, K.; Doyle, R.; Prince, J.; Polis-ner, D. et al. (2001). A controlled clinical trial of bupropion for attention deficit hyperactivity disorder in adults. *Am J Psychiatry* 158:282-288.

Index